BEHAVIORAL EMERGENCIES

BEHAVIORAL EMERGENCIES

An Evidence-Based Resource for
Evaluating and Managing Risk of
Suicide, Violence, and Victimization

EDITED BY

Phillip M. Kleespies

AMERICAN PSYCHOLOGICAL ASSOCIATION
WASHINGTON, DC

Published by
American Psychological Association
750 First Street, NE
Washington, DC 20002
www.apa.org

To order
APA Order Department
P.O. Box 92984
Washington, DC 20090-2984
Tel: (800) 374-2721; Direct: (202) 336-5510
Fax: (202) 336-5502; TDD/TTY: (202) 336-6123
Online: www.apa.org/books/
E-mail: order@apa.org

In the U.K., Europe, Africa, and the Middle East, copies may be ordered from
American Psychological Association
3 Henrietta Street
Covent Garden, London
WC2E 8LU England

Typeset in Goudy by Stephen McDougal, Mechanicsville, MD

Printer: United Book Press, Inc., Baltimore, MD
Cover Designer: Berg Design, Albany, NY
Technical/Production Editor: Devon Bourexis

The opinions and statements published are the responsibility of the authors, and such opinions and statements do not necessarily represent the policies of the American Psychological Association.

Library of Congress Cataloging-in-Publication Data

Behavioral emergencies : an evidence-based resource for evaluating and managing suicidal behavior, violence, and victimization / edited by Phillip M. Kleespies. — 1st ed.
    p. ; cm.
Includes bibliographical references and index.
ISBN-13: 978-1-4338-0406-9
ISBN-10: 1-4338-0406-9
1. Psychiatric emergencies. 2. Crisis intervention (Mental health services)
I. Kleespies, Phillip M. II. American Psychological Association.
[DNLM: 1. Emergency Services, Psychiatric—methods. 2. Crisis Intervention—methods. 3. Evidence-Based Medicine. 4. Suicide—psychology. 5. Violence—psychology. WM 401 B419 2009]
    RC480.6.B438 2009
    362.2'04251—dc22   2008025594

British Library Cataloguing-in-Publication Data
A CIP record is available from the British Library.

Printed in the United States of America
First Edition

CONTENTS

CONTRIBUTORS

Houri Andalibian, JD, MS, Doctoral Candidate, Joint JD–PhD Program in Psychology and Law, Pacific Graduate School of Psychology, Redwood City, CA

Ron E. Acierno, PhD, Associate Professor, National Crime Victims Research and Treatment Center, Department of Psychiatry and Behavioral Sciences, Medical University of South Carolina, Charleston

Bruce Bongar, PhD, ABPP, FAPM, Calvin Professor of Psychology, Pacific Graduate School of Psychology, Redwood City, CA; Consulting Professor of Psychiatry and the Behavioral Sciences, Stanford University School of Medicine, Palo Alto, CA

Randy Borum, PsyD, Professor, Department of Mental Health Law and Policy, University of South Florida, Tampa

Johann Brink, MB, ChB, BA Hons, FCPsych(SA), FRCPC, Clinical and Scientific Director, Forensic Psychiatric Services Commission, BC Mental Health and Addiction Services, Coquitlam, BC, Canada; Clinical Professor, Department of Psychiatry, University of British Columbia, Vancouver, BC, Canada

Jay Callahan, PhD, Adjunct Faculty, Loyola University of Chicago, Chicago, IL

Marie B. Caulfield, PhD, President, Extraordinary Choices Coaching and Consulting, Bethesda, MD

Liliana Cordero, MA, Department of Psychology, Texas Tech University, Lubbock

Pamela J. Deiter-Sands, PhD, Clinical Psychologist and Director, Adult and Adolescent Psychological Services, Glastonbury, CT

Kevin S. Douglas, LLB, PhD, Associate Professor; Coordinator, Law and Forensic Psychology Program; Michael Smith Foundation for Health

Research Career Scholar, Department of Psychology, Simon Fraser University, Burnaby, BC, Canada

Paul Duberstein, PhD, Professor, Department of Psychiatry, Center for the Study and Prevention of Suicide, University of Rochester Medical Center, Rochester, NY

Jill M. Emanuele, PhD, Clinical Psychologist, Bronx Children's Psychiatric Center, Bronx, NY

Kerry Eudy, JD, PhD, Forensic Evaluator, Forensic Health Services, Braintree, MA

Kathryn Fair, PhD, Center for Deployment Psychology, Uniformed Services University of the Health Sciences, Bethesda, MD

Monica M. Fitzgerald, PhD, Assistant Professor, National Crime Victims Research and Treatment Center, Department of Psychiatry and Behavioral Sciences, Medical University of South Carolina, Charleston

Sigmund Hough, PhD, ABPP, Clinical Neuropsychologist, Spinal Cord Injury Service/Psychology, VA Boston Healthcare System; Assistant Professor, Harvard Medical School; Adjunct Assistant Professor, Boston University School of Medicine, Boston, MA

Brooke Howard, PhD, Forensic Psychology Post-Doctoral Fellow, Law and Psychiatry Program, Department of Psychiatry, University of Massachusetts Medical School, Worcester, MA

Thomas E. Joiner Jr., PhD, Professor, Department of Psychology, Florida State University, Tallahassee

Dean G. Kilpatrick, PhD, Distinguished Professor, Department of Psychiatry and Behavioral Sciences; Director, National Crime Victims Research and Treatment Center, Medical University of South Carolina, Charleston

Phillip M. Kleespies, PhD, ABPP, Clinical Psychologist, VA Boston Healthcare System; Assistant Clinical Professor of Psychiatry, Boston University School of Medicine, Boston, MA

Maxine H. Krengel, PhD, Assistant Clinical Professor of Neurology, Boston University School of Medicine; Clinical Neuropsychologist, VISN I Polytrauma Network Site, VA Boston Healthcare System, Boston, MA

Michael R. McCart, PhD, Assistant Professor, Family Services Research Center, Department of Psychiatry and Behavioral Sciences, Medical University of South Carolina, Charleston

Dale E. McNiel, PhD, Professor of Psychology, Department of Psychiatry, School of Medicine, University of California, San Francisco

Alec L. Miller, PsyD, Professor of Clinical Psychiatry and Behavioral Sciences; Chief, Child and Adolescent Psychology, Montefiore Medical Center/Albert Einstein College of Medicine, Bronx, NY

Tonia L. Nicholls, PhD, Michael Smith Foundation for Health Research Career Scholar, BC Mental Health & Addiction Services, Coquitlam,

BC, Canada; Assistant Professor, Department of Psychiatry, University of British Columbia, Vancouver, BC, Canada

Wendy Packman, JD, PhD, Associate Professor of Psychology and Director, Joint JD–PhD Program in Psychology and Law, Pacific Graduate School of Psychology, Redwood City, CA

Laurie Anne Pearlman, PhD, President, Trauma Research, Education, and Training Institute, New Britain, CT

Allison N. Ponce, PhD, Assistant Professor, Department of Psychiatry, Yale University School of Medicine, New Haven, CT

Heidi S. Resnick, PhD, Professor, National Crime Victims Research and Treatment Center, Department of Psychiatry and Behavioral Sciences, Medical University of South Carolina, Charleston

Janet S. Richmond, MSW, Associate Director of Psychiatry, Urgent Care Clinic, VA Boston Healthcare System; Associate Clinical Professor of Psychiatry, Tufts University School of Medicine, Boston, MA

David S. Riggs, PhD, Executive Director, Center for Deployment Psychology, Uniformed Services University of the Health Sciences, Bethesda, MD

Angela M. Romeo, PhD, Postdoctoral Fellow in Rehabilitation Psychology, VA Boston Healthcare System, Boston, MA

M. David Rudd, PhD, ABPP, Professor and Chair, Department of Psychology, Texas Tech University, Lubbock

Jacqueline A. Samson, PhD, Associate Clinical Psychologist, McLean Hospital, Belmont, MA; Assistant Professor of Psychology, Department of Psychiatry, Harvard Medical School, Boston, MA

Harriet Scheft, MD, Psychiatrist, Harvard Vanguard Medical Associates; Assistant Professor of Psychiatry, Tufts-New England Medical Center, Boston, MA

Glenn R. Sullivan, PhD, Assistant Professor, Department of Psychology, Virginia Military Institute, Lexington

Terri Ann Thompson, Intern, Bloomberg School of Public Health, Baltimore, MD

Glenn R. Trezza, PhD, Clinical Psychologist, VA Boston Healthcare System; Assistant Professor of Psychiatry, Boston University School of Medicine, Boston, MA

David Trotter, MA, Department of Psychology, Texas Tech University, Lubbock

Karina Tsatourian, PhD, Clinical Research Manager, Schizophrenia Program, Department of Psychiatry, Massachusetts General Hospital, Boston

Roberta F. White, PhD, ABPP/cn, Associate Dean for Research; Professor and Chair, Department of Environmental Health, Boston University School of Public Health, Boston, MA

Ben Williams, MA, Department of Psychology, Texas Tech University, Lubbock

Tracy K. Witte, MS, Doctoral Candidate, Department of Psychology, Florida State University, Tallahassee

PREFACE

This book was originally conceived as the second edition of another volume I edited, *Emergencies in Mental Health Practice: Evaluation and Management* (1998). During the writing and development stages of the manuscript, however, I realized that the differences between this book and the former book would be substantial enough to merit reconceiving the current one as a new book, rather than a second edition.

In this regard, the former book focused exclusively on the evaluation and management of behavioral emergencies in adults, but it was clear there was also a need to address the evaluation and management of behavioral emergencies in children and adolescents. The current volume does so. In addition, there are other topics that were not covered in my earlier work. The growing evidence that there is a suicide risk associated with the burdens of particular medical illnesses (not simply mental illnesses) was one such topic, and the increased national awareness of the risks of intimate partner or domestic violence was another. Furthermore, my previous book dealt with the evaluation and immediate management of behavioral emergencies but did not address appropriate follow-up treatment (after the emergency has been resolved) to reduce the risk of recurrence. This new book has an entire section devoted to the empirically based treatments available to individuals who, by virtue of having had a behavioral emergency, have shown an increased likelihood of being suicidal, violent, or a victim of violence in the future.

I hope the current volume will provide the mental health clinician with an up-to-date knowledge base, a model for skill development, and a comprehensive resource for particular problems encountered in dealing with patients or clients who engage in life-threatening behaviors or who are the victims of such behaviors when perpetrated by others.

ACKNOWLEDGMENTS

Given the complexities involved in describing this area of practice (i.e., the evaluation and management of patient life-threatening behavior), it seemed necessary to enlist a variety of mental health professionals who have specialized knowledge and skill in discrete areas of emergency-related services. I have been fortunate to bring together a first-rate group of authors who have contributed their knowledge and expertise to this volume, and I would like to thank them. I think the reader will find that they are indeed experts in their field.

The inspiration for this book, as well as for my previous book on this topic, *Emergencies in Mental Health Practice: Evaluation and Management* (1998), came from my many years of clinical experience with patients with serious mental illness and from my supervisory work with psychology interns in emergency room and urgent care clinic settings. I have learned a great deal from patients who presented with a wide range of emergencies and crises, and I have been fortunate to have had the opportunity to work with and instruct many young practitioners in emergency psychological services. Training interns in what can be a volatile setting has prompted considerable thought about what is needed to assist them in gaining competence in this area of practice. I hope that this book reflects that thinking.

My thanks as well to Susan Reynolds, senior acquisitions editor for the American Psychological Association's books department, for her suggestion that I do this book. Last but not least, thanks to my wife, Penelope, for her patience during the long hours I devoted to writing portions of this book and editing the remainder.

BEHAVIORAL
EMERGENCIES

INTRODUCTION

PHILLIP M. KLEESPIES

You are a mental health clinician who has been seeing a young, married couple in therapy for the past several weeks. The woman works for a small company and recently was promoted to a beginning level managerial position. Her husband is a construction worker who has a history of problems with anger and impulse control. He also drinks to intoxication episodically. The couple came to therapy because they have been having intense arguments that seem to be fueled by the husband's feeling that he is being left behind by his wife's success. Late one day, he calls you from a bar. He has been following his wife and has seen her going to dinner with a man who is a higher level manager at her company. He believes they are having an affair, and he plans to confront her about it when she comes home this evening. He states that if there is evidence to support his suspicions, he has thoughts of killing his wife and then himself. Thus far, he has only had thoughts, and he denies that he has made any definite plans or preparations.

It seems believable that such a scenario, or one similar to it, could unfold in any mental health clinician's practice. If you were that clinician, how might you evaluate and manage the situation? Of course, how you respond to such an anxiety-provoking event could have very serious consequences for your patients or clients, and for you. It is a situation that I refer to as a potential *behavioral emergency*.

This is a book about the evaluation and management of behavioral emergencies and the follow-up treatment needed to reduce the risk of their recurrence. A behavioral emergency exists when there is an imminent risk of life-threatening behavior. The term (as used in this book) includes situations in which there is an acute risk of intentional harm or death to self or others, as well as situations in which a vulnerable individual is at acute risk of being seriously harmed or killed. In clinical practice, the situations that qualify as behavioral emergencies include (a) serious suicidal states, (b) potential violence to others, (c) situations of grave risk to a relatively defenseless victim (e.g., a severely battered spouse, an abused child), and (d) states of very impaired judgment in which the individual is endangered.

In this conceptualization, the term *imminent* is taken to mean that there is a risk that the patient will harm or kill him- or herself or others or will be a victim of serious harm, "in the next few minutes, hours, or days" (Pokorny, 1983, p. 249). It is important to acknowledge early in this book, however, that there are in fact no known imminent risk factors for events such as suicide, violence, or interpersonal victimization. This situation results, in part, from the fact that patients who appear to be at imminent risk are typically excluded from research studies for their own protection or the protection of others (Kleespies, Niles, Kutter, & Ponce, 2005). Simon (2006) made this point in a more emphatic way by maintaining that the term *imminence* defies definition (at least in any measurable terms) and that there are no validated short-term risk factors that identify when or whether a patient will, for example, attempt or complete suicide.

Ideally, the mental health clinician knows (or, more accurately, has formed the clinical opinion) that there is imminent risk after doing a thorough evaluation in which he or she uses the available empirical evidence to guide his or her judgment. Yet, it is important to be clear that a statement indicating that a patient is at imminent risk of harm to self or others is a clinical judgment, and as Simon (2006) pointed out, such judgments should not be taken as implying prediction. As discussed later, the prediction of statistically rare events such as suicide or violence or interpersonal victimization eludes our current capabilities.

Nonetheless, behavioral emergencies happen, and when they occur the mental health clinician's skill and coping resources are often seriously tested. Such an emergency scenario prompted Omer and Elitzur (2001) to attempt to provide guidelines for clinicians in an article titled, "What Would You Say to the Person on the Roof?" The events leading up to this article involved two young soldiers, a male adolescent and a female adolescent, who in separate incidents locked themselves up with a gun after declaring their intention to commit suicide. In one case, both professional and laypeople tried for 15 minutes to dissuade the person, and in the other case, for 3 hours. Both adolescents killed themselves.

Omer and Elitzur (2001) spoke with the would-be rescuers and found that they felt helpless and without guidance as to how to communicate with someone who was experiencing such a behavioral emergency. The suicide prevention text that they subsequently developed involved speaking with a hypothetical "person on the roof" about how they (i.e., Omer and Elitzur) understood the individual's pain and how he or she was using "tunnel vision." It prompted a cogent reply from Orbach (2001) titled, "How Would You Listen to the Person on the Roof?" Orbach's major point was that it may not be what you say, but whether you can hear the person's story and reach an empathic understanding of his or her pain that will allow you to break through emotional barriers and help the individual achieve some hope that there may be a solution to his or her problems.

This book is intended to provide guidance and a knowledge base for clinicians who must deal with behavioral emergencies in their practice. The focus of the book is on the first three behavioral emergencies previously noted (i.e., suicide, violence, and interpersonal victimization), because they involve greater potential for direct psychological or behavioral intervention to ameliorate the underlying problems.

In terms of a knowledge base, Bongar, Lomax, and Harmatz (1992) suggested that a model curriculum needed to be developed for the study of suicide; indeed, they cited a curriculum proposed by Lomax (1986) for psychiatry residency programs. Although this recommendation was clearly a good one, it does not go far enough if one considers the need for training among mental health practitioners in assessing and managing behavioral emergencies more broadly (Kleespies, 2000; Kleespies et al., 2000). The field needs a model curriculum and a training sequence for dealing with behavioral emergencies, including those involving suicidal patients, violent patients, and those who are the potential victims of violence. This book is organized according to a proposed curriculum and the following section describes it.

HOW THIS BOOK IS ORGANIZED: A MODEL CURRICULUM

A number of years ago, I proposed a curriculum for acquiring a knowledge base in behavioral emergencies (Kleespies, 1998), and the section on Clinical Emergencies and Crises (Section VII of American Psychological Association's Division 12 [Society of Clinical Psychology]) advocated that such a curriculum be included in the training of psychologists (Kleespies et al., 2000). More recently, Brasch, Glick, Cobb, and Richmond (2004), representing the American Association for Emergency Psychiatry, advocated for the development of a curriculum to accompany emergency training for psychiatric residents.

As noted earlier, this book is organized according to my proposed curriculum. This introduction presents a conceptualization of the domain of behavioral emergencies and a model for training in this area of practice. Thereafter, there are eight parts to the book.

Part I, "Foundations," includes a chapter (i.e., chap. 1) on the basic concepts of behavioral emergencies and behavioral crises and their distinction. Chapter 1 discusses current trends in crisis intervention and demonstrates a new appreciation of resilience in coping with challenging events. It concludes with an integrated model of crisis and emergency intervention that provides guidance in responding to both situations. Chapter 2 presents a model of a clinical interview for evaluating behavioral emergencies. The chapter discusses the difficult task of containing the patient's emotional turmoil so that his or her problem(s) can be clearly defined. It concludes with guidance on how to decide whether the patient can be managed and treated as an outpatient or may require an emergency intervention.

Part II, "Evaluation and Management of Suicide Risk," contains chapters that use an evidence-based approach to inform the clinician about evaluating the risk of suicide and providing immediate management to reduce the risk. Chapter 3 is about evaluating and managing suicidal emergencies in adults, and chapter 4 discusses suicidal emergencies in children and adolescents. Chapter 5 is intended to inform clinicians of the risks of suicide associated with particular medical illnesses and terminal illness. It is especially pertinent for those who work in medical psychology or behavioral medicine.

Part III, "Evaluation and Management of Risk of Violence," provides a section that is parallel to Part II but focuses on an evidence-based approach to evaluating and managing the risk of violence. Thus, chapters 6 and 7 discuss the evaluation and management of the risk of violence in adults and children and adolescents, respectively.

Interpersonal violence, of course, begets victims, and potential victims of violence, as well as those who have recently been victimized and may be at risk of revictimization, often seek clinical assistance. In Part IV, "Evaluation and Management of Interpersonal Victimization," chapter 8 informs the clinician about assessment of the risk of interpersonal victimization and which intervention might be appropriate in its immediate aftermath; chapter 9 provides a more in-depth view of the issue of intimate partner or domestic violence and victimization.

Certain problems or conditions are not behavioral emergencies per se but are often complicating factors that are associated with emergency situations. Part V, "Emergency-Related Crises and Conditions," provides the clinician with a chapter (i.e., chap. 10) on self-injurious behavior in which there is no suicidal intent. These behaviors are often mistakenly seen as suicidal behaviors or suicide attempts, and the practitioner needs to know how to distinguish them. In addition, the section has a chapter (i.e., chap. 11) on alcohol and drug-related crises, because alcohol and drug problems are so frequently present and contribute to suicidal or violent behavior. Chapter 12 discusses the contribution of certain personality disorders (which have often been associated with nonfatal self-injuries) to suicide risk.

Certain medical illnesses and conditions can present with psychological or behavioral symptomatology and precipitate what appears to be a behavioral emergency or crisis. The clinician needs a resource to heighten his or her awareness of such possibilities so appropriate referrals for medical evaluation can be made. Part VI, "Medical Conditions Presenting as Behavioral Emergencies," includes chapters on psychological–behavioral symptoms in neurological disorders (i.e., chap. 13) and psychological–behavioral symptoms in endocrine disorders (i.e., chap. 14).

After a behavioral emergency has been evaluated and immediate management has reduced or eliminated imminent risk to self or others, the patient or client is typically in need of follow-up treatment to reduce the risk of recurrence. The chapters in Part VII, "Follow-Up Treatment of Patients at Risk of Recurrent Emergencies," inform the clinician about available treatments that have empirical support for being effective at reducing such risks. Chapter 15 presents the evidence-based treatments for individuals who are vulnerable to recurring suicidality. Chapter 16 is a similar chapter on treatments for reducing the risk of recurrent violence, and chapter 17 discusses appropriate treatments for those who have been the victims of interpersonal violence and seem vulnerable to revictimization.

In working with patients who present with behavioral emergencies, the practitioner needs to be aware of the ethical and legal issues involved in such high-risk situations. He or she also needs information about the emotional and personal toll that such work can take. Part VIII, "Legal and Psychological Risks in Treating People With Behavioral Emergencies," presents chapters on ethical and legal risk management with behavioral emergencies (i.e, chap. 18) and on the emotional impact of working with patients who are at risk and how the clinician might cope with that impact (i.e., chap. 19).

The curriculum proposed in this book can be taught in a graduate course; however, it ideally should be situated in a broader training context in which clinicians-in-training can learn, firsthand, how to handle behavioral emergencies.

TRAINING IN THE EVALUATION AND MANAGEMENT OF BEHAVIORAL EMERGENCIES

Some time ago, Bongar et al., (1992) pointed out in regard to the assessment of suicide risk, "There is research to support the contention that knowledge of risk factors and the capacity to respond in an effective way to those patients who present as an imminent risk of suicide may be independent areas of clinical competence" (pp. 262–263). It is important that psychologists and other mental health practitioners develop competency in these different components of practice. Although a knowledge base in behavioral emergencies is essential, it is not sufficient for competency. Thus, Lomax (1986) proposed three major areas of emphasis for such training: (a) knowledge, (b) skill, and (c) attitude. This book provides a knowledge base, but training in behavioral emergencies cannot neglect skill and attitude development.

Skill Training in Evaluating and Managing Behavioral Emergencies

Applying a knowledge base in practice with good supervision leads to skill development and true clinical competency. When a patient or client is threatening suicide or is potentially violent, the situation can arouse anxiety in the seasoned professional, let alone in those who are in training and less confident of their clinical abilities and status. A *mentor model* for learning under such conditions seems advisable. In this model, an experienced clinician and intern are paired in settings such as an emergency department or urgent care clinic or on a mobile crisis team. The intern then has the opportunity to observe and work with a professional who has been successfully engaged in this type of clinical work. Cases can be processed on-site and subsequently in a supervisory session. Although initially the intern is more of an observer, the supervisor can gradually shift greater responsibility for the evaluation and management of cases to the professional-in-training. It is during this process of gradual increasing skill and responsibility that some inoculation to the stress involved in these emergency situations occurs—and stress inoculation is very important to clear decision making in situations in which tensions can run high.

As Driskell and Johnston (1998) pointed out, it is important to distinguish between *training* and *stress training*. These authors indicated that most training, which is focused on skill acquisition and retention, takes place under conditions designed to maximize learning (e.g., a quiet classroom, practice under predictable conditions, uniformity of presentation). Some tasks, however, must be performed under conditions that are very different from a training classroom, conditions that include time pressure, ambiguity, a heavy task load, and distractions. The evaluation and management of behavioral emergencies can involve such circumstances, and it can be difficult to maintain effective performance and decision making when there has been no training under such high stress conditions. We discuss stress training and stress inoculation further in the chapter on the emergency interview (see chap. 2, this volume).

Development of a Constructive Attitude

The development of constructive attitudes about work with emergency cases takes root in good program support and in the mentoring previously noted. Clearly, there have been instances in which service pressures have distorted training objectives. As a result, relatively inexperienced trainees have been placed on the front lines, so to speak, with little support. In such an event, emergency work is inevitably seen as trying and burdensome. Good support and supervision, however, can go a long way toward preventing a negative viewpoint and aiding in the development of a sense of competence in dealing with emotionally charged cases. Long ago, Barlow (1974) observed that psychology interns responded initially to emergency department duty with moderate to severe anxiety. He further observed that within approximately 3 months, a second response—of increased clinical confidence and mastery—began to emerge. This sense of mastery was described by interns as one of the more important developments in their training.

Settings for Training in Behavioral Emergencies

Hospital-based internship sites usually have an emergency department where patients with behavioral emergencies are seen. Although this setting is an excellent one for training in evaluating and managing these difficult cases, other sites also have good settings, including an urgent care clinic, mobile crisis team, or even a walk-in clinic where patients who have suicidal ideation or are struggling to control violent impulses can present. This training experience needs to begin with a thorough orientation to this type of work and with the mentor model of supervision previously described. It also needs to be accompanied by supervisory sessions and, ideally, by a brief lecture series on emergency-related topics (e.g., evaluation of suicide risk, evaluation of violence risk, signs and symptoms of alcohol and drug intoxication and withdrawal).

CONCLUSION

Behavioral emergencies confront the mental health clinician or intern with the need to make decisions that can have serious, perhaps irreversible, consequences. The outcomes of such decisions can have far-reaching emotional, ethical, and legal repercussions. Society, through its legal and judicial system, holds psychologists responsible for observing a reasonable standard of care in assessing and managing such emergency situations. Routine and systematic training in the evaluation and management of behavioral emergencies can make for more complete and competent professional practitioners. The professional status of clinical psychology is enhanced when its practitioners are formally trained to respond to and deal with these sometimes frightening, often difficult, and usually trying instances when patients are at risk. I hope that this book will serve as a guide to the provision of this important training.

REFERENCES

Barlow, D. (1974). Psychologists in the emergency room. *Professional Psychology, 5,* 251–256.

Bongar, B., Lomax, J., & Harmatz, M. (1992). Training and supervisory issues in the assessment and management of the suicidal patient. In B. Bongar (Ed.), *Suicide: Guidelines for assessment, management, and treatment* (pp. 253–267). New York: Oxford University Press.

Brasch, J., Glick, R. L., Cobb, T., & Richmond, J. (2004). Residency training in emergency psychiatry: A model curriculum developed by the education committee of the American Association for Emergency Psychiatry. *Academic Psychiatry, 28,* 95–103.

Driskell, J., & Johnston, J. (1998). Stress exposure training. In J. Cannon-Bowers & E. Salas (Eds.), *Making decisions under stress: Implications for individual and team training* (pp. 191–217). Washington, DC: American Psychological Association.

Kleespies, P. M. (1998). The domain of psychological emergencies. In P. M. Kleespies (Ed.), *Emergencies in mental health practice: Evaluation and management* (pp. 9–21). New York: Guilford Press.

Kleespies, P. M. (2000). Behavioral emergencies and crises: An overview. *Journal of Clinical Psychology, 56,* 1103–1108.

Kleespies, P. M., Berman, A., Ellis,T., McKeon, R., McNiel, D., Nock, M., et al. (2000, July). Report on education and training in behavioral emergencies: Abridged version. *APPIC Newsletter, 25*(1), 10, 33–38.

Kleespies, P. M., Niles, B., Kutter, C., & Ponce, A. (2005). Managing behavioral emergencies. In R. Coombs (Ed.), *Family therapy review: Preparing for comprehensive and licensing exams* (pp. 213–231). Hillsdale, NJ: Erlbaum.

Lomax, J. (1986). A proposed curriculum on suicide for psychiatric residency. *Suicide and Life-Threatening Behavior, 16,* 56–64.

Omer, H., & Elitzur, A. (2001). What would you say to the person on the roof? A suicide prevention text. *Suicide and Life-Threatening Behavior, 31,* 129–139.

Orbach, O. (2001). How would you listen to the person on the roof? A response to H. Omer and A. Elitzur. *Suicide and Life-Threatening Behavior, 31,*140–143.

Pokorny, A. (1983). Prediction of suicide in psychiatric patients. *Archives of General Psychiatry, 40,* 249–259.

Simon, R. (2006). Imminent suicide: The illusion of short-term prediction. *Suicide and Life-Threatening Behavior, 36,* 296–301.

I
FOUNDATIONS

1

EMERGENCY INTERVENTION AND CRISIS INTERVENTION

JAY CALLAHAN

In this chapter I provide a foundation for understanding behavioral emergencies and crisis situations. Clinicians frequently use these concepts in ambiguous and ill-defined ways and often use them interchangeably. The lack of clear definitions leads to confusion and hesitation in clinical decision making. Understanding the distinction between a behavioral emergency and a crisis is an important clinical task and can provide clear guidelines about how to proceed in intense and difficult situations.

BEHAVIORAL EMERGENCIES

As described in the Introduction, a *behavioral emergency* is a situation that requires an immediate response to avoid possible harm. The three major behavioral emergencies are suicidal behavior, violent behavior, and interpersonal victimization. The appropriate clinical response to a behavioral emergency is an emergency intervention. Although different chapters in this book describe different types of behavioral emergencies, a consistent concept of intervention applies across all types. An emergency intervention is a single interview conducted on an immediate basis. Its goals are threefold. The first goal is to evaluate the status of the patient and the potential for harm. The second is to intervene in that situation if possible, to reduce the risk of harm. Sometimes simple and straightforward clinical interventions such as providing nonjudgmental active listening and working to clarify a crisis situation can have a major impact on the patient and reduce risk. Sometimes this intervention can make the difference between the need for inpatient versus outpatient treatment. The third goal is the plan, or disposition—what should be done next? In the context of behavioral emergencies, containment or hands-on prevention—hospitalization, intensive residential treatment, continuous family watch, and so forth—is sometimes necessary.

CRISES

The concept of a "crisis" is much less clear, and the word *crisis* is used to describe a wide variety of situations in the psychological and mental health literature. Sometimes it is used as a synonym for emergency. For instance, Johnson et al. (2005) described a crisis as a situation justifying psychiatric admission, specifically one in which psychological deterioration has occurred and the potential for harm exists. This essentially defines a crisis as identical to an emergency. Similarly, Halliday-Boykins, Henggeler, Rowland, and DeLucia (2004) studied youth *psychiatric crisis,* which they defined as a situation that required emergency hospitalization. Kulic (2005) described a "crisis intervention semi-structured interview" that is to be used "with clients in crisis situations who may require emergency psychiatric care" (p. 143).

The term *crisis* is sometimes used also to define any serious or chronic problem. For instance, Castro-Blanco (2005) wrote "Youth Crisis in the Schools," in which he discussed a variety of mental health-related problems adolescents may experience, including depression, anger and aggression, and anxiety disorders. These are certainly problems, but they are not necessarily crises. Similarly, in her book on crisis intervention, Kanel (2007) included a chapter on substance abuse. Drugs and alcohol can certainly precipitate crises, but the disorders of substance abuse and dependence are not crises in themselves. In fact, chronic substance dependence becomes part of an individual's homeostasis and is used in an attempt to cope with life problems.

The term *crisis intervention* is also used to describe intervening in potentially violent situations, which would actually be emergency intervention. Several well-advertised corporations (e.g., Crisis Prevention Institute, Therapeutic Crisis Intervention) offer training for mental health professionals and paraprofessionals in crisis intervention, by which they describe de-escalating and calming agitated and threatening clients.

In other words, there is much confusion about what constitutes a *behavioral emergency* and what constitutes a *mental health crisis.* Many mental health

clinicians use these terms interchangeably, without making a distinction between them. Many publications in psychological, medical, social work, and related literature also interchange the terms *crisis* and *emergency* rather indiscriminately.

Despite this confusion, however, a consensus appears to be forming to define *crisis* in the traditional way that was originally formulated in crisis intervention writings of the 1960s and 1970s (Caplan, 1961; Golan, 1978; Rapoport, 1965). This definition regards a crisis as a loss of psychological equilibrium or a state of emotional instability that includes elements of depression and anxiety. A crisis is precipitated by an external event; it is not a state of endogenous distress. A crisis is also a state of the individual, not the stressor or the precipitating event. The crisis is not the sexual assault, or the bombing, or the airplane crash; the crisis is the state of disequilibrium that may follow one of these stressful events. A crisis implies an inability to cope— a problem of adaptation becomes a crisis because normal coping mechanisms are insufficient, including both primary and secondary (i.e., back-up) methods. In a crisis, an individual's inability to function at his or her usual level is termed *functional impairment*. During a crisis, an individual is often more willing to try new coping methods or accept assistance from others than he or she would in normal circumstances (Aguilera, 1998; Callahan, 1994; Golan, 1978; Roberts, 2005; Slaikeu, 1990). A key element in an individual's vulnerability to crisis is the appraisal or perception of the event, along with the person's perception of her or his ability to cope with that event (Aguilera, 1998; Golan, 1978).

It is frequently pointed out that the Chinese pictogram for *crisis* is made up of the juxtaposition of the two pictograms that represent danger and opportunity (Aguilera, 1998). Arising from the danger of stressful life circumstances, a crisis can be an opportunity for the development of new and constructive coping mechanisms and psychological growth.

Many systems for categorizing types of crises have been proposed, including *developmental* or *maturational* (i.e., crises emerging from normal developmental phases in life) and *situational* (i.e., arising solely from unpredictable stressful situations; Caplan, 1964). Part of this conceptualization includes the idea that most people negotiate these developmental stages without falling into a crisis and that most situational stresses do not trigger a crisis for most people. Many people are very resilient in these situations.

Probably the simplest and most useful categorization is that of dividing crises into those precipitated by normative stress versus traumatic stress. Normative stress is caused by ordinary, commonplace events, such as a job loss or threat of loss, illness of a family member, a flat tire on the morning of a major presentation, or the breakup of a romantic relationship. Traumatic stress, however, is made up of events that involve the threat of life and death. At one time these life-threatening events were described as "outside the range of usual human experience" (American Psychiatric Association, 1987, p. 259).

However, a number of contemporary epidemiologic studies have found that traumatic events are surprisingly common. In a nationwide study of individuals 15 to 54 years old, 19% of the 2,812 men surveyed said they had been threatened with a weapon, held captive, or kidnapped; 35.6% said they had witnessed someone being badly injured or killed. Over 9% of the 3,065 women surveyed said they had been raped, and 15.2% said they had been involved in a fire, flood, or natural disaster (Kessler, Sonnega, Bromet, Hughes, & Nelson, 1995, p. 1050). A subsequent national epidemiologic survey confirmed these findings (Kessler, Berglund, Demler, Jin, & Walters, 2005). Thus, unfortunately, these events are not outside the range of usual human experience. Because of these findings, this phrase was deleted from the *Diagnostic and Statistical Manual of Mental Disorders* (*DSM–IV*; 4th ed.; American Psychiatric Association, 1994).

Crises are substantially similar whether they are triggered by normative or traumatic stress. In both cases, the individual is thrown into a state of emotional disequilibrium, displays symptoms of anxiety and depression, and has difficulty coping. One difference is that many crises precipitated by traumatic stress meet criteria for acute stress disorder (ASD; American Psychiatric Association, 1994), whereas crises precipitated by normative stress usually do not because the stressor does not meet Criterion A (i.e., "an event or events that involved actual or threatened death or serious injury, or a threat to the physical integrity of self or others"; American Psychiatric Association, 1994, p. 427). Another difference is that normative stress rarely causes the dissociative symptoms that are characteristic of ASD. Diagnostically, normative crises can often be diagnosed as episodes of major depression, substance abuse disorders, or adjustment disorders.

Traumatic Stress Versus Posttraumatic Stress Disorder

Because ASD often becomes posttraumatic stress disorder (PTSD), another common misconception is that crisis intervention is an appropriate treatment for PTSD. This is not the case. Crisis intervention is the treatment of choice for a crisis precipitated by traumatic stress, but the crisis is only the initial period of dysfunction.

Various authorities have described the self-limiting quality of a crisis— that it is not possible for a person to continue in the high-arousal state of crisis indefinitely. After about 4 to 6 weeks, the individual inevitably finds a new homeostasis (Golan, 1978; Parad & Parad, 1990). This new equilibrium is often the same level of functioning that was present prior to the crisis; however, in some circumstances the individual might end up functioning at a higher or lower level than previously. These outcomes are often based on how overwhelming the original precipitating event was to an individual, and traumatic events are obviously more overwhelming than normative ones. Another important variable is the nature of the help received, if any. Some individuals receive thoughtful and competent support (i.e., professional or personal) that enables them to adopt new coping abilities; therefore, they are more capable of dealing with future stress after recovery.

Crisis intervention, however, is appropriate only during the period of crisis—usually 4 to 6 weeks. If the dysfunction continues after the crisis is over, which is not uncommon, longer term treatment is indicated. If an individual with PTSD comes for professional help 3 or 6 months after the traumatic event, he or she is no longer in crisis. Some adaptation has occurred, and the period of disequilibrium has passed. The individual is no longer in crisis, and crisis intervention is inappropriate.

Type I Versus Type II Trauma

Terr (1994) described the distinction between Type I and Type II trauma in children, and the distinction is useful for adults as well. Type I is the single traumatic event—the single blow. Examples include rape, assault, natural disasters such as Hurricane Katrina and the 2004 tsunami in Southeast Asia, a motor vehicle accident, or the terrorist attack of September 11, 2001. Type II trauma consists of a series of traumatic events over a period of time that are linked together and perpetrated on victims who are in a situation of physical or psychological captivity. Examples include combat, being a prisoner of war or being held in a concentration camp, many cases of domestic violence, and child abuse and neglect. Type II traumas always include physical or psychological captivity; otherwise, the victim would find a way to escape from the traumatic situation. Individuals who have experienced Type II trauma settle into a new, usually lower level of functioning long before they escape or are able to receive professional assistance. Therefore, they are rarely in a state of crisis when they come to professional attention and require long-term treatment for PTSD (and possibly other posttraumatic disorders), rather than crisis intervention.

RECENT TRENDS IN THE CRISIS INTERVENTION LITERATURE

Traumatic stress has become the new focus of crisis intervention in the early years of the 21st century. This trend began in the 1990s with the development and popularity of *critical incident stress debriefing* (CISD) and the occurrence of a number of natural and man-made disasters, including Hurricane Andrew in 1992 and the bombings of the World Trade Center in 1993 and the Murrah Federal Building in Oklahoma City in 1995. The terrorist attacks of September 11, 2001, however, significantly shifted the focus of crisis intervention to an almost total preoccupation with traumatic stress and disasters. Although some literature continues to explore crises resulting from normative stress, most of the 21st-century crisis literature is about traumatic stress, acute stress disorder, disasters, and critical incidents (e.g., see Bronisch et al., 2006; Chemtob, Nakashima, & Carlson, 2002; Despland, Drapeau, & de Roten, 2005; Reyes & Jacobs, 2006; Ursano, Fullerton, & Norwood, 2003).

Resilience

A particular focus of this recent literature is a new appreciation for resilience and even *posttraumatic growth*. That is, previous literature emphasized the assumption that a sufficiently overwhelming traumatic event produced extensive psychopathology in virtually everyone (Bonanno, 2004). This viewpoint may have developed from thinking about PTSD as essentially a normal adaptation to overwhelming stress, as opposed to a mental disorder. Epidemiologic data, however, have clearly shown that many people who experience traumatic events do not develop PTSD, and a National Institute of Mental Health (NIMH; 2000) consensus document states that "a sensible working principle in the immediate post-incident phase is to expect normal recovery" (p. 2). The National Comorbidity Survey, cited earlier in this chapter (Kessler, Sonnega, et al., 1995), studied a nationally representative sample of over 5,000 individuals from 15 to 54 years old and found a lifetime prevalence of traumatic events of 60.7% for men and 52.1% for women. Over half of the population of the United States from age 15 to age 54 has experienced one or more traumatic events. However, in many or most instances the traumatic event did not lead to PTSD. The overall lifetime rate of PTSD in this sample was 5.0% for men and 10.4% for women (Kessler, Sonnega, et al., 1995). Studies of specific traumatic events have found similar results. For instance, a study of hospitalized survivors of car accidents found a rate of ASD of only 28% (Bryant, Harvey, Guthrie, & Moulds, 2000), and a study of 1991 Gulf War veterans found "minimal psychological distress" in a sample of 775 returnees (Sutker, Davis, Uddo, & Ditta, 1995, p. 447). Not only do victims of trauma survive, in some cases victims experience positive emotions and psychological growth (Calhoun & Tedeschi, 2006; Fredrickson, Tugade, Waugh, & Larkin, 2003).

Controversy Over Critical Incident Stress Debriefing

One of the most controversial issues of the late 1990s and early years of the 21st century is CISD. Originally used in the military, CISD is a single session group crisis intervention technique that emphasizes emotional ventilation, discussion of typical symptoms of traumatic stress, and advice on how to deal with stress (Mitchell & Everly, 1995). CISD has become extremely popular and is one of a number of intervention models that are described as *psychological debriefing*. CISD was developed primarily by Jeffrey Mitchell (1983), a Baltimore paramedic who went on to get a doctorate in psychology. Over the past 20 years numerous CISD and CISM (i.e., critical incident stress management) teams have sprung up around the United States; many of these focus on first responders (i.e., firefighters, police officers, paramedics), but others serve the public. The vast majority of these teams are voluntary organizations consisting of trained police officers, firefighters, paramedics, emergency medical personnel, and mental health professionals.

The controversy centers on whether CISD is an effective intervention in the aftermath of a traumatic event. Advocates argue that a single debriefing 24 to 72 hours after a traumatic event (or critical incident) can substantially reduce subsequent symptomatology and distress (Mitchell, 1983). Randomized controlled studies are few (Kaplan, Iancu, & Bodner, 2001), and findings are equivocal. However, most of the evidence shows little or no effect for psychological debriefing (Deahl, Gillham, Thomas, Searle, & Srinivasan, 1994; Hobbs, Mayou, Harrison, & Worlock, 1996; Lee, Slade, & Lygo, 1996; Marchand et al., 2006; Rose, Brewin, Andrews, & Kirk, 1999; Stallard & Salter, 2003). In two studies the intervention group, which received debriefing, did more poorly than the control group (Bisson, Jenkins, Alexander, & Bannister, 1997; Mayou, Ehlers, & Hobbs, 2000). However, most of these studies have focused on psychological debriefing, which often differs in a variety of ways from Mitchell's (1983; Mitchell & Everly, 1995) CISD. Many of these studies conducted individual, not group, debriefings, and most did not use the seven-stage structure that is characteristic of CISD.

Nonetheless, critics of debriefing point out that CISD not only is of questionable efficacy but also does not fulfill one of Mitchell's earliest claims— that it prevents or mitigates the later development of PTSD (Mitchell & Everly, 1995). Furthermore, several studies seem to suggest that CISD can even be harmful, probably by interfering with some individuals' natural means of coping with extreme stress (Bisson et al., 1997; Mayou et al., 2000).

Other difficulties with CISD have been identified. A common practice in the 1990s was to mandate debriefings for police officers and firefighters after certain extreme traumatic events. This practice was based on the belief that few individuals would come forward, despite a clear need to do so, because of the fear of appearing weak in front of their peers. For example, the entire Oklahoma City Police Department was ordered to undergo CISDs in the aftermath of the Federal Building bombing in 1995. It is not surprising that most reacted negatively to this mandate (Callahan, 2000). An NIMH consensus conference strongly recommended that all interventions be voluntary (NIMH, 2002).

The debate has become contentious, with advocates on both sides arguing about which studies are methodologically rigorous enough to be trusted. One meta-analysis found that "multicomponent CISM are effective interventions" (Roberts & Everly, 2006, p. 10), but one author of this meta-analysis is a former chairman of the board of Mitchell's International Critical Incident Stress Foundation and thus not a neutral observer. One descriptive review found that "debriefing might be an effective intervention" (Kaplan et al., 2001, p. 824). Otherwise, most meta-analyses have found no evidence in support of CISD (McNally, Bryant, & Ehlers, 2003; Rose, Bisson, & Wessely, 2004; van Emmerik, Kamphuis, Hulsbosch, & Emmelkamp, 2002).

Many experts are now calling for practitioners to use *psychological first aid*, a flexible and individualized approach that emphasizes education, reassurance, avoidance of discussing the details of the event, and active intervention for only those showing serious symptoms after 3 to 4 weeks—not 3 to 4 days (McNally et al., 2003; Young, 2006; van Emmerik et al., 2002). In 2001, NIMH sponsored a consensus workshop on early psychological intervention for victims of mass violence. The consensus was that in the aftermath of mass violence, the evidence supports the provision of psychological first aid, screening for morbidity, and follow-up for only specific individuals at risk (NIMH, 2002).

This controversy has highlighted the fact that the published work on crisis intervention is almost wholly concerned with traumatic stress, disasters, and mass violence. In the past decade, little has been written about crisis intervention with normative stress, developmental and maturational crises, and situational stress. Although this development is understandable given the events of the past decade, the field of crisis intervention must not ignore the impact of normative stress on people's lives.

A MODEL OF CRISIS INTERVENTION

Although the majority of the attention in recent years has gone to crises precipitated by traumatic stress, other kinds of crises occur. People lose jobs, family members become ill, and separation and divorce continue to take place. In many of these instances, the stress precipitates a crisis.

There are many models of crisis intervention. In addition to older models by Golan, (1978), Dixon (1979), Puryear (1979), and Hoff (1989), newer models have been proposed by Slaikeu (1990), Janosik (1994), James and Gilliland (2005), and Kanel (2007). Roberts's seven-stage model (2005) is not new but has received renewed attention in recent years. This chapter focuses on a model developed at the Benjamin Rush Center for Problems of Living in Los Angeles, as described by Aguilera (1998; see Figure 1.1). This model describes crisis intervention as brief psychotherapy initiated during a crisis (i.e., a period of psychological disequilibrium caused by an external stressor). This treatment consists of one to six sessions during the crisis period of a few days up to 4 to 6 weeks. In this model, a crisis develops because an individual has difficulties in one or more of the following three areas: (a) his or her coping mechanisms, (b) the availability of adequate social support, and (c) the meaning or perception of the event. Poor coping mechanisms, lack of support, and a malignant perception of the event will more

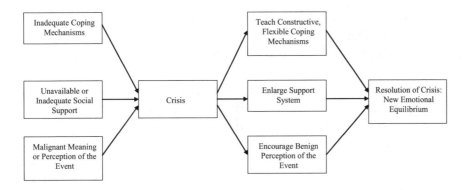

Figure 1.1. Modified model for crisis intervention. This figure was created per the model developed at the Benjamin Rush Center for Problems of Living in Los Angeles, as described by Anguilera (1998).

likely lead to a state of crisis. More constructive and flexible coping, varied sources of support, and a more benign perception of the event will often lead to an individual weathering a stressful event without experiencing a state of crisis (Aguilera, 1998).

The Role of Perception

The perception or meaning of the event is a key element. This characteristic has also been called *appraisal* in the early literature on stress and coping (Lazarus, 1980). The impact of a stressful event, either normative or traumatic, is significantly affected by its appraisal. One person's overwhelming stressor is another person's challenge. A divorce, although stressful for almost everyone, can be overwhelming for one person and merely upsetting for another.

Despite this significant subjectivity, traumatic stress is usually more likely than normative stress to lead to a state of crisis for most people. At first glance it appears that traumatic stress has a more universal or objective meaning. However, even death or the threat of death has diverse meanings to different people.

In general, accidents of nature are perceived as less stressful than traumatic events caused by human error. Trauma caused by human malevolence is the most stressful of all, in part because of the difficulty comprehending that a person could do such terrible things to other people. The events of September 11, 2001, are obvious examples.

Cultural aspects also influence the meaning of traumatic events. As noted by McNally et al. (2003),

> certain norms and beliefs may lead survivors to think that they are irreversibly damaged by the trauma, thereby increasing their risk for PTSD. For example, many Kosovar women who were raped during the recent

Balkan conflict regarded other people's response to their trauma—namely, the belief that they were defiled by the experience—as the worst part of their rape trauma. Culturally based beliefs that worsen the implications of a trauma may complicate treatment. (p. 74)

Many traumatic events lead to a search for explanation. Even though the survivors and victims understand the conventional explanation for a traumatic event, such a conventional explanation is often insufficient. For example, in a memorial service commemorating the 60th anniversary of the liberation of the Auschwitz concentration camp of World War II, a survivor of the camp took the microphone and cried, "Why? Why did they burn my people? Why?" Millions of words have been written about the Holocaust, and yet for a survivor, the search for explanation continues (Fried, 2005).

One explanation for this phenomenon is what Janoff-Bulman (1985) called *violations of basic assumptions* about life and the world. In the aftermath of a traumatic event, an individual's basic beliefs about how the world operates are shattered, and a crisis ensues. These assumptions are (a) a belief in personal invulnerability (i.e., "I never thought this could happen to me"), (b) a perception of the world as meaningful and comprehensible, and (c) a positive view of the self (Janoff-Bulman, 1985). Part of the view that "It'll never happen to me [or my family]" is a belief in a meaningful, and even controllable, world in which events occur for understandable reasons. Indeed, "at a fundamental level, we also believe we are protected against misfortune by being good and worthy people" and that "people deserve what they get and get what they deserve" (Janoff-Bulman, 1985, p. 20). Obviously, this is problematic: When trauma strikes many individuals wonder, "What did I do to deserve this?", and of course there is no answer.

The alternative to this distressing situation is to not find any meaning, which is even more difficult for most people. Many people believe that "everything happens for a reason," which leads them full circle back to "I must have done something to deserve this." Obviously, this is a more malignant meaning to attribute to a traumatic event and makes the crisis more severe and intense. The clinician's role in this dilemma is to engage the patient in a discussion of meaning, keeping in mind that in many instances patients are resistant to changing long-held belief systems.

The function of guilt in the aftermath of a traumatic event is a similar phenomenon. Guilt serves the purpose of giving people the illusion of control. If the victim of a date rape resolves to stop dating entirely or a person hurt in a subway crash refuses to ever take the subway again, each has done something to assure themselves that the terrible event will not happen to them again. Of course, this is a false sense of security, but it is preferable to feeling out of control.

The key issue is that normative or traumatic events have little objective meaning—they are perceived in a wide variety of different ways by different people, and the nature of this perception has a great deal to do with the individual's response to the event as a challenge to be overcome or as a destabilizing crisis.

The Roles of Coping and Support

The nature of one's coping mechanisms is a central issue. *Coping* refers to conscious and habitual methods of solving problems and adapting to demands from the environment. Researchers have found that coping can be categorized as *active problem-focused, passive problem-focused,* and *passive avoidant* (Koopman, Classen, & Spiegel, 1996). In the case of job loss, active problem-solving would include activities focused on obtaining a new job, handling financial matters, and related concerns. Passive problem-solving would include talking with others, quiet contemplation about job and financial issues, and so forth. Passive avoidant coping involves activities that enable the individual to avoid the problem, including escapes into drugs and alcohol. Some passive avoidant coping is not necessarily destructive, but a balance of coping mechanisms is most adaptive.

Social support is the third aspect of crisis. Numerous studies over the past 30 years have demonstrated the benefits of social support on both physical and mental health (Cohen, 2004). Individuals in crisis who have a support system and make use of it, in addition to the support inherent in the therapeutic relationship itself, tend to fare better in crisis situations.

AN INTEGRATED MODEL OF CRISIS AND EMERGENCY INTERVENTION

Now that *crisis, crisis intervention, emergency,* and *emergency intervention* have been defined, they can be combined into an integrated model to respond to both situations. This model is derived from the work of Aguilera (1998) and Puryear (1979), but with added elements of emergency intervention, which takes precedence over crisis intervention. Because a behavioral emergency involves the threat of danger or harm, it always has first priority. Similarly, crisis intervention takes precedence over routine outpatient treatment. If an outpatient comes on a routine visit while experiencing a crisis, the clinician must move away from normal psychotherapeutic activity and use the tools of crisis intervention (see Table 1.1).

If the client experiencing an emergency contacts a clinician or agency for the first time, the clinician's response should be to arrange a face-to-face emergency intervention on an immediate basis. As noted previously, this emergency intervention should include an evaluation of the client's situation as well as a risk assessment of the potential for suicide or violence, an in-session intervention to try to lessen the risk, and a carefully thought out disposition to ensure safety and provide continuity for subsequent care. Many

TABLE 1.1
Goals of Emergency Interventions Versus Crisis Interventions

Type of intervention	Treatment goals
Emergency	An immediate response to perceived imminent risk
	Management to prevent harm or death
	Resolution of the immediate risk within a single encounter
Crisis	A response within 24 to 48 hours
	Therapy to develop or reestablish psychological equilibrium
	Resolution within 4 to 6 weeks

times emergency interventions are carried out in a hospital emergency department, and many agencies and private practitioners routinely refer or even take emergency clients to hospital emergency departments.

Crisis intervention, however, requires a rapid but not immediate response. Much of the crisis intervention literature of the 1960s and 1970s advocated an immediate response to crisis, but this was because of the context of that time. When long-term psychoanalytic psychotherapy was the only treatment available, months-long waiting lists were not uncommon; therefore, immediate attention was not to be taken literally. Newer guidelines suggest seeing a client in crisis within 24 hours (Puryear, 1979). An emergency requires literally an immediate response.

As noted earlier, this model of crisis intervention focuses on perception (i.e., meaning), coping, and support. In the initial session, the clinician provides a safe atmosphere, uses active listening, and is an empathic, nonjudgmental listener. In most cases, open-ended questioning will allow the client to tell his or her story. In this first session, the clinician should listen for the availability and use of support systems, assess the client's coping mechanisms and notice which mechanisms are constructive and which are destructive, and form some preliminary understanding of the meaning of the event to the client. In rare cases of traumatic stress the client may not be able to remember the entire event because of dissociative amnesia (Koopman, Classen, Cardena, & Spiegel, 1995); in some instances, the client may feel the need to avoid discussing certain overwhelming aspects of the situation.

During the first session and periodically throughout the subsequent sessions of the crisis intervention, the clinician must investigate the possibility of a behavioral emergency. Any reason to believe that the client may be potentially suicidal, violent, or a victim of violence constitutes a behavioral emergency, and at that point the crisis intervention is delayed until the emergency is resolved. A risk assessment is carried out. The details of this procedure are beyond the scope of this chapter, but chapters 2 through 9 of this book discuss them in depth. An emergency intervention also includes an in-session attempt to decrease the risk of danger by means of a variety of standard therapeutic techniques. Such techniques include active listening, explicit empathizing, negotiating conflicts with significant others, offering hope, and pointing out the realistic consequences of fantasized actions. As discussed earlier, the emergency intervention includes a specific disposition based on the outcome of the risk assessment, modified by the in-session intervention. If by the end of the session the risk is judged to be low or moderate, the focus can shift back to the crisis intervention. If the risk continues to be high, the session may culminate in a hospitalization or other concrete method of containment and security.

If the risk is low or moderate and the crisis intervention can proceed, certain other aspects must be explored. First is to ascertain that the situation is, in fact, a crisis. As discussed earlier, a crisis is a period of psychological disequilibrium in which the individual experiences anxiety and depression as well as functional impairment. This means the clinician must get a sense of the client's baseline level of functioning to ensure that this period of disequilibrium is an acute episode, not a chronic state. Some individuals who function in a state of constant crisis are not really in crisis at all, because a crisis is defined as different from an individual's baseline. Certain clients with borderline personality disorder, alcohol dependence, or drug dependence can appear to be in crisis, but the chaos they experience is their baseline state. Various questions regarding the individual's functioning prior to the current situation will usually reveal the quality of his or her baseline, especially in terms of impulse control, maturity of relationships, and integrity of ego boundaries (Gerhart, 1990; James & Gilliland, 2005). Crisis intervention, with its rapid intensity of involvement and active style, is not appropriate for these clients and will frequently promote regression (Callahan, 1996; Golan, 1974).

Another important aspect of crisis intervention is the instillation of hope. The clinician must project an attitude of calm optimism, which was described by Puryear (1979) as follows:

> You are attempting to convey by your entire approach your attitude that the client is a capable, decent person who has been temporarily overwhelmed by extreme stresses, and who will use your help to cope with these stresses and get back on the track. (p. 49)

In fact, the instillation of hope may be one of the most crucial and key elements of crisis intervention.

Subsequent sessions in crisis intervention build on the assessment of coping, support, and perception that was conducted in the first session.

- *Coping*. In each subsequent session, the clinician discusses the client's attempts to cope with the situation and reinforces constructive methods of coping while gently confronting and attempting to undermine maladaptive activities. The clinician must be careful, however, because certain coping activities, such as drinking excessively, are usually accompanied by denial and defensiveness. Too intense a confrontation will invariably precipitate a loss of the therapeutic alliance and possibly the client leaving treatment.

- *Support.* In each session, the clinician directly provides support and attempts to enlarge the client's support system. Most people have at least one or two others they can call on for support and the issue is frequently the client's reluctance to use this support, rather than the lack of it. For certain traumatic events and stressful situations, including medical illnesses, support groups are available.
- *Perception.* The clinician elicits the client's perception of the meaning of the event and gently confronts grossly inaccurate depictions such as "I'll never get another job" or "I'll never find anyone else to love again." In crises precipitated by traumatic stress, patients often feel they will never be able to function adequately again. Although chronic PTSD sometimes follows traumatic events, it is also true that many people survive enormously devastating losses and continue to live productive lives.

There are other meanings that some people attach to traumatic events, as described earlier in the discussion of basic assumptions. For instance, a young male patient suffered serious facial burns when the machine he was working on exploded; he later concluded that he was being punished for using drugs and disrespecting his mother. He maintained this belief despite several discussions with his therapist. Similarly, in March 2005, a Chicago judge's husband and mother were murdered; the parishioners at their church were distraught that this could happen, saying, "Don't all these good deeds mean anything?" (Cholo & Ciokajlo, 2005). It is not always possible to influence patients to change the meaning of a horrific event, but when the meaning is particularly malignant or destructive an attempt should be made.

Throughout the course of the crisis intervention, the clinician works to enlarge the patient's support system, promote adaptive coping, and create a more positive and affirming meaning when possible.

In addition, when the precipitating event is traumatic the clinician should also pay attention to the four clusters of symptoms of ASD (American Psychiatric Association, 2000). Although many people experiencing a crisis due to traumatic stress do not meet criteria for ASD, these symptom clusters are a helpful way to conceptualize traumatic reactions. These are (a) reexperiencing phenomena, including flashbacks and intrusive images and thoughts; (b) purposeful avoidance of reminders of the event; (c) dissociative phenomena, including partial amnesia, numbing of emotional responsiveness, a sense of disconnection from life, and so on; and (d) autonomic reactivity and increased tension and anxiety (American Psychiatric Association, 2000). The presence of these reactions in the immediate aftermath of a traumatic event does not necessarily signal a negative outcome—many individuals substantially recover during the 1st month or so. Crisis intervention treatment does not necessarily resolve these reactions but does work toward a new emotional equilibrium with fewer intrusive thoughts, a reduction in dissociative reactions, and decreased anxiety. Some of this improvement is probably directly due to openly discussing the event and one's reactions to it with a nonjudgmental, sympathetic listener. This process can be conceptualized from the cognitive–behavioral perspective as exposure therapy (Rothbaum, Meadows, Resick, & Foy, 2000) or from the psychodynamic perspective as mastering the trauma (Marmar, 1991). Note that this process goes on over a number of sessions, as opposed to the single session of psychological debriefing.

BEHAVIORAL EMERGENCIES THAT ARE NOT PART OF CRISES

A final consideration is that of behavioral emergencies that are not a part of a crisis. As noted earlier, most emergencies (e.g., potential suicide, potential violence, victim of violence) take place in the context of a crisis. For example, a middle-age man loses his job and experiences a crisis. A week later he becomes suicidal, or perhaps he becomes violent toward his former boss. These situations are behavioral emergencies in the context of crises, which happen frequently. In less common situations, however, emergencies can arise in times of stability. Individuals with borderline personality disorder or alcohol or drug dependence often experience chaotic and impulse-ridden lifestyles. In these cases, impulsive suicide attempts can arise during a time of relative stability; borderline patients are sometimes described as having *stable instability*.

Similarly, patients with antisocial personality disorder and perpetrators of domestic battery can become violent not only during the decompensation of a crisis but also during a time of normal, stable functioning.

These acts of potential or actual suicide or violence are behavioral emergencies without crises. The appropriate therapeutic approach is to conduct an emergency intervention, as described earlier, but not crisis intervention. If the risk of harm is low or moderate, the patient can be referred to or continued in routine outpatient treatment; if the risk is high, hospitalization or some other form of containment is the ideal disposition. Either way, this approach avoids the regression that comes about when crisis intervention—with its rapid, intense involvement—is inappropriately applied to a person with a stable personality disorder or substance dependence disorder.

CONCLUSION

Clearly differentiating between a crisis and a behavioral emergency leads to clarity in action and avoids some of the pitfalls of inappropriate interventions. In this chapter I provided definitions for crisis to accompany this book's overall focus on behavioral emergencies and presented a model (not yet empirically tested) to integrate the understanding of both situations. I encourage readers to make use of these concepts in their clinical practice.

REFERENCES

Aguilera, D. C. (1998). *Crisis intervention: Theory and methodology* (8th ed.). St. Louis, MO: Mosby.

American Psychiatric Association. (1987). *Diagnostic and statistical manual of mental disorders* (3rd ed., rev.). Washington, DC: Author.

American Psychiatric Association. (1994). *Diagnostic and statistical manual of mental disorders* (4th ed.). Washington, DC: Author.

American Psychiatric Association. (2000). *Diagnostic and statistical manual of mental disorders* (4th ed., text rev.). Washington, DC: Author.

Bisson, J. I., Jenkins, P. L., Alexander, J., & Bannister, C. (1997). Randomised controlled trial of psychological debriefing for victims of acute burn trauma. *The British Journal of Psychiatry, 171,* 78–81.

Bonanno, G. A. (2004). Loss, trauma, and human resilience: Have we underestimated the human capacity to thrive after extremely aversive events? *American Psychologist, 59,* 20–28.

Bronisch, T., Maragkos, M., Freyer, C., Muller-Cyran, A., Butollo, W., Weimbs, R., & Platiel, P. (2006). Crisis intervention after the tsunami in Phuket and Khao Lak. *Crisis, 27,* 42–47.

Bryant, R. A., Harvey, A. G., Guthrie, R. M., & Moulds, M. L. (2000). A prospective study of psychophysiological arousal, acute stress disorder, and posttraumatic stress disorder. *Journal of Abnormal Psychology, 109,* 341–344.

Calhoun, L. G., & Tedeschi, R. G. (Eds.). (2006). *Handbook of posttraumatic growth: Research and practice.* Mahwah, NJ: Erlbaum.

Callahan, J. (1994). Defining crisis and emergency. *Crisis, 15,* 164–171.

Callahan, J. (1996). A specific therapeutic approach to suicide risk in borderline patients. *Clinical Social Work Journal, 24,* 443–459.

Callahan, J. (2000). Debriefing the Oklahoma City police. *Tulane Studies in Social Welfare, 11–12,* 285–294.

Caplan, G. (1961). *An approach to community mental health.* New York: Grune & Stratton.

Caplan, G. (1964). *Principles of preventive psychiatry.* New York: Basic Books.

Castro-Blanco, D. (2005). Youth crisis in the schools. In A. R. Roberts (Ed.), *Crisis intervention handbook: Assessment, treatment, and research* (3rd ed., pp. 273–290). New York: Oxford University Press.

Chemtob, C. M., Nakashima, J., & Carlson, J. G. (2002). Brief treatment for elementary school children with disaster-related posttraumatic stress disorder: A field study. *Journal of Clinical Psychology, 68*, 99–112.

Cholo, A. B., & Ciokajlo, M. (2005, March 2). Spouse's love, mom's pride remembered. *Chicago Tribune*, p. 1.

Cohen, S. (2004). Social relationships and health. *American Psychologist, 59*, 676–684.

Deahl, M. P., Gillham, A. B., Thomas, J. T., Searle, M. M., & Srinivasan, M. (1994). Psychological sequelae following the Gulf War: Factors associated with subsequent morbidity and the effectiveness of psychological debriefing. *The British Journal of Psychiatry, 165*, 60–65.

Despland, J. N., Drapeau, M., & de Roten, Y. (2005). A naturalistic study of the effectiveness of a four-session format: The brief psychodynamic intervention. *Brief Treatment and Crisis Intervention, 5*, 368–378.

Dixon, S. L. (1979). *Working with people in crisis.* St. Louis, MO: Mosby.

Fredrickson, B. L., Tugade, M. M., Waugh, C. E., & Larkin, G. R. (2003). What good are positive emotions in crises? A prospective study of resilience and emotions following the terrorist attacks on the United States on September 11, 2001. *Journal of Personality and Social Psychology, 84*, 365–376.

Fried, H. (2005, Summer). Holocaust survivor revisits Auschwitz-Birkenau 60 years later. *Trauma StressPoints*, 6–7.

Gerhart, U. C. (1990). *Caring for the chronically mentally ill.* Itasca, IL: Peacock.

Golan, N. (1974). Crisis theory. In F. J. Turner (Ed.), *Social work treatment: Interlocking theoretical approaches* (pp. 420–456). New York: Free Press.

Golan, N. (1978). *Treatment in crisis situations.* New York: Free Press.

Halliday-Boykins, C. A., Henggeler, S. W., Rowland, M. D., & DeLucia, C. (2004). Heterogeneity in youth symptom trajectories following psychiatric crisis: Predictors and placement outcomes. *Journal of Consulting and Clinical Psychology, 72*, 993–1003.

Hobbs, M., Mayou, R., Harrison, B., & Worlock, P. (1996, December 7). A randomised controlled trial of psychological debriefing for victims of road traffic accidents. *BMJ, 313*, 1438–1439.

Hoff, L. A. (1989). *People in crisis: Understanding and helping* (3rd ed.). Redwood City, CA: Addison Wesley.

James, R. K., & Gilliland, B. E. (2005). *Crisis intervention strategies* (5th ed.). Pacific Grove, CA: Brooks/Cole.

Janoff-Bulman, R. (1985). The aftermath of victimization: Rebuilding shattered assumptions. In C. R. Figley (Ed.), *Trauma and its wake* (Vol. 1, pp. 15–35). New York: Brunner/Mazel.

Janosik, E. H. (1994). *Crisis counseling: A contemporary approach* (2nd ed.). Boston: Jones & Bartlett.

Johnson, S., Nolan, F., Hoult, J., White, I. R., Bebbington, P., Sandor, A., et al. (2005). Outcomes of crises before and after introduction of a crisis resolution team. *The British Journal of Psychiatry, 187,* 68–75.

Kanel, K. (2007). *A guide to crisis intervention* (3rd ed.). Belmont, CA: Thomson Brooks/Cole.

Kaplan, Z., Iancu, I., & Bodner, E. (2001). A review of psychological debriefing after extreme stress. *Psychiatric Services, 52,* 824–827.

Kessler, R. C., Berglund, P., Demler, O., Jin, R., & Walters, E. E. (2005). Lifetime prevalence and age-of-onset distributions of *DSM–IV* disorders in the National Comorbidity Survey Replication. *Archives of General Psychiatry, 62,* 593–602.

Kessler, R. C., Sonnega, A., Bromet, E., Hughes, M., & Nelson, C. B. (1995). Posttraumatic stress disorder in the National Comorbidity Survey. *Archives of General Psychiatry, 52,* 1048–1060.

Koopman, C., Classen, C., Cardena, E., & Spiegel, D. (1995). When disaster strikes, acute distress disorder may follow. *Journal of Traumatic Stress, 8,* 29–46.

Koopman, C., Classen, C., & Spiegel, D. (1996). Dissociative responses in the immediate aftermath of the Oakland/Berkeley firestorm. *Journal of Traumatic Stress, 9,* 521–540.

Kulic, K. R. (2005). The crisis intervention semi-structured interview. *Brief Treatment and Crisis Intervention, 5,* 143–157.

Lazarus, R. S. (1980). The stress and coping paradigm. In L. A. Bond & R. C. Rosen (Eds.), *Competence and coping during adulthood* (pp. 28–74). Hanover, NH: University Press of New England.

Lee, C., Slade, P., & Lygo, V. (1996). The influence of psychological debriefing on emotional adaptation in women following early miscarriage: A preliminary study. *British Journal of Medical Psychology, 69,* 47–58.

Marchand, A., Guay, S., Boyer, R., Iucci, S., Martin, A., & St.-Hilaire, M.-H. (2006). A randomized controlled trial of an adapted form of individual critical incident stress debriefing for victims of an armed robbery. *Brief Treatment and Crisis Intervention, 6,* 122–129.

Marmar, C. R. (1991). Brief dynamic psychotherapy of post-traumatic stress disorder. *Psychiatric Annals, 21,* 405–414.

Mayou, R. A., Ehlers, A., & Hobbs, M. (2000). Psychological debriefing for road traffic accident victims: Three-year follow-up of a randomised controlled trial. *The British Journal of Psychiatry, 176,* 589–593.

McNally, R. J., Bryant, R. A., & Ehlers, A. (2003). Does early psychological intervention promote recovery from posttraumatic stress? *Psychological Science in the Public Interest, 4,* 45–79.

Mitchell, J. T. (1983). When disaster strikes . . . the critical incident stress debriefing process. *Journal of Emergency Medical Services, 8,* 36–39.

Mitchell, J. T., & Everly, G. S. (1995). *Critical incident stress debriefing: An operations manual for the prevention of traumatic stress among emergency services and disaster workers* (2nd ed.). Ellicott City, MD: Chevron.

National Institute of Mental Health (2002). *Mental health and mass violence: Evidence-based early psychological intervention for victims/survivors of mass violence.* (NIH Publication No. 02-5138). Washington, DC: U.S. Government Printing Office.

Parad, H. J., & Parad, L. G. (1990). Crisis intervention: An introductory overview. In H. J. Parad & L. G. Parad (Eds.), *Crisis intervention: Book 2. The practitioner's sourcebook for brief therapy* (pp. 3–31). Milwaukee, WI: Family Service America.

Puryear, D. A. (1979). *Helping people in crisis.* San Francisco: Jossey-Bass.

Rapoport, L. (1965). The state of crisis: Some theoretical considerations. In H. J. Parad (Ed.), *Crisis intervention: Selected readings* (pp. 22–31). New York: Family Service Association of America.

Reyes, G., & Jacobs, G. A. (Eds.). (2006). *Handbook of international disaster psychology: Interventions with special needs populations* (Vol. 4). Westport, CT: Praeger Publishers.

Roberts, A. R. (2005). Bridging the past and present to the future of crisis intervention and crisis management. In A. R. Roberts (Ed.), *Crisis intervention handbook: Assessment, treatment, and research* (3rd ed., pp. 3–34). New York: Oxford University Press.

Roberts, A. R., & Everly, G. S. (2006). A meta-analysis of 36 crisis intervention studies. *Brief Treatment and Crisis Intervention, 6,* 10–21.

Rose, S., Bisson, J., & Wessely, S. (2004). Psychological debriefing for preventing post traumatic stress disorder (PTSD). *The Cochrane Library, 1.* Chichester, England: Wiley.

Rose, S., Brewin, C. R., Andrews, B., & Kirk, M. (1999). A randomized controlled trial of individual psychological debriefing for victims of violent crime. *Psychological Medicine, 29,* 793–799.

Rothbaum, B. O., Meadows, E. A., Resick, P., & Foy, D. W. (2000). Cognitive–behavioral therapy. In E. B. Foa, T. M. Keane, & M. J. Friedman (Eds.), *Effective treatments for PTSD: Practice guidelines from the International Society for Traumatic Stress Studies* (pp. 60–83). New York: Guilford Press.

Slaikeu, K. A. (1990). *Crisis intervention: A handbook for practice and research* (2nd ed.). Boston: Allyn & Bacon.

Stallard, P., & Salter, E. (2003). Psychological debriefing with children and young people following traumatic events. *Clinical Child Psychology and Psychiatry, 8,* 445–457.

Sutker, P. B., Davis, J. M., Uddo, M., & Ditta, S. R. (1995). War zone stress, personal resources, and PTSD in Persian Gulf War returnees. *Journal of Abnormal Psychology, 104,* 444–452.

Terr, L. (1994). *Unchained memories: True stories of traumatic memories, lost and found.* New York: Basic Books.

Ursano, R. J., Fullerton, C. S., & Norwood, A. E. (Eds.). (2003). *Terrorism and disaster: Individual and community mental health interventions.* Cambridge, England: Cambridge Press.

van Emmerik, A. A. P., Kamphuis, J. H., Hulsbosch, A. M., & Emmelkamp, P. M. G. (2002, September 7). Single session debriefing after psychological trauma: A meta-analysis. *The Lancet, 360,* 766–771.

Yeager, K. R., & Roberts, A. R. (2005). Differentiating among stress, acute stress disorder, acute crisis episodes, trauma, and PTSD: Paradigm and treatment goals. In A. R. Roberts (Ed.), *Crisis intervention handbook: Assessment, treatment, and research* (3rd ed., pp. 90–119). New York: Oxford University Press.

Young, B. H. (2006). The immediate response to disaster: Guidelines for adult psychological first aid. In E. C. Ritchie, P. J. Watson, & M. J. Friedman (Eds.), *Interventions following mass violence and disasters: Strategies for mental health practice* (pp. 134–154). New York: Guilford Press.

2

EVALUATING BEHAVIORAL EMERGENCIES: THE CLINICAL INTERVIEW

PHILLIP M. KLEESPIES AND JANET S. RICHMOND

Evaluating a patient or client who may be at imminent risk of life-threatening behavior requires skills that go beyond those needed for the traditional clinical interview. With a patient or client who is in a volatile emotional state, the interview process often takes place in a charged atmosphere. The patient is stressed and the clinician may be stressed as well. The clinician needs to be concerned about dealing with and attempting to modulate the emotional state of an individual who may be hostile, agitated, paranoid, or impulsive. The patient or client may provide incomplete and conflicting information. There may be pressure to arrive at an assessment of the problem and a decision about management in a very limited period of time.

There may be other workload demands to which the clinician feels that he or she needs to attend. If the patient begins to lose behavioral control, the interviewer must be thinking about what he or she may need to do to prevent the patient from harming him- or herself, or others. Decision making under such conditions can be compromised, and errors in judgment can occur that may have serious consequences for the patient, the clinician, and for others (Cannon-Bowers & Salas, 1998b).

As noted in the introduction to this book, instruction in the classroom or in workshops with simulated interviews cannot fully prepare one to be an effective interviewer and decision maker under such anxiety provoking circumstances. Rather, these skills are ultimately learned under naturalistic conditions in which one goes through the process of stress exposure and inoculation with the aid of a mentor or supervisor (Cannon-Bowers & Salas, 1998a). This is not to say that lectures, workshops, and readings (such as this chapter) are not valuable components of the learning process. They clearly are. In the final analysis, however, the skills needed to evaluate and manage behavioral emergencies are assimilated and integrated in the performance of the task.

The interview discussed in this chapter is intended to provide structure and guidance to the clinician who is being trained in evaluating behavioral emergencies. The major tasks in an emergency interview are to (a) contain the patient's emotional turmoil (if necessary), (b) define the problem(s), (c) estimate the risk to self or others, and (d) provide appropriate care and treatment (Gerson & Bassuk, 1980; Kleespies, Deleppo, Mori, & Niles, 1998). In the sections that follow, these major tasks are explored in greater depth. The initial focus is on methods of encouraging the patient's cooperation and, when necessary, on methods of dealing with the patient's or client's emotional turmoil. Not all cases require such an emphasis; however, if a patient is distraught or agitated, it is essential to help the patient gain better self-control if the remainder of the interview is to proceed.

CONTAINING THE PATIENT'S EMOTIONAL TURMOIL

Although an interview under emergency or crisis conditions requires an evaluative approach, one should not ignore the potential need to form a cooperative or working alliance with the client or patient. In this regard, the less experienced interviewer can run the risk of two types of errors: (a) assuming too readily that there is an alliance with a patient when none exists and (b) dwelling too long on establishing a relationship when it is already assumed by the patient. As Echterling and Hartsough (1989) demonstrated, the patient usually expects that the role of the interviewer in an emergency or crisis is a helping one and that part of this role is doing an evaluation of the problem. The sections that follow discuss how to help the patient or client with his or her distress so a productive evaluation and recommendation for follow-up care can be made.

General Principles in the Engagement Process

Engaging a patient or client in a working alliance for the purpose of conducting a clinical interview under crisis or emergency conditions can be challenging. Regardless of where the interview takes place, certain elements must be present for the patient to develop a sense of trust and safety.

A major element in engaging the patient in the evaluative process is the ability of the clinician to convey empathy. Shea (1998) emphasized the use of a gradation of basic to complex empathic statements, in which the clinician reflects degrees of certainty regarding what the patient is experiencing: The more certainty, the more incisive the empathic comment. Basic empathic statements are usually made in the early part of the interview, when rapport is first developing and the clinician is less knowledgeable about the patient's presenting issues and mental status. On the one hand, a basic empathic comment such as, "It sounds as though things have gotten more difficult to manage since the loss of your wife," is general and open and less likely to be threatening to the patient. On the other hand, when the clinician feels more confident about having an alliance with the patient and has a better understanding of the issues and corresponding affect, a more pointed empathic comment, such as "You are feeling quite sad and are having more difficulty managing since the loss of your wife," can be timely and may facilitate greater verbal material and emotional expression.

A second major element in engaging the patient is authenticity. It comes from the capacity of the interviewer to be real and genuine in his or her interactions with the patient or client. If the patient shows humor, a clinician's smile can allay some of the patient's anxiety and also convey the message that the clinician is human and can enjoy things as others do. The interviewer who can be spontaneous, nondefensive, and flexible is role-modeling that it is acceptable to be responsive and expressive about one's feelings and problems. As Shea (1998) pointed out, however, spontaneity and nondefensiveness do not imply sharing whatever comes to mind or violating clinician–patient boundaries. Rather, the skilled clinician continuously assesses the potential impact of his or her statements and can exhibit spontaneity when it is appropriate. An alliance between the clinician and patient comes from the patient's or client's perception that the clinician is caring, available, and skilled in pursuing the issues.

Special Issues in Forming a Working Alliance

Many different factors can affect the development of a working alliance with the patient. These issues include patient demographic and cultural variables, difficult patient emotional states or behaviors, and the clinician's own reactions to the interaction.

Patient Demographic Variables

It is clearly important that clinicians be aware of possible group differences to minimize the potential negative impact of misinterpretation. In some instances, it may be helpful to consult with or bring into the interview a clinician of the same race, ethnic group, or gender as the patient or client.

Ethnicity and Race. Being sensitive to how ethnic and racial factors affect the patient's values, norms, and perceptions is critical. African Americans, for example, have experienced unequal access to health care (Ayanian, Cleary, Weissman, & Epstein, 1999) and, not surprisingly, have been found to be less trusting of the health care system (Caralis, Davis, Wright, & Marcial, 1993). Moreover, clinicians can misunderstand or misinterpret culture- or race-specific behavior patterns; for example, in Japanese culture direct eye contact can be considered aggressive or disrespectful, but to a Western clinician lack of eye contact might be seen as a sign of low self-esteem or furtiveness (Shea, 1998; Turner & Hersen, 1994). Such instances of cultural misunderstanding may have contributed to the finding that minority populations are often overpathologized and misdiagnosed (Jones & Gray, 1986; Lopez & Hernandez, 1986). It appears that race can also play a role in treatment decisions. Thus, Segal, Bola, and Watson (1996) found that emergency service clinicians, most of whom were European Americans, "prescribed more psychiatric medications to African Americans than to other patients and devoted less time to their evaluation" (p. 282).

Gender. Evidence suggests that a patient's gender can influence diagnostic decisions and disposition outcomes (Loring & Powell, 1988). Tudor, Tudor, and Gove (1977) found, for example, that men are more likely to be hospitalized than are women, and at a younger age. There are also studies indicating that women are more likely to be diagnosed with histrionic personality disorder when they are seen by male clinicians (Loring & Powell, 1988).

Difficult Patient Conditions

A number of difficult patient conditions can make an emergency evaluation challenging. Knowing how to work with the patient who has behavioral problems can help the clinician feel more confident and achieve a better outcome. Here are a few potential patient conditions that can be hard to manage.

The Agitated or Hostile Patient. An agitated, angry patient may be at risk of acting out when feeling disempowered and out of control. It is important that the clinician maintain a clinical perspective and not take hostile statements personally. It can be helpful to keep in mind that the patient is behaving in a difficult way because of his or her psychopathology. If the patient becomes threatening, acknowledging his or her anger while setting empathic but firm limits on potential violence can be an effective way to diffuse the tension. It is appropriate for the patient to express anger verbally, but the physical expression of anger cannot be allowed. As Guy and Brady (1998) noted, less experienced clinicians seem to be at greater risk of being assaulted, and one hypothesis is that they may be more hesitant to set limits and therefore are more likely to allow threatening behavior to escalate.

The Paranoid Patient. Patients who are paranoid are often defensive, secretive, irritable, and quick to react in a hostile fashion to a perceived threat. These patients are frequently reassured if clinicians remain professionally confident and in control (Dubin, 1990). Interviewers should maintain a professional demeanor and treat such patients respectfully, without being overly familiar or friendly. In fact, Shea (1998) reported that overly empathic statements served to disengage the guarded or paranoid patient who is uncomfortable with intimacy. By acknowledging the patient's difficulty with trust, the interviewer can at times elicit some capacity to participate in the evaluation (Jesse & Anderson, 1990). It is important, however, to be sensitive to the patient's limitations in regard to questions that may be perceived as too intrusive or invasive.

The Disorganized or Psychotic Patient. The psychotic patient's thinking can become loose and tangential. When interviewing acutely psychotic patients, the clinician should assess symptoms without attempting to use logic or convince the patient that his or her perceptions are wrong (Dubin, 1990; Jesse & Anderson, 1990). If there is a question about how fixed a patient's delusional thinking may be, the clinician might test to see whether the patient would consider an alternative explanation. This testing, however, should not be done in a vain effort to refute the irrational nature of the patient's thinking. If the patient is disorganized, the clinician will need to provide structure by redirecting the patient's thought back to the task at hand.

The Intoxicated Patient. Patients who abuse substances appear frequently in emergency departments and, on occasion, in outpatient clinic settings. Depending on the level of intoxication, an interview may not be immediately possible. It may be necessary to simply arrange for the patient to be monitored for safety while he or she sobers up. If the patient has symptoms such as slurred speech and an unsteady gait, it is important to have the patient seen in an emergency department or urgent care clinic where a breathalyzer test or blood alcohol level and vital signs can be used to monitor the patient's condition. High blood alcohol levels can become medical emergencies (Trezza & Popp, 1998). For the patient who has been a heavy drinker but has cut back or stopped drinking in the past few days, it is important to be familiar with the symptoms of withdrawal and delirium tremens. The latter can be a potentially life-threatening condition that requires immediate medical attention (Dubin, 1990; Trezza & Popp, 1998). Although intoxicated patients can become a behavioral nuisance, the clinician needs to keep in mind that such patients are often disinhibited and can be a risk to themselves and others by virtue of their poor judgment. Alcoholic patients who express suicidal ideation can be particularly worrisome because alcoholic patients who commit suicide typically do so during a period of active drinking (Conwell et al., 1996). See chapter 11 of this volume for a detailed discussion of treating patients who are abusing substances.

Clinician Reactions That Affect the Interaction

Managing a behavioral emergency competently can be very rewarding. Emergency or crisis work, however, can also expose the clinician to difficult and uncooperative patients or clients. Hanke (1984) reported that clinicians may respond to the difficulties of this work with a range of feelings, including anger, anxiety, discouragement, and avoidance. It can be difficult to acknowledge such feelings but if not dealt with adequately, clinical judgment and decision making can be compromised (Dubin, 1990; Pope & Tabachnick, 1993). For example, patients who are manic or have narcissistic features can be very good at finding the sensitivities of the interviewer and devaluing him or her. One way to manage the impact of such remarks is to observe your reactions and use them as a therapeutic resource for understanding the patient (Pope & Tabachnick, 1993). Thus, if you feel the patient is devaluing you, it is likely that he or she is attempting to bolster self-esteem or to compensate for a perceived narcissistic injury.

Responding When a Patient Is at Risk of Losing Self-Control

Despite the best of efforts, there are times when a patient is unable to be cooperative or to form a working alliance with the clinician. Signs and symptoms of loss of self-control and potential for dangerousness include the following: (a) psychomotor activity such as sweating, pacing, fidgeting, clenching fists, grinding teeth, or being unable to sit down; (b) affective and facial changes that reflect either hostility, fear, or paranoia; and (c) the tone and content of the patient's speech. Other signs include verbal expressions of impatience or frustration, subtle indications of anger, or a defiant demeanor. Psychotic patients may show signs of responding to internal stimuli such as command hallucinations. The clinician needs to attend to and make a mental note of each factor on a minute-by-minute basis during the examination. Additionally, the clinician must pay careful attention to his or her own negative reactions, as they can contribute to an escalating and unsafe situation (Hillard, 1990; Kaplan & Sadock, 1993).

The sections that follow briefly discuss the types of patients who may become dangerous and ways to decrease the risk of harm, including both preventive measures before the interview and intervention during the interview.

Types of Patients Who May Be at Risk

Evaluation and management of the potentially violent patient are dealt with at greater length in chapters 6 and 7. For the purposes of this chapter, it is assumed that patients who are acutely psychotic, neurologically compromised, intoxicated, delirious, or in an extreme state of agitation can be more susceptible to behaving in a violent manner. Antisocial, borderline, and narcissistic personality disorder patients have, of course, also been associated with risk of violence. One should take particular care with patients for whom the need to seek help is considered humiliating and shameful.

In dealing with patients who have the potential to lose control, the safety of the patient, clinician, other patients, and staff are of critical importance. Although the clinician is working to respect the patient's autonomy and civil rights as much as possible, she or he must be prepared to help the patient maintain self-control and become more collaborative (Hillard 1990; Kaplan & Sadock, 1993).

Ways to Decrease Risk of Harm

If the clinician has observed some of the behavioral or emotional cues noted earlier or has a gut feeling that the patient may be dangerous, he or she should not become isolated in a room with the patient. It is recommended that the interview room be arranged so the clinician will have easy access to an exit and can obtain help in the event of a serious threat to safety. Panic buttons can also be useful. With the intensely paranoid patient who might become aggressive if feeling trapped, it may make sense to arrange the room so both the interviewer and the patient have an exit or perhaps have equal access to a single exit. In some settings, it may be possible to alert the police or security team that they need to respond quickly.

Finding ways to decrease the risk of harm from a patient may include the use of verbal limits. This can be a simple yet effective way to defuse the patient's aggressive feelings by using nonjudgmental, empathic statements.

Verbal Limits

Asserting verbal limits can be an effective way to decrease risk. Verbal limits might include empathic, observational statements about the fact that the patient appears upset. It is often helpful to ask whether he or she can talk about what's so upsetting. Appealing to the patient's rational side may be useful. For example, statements such as "As you know there are some very distressed people here who need things to be quiet" can decrease a patient's boisterousness. If there is a concern about loss of control, one effective technique is to ask the patient whether the clinician should be worried about his or her own safety. Another technique is to use a degree of self-disclosure stating, for example, "If you do things that make me tense and nervous, I can't help you as well as I might." Multiple short interviews may be necessary to defuse some situations; therefore, statements such as "OK, let's take a break for a few minutes" or "It seems like we're getting annoyed or frustrated with each other; let's both calm down and resume our discussion in 10 minutes" can be extremely helpful.

When Verbal Limits Fail

If a patient or client is not responsive to verbal limit setting and persists or escalates his or her agitated or threatening behavior, the next step will likely depend on the environment and the availability of assistance. Clinicians who work in a counseling center or private practice setting may wish to consider the options of terminating the interview (if it is safe to do so), summoning security officers, or if necessary, calling the local police and ambulance to take the patient to a secure setting such as a hospital emergency department for further evaluation. In these instances it is helpful to be working with a colleague who can assist either by calling or by staying with the patient while the clinician calls. The private practitioner needs to plan ahead for emergency situations that might arise in his or her setting.

Those working in an emergency department, hospital, or urgent care clinic setting usually have more options than do those in less secure environments. In particular, medical staff can offer the patient tranquilizing medication and, if necessary, have the patient voluntarily or involuntarily restrained.

Pharmacologic Intervention. For short-term control of agitated or potentially violent behavior, benzodiazepines and antipsychotics have been the medications of choice (Hillard, 1990; Kaplan & Sadock, 1993; Tardiff, 1989). Although benzodiazepines have been reported to increase aggressive behavior, it is a relatively rare phenomenon. If a patient is already prescribed an antipsychotic medication, more of the same medication can usually be offered. Otherwise, haloperidol (i.e., Haldol) 5 mg by mouth or intramuscularly, along with a benzodiazepine such as lorazepam (i.e., Ativan) 1 to 2 mg by mouth or intramuscularly, is customary for an initial trial. These dosages can be repeated in 30 to 60 minutes if the patient is still agitated. Benztropine (i.e., Cogentin) is sometimes added as a prophylactic against dystonias and extrapyramidal side effects. Cardiac irregularities or changes in heart rhythm can also be a rare side effect of haloperidol.

In recent years, the benefits of using atypical antipsychotics (e.g., risperidone, olanzapine, ziprasidone) in emergency situations have been promoted because these medications were believed to have lower risks of extrapyramidal side effects and greater cardiac safety (Allen, Currier, Carpenter, Ross, & Docherty, 2005). Further experience with atypicals, however, has indicated that they too can create cardiac irregularities. Moreover, the atypicals may induce unpleasant or dangerous drug interactions if combined with certain other medications (Ciraulo, Shader, Greenblatt, & Creelman, 2005).

Most patients can be managed well with the established regimen of haloperidol and lorazepam. These medications have the advantage of being readily available in emergency and urgent care settings, and emergency personnel are familiar with their use. The risk of extrapyramidal side effects decreases dramatically after age 40, so the use of an atypical or of benztropine prophylaxis is indicated only for younger patients. It is recommended that patients with liver disease be given lorazepam or oxazepam as the benzodiazepines of choice because they metabolize quickly and are eliminated by the kidney (Saitz, Ciraulo, Shader, & Ciraulo, 2003). It is important to note that benzodiazepines such as lorazepam are considered less effective for those who have developed a tolerance to them—for example, through excessive use of the medication or through the excessive use of alcohol—because both alcohol and benzodiazepines work on the same neural receptors.[1]

Physical Restraint and Seclusion. It is important to remember that for patients with a history of being traumatized by violence or abuse, the prospect of physical restraint or seclusion can reawaken painful and frightening memories. Restraint or seclusion should be avoided, if possible, with such patients. At times, a show of force including nursing staff, police, or security officers can help to calm and contain an escalating situation and obviate the need for restraint. Nonetheless, for the agitated and threatening patient who is unable to respond to verbal limits or to a show of force and refuses medication or who has clearly lost behavioral control, physical restraint or seclusion is necessary as an effective and humane response to a situation that could lead to serious injury to others or to the patient (Kleespies et al., 1998). The frustration and confusion of being restrained or secluded is a temporary stressor for the patient, but the consequences of uncontained violence can be irreversible (Kaplan & Sadock, 1993).

It is also important to note that the restraint procedure itself (or the act of placing someone in a seclusion room) can be dangerous for both patient and staff. These procedures should be done with a clear plan for maintaining safety, and only trained staff should carry them out. Negotiations regarding restraint or seclusion should occur before the procedure is initiated—not during the procedure (Hillard, 1990; Kaplan & Sadock, 1993; Tardiff, 1989). After the decision has been made to restrain or seclude the patient, reengaging in negotiation can be confusing to the staff team and place them at greater risk.

Whereas some patients are cooperative or even request restraints or seclusion, many patients resist. A limited number of staff is needed to manage a resistant patient—one trained person to control each limb and one to protect and control the head. A sixth person should be available to coordinate the procedure and talk to the patient while the other team members are placing him or her in restraints or in the seclusion room. Vital signs as well as agitation are likely to increase for the first few minutes after a patient is placed in restraints or seclusion. In the case of restraints, the positioning of the patient needs to be considered. Most patients are restrained in the face

---

[1]We, the chapter authors, wish to thank Edward P. Monnelly, MD, Psychiatry Service, VA Boston Healthcare System, for his review of this section on pharmacologic interventions.

up position; some patients, particularly those with histories of sexual trauma, may become more agitated and frightened by being placed in such a vulnerable position. For these patients, restraint while lying on their side may be preferred.

Of course, after a patient is restrained, a staff member needs to sit with the patient to monitor his or her emotional and physical condition. As is done with seclusion, a staff member should be seated outside the door of the room. Legal requirements and hospital policies typically require that leather restraints be checked every 15 minutes to ensure that there is no interference with circulation. Providing it is safe to do so, each limb is to be removed from restraint for exercise once per hour. Many patients become calmer after they are in restraints or seclusion and control has been established. Others, however, may continue to be agitated or may become more so. In such cases, it may be necessary to request that medication be prescribed to ease the patient's distress and turmoil. Restraints or seclusion are to be maintained for the minimum time necessary for the patient to regain self-control.

DEFINING THE PROBLEM

At times in the setting of a clinical emergency, the problem is evident or clearly stated. Often, however, the patient or client is too stressed or decompensated to present his or her difficulties in an organized, coherent manner. To gather the essential information needed to formulate the problem or problems, the clinician must have a framework available that will provide guidance to his or her interview.

A General Framework and Strategy

We suggest a general framework that has two components: (a) a biopsychosocial approach that enables one to appreciate the multidimensional nature of many emotional and mental disorders or conditions and (b) a hypothesis testing strategy that will allow one to probe for a better understanding of the issues involved.

Biopsychosocial Approach

The biopsychosocial approach to understanding human problems is complex and multidetermined. It encourages the interviewer to examine the patient in terms of possible biological, psychological–behavioral, and social contributions to his or her distress or dysfunction. It discourages reductionistic or overly simplistic formulations. Thus, biological factors involved in mental disorders such as schizophrenia or bipolar disorder are considered. Psychological factors such as the patient's limited coping resources, poor ability to regulate emotion, or impoverished self-esteem are reviewed. The patient's social network, which might include his or her family system, marital or partner relationship, and current living arrangement, is examined. Each of these potential spheres of influence is given weight in understanding the client's condition.

Hypothesis Testing Strategy

Confronted with the complex array of material generated by a biopsychosocial perspective, the clinician must attempt to determine the key factors contributing to the patient's or client's problem. This effort can be aided by a hypothesis testing strategy in which the clinician takes particularly salient factors presented by the patient and tests them for relevance. By way of example, a clinician is asked to evaluate a patient who has presented to an emergency department or urgent care clinic with a complaint of depression and suicidal ideation. A review of the patient's record indicates that he presented in a similar fashion a year ago and was hospitalized with diagnoses of major depression and posttraumatic stress disorder. He was treated with an antidepressant medication and psychotherapy and responded well to this regimen. On the basis of this information, the clinician generates some hypotheses or questions about possible precipitants to the current episode. Is this an anniversary reaction to the time of the patient's original trauma? Did the patient discontinue his or her medication or follow-up treatment prematurely? Has there been some new reversal that has negatively affected the patient's self-esteem?

The clinician begins by eliciting the patient's presentation of the problem. In this case, the patient states that he has been feeling anxious and depressed and has had an increased frequency of trauma-related nightmares for the past several weeks. He is not sure what brought these problems on, but they have been severe enough that he feels as though he might want to end it all by committing suicide. The clinician's questions and hypotheses are investigated with the patient as he or she proceeds through the interview. The patient denies any recent psychosocial stressors, but he reports that he often seems to have difficulty with depression at this time of year. When questioned further about this issue, he reveals that it was at this time of year that he experienced his most severe combat-related trauma that involved a fellow soldier dying in his arms while begging the patient not to let him die. He has longstanding survivor guilt relative to this loss. He also reports that he stopped taking his antidepressant medication because he did not like the side effect of sexual dysfunction. In an effort to cope with his anxiety and depression, he has started to abuse alcohol.

At the end of such an interviewing process, the clinician can arrive at a formulation based on several biopsychosocial findings. Factors contributing to the patient's presenting condition include recurrent anxious depression precipitated by a trauma-related anniversary reaction that involves unresolved survivor guilt, the discontinuation of antidepressant medication that might have been preventive, and the initiation of a maladaptive effort to cope by self-medicating with alcohol.

Putting Theory Into Practice: Using a Semistructured Emergency Interview

Open-ended questions (e.g., "What brings you here today?") are most appropriate in the early stages of an emergency interview. After initial data have been collected, the interviewer can begin to formulate further questions and generate hypotheses. Questioning can become increasingly specific as the interviewer attempts to confirm or negate the validity of the data and engage in hypothesis testing.

ESTIMATING RISK TO SELF OR OTHERS

Under the pressure of emergency or crisis conditions, a premium is placed on the rapid acquisition of information that is essential to reaching a decision about whether an emergency intervention will be needed to prevent harm to self or others. We propose that there are several categories of information that should be covered in virtually all emergency interviews, except perhaps those in which a patient's condition will not permit it. These categories include the chief complaint, precipitating factors, current functional status, mental health and substance abuse history, acute or chronic medical problems, medications with dosages and compliance, and of course, an assessment of lethality.

Chief Complaint

Interviews typically begin with a request for the patient's or client's chief complaint; that is, his or her explanation of what has brought him or her to seek help. It is also wise to ask what outcome the patient wants from the evaluation. Of course, there can be instances when the patient is unable or unwilling to provide this information and it must be sought through collateral sources (e.g., the referring practitioner or a family member who has accompanied the patient).

Precipitating Factors

After the chief complaint or presenting problem has been elicited, the interviewer can focus on events or issues that the patient feels may have contributed to his or her complaint or problem. It is useful to know how long the patient or client has had a particular problem or problems, and what the course of the problems may have been. Have there been recent stressors, losses, or changes in circumstance that may have contributed? What, if anything, has the patient done to remedy the problem?

Current Functional Status

Information about the patient's current familial, social, and occupational functioning is necessary for the formulation of the problem and for the development of a plan of action. The clinician should assess how well the patient or client interacts with family and friends, performs tasks of daily living, or is able to work or attend school. Does the patient have housing? The quality of the patient's social network, or the lack of a social network, may be particularly important in arriving at a disposition.

Mental Health and Substance Use History

Because past behavior is one of the best predictors of future behavioral problems, the patient's history of suicide attempts and violence or threats of violence is vital information. A brief history of previously conferred diagnoses and of inpatient and outpatient courses of treatment is also useful in formulating the current problem as well as the plan of action. Assessment of any current and past alcohol and drug abuse is clearly important. Such an assessment should include the amount typically used on a daily or weekly basis, the last use plus the amount, and any history of withdrawal symptoms (which for alcohol should include an inquiry about past withdrawal seizures and episodes of delirium tremens).

Acute or Chronic Medical Problems

Some acute and chronic medical problems can add to the burden that the patient or client must bear. Acute or chronic pain, for example, can lower frustration tolerance. Certain endocrine disorders and neurological disorders can cause anxiety and depression (see chaps. 13 and 14). Some medical illnesses, such as HIV/AIDS and multiple sclerosis, have been associated with an increased risk of suicide (see chap. 5). If a patient has a medical illness, it is important to consider whether it may be a factor in his or her presentation.

Medications

Ideally, the interviewer will have a list of the patient's medications and their dosages available. Whether the patient has been compliant or noncompliant with medication will have a bearing on how one thinks about the patient's condition. Is it occurring despite compliance or as a result of noncompliance? Of course, medications such as steroids can cause serious mental status changes, and the SSRI (i.e., selective serotonin reuptake inhibitor) antidepressants as well as many antihypertensive medications can cause sexual dysfunction. Drug interactions can also cause emotional or behavioral changes. These would clearly be factors to consider in assessing the patient's mental and emotional state.

Lethality Assessment

An assessment of the patient's potential lethality toward self or others is at the heart of the emergency interview. Risk of suicide, potential for violence, and inability to protect oneself from interpersonal victimization are topics covered in detail in other sections of this book (see chaps. 3–9). They cannot be adequately addressed in this chapter, but a few guidelines can be offered.

In a lethality assessment, the interviewer should ask about suicidal or violent ideation in a straightforward manner. There is no known evidence that asking will increase the chances of suicidal or violent behavior occurring. Rather, an inquiry into the patient's ideation may allow the clinician to take the steps necessary to ensure safety. Patients may be hesitant to reveal their suicidal or violent thoughts for various reasons. They may wish to avoid appearing "crazy" or avoid being hospitalized, or they may feel it is inappropriate to burden others with their troubles. In such cases, the clinician needs to be sensitive to subtle expressions of despair or frustration, and to follow up on indirect communications. For example, a patient may simply report, "I'm just so tired of all the hassles." Further questioning of this patient may reveal a wish to die or to commit suicide.

After it is determined that a patient or client has suicidal or violent ideation, the interviewer will want to inquire about the level of intent and whether the patient has a plan of action or is likely to act impulsively. Level of intent (or degree of ambivalence) can be assessed by asking about those factors that might incline the patient to act and those that might attenuate action. One might have the patient rate intent on a scale. For example, he or she might be asked, "On a scale from 1 to 10—on which 1 means that you definitely will not carry through on your suicidal (or violent) thoughts and 10 means that you definitely will—where would you rate yourself now?" The interviewer can then follow up on the meaning of such a rating. The patient's likelihood of acting impulsively might be ascertained by asking about similar situations in the past and how the patient handled them. Thus, he or she might be asked, "Have you ever been this angry at someone before? What did you do then?"

In addition to evaluating for ideation and intent, however, the interviewer will want to consider the larger context of the patient's condition. Such a consideration might include determining whether the patient has a diagnosis or diagnoses that are associated with a high risk of suicide or violence and whether he or she may have evidence-based risk factors that are associated with that particular diagnosis (Clark, 1998; Clark & Fawcett, 1992). Moreover, a general review of known risk factors and protective or attenuating factors would be warranted. The clinician will then need to exercise judgment that is guided by the available empirical evidence and his or her own clinical acumen.

Validity

After gathering all the critical information from the patient, it is then necessary to determine how valid this information really is. Validity in the clinical interview has to do with the accuracy of the data elicited from the patient. It is obviously a critical factor in an emergency situation in which decisions about disposition can have very serious implications. Shea (1998) suggested two ways to test for validity. One method is to ask the patient or client to describe specific details of events rather than asking for opinions about these events. For example, the interviewer might ask a female patient what sorts of things her husband actually did to provide emotional support rather than whether she felt satisfied with his support. A second method of establishing validity is to seek verification of information from family and friends, provided that they are available and that the patient gives the clinician permission to seek their input.

Assessing Current Functioning and Mental Status

Although the first part of the emergency interview is an examination of relevant aspects of the patient's recent and past history, the mental status exam (MSE) gives the interviewer a cross sectional view of the patient's current mental and emotional functioning. In its more comprehensive form (e.g., see Pruyser, 1979), the MSE covers all areas of mental, emotional, and behavioral functioning needed for diagnostic classification. An MSE that is so inclusive may be unwieldy in the context of a behavioral emergency, however, and is usually unnecessary. A skilled clinician can glean a good deal of information about current functioning from his or her observations of the patient or from deductive reasoning throughout the interview.

Nonetheless, the interviewer should be sufficiently thorough in his or her evaluation to be able to report on the following aspects of the patient's presentation and functioning: general appearance, attitude toward the examiner, orientation, attention and concentration, immediate and delayed recall, fund of information, mood and affect, psychomotor activity, risk to self or others, symptoms of anxiety or posttraumatic stress, intelligence, speech, thought content and process, psychotic symptoms (i.e., hallucinations and delusions), substance abuse, judgment, and insight. A sample MSE form cov-

TABLE 2.1
Elements of a Mental Status Examination

Elements	Descriptors/Measures
Appearance	Neat, disheveled, inappropriately dressed, diaphoretic, ruddy-faced, emaciated, obese, well-developed and well-nourished, glasses or hearing aid
Behavior	Psychomotor retardation, agitation, fidgeting, abnormal motor movements (e.g., ticks, contractures of limbs, akathisia, akinesia, grimaces, blephorospasm)
Attitude	Cooperative and friendly, intrusive, guarded, vague, hypervigilant, suspicious, seductive, ingratiating, controlling, good or poor eye contact
Level of arousal	Alert, hyperalert, sedated, sluggish, drowsy, minimally responsive, comatose (completely nonresponsive to external stimuli—e.g., to noise, pain, temperature)
Orientation	Time, place, person, purpose
Memory	Registration delayed recall (give three unassociated words—e.g., *baby pen tree*—and ask patient to immediately repeat them back and then ask the patient to repeat them after 3 to 5 minutes [immediate and short-term memory]). Where was patient born? (remote)
Concentration	Serial 7s or 3s; adding, subtracting, and multiplying simple numbers; give months of year in backward order; spell *world* backward
Visual–spatial organization	Draw-a-clock, copy intersecting shapes
Fund of information	Major news event, last 8 to 10 presidents, 6 northeastern states
Abstraction	Similarities (e.g., apple and banana, table and chair); proverbs (e.g., book by cover, stitch in time, bird in hand)
Social judgment	What would you do if you found a stamped, addressed envelope on the street? What would you do if you saw smoke and fire in a crowded movie theater?
Insight	Does the patient understand that he or she is ill or has a problem?
Affect	Objective description of moment by moment shifts in affect—emotional tone (e.g., labile, expensive, constructed, isolated, flat, bland, blunted). Appropriateness to thought content or congruent with topic and mood?
Mood	Overall, sustaining emotional tone of the patient (e.g., elated, exuberant, hypomanic, manic, angry, petulant, irritable, anxious, fearful, happy sad, depressed [with neurovegetative signs of depression], dysphoric, bland, bereaved, grief-stricken)
Risk to self or others	Suicidal ideation, prior suicide attempts, homicidal or otherwise violent ideation, history of violence
Illusions or hallucinations	Misperceptions, illusions, hallucinations (e.g., auditory, visual, olfactory, gustatory, tactile)
Speech	Tone, rate modulation, articulation, dysarthric, aphasic, lisp, stutter, pressure, echolalia, coherent, lucid
Thought process	Associations intact, thoughts goal directed; illogical; derailed; circumstantial; tangential; loosening of associations; flight of ideas; perseveration; clang associations; word salad;

	punning and rhyming; neologisms; thought blocking; mutism (deliberate or nondeliberate)
Thought content	Obsessions, somatizations, ESP, thought insertion, mind control, special messages from TV or radio, ideas of reference, paranoia, delusions (e.g., grandiose, nihilistic, persecutory, paranoid), thought broadcasting
Reasoning	Does the patient have a rational plan for taking care of his or her illness?

ering these areas is provided in Table 2.1. There are also standardized MSEs that can be used as brief screening instruments. Both the Mini-Mental State Exam (Folstein, Folstein, & McHugh, 1976) and the St. Louis University Mental Status, for example, are easily administered and can be used to obtain an assessment of cognitive functioning. Given that they tend to be limited to the assessment of cognition and memory, however, they should be used as only a part of a more comprehensive MSE in an emergency interview.

Developing a Case Formulation

One objective of an emergency interview is to establish a working diagnosis for the patient's or client's presenting problem(s). Although arriving at a diagnosis or a set of diagnoses is an important and necessary step in organizing and making sense of the data gathered in the interview, it is typically not sufficient for a more complete understanding of the patient. A case formulation is a more encompassing level of organization that takes into account not only clinical syndromes (i.e., Axis I and Axis II diagnoses) but also precipitating events, predisposing vulnerabilities, coping resources, family system and social network factors, and so forth.

When the interview is completed, the clinician must examine the biopsychosocial data to see not only which diagnoses are supported and which are refuted but also what case formulation makes most sense of the data. For example, the interviewer may have found that a male patient's thinking is loose and tangential, for the past month he has been having auditory hallucinations of voices telling him not to trust anyone, and during that same time frame he has had the delusional belief that his neighbor is attempting to poison him. These data are consistent with the interviewer's diagnostic hypothesis that the patient is having an acute episode of paranoid schizophrenia. The interviewer has also learned that (a) the patient's family recently moved out of the area and has less contact with him; (b) the patient has become increasingly angry and isolated; (c) the patient threatened his neighbor and told him he had "better stop messing" with him; and (d) the patient stopped taking his neuroleptic medication approximately 6 weeks ago, shortly after his family's departure. The interviewer's formulation is thus that the patient is having an acute psychotic episode precipitated by feeling abandoned by those whom he trusted, losing a crucial part of his support system, feeling more vulnerable, and discontinuing his medication in protest. He is also at possible risk of harming his neighbor.

As one can see, the clinician must use his or her clinical judgment in weighing the many possible contributing factors and risk indicators. Whether his or her clinical opinion suggests mild, moderate, or severe risk, it is seldom a matter of a single cause but involves the consideration of multiple possible determinants.

The Limits of Risk Prediction and Estimation

It is important to recognize that even the best of clinicians, using the best interviewing methods and aided by the best standardized risk assessment instruments, are not able to predict suicide or violence with any great degree of accuracy (Kleespies & Dettmer, 2000). In 2005, the base rate of suicide was approximately 11 per 100,000 in the general U.S. population (American Association of Suicidology, 2008). The rate for the psychiatric population is approximately 5 to 6 times that rate for the general population, or 55 to 66 per 100,000 (Hillard, 1995; Tanney, 1992). In 2005, the base rate of homicide was 5.6 per 100,000 for adults in the general U.S. population (Bureau of Justice, 2008). There is a modest relationship between mental disorder and violence (Monahan et al., 2001), but one would not expect the homicide rate among those with mental illness to be dramatically higher than that among the general population. The risk assessment and evaluation methods that are available do not have the sensitivity and specificity for accurate prediction when base rates are this low. As a result, the field has shifted to the more modest and realistic goal of attempting to improve the ability to estimate levels or probabilities of risk (Motto, 1992). The remaining chapters in this book present the available empirical evidence that can assist the clinician in arriving at such an estimate of risk.

PROVIDING APPROPRIATE CARE AND TREATMENT

Even after a patient's problem has been defined, there is no absolute rule for when a patient at risk can be treated on an outpatient basis or when one must make an emergency intervention, something that often results in hospitalization. Yet, this is a decision that must be made when clinicians are faced with a patient or client who presents as a potential danger to self or others.

When Is Outpatient Management Feasible?

Clinicians may be disposed to hospitalize patients who are at risk because they feel it is safer and because they have a high index of concern about liability issues. Many patients with suicidal ideation or violent ideation, however, can be managed successfully on an outpatient basis. Of course, level of risk is the key issue in making this decision. Generally, outpatient management for patients at mild or even moderate risk has been found to be feasible and often preferable to inpatient hospitalization. More detailed information about arriving at an estimate of the level of risk of suicidal behavior or for violence is available in chapters 3 through 9. Suffice it to say that if a patient or client is evaluated as at mild or moderate risk, there are a number of outpatient management strategies that could be used.

For the patient who is at mild to moderate risk of suicidal behavior, Rudd and Joiner (1998) suggested the following contingencies in outpatient treatment planning: (a) an increase in outpatient visits or telephone contacts, (b) frequent assessment of suicide risk, (c) recurrent evaluation for hospitalization, (d) 24-hour emergency availability, (e) consideration of changes in the medication regimen, (f) reevaluation of the treatment plan as needed, and (g) use of professional consultation as warranted. For the patient who is at mild to moderate risk of violent behavior, Otto (1998) suggested the following possible outpatient treatment and environmental interventions: (a) the monitoring of symptoms associated with aggression by the patient and by significant others, (b) anger management and stress management training, (c) substance abuse treatment (if substance abuse has contributed to disinhibition), and (d) psychotropic medication to decrease anger and impulsivity.

When Is Emergency Intervention and Hospitalization Necessary?

Emergency intervention is necessary when the level of risk is considered severe and imminent; that is, when the clinician's considered opinion is that serious injury or death could occur in the next few minutes, hours, or days. Typically, hospitalization is indicated when it is not possible to establish a treatment alliance, when crisis intervention techniques fail, when the patient or client continues to indicate intent to commit suicide or seriously harm others in the immediate future, and in the case of violence risk, when warning the intended victim may not be sufficient to protect him or her from harm (Comstock, 1992; Otto, 1998). Because most patients who are a risk to self or others have some ambivalence about what they intend to do, many will agree to voluntary hospitalization. When patients evaluated at imminent risk refuse hospitalization, however, the clinician is confronted with a decision about involuntary temporary commitment. This decision can be difficult because we know that risk estimation is not always reliable, and involuntary hospitalization can create barriers to an effective treatment alliance in the future. In the final analysis, the decision to hospitalize involuntarily must be based on sound clinical judgment that considers the risk–benefit ratio. In making such decisions, it may be helpful to keep in mind that once hospitalization has occurred, resistant patients often begin to perceive the caring nature of the clinician's actions and are willing to reestablish a treatment alliance.

CONCLUSION

In this chapter we discussed the major tasks of an emergency interview, that is, to (a) contain the patient's emotional turmoil (if necessary), (b) define the problem(s), (c) estimate the risk to self or others, and (d) provide appropriate care and treatment. We also presented a semistructured interview format for carrying out such an evaluation. In practice, however, an interview format comes to life through the skill and knowledge of the interviewer. In the chapters that follow, we hope that a sound knowledge base for dealing with behavioral emergencies is made available to the interested clinician.

REFERENCES

Allen, M., Currier, G., Carpenter, R., Ross, R., & Docherty, J. (2005). Expert consensus panel for behavioral emergencies. *Journal of Psychiatric Practice, 11*(Suppl. 1), 5–108.

American Association of Suicidology. (2008). *U.S.A. suicide: 2005 official final data.* Retrieved February 21, 2008, from http://www.suicidology.org/associations/1045/files/SuicideintheU.S.pdf

Ayanian, J., Cleary, P., Weissman, J., & Epstein, A. (1999). The effect of patients' preferences on racial differences in access to renal transplantation. *The New England Journal of Medicine, 341,* 1661–1669.

Bureau of Justice. (2008). *Homicide trends in the U.S.* Retrieved February, 21, 2008 from http://www.ojp.usdoj.gov/bjs/homicide/tables/totalstab.htm

Cannon-Bowers, J. A., & Salas, E. (1998a). Individual and team decision making under stress: Theoretical underpinnings. In J. A. Cannon-Bowers and E. Salas (Eds.), *Making decisions under stress: Implications for individual and team training* (pp. 17–38). Washington, DC: American Psychological Association.

Cannon-Bowers, J. A., & Salas, E. (1998b). *Making decisions under stress: Implications for individual and team training.* Washington, DC: American Psychological Association.

Caralis, P., Davis, B., Wright, K., & Marcial, W. (1993). The influence of ethnicity and race on attitudes toward advance directives, life-prolonging treatments, and euthanasia. *The Journal of Clinical Ethics, 4,* 155–165.

Ciraulo, D., Shader, R., Greenblatt, D., & Creelman, W. (2005). *Drug interactions in Psychiatry* (3rd ed.). Philadelphia: Lippincott Williams & Wilkins.

Clark, D. (1998). The evaluation and management of the suicidal patient. In P. M. Kleespies (Ed.), *Emergencies in mental health practice: Evaluation and management* (pp. 75–94). New York: Guilford Press.

Clark, D., & Fawcett, J. (1992). Review of empirical risk factors for evaluation of the suicidal patient. In B. Bongar (Ed.), *Suicide: Guidelines for assessment, management, and treatment* (pp. 16–48). New York: Oxford University Press.

Comstock, B. (1992). Decision to hospitalize and alternatives to hospitalization. In B. Bongar (Ed.), *Suicide: Guidelines for assessment, management, and treatment* (pp. 204–217). New York: Oxford University Press.

Conwell, Y., Duberstein, P., Cox, C., Hermann, J., Forbes, N., & Caine, E. (1996). Relationships of age and Axis I diagnoses in victims of completed suicide: A psychological autopsy study. *American Journal of Psychiatry, 153,* 1001–1008.

Dubin, W. (1990). Psychiatric emergencies: Recognition and management. In A. Stoudemire (Ed.), *Clinical psychiatry for medical students* (pp. 497–526). Philadelphia: Lippincott Williams & Wilkins.

Echterling, L., & Hartsough, D. (1989). Phases of helping in successful crisis telephone calls. *Journal of Community Psychology, 17,* 249–257.

Folstein, M., Folstein, S., & McHugh, P. (1976). Mini-mental state: A practical method for grading the cognitive state of patients for the clinician. *Journal of Psychiatric Research, 12,* 189–198.

Gerson, S., & Bassuk, E. (1980). Psychiatric emergencies: An overview. *American Journal of Psychiatry, 137,* 1–11.

Guy, J., & Brady, J. L. (1998). The stress of violent behavior for the clinician. In P. M. Kleespies (Ed.), *Emergencies in mental health practice: Evaluation and management* (pp. 398–417). New York: Guilford Press.

Hanke, N. (1984). *Handbook of emergency psychiatry.* Lexington, MA: Collamore Press.

Hillard, J. (1990). *Manual of clinical emergency psychiatry.* Washington, DC: American Psychiatric Press.

Hillard, J. (1995). Predicting suicide. *Psychiatric Services, 46,* 223–225.

Jesse, S., & Anderson, G. (1990). Emergency services. In S. Levy & P. Ninan (Eds.), *Schizophrenia: Treatment of acute psychotic episodes* (pp. 27–43). Washington, DC: American Psychiatric Press.

Jones, B., & Gray, B. (1986). Problems in diagnosing schizophrenia and affective disorders among Blacks. *Hospital and Community Psychiatry, 37,* 61–65.

Kaplan, H., & Sadock. B. (1993). *Pocket handbook of emergency psychiatric medicine.* Baltimore: Lippincott Williams and Wilkins.

Kleespies, P. M., Deleppo, J., Mori, D., & Niles, B. (1998). The emergency interview. In P. M. Kleespies (Ed.), *Emergencies in mental health practice: Evaluation and management* (pp. 41–72). New York: Guilford Press.

Kleespies, P. M., & Dettmer, E. (2000). An evidence-based approach to evaluating and managing suicidal emergencies. *Journal of Clinical Psychology, 56,* 1109–1130.

Kleespies, P. M., Hughes, D., & Gallacher, F. (2000). Suicide in the medically and terminally ill: Psychological and ethical considerations. *Journal of Clinical Psychology, 56*, 1153–1171.

Lopez, S., & Hernandez, P. (1986). How culture is considered in evaluations of psychopathology. *The Journal of Nervous and Mental Disease, 176*, 598–606.

Loring, M., & Powell, B. (1988). Gender, race, and *DSM–III*: A study of the objectivity of psychiatric diagnostic behavior. *Journal of Health and Social Behavior, 29*, 1–22.

Monahan, J., Steadman, H., Silver, E., Appelbaum, P., Robbins, P., Mulvey, E., et al. (2001). *Rethinking risk assessment: The MacArthur study of mental disorder and violence*. New York: Oxford University Press.

Motto, J. (1992). An integrated approach to estimating suicide risk. In R. Maris, A. Berman, J. Maltsberger, and R. Yufit (Eds.), *Assessment and prediction of suicide* (pp. 625–639). New York: Guilford Press.

Otto, R. (1998). Assessing and managing violence risk in outpatient settings. *Journal of Clinical Psychology, 56*, 1239–1262.

Perlmutter, A., & Jones, J. (1985). Assessment of families in psychiatric emergencies. *American Journal of Orthopsychiatry, 55*, 130–139.

Pope, K., & Tabachnick, B. (1993). Therapists' anger, hate, fear, and sexual feelings: National survey of therapist responses, client characteristics, critical events, formal complaints, and training. *Professional Psychology: Research and Practice, 24*, 142–152.

Pruyser, P. (1979). *The psychological examination: A guide for clinicians*. New York: International Universities Press.

Rudd, M. D., & Joiner, T. E., Jr. (2000). The assessment, management, and treatment of suicidality: Toward clinically informed and balanced standards of care. *Clinical Psychology: Science and Practice, 5*, 135–150.

Saitz, R., Ciraulo, D., Shader, R., & Ciraulo, A. (2003). Treatment of alcohol withdrawal. In R. Shader (Ed.), *Manual of psychiatric therapeutics* (3rd ed., pp. 127–168). Philadelphia: Lippincott Williams & Wilkins.

Segal, S., Bola, J., & Watson, M. (1996). Race, quality of care, and antipsychotic prescribing practices in psychiatric emergency services. *Psychiatric Services, 47*, 282–286.

Shea, C. (1998). *Psychiatric interviewing: The art of understanding* (2nd ed.). Philadelphia: Saunders.

Tanney, B. (1992). Mental disorders, psychiatric patients, and suicide. In R. Maris, A. Berman, J. Maltsberger, and R. Yufit (Eds.), *Assessment and prediction of suicide* (pp. 277–320). New York: Guilford Press.

Tardiff, K. (1989). *Concise guide to assessment and management of violent patients*. Washington, DC: American Psychiatric Press.

Trezza, G., & Popp, S. (1998). The evaluation and management of alcohol- and drug-related crises. In P. M. Kleespies (Ed.), *Emergencies in mental health practice: Evaluation and management* (pp. 258–279). New York: Guilford Press.

Tudor, W., Tudor, J., & Gove, W. (1977). The effect of sex role differences on the social control of mental illness. *Journal of Health and Social Behavior, 18*, 98–112.

Turner, S., & Hersen, M. (1994). The interviewing process. In M. Hersen & S. Turner (Eds.), *Diagnostic interviewing* (2nd ed., pp. 3–24). New York: Plenum Press.

II

EVALUATION AND MANAGEMENT OF SUICIDE RISK

3

ASSESSING SUICIDE RISK IN THE ADULT PATIENT

GLENN R. SULLIVAN AND BRUCE BONGAR

Suicidal patients are ubiquitous in mental health practice. A clinical practices survey (Sullivan, 2004) revealed that the typical clinical psychologist sees more than five patients each month for whom suicide is an issue. Only 5% of clinical psychologists reported that they never treated suicidal patients. Furthermore, nearly 36% indicated that they had lost a patient under their care to suicide at some point during their careers. For professional counselors, a rate of nearly 24% has been reported (McAdams & Foster, 2000). The odds of a psychiatrist losing a patient to suicide over the course of his or her career are about 1:2 (Chemtob, Bauer, Hamada, Pelowski, & Muraoka, 1989). As many as 11% to 17% of clinical psychology graduate students experience a patient suicide before they complete their training (Kleespies, Penk, & Forsyth, 1993; Kleespies, Smith, & Becker, 1990), and 97% report treating at least one patient with suicidal ideation or behavior during their training years (Kleespies et al., 1993).

After the landmark study by Pokorny (1983), it has become increasingly clear that the critical issue for clinicians and researchers is not the prediction of suicide but rather the assessment of suicide risk. For a variety of reasons, the low base rates of completed suicide in both clinical and general populations make it statistically impossible to develop a psychological test, scale, or interview strategy that can accurately predict whether a given individual will commit suicide over the long term. Despite this, the ability to predict suicide is perceived by the courts and public to be a prime competency of mental health practitioners and perhaps their most salient duty. In this chapter we review the empirical evidence pertaining to suicide risk assessment and offer practice-friendly suggestions regarding the improvement of clinical practice in this critical area.

The actual rate of suicide risk assessment by mental health practitioners and the quality of those assessments are largely unknown. What evidence there is, however, suggests that adherence to even the most basic standard of care is often suboptimal. Sullivan (2004) found that only 77% of clinical psychologists registered with the American Psychological Association's Practice Directorate reported performing suicidal ideation inquiries during initial sessions with new patients. In a study of physicians who had lost a patient to suicide, it was found that suicide risk assessments had been completed in only 38% of cases (Milton, Ferguson, & Mills, 1999).

Lack of formal training at the graduate level is a partial explanation for suboptimal rates of suicide risk assessment (Bongar & Harmatz, 1991). Less than 70% of psychologists report receiving at least some formal training in suicide, either at the predoctoral level or postlicensing (Greaney, 1996). Making direct inquires regarding past and current suicidal behavior often provokes intense anxiety in clinical trainees. This anxiety often manifests as (a) *resistance* (to proposed risk assessment approaches), (b) *denial* (that suicide is a concern for a particular patient or patient population), or (c) *helpless dependence* (in the form of requests for direct or increased supervision or, more commonly, detailed scripts to follow when conducting suicide risk assessments).

A primary source of this anxiety among trainees (and licensed clinicians) is that no clinical consensus or authority has ever defined the elusive standard of care for suicide risk assessment (Simon & Shuman, 2006). It has been almost 2 decades since Motto (1989) noted that we have "no established and generally accepted procedure to guide us" (p. 245) in the assessment of suicide risk. More recently, Simon (2002) reminded us that "no suicide risk assessment method has been empirically tested for reliability and validity" (p. 342). The American Psychiatric Association (2003) practice guidelines for assessing patients with suicidal behaviors are a significant contribution, but even they do not constitute a commonly accepted standard of care for this challenging procedure. It is our opinion that mental health clinicians should perform, at a minimum, the procedures outlined in Exhibit 3.1 with all their patients.

We now consider the various elements of this outline while simultaneously enjoining clinicians to avoid a checklist approach to suicide risk assessment. The checklist approach focuses on a (usually quite lengthy) list

EXHIBIT 3.1
Procedures for Mental Health Clinicians Assessing Patients
With Suicidal Behaviors

---

1. Perform a thorough diagnostic evaluation.
   a. Assess the presence of psychiatric disorders.
   b. Assess suicide accelerants: hopelessness, psychological pain, recent losses, substance use, firearm access, insomnia, and so on.
   c. Use psychological testing.
2. Directly inquire about suicide.
   a. Assess current suicidal ideation.
   b. Assess history of suicidal behaviors.
   c. Evaluate patient's risk factors and protective factors.
   d. Determine current level of suicide risk.
3. Develop a treatment plan.
   a. Consider referral for psychiatric medication evaluation.
   b. Consider psychiatric hospitalization.
   c. Involve others in the patient's care.

---

of risk factors and neglects clinical judgment and the building of a therapeutic relationship. Suicide risk assessment is in many respects similar to other areas of clinical mental health work, in that it demands the effort and empathy to comprehend the unique features and circumstances of the patient sitting before you. Suicide risk assessment integrates a careful clinical history, mental status examination, ongoing clinical evaluations, consultations, information from significant others, and data from psychological assessment into a broad-spectrum information gathering procedure for systematic assessment and management of detected risk.

BIOPSYCHOSOCIAL RISK FACTORS

The review of a patient's suicide risk factors is only the beginning of a comprehensive suicide assessment. Assessment of a patient's basic personality traits, communication patterns, attachment history, psychological needs, and character strengths will significantly enhance any evaluation of risk. Clinicians should also consider potential interactions among a patient's various risk factors.

Psychiatric Diagnosis

Suicidality is not a *Diagnostic and Statistical Manual of Mental Disorders* (*DSM–IV–TR*; 4th ed., text rev.; American Psychiatric Association, 2000) category. Indeed, major depression disorder and borderline personality disorder are the only diagnoses in the *DSM–IV–TR* for which suicidality is among the listed criteria. Nevertheless, the association between mental illness and completed suicide is very strong, with some researchers estimating that over

90% of all individuals who commit suicide have a diagnosable mental disorder, usually an affective disorder (Maris, Berman, Maltsberger, & Yufit, 1992).

Harris and Barraclough (1997) calculated standard mortality ratios for a wide range of psychiatric disorders and reported that diagnoses of eating disorders, mood disorders, substance abuse, obsessive–compulsive disorder, panic disorder, and schizophrenia all presented a substantial increase in suicide risk. In fact, one implication of their findings is that the presence of any mental disorder (with the exception of mental retardation) elevates an individual's suicide risk.

Depressive symptoms and suicide are closely associated; however, as Linehan (1997) observed, it is important to remember that the presence of the former is neither necessary nor sufficient for the latter to occur. The lifetime risk of suicide for patients with untreated depressive symptoms is 15% (Isometsä, Henriksson, Hillevi, Kuopposalmi, & Lönnqvist, 1994). Psychotic depression itself does not appear to increase suicide risk relative to less severe forms of depression (Simon, 2006). However, specific psychotic symptoms such as delusions of grandeur, mind reading, and thought insertion do appear to increase suicide risk in patients with affective disorders (Fawcett et al., 1990). Other clinical features that increase risk of suicide within 1 year in patients with affective disorders are panic attacks, severe anxiety, diminished concentration, global insomnia, alcohol abuse, and anhedonia (Fawcett et al., 1990).

Recent discharge from a psychiatric hospital has long been recognized as a risk factor for suicide (Simon, 1988). This risk is greater for patients who reported command hallucinations related to self-harm during their hospitalization. In one study (Zisook, Byrd, Kuck, & Jeste, 1995), 10% of inpatients (2 out of 20) with self-harming command hallucinations died of suicide while hospitalized. In another sample (P. Rogers, Watt, Gray, MacCulloch, & Gournay, 2002), 5.4% of inpatients (2 out of 37) with self-harming command hallucinations committed suicide within 3 months postdischarge. Diagnostic categories in which command hallucinations to self-harm may be present include but are not limited to schizophrenia, mood disorders, borderline personality disorder, and antisocial personality disorder.

Suicide Accelerants and Other Risk Factors

A great number of risk factors have been identified as contributing to suicide risk. Few patients will demonstrate all or even most risk factors; some who commit suicide will demonstrate few or no risk factors. Hall, Platt, and Hall (1999) studied the clinical case histories of 100 patients admitted to a hospital after a serious suicide attempt. They identified a number of risk factors that appeared with relative frequency in their sample, including partial insomnia (92%), severe anxiety (92%), depressed mood (80%), panic attacks (80%) and recent loss of a close personal relationship (78%). Somewhat less frequent but still common were the following: a chronic deteriorating medical illness (41%), inability to maintain job or student status (36%), feelings of worthlessness (29%), and recent onset of impulsive behavior (29%). Data from this study are mentioned in this chapter not because they are definitive, nor because they compose a set of universal critical risk factors, but because the study illustrates the difference between evidence-based approaches to identifying suicide risks and the more prevalent expert opinion approach.

Recent research has suggested that from the perspective of clinicians, the relative importance of the multitude of suicide risk factors varies considerably across diagnostic and demographic categories (Bongar, 2002). A preliminary clinical consensus regarding critical risk factors for major depression, alcohol dependence, and schizophrenia is presented in Table 3.1, and for adolescent and older adult patients, in Table 3.2. In this chapter we do not attempt to present a comprehensive list of suicide risk factors; rather, we comment briefly on factors that appear to be most strongly related to suicidal behavior (i.e., *suicide accelerants*), cite empirical evidence where it exists, and comment on other factors that are often the focus of clinical attention.

Psychache and Hopelessness

Edwin Shneidman (1993), the founder of American suicidology, believed that the central feature of suicide is pain, and that the key to suicide prevention lies in the reduction of that individual's psychological pain (i.e., *psychache*). All else—demographic variables, family history, previous suicidal history—is peripheral except as those factors bear on the presently felt pain. Ultimately, suicide occurs when there is the coexistence of (a) intolerable psychological *pain*, often related to thwarted psychological needs such as autonomy, achievement, or avoidance of humiliation; (b) intense negative *press* (i.e., actual or imagined events that affect the individual and to which he or she reacts); and (c) extreme *perturbation* accompanied by perceptual and cognitive constriction and a penchant for life-ending action (Shneidman, 1988, pp. 176–177). Under this conceptual framework, the management of suicide risk could be thought of as psychological pain management.

The idea that death may appear to provide relief from terrible psychological pain—that cessation of consciousness may seem preferable to one's current (or anticipated) level of subjective distress—is central to the understanding of suicidal behavior (Shneidman, 1989). For many tormented patients, suicide itself becomes their "last best hope." The loss of all other hope for succor or remediation is a common feature of suicidal crises. Beck, Steer, Kovacs, and Garrison (1985) found that hopelessness is a better predictor of suicide than severity of depressive symptoms. Hopelessness can contribute to dichotomous thinking and cognitive rigidity, which can make it extremely difficult for a patient to perceive alternatives to suicide.

TABLE 3.1
Risk Factors Across Diagnostic Categories (as Ranked By Clinicians)

Rank	Major Depression	Alcohol Dependence	Schizophrenia
1	Seriousness of previous attempt(s)	Seriousness of previous attempt(s)	Seriousness of previous attempt(s)
2	History of attempts	History of attempts	History of attempts
3	Acute suicidal ideation	Feelings of hopelessness	Acute suicidal ideation
4	Severe hopelessness	Suicidal communication	Substance abuse
5	Attraction to death	Impulsivity	Hopelessness
6	Family history of suicide	Family history of suicide	Impulsivity
7	Acute overuse of alcohol	Currently drinking	Family history of suicide
8	Loss/separations	Depressive episode	Command hallucinations
9	—	Recent interpersonal loss	Medication noncompliance
10	—	Lack of social support	Depressed mood
11	—	Anticipated loss	Increased agitation
12	—	Illicit drug use	Lack of family support
13	—	Living alone	—

Note. Data from Bongar, Brown, Cleary, Sullivan, and Crawford (2002).

Recent Losses, Stress, and Life Events

Suicide can be precipitated by undesirable life events or stress over fairly long periods of time (Bongar, 2002). Alternatively, it can result from a sudden, unexpected reversal or loss. Examples of life events that have been associated with increased risk of suicide are arrest and incarceration (even for relatively minor offenses) and the end of interpersonal relationships. Narcissistic injury, feelings of shame, guilt, or humiliation, and perceived financial strain might contribute to the development of a suicidal crisis. It is incumbent on the clinician to elicit a detailed history of recent psychosocial stressors from the patient and to gauge the patient's capacity to cope with existing and potential stressors.

Substance Use

Merrill, Milner, Owens, and Vale (1992) found that alcohol had been consumed at the time of the suicide attempt by between 15% to 25% of those who completed suicide and by approximately 55% of individuals who attempted suicide. Alcohol and other drugs may have a disinhibiting effect on the suicidal patient and therefore make a suicide attempt more likely. The suicide rate among people with a diagnosis of alcohol dependence is 50 times greater than that of people without alcohol dependence (Roy, 1998).

TABLE 3.2
Critical Risk Factors Ranked Across Demographic Categories

Rank	Adolescents	Older Adults
1	Previous suicide attempt	History of suicide attempts
2	Severe hopelessness	Severe hopelessness
3	Medical seriousness of previous attempt	Medical seriousness of previous attempt
4	Acute suicidal ideation	Acute suicidal ideation
5	Family history of completion	Drinking toxic liquid
6	Family history of suicidal behavior	Major depressive disorder
7	Major depressive disorder	Socially isolated
8	Bipolar I disorder	Family history of suicide
9	Presence of firearm in home	Presence of firearm in home
10	Recent suicide of peer	Cutting self with sharp object
11	Impulsivity	Alcohol abuse
12	Suicidal communication	Overdosing with medication
13	Withdrawn/socially isolated	Refusing to eat
14	History of sexual abuse/assault	Loss/separations
15	Chronic alcohol abuse	Loneliness
16	Recent interpersonal loss	Presence of physical pain
17	Acute overuse of alcohol	History of psychiatric illness
18	Imitation of other suicides	—

Note. Data from Bongar, Brown, Cleary, Sullivan, and Crawford (2002).

Substance use may intensify depressive symptoms, exacerbate work problems, and unleash aggression directed at the self and others.

Firearms Access

In the United States, more people die by self-inflicted gunshot than by all other suicide methods combined (Miller, Azrael, & Hemenway, 2002). There are more firearm suicides in the United States than firearm homicides. Whether or not a patient has access to a firearm can determine the outcome of a suicidal crisis. Deficient clinical screening for firearms access increases the risk of suicide completion (M. S. Kaplan, Adamek, & Rhoades, 1998). However, only about 20% of patients evaluated by clinical psychologists are asked about their access to firearms (Sullivan, 2004). Inquiries regarding firearms access should be routinized because all patients seeking mental health care represent some magnitude of suicide risk, firearm ownership is common in the United States (up to 40% of households), and self-inflicted gunshot is a highly lethal suicide method.

Medical Illness

Generally, the presence of a medical illness increases the risk of suicide. Chronic, incurable, and painful conditions seem to be associated with the greatest risk, specifically, HIV/AIDS, cancer, spinal cord injury, Huntington's chorea, and head injury (Mackenzie & Popkin, 1990; also see chap. 5, this volume). Harris and Barraclough (1994) added multiple sclerosis, peptic ulcer, renal disease, and systemic lupus erythematosus to that grim list. Hendin (1999) noted that medical illness plays a critical role in approximately 25% of those who commit suicide and that this percentage increases with age, from nearly 50% in persons over age 50 to over 70% in persons age 60 and older. A pattern of high utilization of medical care may indicate increased suicide risk. In a study by Conwell (1994), 20% of older patients who committed suicide had visited their primary care physician *on the same day* as their suicide. Forty percent had seen a physician within 1 week (and 70% within 1 month) of their deaths. More recently, Juurlink, Herrman, Szalai, Kopp, and Redelmeier (2004) found that nearly half of suicide completers age 66 or older had visited a physician within 1 week of their deaths. In these elderly patients, the presence of severe physical pain increased suicide risk more than diagnoses of depression, psychosis, or anxiety (Juurlink et al., 2004).

Prior Suicide Attempts and Current Suicidal Ideation

A history of a life-threatening suicide attempt may be the best single predictor of eventual completed suicide (Moscicki, 1997). Approximately 15% of all nonfatal suicide attempters will eventually die by suicide (Maris, 1981). Risk is greatest during the first 3 months after an attempt (Roy, 1998). Nevertheless, the modal number of prior attempts among suicide completers is zero; two thirds of completed suicides occur on the first attempt (Mann, 2002).

Methods of higher lethality (e.g., using firearms, hanging, jumping from high places) are associated with higher rates of completed suicide. Although every effort should be made to decrease the lethality of a suicidal patient's environment, it should always be remembered that the means to self-annihilation are never remote. As long as a patient has access to an automobile, a nonbarriered building at least six stories tall, a railroad track, or a body of water, his or her environment must be described as potentially lethal.

Suicidal ideation is neither necessary nor sufficient for a completed suicide to occur. The presence of suicidal ideation increases a patient's suicide risk, but the high prevalence of suicidal ideation among people seeking mental health care and the low base rate of completed suicide significantly weakens the relationship between the two variables. Prevalence data from Kessler, Borges, and Walters (1999) suggested that suicide attempts are as likely to be unplanned as planned. However, 72% of persons who report having a suicide plan do go on to attempt suicide. However, even among patients with articulated suicide plans, there is evidence of substitution of method from one attempt to another (Isometsä & Lönnqvist, 1998). The evidence is lacking regarding the strength of the association between suicide methods contemplated during the suicidal crisis and the method ultimately used.

Demographic Factors

In any discussion of demographic risk factors, no matter how cursory, it is useful to recall Hirschfeld and Davidson's (1988) cautionary dictum to mental health professionals: "On the other hand, one cannot dismiss the possibility of suicide in, say, a thirty-year-old, married black woman simply because she doesn't fit the epidemiological profile of a high-risk patient" (p. 307) In the United States, approximately 70% of all suicide completers are Caucasian males and an additional 20% are Caucasian females. Although suicide rates for Caucasian males increase dramatically with age, it is crucial not to conceive of suicide as primarily the domain of older Caucasian men.

In recent years approximately 50% of completed suicides have been in individuals under age 45. Adolescents represent a unique risk group because their suicides are often highly impulsive, subject to the effects of suicide contagion, and often occur in the absence of a diagnosed mental illness. For non-Caucasian males, suicide risk tends to peak between the ages of 15 and 29.

The fact of being a psychiatric patient tends to skew demographic risk factors. Male psychiatric patients tend to commit suicide between the ages of 25 and 40, whereas female psychiatric patients who kill themselves tend to be older, between 35 and 50 (Bongar, 2002). In the general population, men are more at risk of completed suicide (4.5:1). However, for psychiatric patients, the male–female ratio is smaller (1.5:1).

Suicidal Communication

It is estimated that 50% to 80% of all people who commit suicide communicate presuicidal clues about their suicidal intention (Fawcett, 1988). High suicide risk group members often communicate their intent only to their significant others. Moderate suicide risk group members may frequently threaten suicide to family group members and/or health care providers. Ongoing communication between the clinician and the family and intimates of the suicidal patient could provide early warning of a suicide attempt. There are also a variety of social clues to suicidal intent, including the patient putting his or her affairs in order, giving away prized possessions, behaving in any way that is markedly different from his or her usual pattern of living, saying good-bye to friends or psychotherapists, and settling estates (Shneidman, 1985).

Social Isolation

One study by Maris (1981) found that 50% of suicide completers had no close friends. Many studies have found that being single, divorced, widowed, separated, or living alone increased the risk of suicide. Alternatively, people may be at increased risk of suicide if they report feeling like a burden to their partners or family. Marriage and having a family are associated with lower rates of suicide. A more powerful indicator may be responsibility for children under age 18 (Maris et al., 1992). In at least one study, having recently given birth constituted a protective factor against suicidal behaviors. Uncharacteristic social withdrawal may signal depression or even the onset of a psychotic disorder.

Biological–Genetic–Dispositional

Maris (1981) found that 11% of suicides had a history of at least one other suicide among their first degree relatives. A history of suicide (or attempted suicide) in the patient's close biological relations and a family history of affective disorders are commonly considered risk factors for suicide (Moscicki, 2001). It remains unclear whether genetic or social modeling influences play the larger role. The social contagion effect, whereby suicide risk increases after the suicide of a nonrelated peer or even of a celebrity or stranger, argues against a purely genetic explanation. Physical signs of depression (e.g., loss of appetite, sleep disturbance, change in weight, fatigue) should be considered possible contributors to suicide risk.

Lack of Protective Factors

Relatively little is known about protective factors that may increase a patient's resilience to suicidal crises. Family and social support are often cited as protective, but it is the quality of these interpersonal relationships, not just their existence, that matters. Toxic or high-conflict relationships or family histories marked by early maltreatment may increase, rather than reduce, suicide risk. Similarly, religious belief in and of itself does not constitute a protective factor: In all cases the patient's belief system and his or her quite possibly idiosyncratic views of the moral and spiritual meaning of suicide should be explored. Even a person who describes himself as a devout Roman Catholic (i.e., a member of a religion that prohibits suicide) may harbor the belief that God has provided him with suicide as a means of escaping persistent psychological torment or intolerable earthly humiliation.

Wealth and status clearly are not protective factors against suicide, but they do not increase suicide risk either. It is a persistent myth, even among many clinicians, that suicide is a "disease of the rich" (or, conversely, a "disease of the poor"). Both the medical and the legal professions have high suicide rates, but so do less highly paid public safety occupations such as law enforcement and fire fighting. Income and education may provide buffers against mental disorders in general, but not suicide in particular.

The most reliable protective factor against suicide may prove to be effective clinical intervention for mental anguish, physical illness, and substance abuse. The positive impact of therapeutic concern on suicide risk is illustrated by a remarkable study of the effects of long-term contact with persons discharged after treatment for a suicide attempt (Motto & Bostrom,

EXHIBIT 3.2
Direct Inquiries for Evaluating Risk of Suicide

1. Do you ever have periods of feeling sad or depressed about how your life is going?
2. How long do such periods last? How frequent are they? How bad do they get? Have you found yourself crying more often than is usual for you? Do you find it harder to concentrate, perform your daily activities, or just get through your day? Have you noticed any changes in your sleep habits, sex drive, or appetite?
3. Do you ever feel hopeless, discouraged, or self-critical? Do these feelings ever get so intense that life does not seem worthwhile?
4. People who feel depressed often have thoughts about suicide; how often do thoughts of suicide come to mind? How persistent are such thoughts? How strong have they been? Does it require much effort to resist them? Have you had any impulses to carry them out?
5. Have you made any plans to end your life? How would you go about doing it? Have you taken any initial steps to execute this plan, such as scouting locations, investigating the lethality of various medications, or buying a gun?
6. Are there any firearms in your home? If you wanted to, how quickly could you get hold of a gun? Where would you get it? Are you satisfied that this situation is safe for you? If not, how can it be made safer?
7. Can you manage these feelings if they come back? If you cannot, is there a support system for you to turn to in helping to manage these feelings? What is your plan for getting through the next down period? Who should you tell when you have these feelings?

Note. Data from Motto (1989).

2001). The researchers found that sending regular follow-up letters to this high-risk group significantly reduced the rate of subsequent suicide attempts.

EVALUATING RISK

Most clinicians rely primarily on the clinical interview and certain valued questions and observations to assess suicide risk. Motto (1989) noted that the most straightforward way to determine the probability of suicide is to ask the patient directly. This approach should emphasize matter-of-factness, clarity, and freedom from implied criticism. A typical sequence might be to ask the questions presented in Exhibit 3.2. In all cases, we recommend that the history-taking clinician invite the patient to consider the broadest definition of dangerousness, such as by asking, "Have you, at any time in your life, ever done anything that anyone could possibly have interpreted as self-destructive or even suicidal?"

Motto (1989) pointed out that such an inquiry, carried out in an empathic and understanding way, will provide the clinician with a preliminary estimate of risk. The approach rests on the premise that "going directly to the heart of the issue is a practical and effective clinical tool, and patients and collaterals will usually provide valid information if an attitude of caring concern is communicated to them" (p. 247). As always, however, the clinician should remember that the absence of reported suicidal thoughts or behaviors does not rule out the presence of suicide risk.

Psychological Testing

The ultimate challenge and responsibility of suicide risk assessment is the elimination of false negatives, that is, the misclassification of suicidal people as nonsuicidal. Psychological tests and scales can be used effectively to assist clinicians in the identification of individuals at increased risk of imminent self-harm. It must be noted, however, that suicide is too complex a behavior to be adequately captured by a single sign or score (Eyman & Eyman, 1991). The assessment of a patient's risk of suicide should never be based solely on the results of psychological testing. A complete evaluation of risk factors should be considered in conjunction with psychological assessment results (Maris et al., 1992). We now briefly review a handful of the most commonly used psychological tests.

Minnesota Multiphasic Personality Inventory—2

The Minnesota Multiphasic Personality Inventory—2 (MMPI–2) is the most widely used instrument for assessing psychopathology in clinical practice (Greene, 2000). Used properly, the MMPI–2 can be an important tool in the assessment of suicide risk, if not the prediction of actual completed or attempted suicide. The 567-item MMPI–2 can provide important data about a patient's subjective experience that might not be collected in a standard clinical interview.

Meyer (1993) pointed out that the likelihood of suicidal ideation resulting in an attempt increases as scores on Clinical Scales 4 (Psychopathic Deviancy), 8 (Schizophrenia), and 9 (Hypomania) rise. The increased elevations on these scales reflect greater impulsivity or resentment (Scale 4), heightened alienation from self and others (Scale 8), and increased energy to carry out a suicide attempt (Scale 9).

M. L. Kaplan, Asnis, Sanderson, and Keswani (1994) found that many patients tend to disclose more information regarding recent suicidal ideation on self-report forms than they do in clinical face-to-face interviews. Glassmire, Stolberg, Greene, and Bongar (2001) found that psychotherapy outpatients who failed to endorse suicidal ideation or behaviors during direct clinical inquiry often endorsed suicide-related items on the MMPI–2. This suggests that certain MMPI–2 items (e.g., items 150, 303, 506, 520, 524, and 530) may have greater sensitivity for the detection of suicide potential than even direct oral inquiry. These findings have important risk management implications because they suggest that clinicians should always review the six MMPI–2 suicide items, particularly items 506 and 520, even when clients do not report depressed mood, current suicidal ideation, or past suicidal behavior. Sepaher, Bongar, and Greene (1999) referred to Items 506 and 520 as the "I mean business" items because the unmistakable content of both items is simply a variation of the direct clinical inquiry, "Have you recently considered killing yourself?"

We strongly caution clinicians to remember that a raw score of 0 on any MMPI–2 scale associated with increased suicide risk, or a negative finding on any other suicide scale or indicator, does not indicate the absence of suicide risk. For some patients, refusal to acknowledge suicidal ideation or intent on psychological testing may actually represent a strong determination to die.

Rorschach Inkblot Method

Among the recent additions to the Rorschach Comprehensive System (Exner, 2003) is the inclusion of a Suicide Constellation (S-CON) among the Rorschach special indexes. The S-CON consists of 12 variables and highlights certain features that are common in the Rorschach protocols of individuals who completed suicide within 60 days of the test administration. The S-CON dataset now comprises 101 individual protocols.

Exner (2000) stated that proper interpretation of the Rorschach protocol of any person age 15 or older must begin with the scoring and review of the S-CON index. The endorsement of 8 of the 12 variables of the S-CON can serve as a red flag to warn a psychologist that commonalities exist between the patient being tested and the 101 suicide completers. Exner cautioned strongly that a score of less than 8 does not ensure that an individual will not attempt or complete suicide. In fact, the suicide sample was found to contain approximately 20% to 25% false-negative records.

A discussion of the conceptual foundations of the Rorschach variables that are indicative of potential suicide risk is beyond the scope of this chapter. For a detailed review, see Exner (2003), Eyman and Eyman (1991), and Meyer (1993). Whenever overt suicidal content (e.g., "It looks like a man hanging from a bridge") or covert suicidal content (e.g., "A broken down wreck of something") is provided during the administration of the Rorschach or any other projective personality test, it should be taken seriously as a possible indication of self-destructive intent. In these cases it should be assumed that the patient has used the testing situation to communicate suicidal intent or feelings. As with other projective personality tests, the investment of time and skill required for the proper administration and interpretation of the Rorschach cannot be justified if the purpose of assessment is solely to gauge more immediate suicide risk potential.

Suicide Assessment Measures

An abundance of suicide assessment measures is available to clinicians. One recent review included over 35 suicide assessments (J. R. Rogers & Oney, 2005). None of these (with the possible exception of the revised Beck Depression Inventory [BDI–II]), however, has attained common and widespread use. The following examples are meant to be representative of this approach to the assessment of suicide, rather than an exhaustive list of all available instruments.

Beck Depression Inventory and Beck Hopelessness Scale

The BDI–II consists of 21 items designed to assess the severity of depression in adolescents and adults (Beck, Steer, & Brown, 1996). Each item is rated on a 4-point scale (0–3), so total scores can range from 0 (*no reported symptoms of depression*) to 63 (*extreme symptom endorsement*). Scores from 0 to 13 indicate minimal depression; 14 to 19, mild depression; 20 to 28, moderate depression; and 29 to 63, severe depression (Beck et al., 1996). The BDI–II is a clear and concise instrument that enables patients to self-report depressive symptoms in less than 10 minutes. Two items on the BDI–II have a direct bearing on suicide risk assessment: Item 2 (pessimism) and Item 9 (suicidal thoughts or wishes). Clinicians should review patients' responses to these items, and follow up on and document any patient ratings of 2 or 3.

The possible mediating effect of hopelessness on suicidality contributed to the development of the Beck Hopelessness Scale (BHS; Beck & Steer, 1988). Beck et al. (1985) reported that Beck Hopelessness Scale scores of 9 or more were predictive of eventual suicide in 10 out of 11 depressed suicide ideators who were followed for 5 to 10 years after discharge from the hospital. In a subsequent study of outpatients (Beck, Brown, Berchick, Stewart, & Steer, 1990), a BHS cutoff score of 9 or above identified 16 of the 17 eventual suicides (94.2%). The high-risk group identified by this cutoff score was 11 times more likely to commit suicide than the rest of the outpatients. In most clinical settings, this cutoff score results in large numbers of false positive results.

Linehan Reasons for Living Inventory

The Reasons for Living Inventory (LRFL; Linehan, Goodstein, Nielsen, & Chiles, 1983) assesses the strength of an individual's commitment not to die. The 48-item self-report measure takes about 10 minutes to administer; a 72-item version is also available. Internal consistency is high, and test–retest reliability over 3 weeks is moderately high. The LRFL has been noted to be sensitive to reductions in depression, hopelessness, and suicidal ideation in female patients receiving treatment for borderline personality disorder (Linehan, Armstrong, Suarez, Allman, & Heard, 1991).

Conceptually, the basis for the LRFL is that the lack of positive reasons to live is as strong a contributor to suicide as the wish to die. Patients are asked to rate a series of reasons for not killing themselves, using a 6-point Likert-type scale (1 = *not at all important*; 6 = *extremely important*). Subscales include Responsibility to Family (e.g., "My family depends on me and needs me"), Fear of Suicide (e.g., "I am afraid of the unknown"), and Moral Objections (e.g., "I believe only God has the right to end life"). The LRFL appears most appropriate as a means of monitoring chronic suicidality in high-risk patients and measuring the effectiveness of suicide-focused treatment interventions, rather than as an initial assessment of suicide risk.

False Positives

At this point, it is appropriate to comment on the production of false positives in the assessment of suicide risk. Historically, much concern has been expressed regarding the importance of minimizing the number of false positive identifications, that is, the percentage of nonsuicidal patients misclassified as suicidal. In our opinion, it is possible for this concern to be overstated. Realistically, the negative consequences for a patient who completes a psychological test or screen in a manner similar to that of patients who report suicidal thoughts or intent are limited.

It is highly unlikely that an unjustified involuntary hospitalization or inappropriate psychopharmacological intervention would result solely from a score on a suicide risk scale. If delivered frankly and within the context of the clinician's concern for the patient's safety, the communication of positive test findings should not damage the therapeutic alliance. A conservative stance on the matter of false positives acknowledges that the purpose of testing is the assessment of risk, not the prediction of suicide and that all patients who seek the services of mental health professionals are to varying degrees at elevated risk of suicide.

MANAGING RISK

All patients should be categorized on the basis of their current level of suicide risk (see Joiner, Walker, Rudd, & Jobes, 1999, for a useful approach to risk categorization). This categorization is dynamic, not static, and should account for potential changes in the patient's psychiatric condition or life stressors. Furthermore, the categorization should have an explicit expiration date—the length of time beyond which it is not reasonable to attempt to foresee, and after which another suicide risk assessment should be performed. For patients with the lowest risk, a 6-month time frame may be appropriate; for patients with a higher risk, suicide risk assessment may need to be conducted several times daily and certainly at every treatment transition (e.g., transfer from emergency department to psychiatric inpatient unit; granting of passes; discharge). The best estimation of risk comes from repeated assessments over time on a broad array of clinical variables (Clark, Young, Scheftner, Fawcett, & Fogg, 1987).

A possible risk category range could be low, low–moderate, moderate, moderate–high, high. It seems prudent never to deem a patient's suicide risk "none" or "nonexistent"; as noted previously, the suicide risk of most patients seeking mental health care is elevated above the population mean. Future research may determine the utility and feasibility of developing actuarial anchors for risk categories (e.g., high = *in the absence of clinical intervention, 10% of patients with similar symptoms and life stressors will die by suicide within 12 months*).

Suicide risk assessments should be thoroughly documented: In the legal aftermath of a patient suicide, an undocumented suicide risk assessment may as well have never taken place (at least from the perspective of the attorney representing the deceased patient's survivors). When suicide risk increases, so should the amount of peer and expert consultation and the level of documentation.

For patients deemed at high or moderate–high suicide risk (or their local equivalents), the mental health practitioner must consider the appropriateness of intensified outpatient treatment, interventions aimed at reducing patient access to firearms, hospitalization (either voluntary or involuntary), and psychiatric medication evaluation. The appropriateness of electroconvulsive therapy to treat severe depressive symptoms should also be considered. Supportive family members should be included in the treatment planning, and clinicians should adopt a team approach. The use of no-harm contracts has no empirical support and may actually lull clinicians into a false sense of security. Failure to establish a solid therapeutic alliance may increase suicide risk.

CONCLUSION

The most critical question for any mental health practitioner is, "Is this patient, sitting here with me now, about to commit suicide?" (Maltsberger, 1988, p. 47). Unfortunately, none of the approaches suggested and risk factors discussed in this chapter will enable clinicians to accurately predict suicidal behavior. After almost 50 years of suicide research in the United States, psychologists still lack an established standard of care for suicide risk assessment, and our evaluative strategies are generally based more on professional judgment than on evidence-based approaches. Clinicians should realize that reasonable and prudent practice activities—those grounded in a realistic understanding of the current knowledge base—reflect the reality that each clinical decision point is a probabilistic determination, a decision involving a contemporaneous calculation of risk, rather than a determination of any clinical certainty.

REFERENCES

American Psychiatric Association. (2000). *Diagnostic and statistical manual of mental disorders* (4th ed., text rev.). Washington, DC: Author.

American Psychiatric Association. (2003). Practice guidelines for the assessment and treatment of patients with suicidal behaviors. *American Journal of Psychiatry, 160*, 1–60.

Beck, A. T., Brown, G., Berchick, R. J., Stewart, B. L., & Steer, R. A. (1990). Relationship between hopelessness and ultimate suicide: A replication with psychiatric outpatients. *American Journal of Psychiatry, 147*, 190–195.

Beck, A. T., & Steer, R. A. (1988). *Manual for the Beck Hopelessness Scale.* San Antonio, TX: The Psychological Corporation.

Beck, A. T., Steer, R. A., & Brown, G. (1996). *Beck Depression Inventory—II manual.* San Antonio, TX: The Psychological Corporation.

Beck, A. T., Steer, R. A., Kovacs, M., & Garrison, B. (1985). Hopelessness and eventual suicide: A 10-year prospective study of patients hospitalized with suicidal ideation. *American Journal of Psychiatry, 142*, 559–563.

Bongar, B. (2002). *The suicidal patient: Clinical and legal standards of care* (2nd ed.). Washington, DC: American Psychological Association.

Bongar, B., Brown, L. M., Cleary, K., Sullivan, G. R., & Crawford, E. (2002, August). *Treating suicide risk factors among various age and diagnostic populations.* Paper presented at the 110th Annual Convention of the American Psychological Association, Chicago, IL.

Bongar, B., & Harmatz, M. (1991). Clinical psychology graduate education in the study of suicide: Availability, resources, and importance. *Suicide and Life-Threatening Behavior, 21*, 231–244.

Chemtob, C. M., Bauer, G. B., Hamada, R. S., Pelowski, S. R., & Muraoka, M. Y. (1989). Patient suicide: Occupational hazard for psychologists and psychologists. *Professional Psychology: Research and Practice, 20*, 294–300.

Clark, D. C., Young, M. A., Scheftner, W. A., Fawcett, J., & Fogg, L. (1987). A field test of Motto's risk estimator for suicide. *American Journal of Psychiatry, 144*, 923–926.

Conwell Y. (1994). Suicide in elderly patients. In L. S. Schneider, C. F. Reynolds, B. D. Lebowitz, & A. J. Friedhoff (Eds.), *Diagnosis and treatment of depression in late life: Results of the NIH Consensus Development Conference* (pp. 397–418). Washington, DC: American Psychiatric Press.

Exner, J. E. (2000). *A primer for Rorschach interpretation.* Asheville, NC: Rorschach Workshops.

Exner, J. E. (2003). *The Rorschach: A comprehensive system: Vol. 1. Basic foundations* (4th ed.). New York: Wiley.

Eyman, J. R., & Eyman, S. K. (1991). Personality assessment in suicide prediction. *Suicide and Life-Threatening Behavior, 21*, 37–55.

Fawcett, J. (1988). Predictors of early suicide: Identification and appropriate intervention. *Journal of Clinical Psychiatry, 49*(Suppl.), 7–8.

Fawcett, J., Scheftner, W. A., Fogg, L., Clark, D. C., Young, M. A., Hedeker, D., & Gibbons, R. (1990). Time-related predictors of suicide in major affective disorder. *American Journal of Psychiatry, 147*, 1189–1194.

Glassmire, D. M., Stolberg, R. A., Greene, R. L., & Bongar, B. (2001). The utility of MMPI–2 suicide items for assessing suicidal potential: Development of a suicidal potential scale. *Assessment, 8*, 281–290.

Greaney, S. A. (1996). Psychologists' behaviors and attitudes when working with the nonhospitalized suicidal patient. *Dissertation Abstracts International, 56*, 10-B.

Greene, R. L. (2000). *The MMPI–2: An interpretive manual*. Boston: Allyn & Bacon.

Hall, R. C. W., Platt, D. E., & Hall, R. C. W. (1999). Suicide risk assessment: A review of risk factors for suicide in 100 patients who made severe suicide attempts. *Psychosomatics, 40*, 18–27.

Harris, E. C., & Barraclough, B. M. (1994). Suicide as an outcome for medical disorders. *Medicine, 73*, 281–296.

Harris, E. C., & Barraclough, B. M. (1997). Suicide as an outcome for mental disorders: A meta-analysis. *The British Journal of Psychiatry, 170*, 205–228.

Hendin, H. (1999). Suicide, assisted suicide, and medical illness. *Journal of Clinical Psychiatry, 60*(Suppl. 2), 46–50.

Hirschfeld, R. M. A., & Davidson, L. (1988). Risk factors for suicide. In A. J. Frances & R. E. Hales (Eds.), *Review of psychiatry* (Vol. 7, pp. 307–333). Washington, DC: American Psychiatric Press.

Isometsä, E. T., Henriksson, M. M., Hillevi, M. E., Kuoppasalmi, K. I., & Lönnqvist, J. K. (1994) Suicide in major depression. *American Journal of Psychiatry, 151*, 530–536.

Isometsä, E. T., & Lönnqvist, J. K. (1998). Suicide attempts preceding completed suicide. *The British Journal of Psychiatry, 173*, 521–535.

Joiner, T. E., Jr., Walker, R. L., Rudd, M. D., & Jobes, D. A. (1999). Scientizing and routinizing the assessment of suicidality in outpatient practice. *Professional Psychology: Research and Practice, 30*, 447–453.

Juurlink, D. N., Herrman, N., Szalai, J. P., Kopp, A., & Redelmeier, D. A. (2004). Medical illness and the risk of suicide in the elderly. *Archives of Internal Medicine, 164*, 1179–1184.

Kaplan, M. L., Asnis, G. M., Sanderson, W. C., & Keswani, L. (1994). Suicide assessment: Clinical interview versus self-report. *Journal of Clinical Psychology, 50*, 294–298.

Kaplan, M. S., Adamek, M. E., & Rhoades, J. A. (1998). Prevention of elderly suicide: Physicians' assessment of firearm availability. *American Journal of Preventive Medicine, 15*, 60–64.

Kessler, R. C., Borges, G., & Walters, E. E. (1999). Prevalence of and risk factors for lifetime suicide attempts in the National Comorbidity Study. *Archives of General Psychiatry, 56*, 617–626.

Kleespies, P. M., Penk, W. E., & Forsyth, J. P. (1993). The stress of patient suicidal behavior during clinical training: Incidence, impact, and recovery. *Professional Psychology: Research and Practice, 24*, 293–303.

Kleespies, P. M., Smith, M. R., & Becker, B. R. (1990). Psychology interns as patient suicide survivors: Incidence, impact, and recovery. *Professional Psychology: Research and Practice, 21,* 257–263.

Linehan, M. M. (1997). Behavioral treatments of suicidal behaviors. In D. M. Stoff & J. J. Mann (Eds.), *The neurobiology of suicidal behavior* (pp. 302–328). New York: New York Academy of Sciences.

Linehan, M. M., Armstrong, H. E., Suarez, A., Allman, D., & Heard, H. L. (1991). Cognitive–behavioral treatment of chronically parasuicidal borderline patients. *Archives of General Psychiatry, 48,* 1060–1064.

Linehan, M. M., Goodstein, J. L., Nielsen, S. L., & Chiles, J. A. (1983). Reasons for staying alive when you are thinking of killing yourself: The Reasons for Living Inventory. *Journal of Consulting and Clinical Psychology, 51,* 276–286.

Mackenzie, T. B., & Popkin, M. K. (1990). Medical illness and suicide. In S. J. Blumenthal & D. J. Kupfer (Eds.), *Suicide over the life cycle: Risk factors, assessment, and treatment of suicidal patients* (pp. 205–234). Washington, DC: American Psychiatric Press.

Maltsberger, J. T. (1988). Suicide danger: Clinical estimation and decision. *Suicide and Life-Threatening Behavior, 18,* 47–54.

Mann J. J. (2002). A current perspective of suicide and attempted suicide. *Annals of Internal Medicine, 136,* 302–11.

Maris, R. W. (1981). *Pathways to suicide: A survey of self-destructive behaviors.* Baltimore: Johns Hopkins University Press.

Maris, R. W., Berman, A. L., Maltsberger, J. T., & Yufit, R. (Eds.). (1992). *Assessment and prediction of suicide.* New York: Guilford Press.

McAdams, C. R., & Foster, V. A. (2000). Client suicide: Its frequency and impact on counselors. *Journal of Mental Health Counseling, 22,* 107–121.

Merrill, J., Milner, G., Owens, J., & Vale, A. (1992). Alcohol and attempted suicide. *British Journal of Addiction, 87,* 83–89.

Meyer, R. G. (1993). *The clinician's handbook: Integrated diagnostics, assessment, and intervention in adult and adolescent psychopathology* (3rd ed.). Boston: Allyn & Bacon.

Miller, M., Azrael, D., & Hemenway, D. (2002). Household firearm ownership and suicide rates in the United States. *Epidemiology, 13,* 514–524.

Milton, J., Ferguson, B., & Mills, T. (1999). Risk assessment and suicide prevention in primary care. *Crisis, 20,* 171–177.

Moscicki, E. K. (1997). Identification of suicide risk factors using epidemiologic studies. *Psychiatric Clinics of North America, 20,* 499–517.

Moscicki, E. K. (2001). Epidemiology of completed and attempted suicide: Toward a framework for prevention. *Clinical Neuroscience Research, 1,* 310–323.

Motto, J. A. (1989). Problems in suicide risk assessment. In D. G. Jacobs & H. N. Brown (Eds.), *Suicide: Understanding and responding: Harvard Medical School perspectives on suicide* (pp. 129–142). Madison, CT: International Universities Press.

Motto, J. A., & Bostrom, A. G. (2001). A randomized controlled trial of postcrisis suicide prevention. *Psychiatric Services, 52,* 828–833

Pokorny, A. D. (1983). Prediction of suicide in psychiatric patients: Report of a prospective study. *Archives of General Psychiatry, 40,* 249–257.

Rogers, J. R., & Oney, K. M. (2005). Clinical use of suicide assessment scales: Enhancing reliability and validity through the therapeutic relationship. In R. I. Yufit & D. Lester (Eds.), *Assessment, treatment, and prevention of suicidal behavior* (pp. 7–27). New York: Wiley.

Rogers, P., Watt, A., Gray, N. S., MacCulloch, M., & Gournay, K. (2002). Content of command hallucinations predicts self-harm but not violence in a medium secure unit. Journal of *Forensic Psychiatry, 13,* 251–262.

Roy, A. (1998). Suicide. In H. I. Kaplan & B. J. Sadock (Eds.), *Synopsis of psychiatry* (8th ed., pp. 867–872). Baltimore: Lippincott Williams & Wilkins.

Shneidman, E. S. (1985). *Definition of suicide.* New York: Wiley.

Shneidman, E. S. (1988). A psychological approach to suicide. In G. R. VandenBos & B. K. Bryant (Eds.), *Cataclysms, crises, and catastrophes: Psychology in action* (pp. 147–183). Washington, DC: American Psychological Association.

Shneidman, E. S. (1989). Overview: A multidimensional approach to suicide. In D. G. Jacobs & H. N. Brown (Eds.), *Suicide: Understanding and responding: Harvard Medical School perspectives on suicide* (pp. 1–30). Madison, CT: International Universities Press.

Shneidman, E. S. (1993). Suicide as psychache. *The Journal of Nervous and Mental Disease, 181,* 145–147.

Simon, R. I. (1988). *Concise guide to clinical psychiatry and the law.* Washington, DC: American Psychiatric Press.

Simon, R. I. (2002). Suicide risk assessment: What is the standard of care? *Journal of the American Academy of Psychiatry and the Law, 30,* 340–344.

Simon, R. I. (2006). Suicide risk assessment: Is clinical experience enough? *Journal of the American Academy of Psychiatry and the Law, 34,* 276–278.

Simon, R. I., & Shuman, D. W. (2006). The standard of care in suicide risk assessment: An elusive concept. *CNS Spectrum, 11,* 6–9.

Sepaher, I., Bongar, B, & Greene, R. L. (1999). Codetype base rates for the "I mean business" suicide items on the MMPI–2. *Journal of Clinical Psychology, 55,* 1167–1173.

Sullivan, G. R. (2004). Suicide-by-firearm and the clinical assessment of firearm access. *Dissertation Abstracts International, 65,* 04B.

Zisook, S., Byrd, D., Kuck, J., & Jeste, D. (1995). Command hallucinations in outpatients with schizophrenia. *Journal of Clinical Psychiatry, 56,* 462–465.

4

CHILDREN AND ADOLESCENTS
AT RISK OF SUICIDE

ALEC L. MILLER AND JILL M. EMANUELE

Suicide in children and adolescents is a major public health problem and accounts for at least 100,000 annual deaths in young people worldwide (World Health Organization, 2002). In the United States suicide accounts for more adolescent deaths than all natural causes combined, with approximately 4,000 young people ages 15 to 24 dying by suicide in 2002 (Kochanek, Murphy, Anderson, & Scott, 2004). The American Association of Suicidology (2003) estimated that in the United States a teenager kills him- or herself every 2 hours. Suicide ranks as the third leading cause of death in the United States among the 10- to 14-year-old and 15- to 19-year-old age groups, exceeded by only accidents and homicide (Anderson, 2002).

The Centers for Disease Control and Prevention's Youth Risk Behavior Survey found that of 1 million teenagers surveyed, nearly 20% seriously considered suicide in the past year, 15% made a specific plan to attempt suicide, and 9% reported an attempt; approximately 700,000 received medical attention for their attempt (Grunbaum et al., 2002). These results are consistent with those cited in other epidemiological studies in the United States (e.g., see Wichstrom, 2000).

Although suicide attempts are less common before adolescence, they increase significantly during adolescence, with a peak between ages 16 and 18 (Lewinsohn, Rohde, & Seeley, 1996). After age 18 the frequency of suicide attempts declines markedly, especially for young women (Kessler, Borges, & Walters, 1999; Lewinsohn, Rohde, Seeley, & Baldwin, 2001). As a result, the rate of suicide attempts across the life span is highest during adolescence, whereas the rate of completion is highest among persons older than age 65. For each youth suicide, there are approximately 100 to 200 youth suicide attempts (American Association of Suicidology, 2003). Researchers found that 31% to 50% of adolescents who attempt suicide reattempt suicide (Shaffer & Piacentini, 1994), with 27% of boys and 21% of girls reattempting within 3 months of the first attempt (Lewinsohn et al., 1996). Strikingly, 50% of adolescents who attempt suicide fail to receive any follow-up mental health treatment (Spirito, Brown, Overholser, & Fritz, 1989); of those who do receive treatment, up to 77% do not attend therapy appointments or fail to complete treatment (Trautman, Stewart, & Morishima, 1993). Suicidal behavior is the leading reason for admission to adolescent inpatient psychiatric units in the United States and abroad. With shorter lengths of stay mandated by managed care companies, psychiatric hospitals have become revolving doors for highly troubled youth. These data have major treatment implications, including the need for evidence-based treatments that effectively engage and retain high-risk suicidal youth in outpatient settings.

The evidence-based assessment and management of suicidality in children and adolescents is critical and complex for even the most seasoned clinician. In this chapter we offer a guide for working with this significantly at-risk population. First, we provide an overview of risk factors that inform the clinician's decision making between referring a patient for hospitalization versus continuing to treat the adolescent as an outpatient. Second, we offer strategies for evaluating suicide risk in children and adolescents. Third, we discuss managing this risk. The discussion of risk management includes a hypothetical case example to illustrate the key points.

Note that adolescent suicide attempts often have ambivalent—rather than certain—intention, further complicating their accurate assessment (King et al., 1995). Therefore, for our purposes we define a suicide attempt as self-injurious behavior with either ambivalent or certain intent to die.

BIOPSYCHOSOCIAL RISK FACTORS

Suicidologists have worked vigorously to identify risk factors for suicidal behavior in youth. One of the greatest frustrations for clinicians, researchers, school personnel, family members, and friends is the inability to predict suicidal behavior among individual children and adolescents because it is a low base rate behavior (see chap. 3 for a discussion about suicide prediction vs. suicide risk assessment). Research is limited by ethical problems, such as determining whether predictions are accurate. The best that can be done is to describe the characteristics of populations in which rates of suicide are higher than in the population as a whole. Thus, evidence-based assessment is helpful to evaluate risk factors commonly associated with suicide, rather than enabling one to say with conviction or certainty that an individual will commit suicide.

The research has clearly demonstrated the presence of certain distal (i.e., underlying vulnerabilities) and proximal (i.e., precipitating events) risk factors that when combined increase the probability of suicidal behavior. Suicide risk increases when these precipitating events occur in the context of the distal risk factors. Hence, Lewinsohn et al. (1996) hastened to point out that stressful life events should be considered red flags for clinicians. By the same token, experiencing one or more of these stressful life events by themselves need not alarm a clinician. Assessment of risk is complicated by the fact that some risk factors can be considered both distal and proximal. For example, social and environmental factors, such as family conflict and parental psychopathology, can function as proximal factors that cause or exacerbate existing mental disorders or psychological pain, which in turn increase the risk of suicide. Exhibit 4.1 lists the major distal and proximal risk factors that are highlighted.

Distal Risk Factors

Prior Suicide Attempts

It has become well established that a prior suicide attempt is one of the single most important predictors of completed suicide (Gould, Greenberg, Velting, & Shaffer, 2003), with a thirtyfold increased risk for boys and a threefold increased risk for girls (Shaffer et al., 1996). Numerous autopsy studies of adolescents who committed suicide have found high rates of previous suicide attempts, ranging between 10% and 44% (Marttunen, Aro, & Lönnqvist, 1992). Furthermore, in a study of adolescents who attempted suicide evaluated in an emergency department, researchers discovered 8.7% of the boys and 1.2% of the girls committed suicide within 5 years (Kotila, 1992).

Mental Disorders

Clinical researchers agree that suicidal behaviors among adolescents are clearly associated with diagnosable mental disorders (e.g., see Kovacs, Goldston, & Gatsonis, 1993; Lewinsohn et al., 1996). Psychological autopsy studies have reported greater than 90% of adolescent suicide victims with a mental illness at the time of their death, although younger adolescent suicide victims tend to have lower rates of mental illness, averaging around 60% (e.g., see Beautrais, 2001; Brent, Baugher, Bridge, Chen, & Chiappetta,

EXHIBIT 4.1
General Risk Factors for Adolescent Suicidal Behavior

Distal risk factors underlying vulnerabilities	Proximal risk factors precipitating events
Prior suicide attempts	Suicidal ideation
Mental disorders	Accessible means to suicide
Affective and anxiety disorders	Stressful adverse life events
Disruptive and antisocial disorders	Suicide in the social milieu
Alcohol and substance use disorders	Academic difficulties
Personality disorders	Childhood sexual and physical
Comorbid disorders	abuse
Demographic risk factors	Functional impairment from
Gender	physical disease and injury
Sexual orientation	
Ethnicity	
Socioeconomic status	
Family dysfunction and parental	
psychopathology	

Note. From *Dialectical behavior therapy with suicidal adolescents* (p. 12), by A. L. Miller, J. H. Rathus, and M. M. Linehan, 2007, New York: Guilford Press. Copyright 2007 by The Guilford Press. Reprinted with permission.

1999). Although a variety of mental disorders exist among adolescents who committed suicide, adolescents internationally are diagnosed with one of three classes of Axis I disorders: (a) affective and anxiety disorders, (b) disruptive and antisocial behavior disorders, or (c) alcohol and substance use disorders (e.g., see Fergusson & Lynskey, 1995; Gould et al., 2003).

Affective and Anxiety Disorders. Depressive disorders have been reported among adolescents who attempted suicide and those who committed suicide, ranging from 49% to 64% (Brent, Perper, et al., 1993; Shaffer et al., 1996), with rates highest among psychiatric inpatients (Spirito et al., 1989). Suicidal behaviors are common among adolescents with early-onset depressive disorders (Brent, Perper, et al., 1993). Kovacs et al. (1993) found a four- to fivefold increase in suicidal ideation and behavior among adolescents with affective disorders compared with adolescents with other mental disorders. These statistics are noteworthy because the risk of developing a depressive disorder increases as one gets older but rises dramatically between ages 9 and 19 (King, 1997). In addition, although bipolar disorder is less prevalent among adolescents, it has been considered a significant risk factor in many studies (e.g., see Brent et al., 1988; Geller et al., 2002).

Lewinsohn et al. (1996) identified anxiety disorders as a risk factor for suicidal behavior among adolescents. Goldston et al. (1999) reported trait anxiety to be predictive of posthospitalization suicide attempts, independent of mental disorder. In another study, investigators found that adolescents with a history of panic attacks were 3 times more likely to express suicidal ideation and 2 times more likely to report suicide attempts than those without a history (Pilowsky, Wu, & Anthony, 1999). Moreover, posttraumatic stress disorder has also been associated with adolescent suicidal behavior (Giaconia et al., 1995; Mazza, 2000).

Disruptive and Antisocial Disorders. Several researchers have suggested that most completed suicides by adolescents are impulsive, with only about 25% providing evidence of planning (Hoberman & Garfinkel, 1988). Aggression with impulsivity has also been linked with suicidal behavior in children and adolescents (e.g., see Apter et al., 1995; Brent et al., 1994). A study of suicidal adults suggested that a personality style marked by pronounced impulsivity and aggression characterized individuals at risk of suicide attempts regardless of mental disorder (Mann, Waternaux, Haas, & Malone, 1999). It should not be a surprise that disruptive behavior disorders are a common diagnosis among suicidal adolescents (e.g., Kovacs et al., 1993), especially boys (Brent, Johnson, et al., 1993; Shaffer et al., 1996). Furthermore, Apter et al. (1995) suggested that aggression, a large component of conduct disorder, may be as important a risk factor as depression in some kinds of suicidal behavior.

Alcohol and Substance Use Disorders. Drug and alcohol use and abuse have been found with great frequency among those adolescents who attempted suicide and those who committed suicide and, consequently, are considered primary risk factors (e.g., see Shaffer et al., 1996). In a study of adolescent substance users, suicide attempts occurred at rates threefold those of nonsubstance using adolescents, with the wish to die increasing dramatically after the onset of substance use (Berman & Schwartz, 1990).

Personality Disorders. There is a reluctance to diagnose personality disorders in adolescents because of the commonly held belief that the adolescent personality is still evolving (Miller, Rathus, & Linehan, 2007). However, personality disorders and the tendency to engage in impulsive acts have become critical risk factors for completed suicide among adolescents (Brent et al., 1994). Completed suicide occurs in 8% to 10% of persons diagnosed with borderline personality disorder (BPD), and self-mutilative acts and suicidal threats and attempts are extremely common (American Psychiatric Association, 2000). Brent, Johnson, et al. (1993) compared inpatient adolescents who had attempted suicide with inpatient control participants who were never suicidal and found that suicidal clients were more likely than control participants to have personality disorders or features, particularly those of the borderline type. In addition, Velting, Rathus, and Miller (2000) found that adolescents who attempted suicide had higher levels of borderline behavioral criteria on the Millon Adolescent Clinical Inventory (Millon, Millon, & Davis, 1993).

Comorbid Disorders. Comorbidity of mental disorders is the rule rather than the exception among adolescents (Volkmar & Woolsten, 1997), and comorbid disorders are often present in adolescents who commit suicide (Miller et al., 2007). Depressed teenagers with comorbid alcohol and substance abuse, conduct problems, or BPD represent a particularly high-risk profile for suicidal behavior and completed suicide among teenagers (Kovacs et al., 1993; Marttunen et al., 1995). Although most adolescents who make a suicide attempt have a diagnosable mental disorder, it is important to note that most adolescents with a mental disorder do not make a suicide attempt (Lewinsohn et al., 1996). Adolescents at highest risk for suicide tend to have high rates of comorbidity of both Axis I and Axis II disorders.

Demographic Risk Factors

Gender. Although suicidal ideation and attempts are more common among females in the United States (Gould et al., 1998; Grunbaum et al., 2002), completed suicide is 5 times more common among 15- to 19-year-old males (Anderson, 2002). Studies have consistently found gender differences among adolescents who attempted suicide (Gould et al., 2003). Approximately 10% to 20% of girls versus 4% to 10% of boys report having made a suicide attempt during their lifetime. Hence, girls report attempting suicide 2 to 4 times as frequently as boys.

Sexual Orientation. Cross-sectional and longitudinal epidemiological studies found homosexual adolescents of both sexes to be 2 to 6 times more likely to attempt suicide than their heterosexual peers (Blake et al., 2001; Russell & Joyner, 2001). Garofalo, Wolf, Wissow, Woods, and Goodman (1999) found that self-identified gay, lesbian, and "not sure" youth were 3.41 times more likely to report a suicide attempt than their peers. In addition, they found sexual orientation to have an independent association with suicide attempts for male adolescents. For female adolescents, the association of sexual orientation with suicidality may be mediated by drug use and violence–victimization behaviors.

Ethnicity. In the United States, youth suicide is most common among Native Americans (Middlebrook, LeMaster, Beals, Novins, & Manson, 2001). Caucasian youth have higher rates than African American youth, with Asian/Pacific Islanders having the lowest rates. It is important to note that since the mid-1990s suicide rates have gradually declined among both Caucasian and African American male and female adolescents (Gould et al., 2003). Latinos have a relatively low suicide completion rate but are significantly more likely than either Caucasian or African American adolescents to report suicidal ideation and to have made a suicide attempt (Kann, Kinchen, Williams, & Ross, 2000; Tortolero & Roberts, 2001).

Socioeconomic Status. The data are mixed regarding the effect of socioeconomic status and suicide (Miller et al., 2007). Several studies have found that youth who have attempted suicide have higher rates of socioeconomic disadvantage than community control participants, even after controlling for other social and mental health risk factors (e.g., see Fergusson, Woodward, & Horwood, 2000). Other studies have found little effect of socioeconomic disadvantage on suicide victims generally after adjusting for family history of mental illness or suicide (Agerbo, Nordentoft, & Mortensen, 2002).

Family Dysfunction and Parental Psychopathology

Various theories, coupled with research data, suggest that family functioning plays an important role in the etiology and maintenance of adolescent suicidal ideation and behavior (e.g., see Adams, Overholser, & Lehnert, 1994). A family history of suicidal behavior significantly increases the risk of completed suicide (Gould, Fisher, Parides, Flory, & Shaffer, 1996) and attempted suicide (Bridge, Brent, Johnson, & Connolly, 1997). Agerbo et al. (2002) found youth suicide to be nearly 5 times more likely in the offspring of mothers who have completed suicide and twice as common in the offspring of fathers, even after adjusting for parental mental disorder. Furthermore, parental depression and substance abuse have been associated with suicidal ideation, attempts, and completed suicide in adolescents (e.g., see Gould et al., 1996). Impaired parent–child communication and low levels of emotional support and expressiveness are also associated with adolescent suicidal behavior (e.g., see Wagner, 1997).

Proximal Risk Factors

Suicidal Ideation

Suicidal ideation is a strong, if not one of the best, predictors of suicide attempts (Gould et al., 2003). Suicidal ideation generally requires that the adolescent has current thoughts of death, of killing himself, or of being killed. Some adolescents may present with passive suicidal ideation (e.g., "I wish I were dead") but report having no plan or intent to kill themselves. In contrast, some adolescents report active suicidal ideation that is more alarming (e.g., "I feel like killing myself"). When asked, these clients may report having a specific plan to kill themselves. A suicidal plan involves identifying a specific method and possibly a given time frame, in which an adolescent plans to kill him- or herself. After an adolescent reports having a plan the clinician must assess for suicidal intent, which characterizes the adolescent's level of commitment in carrying out the plan. Hence, adolescents may report having a specific plan but have no intent to die (e.g., "I thought about jumping, but I would never do it"). Others may describe their intent as ambivalent (e.g., "I think about taking an overdose, but I am not sure whether I can do it"), and still others may have full intent to kill themselves (e.g., "I intend to shoot myself this Sunday when my parents leave town"). Further complicating matters is the inconsistency across assessments in adolescents' reports of their own suicidal behavior (Velting, Rathus, & Asnis, 1998).

Accessible Means of Suicide

Accessibility to the means of suicide is a significant proximal risk factor. The most common method of suicide in the United States, regardless of age, race, or gender, is firearms (Minino, Arias, Kochanek, Murphy, & Smith,

2002). In 2001, firearms were used in 54% of completed youth suicides (Anderson & Smith, 2003). The probability of suicide increases 5 times when a firearm is kept in the home (Brent et al., 1991). Other common methods used by male adolescents for completed suicide in the United States include jumping, hanging, and carbon monoxide poisoning. For female adolescents, the next most frequent methods include overdosing on pills or ingesting solid and liquid poisons (Minino et al., 2002).

The overwhelming majority of adolescent suicide attempts in the United States and the United Kingdom involve intentional overdose (Berman, Jobes, & Silverman, 2006). Lewinsohn et al. (1996) found that ingestion and self-cutting accounted for 86% of the suicide attempts reported by girls and 45% of those reported by boys. In addition to ingestion (20%) and self-cutting (25%), they found that other common methods used by boys were gun use (15%), hanging (11%), and other (22%), which included activities such as shooting air into one's veins and running into traffic.

Medical lethality of method and suicide intent has been found to be highly correlated (e.g., see Robbins & Alessi, 1985), although certainly not synonymous. However, Harris and Myers (1997) found that adolescents who overdose without intent to die seriously underestimated the dangerousness of their actions. These data confirm that many teens have little understanding of the medical–biological consequences of their actions; some adolescents assume taking five extra strength Tylenol will kill them, whereas others believe that ingesting 100 of the same pills will merely help them sleep better.

Stressful Adverse Life Events

Historically, interpersonal conflicts and separations are considered the most common precipitants to adolescent suicide (Miller & Glinski, 2000). Breakup of a romantic relationship, disciplinary or legal problems, and arguments are some of the stressful life events identified in attempted and completed suicide of youth worldwide, even after adjusting for family, personality factors, and psychopathology (e.g., see Beautrais, 2001). Specific stressors may vary depending on age. For example, romantic difficulties are common precipitants among older adolescents, and parent–child conflicts are common among younger adolescents (Miller & Glinski, 2000).

Suicide in the Social Milieu

Exposure to the suicidal behavior of others, including through the media, can precipitate imitative suicidal behavior, at least in some individuals (Velting & Gould, 1997). Adolescents are highly susceptible to suggestion and imitative behavior, as these are primary modes of social learning and identity formation. Velting and Gould (1997) proposed that modeling cues through personal acquaintance, community exposures, and exposure to media coverage may all play a role in imitative suicidal behavior. Numerous studies have found significantly more peers, friends or family members had attempted or completed suicide in the social networks or families of those who ideated about, attempted, and committed suicide than in control groups.

In addition to increased rates of suicidal behavior in the relatives and friends of suicide victims, suicidologists have examined cluster suicides. A suicide cluster may be defined as a group of suicide attempts that occur closer together in time and space than would normally be expected in a given community (Centers for Disease Control and Prevention, 1988). In a review of the suicide cluster literature, Velting and Gould (1997) argued that suicide contagion is a real effect, even though it appears to be a less potent risk factor than other psychiatric and psychosocial risk factors for suicide. In addition, adolescents are at highest risk for a cluster suicide.

Academic Difficulties

School difficulties, not working or attending school, and dropping out of high school have been identified as risk factors for attempted and completed suicide in several countries, even after controlling for psychopathology and social risk factors (e.g., see Wunderlich, Bronish, & Wiichen, 1998).

Sexual and Physical Abuse

Researchers have found that childhood sexual and physical abuse are also associated with suicidal behavior in adolescents, even after controlling for a variety of potentially confounding variables, including the adolescent's psychopathology, parental psychopathology, and demographics (Gould et al., 2003; Johnson et al, 2002).

Functional Impairment From Physical Disease and Injury

Physical diseases and injury and related functional impairment have been found to increase the risk of future suicide attempts in adolescents (Lewinsohn et al., 1996). Nevertheless, certain diseases require more attention in this population. For example, a diagnosis of HIV/AIDS, although considered a more definitive risk factor among adults, has not received adequate empirical study among adolescents.

EVALUATING RISK

To assess a new suicidal patient effectively, particularly in an outpatient setting, it is critically important to first conduct a thorough diagnostic evaluation, as certain mental disorders are clear risk factors for adolescent suicidal behavior. One of the most commonly used semistructured diagnostic interviews to assess Axis I disorders in children and adolescents is the Schedule for Affective Disorders and Schizophrenia for School-Age Children, Present and Lifetime Version (Kaufman, Birmaher, Brent, Rao, & Ryan, 1997). Both the adolescent and the parent or guardian are interviewed separately to obtain diagnostic information. It must be noted that in certain settings, such as a hospital emergency department, acute care facility, or urgent care outpatient appointment, it may not be feasible to conduct a thorough evaluation because of the time required. In these cases, one must rely on diagnoses obtained from a standard clinical interview. Regardless, one needs to obtain specific information about the adolescent's suicidal ideation, plan, and intent. Sometimes an adolescent directly informs the therapist that he or she is feeling suicidal. The patient may be thinking or even planning a suicide attempt without directly informing the therapist. Should a therapist raise the question if the patient has not directly brought it up? The answer is a definitive *yes*. Ask questions about ideation, plan, and intent directly. The following are several occasions that may prompt a therapist to ask whether the adolescent is having thoughts about suicide: (a) the occurrence of an event that was a precipitant to a prior suicide attempt or serious suicidal ideation; (b) worsening of psychiatric symptomatology, especially depressive symptoms, panic attacks, or psychotic symptoms; (c) increasing amounts of alcohol or drug use; and (d) statements made by the adolescent, such as she wishes she were dead or she believes her family would be better off without her. Key questions about suicidal behavior include the following:

1. Given what you are saying about your current life circumstances, are you feeling hopeless or discouraged right now?
2. Have you been feeling so unhappy lately that you are having thoughts about death or of killing yourself? If *yes*,
3. Do you have a plan for how you would do this? What is it and do you have the means to carry this out (i.e., accessibility of instrument)? If *yes* to plan,
4. How intent are you on carrying out this plan? What is the likelihood of your actually doing it?
5. What reasons do you have to live right now (i.e., assessing for intent and protective factors)?
6. Have you ever attempted suicide before?
7. Have you ever injured yourself without intent to die? What about now (i.e., assessing nonsuicidal self-injurious behavior, which is an important risk factor for suicide)?

Research suggests that suicidal clients are more likely to disclose current suicidal ideation on a self-report measure than in a clinical interview (Kaplan et al., 1994; Velting et al., 1998). Nevertheless, it is equally important not to rely exclusively on self-report measures. A clinical interview yields important information that cannot be obtained through questionnaires, such as the adolescent's quality of affect and compliance with the interviewer (Velting et al., 1998). Some adolescents are reluctant to actively engage in the evaluation process. At times, it is critical to check in with them, potentially validate their feelings that this is a difficult process, and then either take a break or establish a commitment that they will work with you to complete the evaluation.

When possible, a comprehensive assessment battery that includes semistructured diagnostic interviews in addition to parent, teacher, and adolescent self-reports is recommended. Examples of commonly used self-report inventories of suicidal ideation and behavior include the Suicidal Ideation Questionnaire (W. M. Reynolds, 1987), the Scale for Suicide Ideation (Beck, Steer, & Ranieri, 1988), and the Harkavy-Asnis Suicide Survey (Harkavy-Friedman & Asnis, 1989). Nock, Holmberg, Photos, and Michel, (2007) developed a new instrument called the Self-Injurious Thoughts and Behaviors Interview, which has strong psychometric properties to assess suicidal ideation and behavior as well as nonsuicidal self-injurious urges and behaviors among an adolescent population. One may also consider administering another self-report measure that approaches suicide from a different vantage point. The Reasons for Living Inventory for Adolescents (Osman et al., 1998), is a modified version of the adult questionnaire of the same name that taps expectancies about the consequences of living versus killing oneself and assesses the importance of reasons for living. This instrument functions to identify protective factors against suicide. Several additional self-report measures may be useful to use when working with this population, including the Beck Depression Inventory—II (Beck, Steer, Ball, & Ranieri, 1996), Symptom Checklist-90—Revised (Derogatis, 1975), and the Behavioral Assessment Scales for Children (C. R. Reynolds & Kamphaus, 2004).

MANAGING RISK

In real-life clinical practice, it is rare to completely separate assessment from treatment when engaging in ongoing work with a suicidal adolescent. It feels necessary when writing about these issues to describe them in a more linear fashion. However, when evaluating an adolescent for the first time, it is usually best to first conduct a diagnostic evaluation and suicide risk assessment (through clinical interview and self-report measures) and then implement interventions that are known to effectively manage suicidal behaviors in youth. In this section we discuss the clinical management of suicidal behavior through the use of a youth suicide emergency protocol. Many of these principles derive from Linehan's (1993) work with suicidal adults and are equally applicable to teens.

To help clarify the protocol, we start by briefly describing an adolescent client referred for therapy to our outpatient adolescent depression and suicide program. Donna is a fictionalized 15-year-old African American girl who was referred by the psychiatric emergency department after expressing suicidal ideation to her guidance counselor at school. At the time of the intake evaluation, Donna reported that she had been experiencing suicidal thoughts, sad mood, decreased appetite, anhedonia, and irritability for the past year. She stated that she had thoughts of killing herself by ingesting a large quantity of her mother's antidepressant medication and sleeping pills; however, she had not experienced any thoughts during the past week and a half, which she attributes to recently beginning a relationship with a boy in her school. Upon returning for the follow-up appointment, Donna tearfully reported to the intake therapist that her boyfriend broke up with her that morning and that she had gotten into a physical altercation with a girl at school the day before. She stated that she did not want to attend the appointment because "it won't help."

In Donna's case, the therapist was aware of her history of significant suicidal thoughts and depressive symptoms. Although Donna did not offer the information, the therapist directly asked about Donna's current level of suicidal ideation, plan, and intent. After the therapist's inquiry, Donna did indicate that she had been thinking about killing herself by overdosing on pills but was uncertain if she could carry out the act.

Delay Impulses and Restore Hope

One of the greatest problems for suicidal youth is that they cannot see a way out of the pain they are experiencing. In these circumstances, therapists need to simultaneously use assessment and intervention strategies. Many suicidal patients describe their current experience as though there is a mountain of accumulated problems in front of them that appears insurmountable. Thus, the challenge for the therapist is to model how to break down this mountain into manageable problems that can be solved in the present. A protective factor for suicide is when the patient can identify reasons for living. The therapist can ask the suicidal patient, "What reasons do you have for living right now?" The therapist hopes that the patient does not require significant prompting. However, because suicidal patients are often in acute emotional distress, the therapist might prompt with statements such as, "What about your family and friends?"; "How would they feel if you killed yourself?"; "What about your future?"; "What do you want to be when you grow up?"; and "What about your religion?" If these reasons for living are significant, they can serve as a protective factor against imminent suicidal behavior.

With minor prompting, Donna was able to acknowledge the painful feelings she had when she considered how hurt her mother and family would be if she killed herself. The therapist was able to provide validation for the anguish Donna was feeling and help her recognize that she now had another advocate to help her to decrease her pain. In addition, the therapist told Donna that despite feelings to the contrary, she could make it through this difficult period if she gave the therapist a chance to help. The therapist reminded her of prior occasions that Donna had *stuck it out* and came out on the other side feeling better. If recalling past coping successes is ineffective, the therapist can use irreverent statements such as, "How do you know you will feel less upset after you kill yourself?"; "Why don't you give us a chance to work on solving your problems and lessen your pain?"; and "What do you have to lose?"

If the patient cannot identify any reasons for living and is unable to demonstrate any future perspective in terms of goals, the therapist must recognize this as an absence of protective factors that needs to be factored into the decision about psychiatric hospitalization.

Problem-Solve the Current Problem

Frequently, the adolescent's assumptions about the outcomes of his or her behavioral choices are unrealistic and need to be gently but directly confronted. Ideally, therapists help patients generate their own solutions to their problems. However, in an emergency there are times when the patient does not know what to do. In these circumstances it is advisable for the therapist to give direct, concrete suggestions about how to manage specific situations (Miller, Nathan, & Wagner, in press). Therapists should be careful not to assume that a patient who generates a solution also knows exactly how to carry it out. Thus, therapists should pay attention to these details and generate solutions for the patient to try.

The therapist was able to recognize that Donna was overwhelmed by her emotions and suicidal thoughts. The therapist helped Donna identify that she had survived these thoughts and feelings before by using specific strategies, including talking with her mother, listening to music, and writing poetry. For Donna, the long-term goal of therapy was to learn to affiliate with people, particularly boyfriends, who would treat her respectfully. The therapist, however, helped Donna focus on the short-term goal, which was to get through this suicidal emergency situation. As a result, in addition to helping Donna identify strategies for managing her emotions, the therapist also made herself available by pager 24 hours a day and added an additional session later in the week to increase social support.

Reduce High Risk Behavioral Factors

Regardless of whether the lethal means is a gun, liquid poison, or pills of some sort, it is imperative that the therapist spend a portion of the emergency session ensuring that the removal of lethal means has occurred or will occur. Depending on the acute nature of the emergency, the therapist may instruct the patient to bring the lethal items to the next session or insist that the patient go home and bring in the items immediately. In other cases, when the patient calls the therapist in a suicidal emergency, the therapist may instruct the patient to flush the pills down the toilet and should wait on the phone while the patient complies. In other cases, family members, significant others, or roommates may be enlisted to facilitate the removal of lethal means from the patient's home. Locking up a firearm in the home or separating the ammunition from the gun is not sufficient. The weapon needs to be secured outside of the home.

Because Donna is a minor, the therapist brought Donna's mother into the session to inform her of Donna's suicidal thoughts, plan, and possible intent. The therapist specifically asked Donna's mother whether all the medications in the house were locked away and told her that if they were not, she should insure they were as soon as they returned home. Donna agreed to this plan, stating that she did not trust herself with access to the pills.

If the adolescent refuses to consent and is noncompliant with the therapist's recommendations to remove lethal items herself, it is typically a bad prognosis regarding the adolescent's willingness and capacity to maintain safety and thus may require an inpatient admission. Either way, because suicidal behavior is at issue, the therapist is justified in breaking confidentiality by contacting a family member to remove the lethal means. In addition, some patients self-medicate with drugs or alcohol. During a suicidal emergency, the patient needs to be instructed to discontinue any alcohol or drug use because of their disinhibiting properties. If the adolescent is unwilling to discontinue drug or alcohol use, the therapist must factor this high-risk behavior into the decision about psychiatric hospitalization.

Commit to a Plan of Action

After a sufficient number of solutions are generated, the therapist asks the patient to commit to a plan of action. Considerable evidence suggests that the commitment to behave in a particular way, especially when the commitment is made publicly instead of privately, is strongly related to future performance (Linehan, 1999). First and foremost is obtaining the patient's commitment to not engage in any suicidal or self-harm behaviors until the next session.

Donna, with the therapist's assistance, identified the specific strategies she would use to survive this emergency situation. She committed to staying alive until the next scheduled session and agreed to tell her mother if her suicidal thoughts became unbearable. She also agreed to tolerate distress by listening to music, writing poetry, and calling her friends on the phone. Donna informed her mother about the plan.

Troubleshoot the Plan—Tolerate Distress

Therapists working with suicidal patients need to suggest that one additional solution to their problems is to simply tolerate the painful consequences, including the negative affect, that the situation has generated. At first blush, many suicidal patients have trouble grasping the value and function of this solution. However, with practice, patients begin to recognize and appreciate the idea of tolerance as a solution.

In Donna's case, the therapist validated her pain and normalized that anyone would feel this way after an abrupt breakup of a romantic relationship. The therapist noted that although it sounded strange, "Learning how to tolerate pain and disappointment is a difficult and important life lesson. I don't wish pain and disappointment on anyone, especially you, Donna, but I actually think this is an opportunity for me to help you learn how to soothe yourself during difficult times in your life."

TROUBLESHOOTING AND RELAPSE PREVENTION

Despite the therapist's best efforts to effectively deliver interventions and the patient's apparent commitment to follow through, it is inevitable that obstacles will arise. Troubleshooting refers to anticipating obstacles before they occur and proposing solutions for managing them. When working with suicidal patients, it is even more imperative to troubleshoot the solutions, as it can be a matter of life and death.

The therapist asked Donna, "So what might interfere in your ability to write poetry, listen to music, or reach out to me or your mother if and when you feel suicidal later tonight or tomorrow? Might you be afraid to 'bother me' or not be in the mood to write? What then?" The therapist and Donna problem-solved how to manage these potential obstacles.

Anticipate Recurrence of Emergency Response

The therapist anticipated that, for Donna, thinking of the boyfriend or focusing on her feelings of rejection might exacerbate her suicidal response. Although this is predictable, the therapist wanted to review with Donna how she will manage the situation (see previous troubleshooting discussion).

Reassess Suicide Potential

Although the protocol for handling suicidal emergencies is basically the same regardless of whether they occur at the beginning or during the course of treatment, there are important differences: At the initial evaluation, there is not yet a therapeutic alliance to use in handling the situation, and the therapist does not know the patient or his or her biggest vulnerability factors or strengths. Although these differences may seem to suggest higher risk and a necessarily poorer outcome, the converse may actually be true:

Evidence indicates that youth and their parents may be more likely to follow through with treatment when presenting in a more acute state of distress (e.g., see Kendall & Sugarman, 1997).

Intersession Contact

Interpersonal supports are a protective factor for the suicidal patient. Thus, in addition to coaching the patient on enlisting her family members and friends for support whenever possible, therapists must also make themselves available during these potential emergencies. The general rule is to stay in contact with the patient, either in person or by phone, until the therapist is convinced that the patient will be safe after the contact is broken off (Linehan, 1999). At these times, therapy sessions or phone calls may need to be extended until a safety plan is established and the patient is committed to comply. We suggest that therapists who carry pagers encourage their patients to make use of this method of contact. All therapists who work with suicidal patients should keep the names, phone numbers, and addresses of their clients handy in case of an emergency in which they may need to send an ambulance to their home.

Depending on the imminent nature of the emergency, the therapist may contact the parents or guardians and other treatment providers. The therapist should attempt to select the least intrusive intervention necessary (i.e., notify the fewest number of additional parties) to ensure the patient's safety. That is often a challenging judgment call to make when the issue of suicidality arises. Naturally, contacting an adolescent's parent or parents is a necessity when an acute suicidal emergency occurs or when an adolescent's low-level chronic suicidality worsens. Moreover, a nonmedical therapist should always notify the adolescent's prescribing doctor (if there is one) regarding the patient's increased risk of overdose. In addition, suicidal adolescents and their significant others (if appropriate) are always referred to their local psychiatric emergency department or told to call 911 if the suicidal impulses escalate and they are unable or unwilling to contact their therapist. In Donna's case, the therapist offered Donna an additional session later that week and reviewed the fact that Donna could page the therapist any time, day or night, for skills coaching to manage suicidal impulses.

Give Emergency Card

All suicidal patients should receive an emergency card by the time they leave the session. At a minimum, the emergency card contains important telephone and pager numbers for all designated people. Additionally, some emergency cards contain a list of personalized coping skills.

WHEN SHOULD INPATIENT PSYCHIATRIC HOSPITALIZATION BE RECOMMENDED OR CONSIDERED?

Although more suicides occur in the community than in hospitals, there are no empirical data to date that support the notion that acute, inpatient hospitalization is effective at preventing suicide. Moreover, no studies have found inpatient hospitalization to be the treatment of choice for the chronically suicidal patient (Linehan, 1999). However, on the basis of clinical experience, there are situations in which the therapist should consider recommending brief, inpatient hospitalizations. The following is a list of potential circumstances that may warrant this type of recommendation; the first five are adapted from Linehan (1993):

1. The patient is psychotic and is threatening suicide or having command auditory hallucinations to kill himself or someone else.
2. The patient is on psychotropic medications, has a history of overdose on these medications, and is having problems that require close monitoring of medication or dose.
3. The relationship between therapist and patient is severely strained, which is contributing to the suicidal emergency. The inpatient staff might be helpful in repairing the relationship by facilitating a meeting with both parties.
4. The patient is not responding to outpatient therapy and there is severe depression or debilitating anxiety.
5. Operant suicide threats are escalating and hospitalization is considered aversive by the patient.
6. The patient is actively abusing alcohol or drugs and is refusing to reduce usage during the emergency.
7. The patient refuses to remove lethal items from the home or refuses to use an emergency card to call the therapist or others if suicidal ideation returns.
8. The patient is profoundly hopeless and unable to identify any reasons for living, even with prompting.
9. The patient cannot identify any social supports that she is willing to use for help during the emergency period.

This list is not meant to be exhaustive but merely represents several common situations that may, individually or in combination, warrant inpatient admission for the suicidal patient. Of course, each of these situations needs to be considered in a fuller clinical context. The therapist must always take into account the patient's prior history of suicidal behavior, current suicidal ideation, plan, and intent, as well as the myriad of environmental and behavioral high-risk factors.

CONCLUSION

The field of adolescent suicidology is advancing. In this chapter we highlighted the expanding list of evidence-based suicide risk and protective factors useful for evaluating the at-risk youth as well as managing suicidal crises. Although we did not focus on the ongoing treatment of suicidal youth, we presented a crisis protocol to be used during an acute 1- or 2-day suicidal crisis period with a clinical vignette to illustrate the principles. In addition, we offered recommendations about when to hospitalize a suicidal teen. Although the evaluation and management of suicidal children and adolescents can be stressful and overwhelming to even the most seasoned therapists, knowledge about and practice with a protocol focused on decreasing suicidal behaviors and increasing effective coping strategies can provide significant short- and long-term benefits for these youth and their families.

REFERENCES

Adams, D. A., Overholser, J. C., & Lehnert, K. L. (1994). Perceived family functioning and adolescent suicidal behavior. *Journal of the American Academy of Child & Adolescent Psychiatry, 33,* 498–507.

Agerbo, E., Nordentoft, M., & Mortensen, P. B. (2002, July 13). Familial, psychiatric, and socioeconomic risk factors for suicide in young people: Nested case-control study. *BMJ, 325,* 74–77.

American Association of Suicidology. (2003). *Year 2003: Official final data on suicide in the United States.* Retrieved September 15, 2006, from http://www.suicidology.org/associations/1045/files/2003datapgb.pdf

American Psychiatric Association. (2000). *Diagnostic and statistical manual of mental disorders* (4th ed., text revision). Washington, DC: Author.

Anderson, R. N. (2002). Deaths: Leading causes for 2000. *National Vital Statistics Reports, 50*(16). Hyattsville, MD: National Center for Health Statistics.

Anderson, R. N., & Smith, B. L. (2003). Deaths: Leading causes for 2001. *National Vital Statistics Report, 52*(9). Hyattsville, MD: National Center for Health Statistics.

Apter, A., Gothelf, D., Orbach, I., Weizman, R., Ratzoni, G., Har-Even, D., & Tyano, S. (1995). Correlation of suicidal and violent behavior in different diagnostic categories in hospitalized adolescent patients. *Journal of the American Academy of Child & Adolescent Psychiatry, 34,* 912–918.

Beautrais, A. L. (2001). Child and young adolescent suicide in New Zealand. *Australian and New Zealand Journal of Psychiatry, 35,* 647–653.

Beck, A. T., Steer, R. A., Ball, R., & Ranieri, W. F. (1996). Comparison of Beck Depression Inventories–IA and –II in psychiatric outpatients. *Journal of Personality Assessment, 67,* 588–597.

Beck, A. T., Steer, R. A., & Ranieri, W. F. (1988). Scale for suicide ideation: Psychometric properties of a self-report version. *Journal of Clinical Psychology, 44,* 499–505.

Berman, A. L., Jobes, D. A., & Silverman, M. M. (2006). *Adolescent suicide: Assessment and intervention* (2nd ed.). Washington, DC: American Psychological Association.

Berman, A. L., & Schwartz, R. (1990). Suicide attempts among adolescent drug users. *American Journal of Diseases of Children, 144,* 310–314.

Blake, S. M., Ledsky, R., Lehman, T., Goodenow, C., Sawyer, R., & Hack, T. (2001). Preventing sexual risk behaviors among gay, lesbian, and bisexual adolescents: The benefits of gay- sensitive HIV instruction in schools. *American Journal of Public Health, 91,* 940–946.

Brent, D. A., Baugher, M., Bridge, J., Chen, T., & Chiappetta, L. (1999). Age and sex-related risk factors for adolescent suicide. *Journal of the American Academy of Child & Adolescent Psychiatry, 38,* 1497–1505.

Brent, D. A., Johnson, B., Bartle, S., Bridge, J., Rather, C., Matta, J., et al. (1993). Personality disorder, tendency to impulsive violence, and suicidal behavior in adolescents. *Journal of the American Academy of Child & Adolescent Psychiatry, 32,* 69–75.

Brent, D. A., Johnson, B. A., Perper, J. A., Connolly, J., Bridge, J., Bartle, S., et al. (1994). Personality disorder, personality traits, impulsive violence, and completed suicide in adolescents. *Journal of the American Academy of Child & Adolescent Psychiatry, 33,* 1080–1086.

Brent, D. A., Perper, J. A., & Allman, C. J. (1987). Alcohol, firearms, and suicide among youth. *Journal of the American Medical Association, 257,* 3369–3372.

Brent, D. A., Perper, J. A., Allman, C. J., Moritz, G. M., Wartella, M. E, & Zelenak, J. P. (1991). The presence and accessibility of firearms in the homes of adolescent suicides. *Journal of the American Medical Association, 266,* 2989–2995.

Brent, D. A., Perper, J. A., Goldstein, C. E., Kolko, D. J., Allan, M. J., Allman, C. J., et al. (1988). Risk factors for adolescent suicide. A comparison of adolescent suicide victims with suicidal inpatients. *Archives of General Psychiatry, 445,* 581–588.

Brent, D. A., Perper, J. A., Moritz, G., Allman, C., Friend, A., Roth, C., et al. (1993). Psychiatric risk factors for adolescent suicide: A case-control study. *Journal of the American Academy of Child & Adolescent Psychiatry, 35,* 521–529.

Bridge, J. A., Brent, D. A., Johnson, B. A., & Connolly, J. (1997). Familial aggregation of psychiatric disorders in a community sample of adolescents. *Journal of the American Academy of Child & Adolescent Psychiatry, 36,* 628–636.

Centers for Disease Control and Prevention. (1988). Recommendations for a community plan for the prevention and containment of suicide clusters. *Morbidity and Mortality Weekly Reports, 37,* 1–11.

Derogatis, L. R. (1975). *The SCL-90-R.* Baltimore: Clinical Psychometric Research.

Fergusson, D. M., & Lynskey, M. T. (1995). Suicide attempts and suicidal ideation in a birth cohort of 16-year-old New Zealanders. *Journal of the American Academy of Child & Adolescent Psychiatry, 34,* 1308–1317.

Fergusson, D. M., Woodward, L. J., & Horwood, L. J. (2000). Risk factors and life processes associated with the onset of suicidal behavior during adolescence and early adulthood. *Psychological Medicine 30*, 23–39.

Garofalo, R., Wolf, R. C., Wissow, L. S., Woods, E. R., & Goodman, E. (1999). Sexual orientation and risk of suicide attempts among a representative sample of youth. *Archives of Pediatrics & Adolescent Medicine, 153*, 487–493.

Geller, B., Zimmerman, B., Williams, M., DelBello, M. P., Frazier, J., & Beringer, L. (2002). Phenomenology of prepubertal and early adolescent bipolar disorder: Examples of elated mood, grandiose behaviors, decreased need for sleep, racing thoughts and hypersexuality. *Journal of Child & Adolescent Psychopharmacology, 12*, 3–9.

Giaconia, R. M., Reinherz, H. Z., Silverman, A. B., Pakiz, B., Frost, A. K., & Cohen, E. (1995). Traumas and posttraumatic stress disorder in a community population of older adolescents. *Journal of the American Academy of Child & Adolescent Psychiatry, 34*, 1369–1380.

Goldston, D. B., Daniel, S. S., Reboussin, D. M., Reboussin, B. A., Frazier, P. H., & Kelley, A. E. (1999). Suicide attempts among formerly hospitalized adolescents: A prospective naturalistic study of risk during the first 5 years after discharge. *Journal of the American Academy of Child & Adolescent Psychiatry, 38*, 660–671.

Gould, M. S., Fisher, P., Parides, M., Flory, M., & Shaffer, D. (1996). Psychosocial risk factors of child and adolescent completed suicide. *Archives of General Psychiatry, 53*, 1155–1162.

Gould, M. S., Greenberg, T., Velting, D. M., & Shaffer, D. (2003). Youth suicide risk and preventive interventions: A review of the past 10 years. *Journal of the American Academy of Child & Adolescent Psychiatry, 42*, 386–405.

Gould, M. S., King, R., Greenwald, S., Fisher, P., Schwab-Stone, M., Kramer, R., et al. (1998). Psychopathology associated with suicidal ideation and attempts among children and adolescents. *Journal of the American Academy of Child & Adolescent Psychiatry, 37*, 915–923.

Grunbaum, J. A., Kann, L., Kinchen, S. A., Williams, B., Ross, J. G., & Lowry, R. (2002). Youth risk behavior surveillance: United States, 2001. *Morbidity and Mortality Weekly Report Surveillance Summary, 51*, 1–64.

Harkavy-Friedman, J. M., & Asnis, G. M. (1989). Assessment of suicidal behavior: A new instrument. *Psychiatric Annals, 19*, 382–387.

Harris, H. E., & Myers, W. C. (1997). Adolescents' misperception of the dangerousness of acetaminophen in overdose. *Suicide and Life-Threatening Behavior, 27*, 274–277.

Hoberman, H. M., & Garfinkel, B. D. (1988). Completed suicide in children and adolescents. *Journal of the American Academy of Child & Adolescent Psychiatry, 27*, 689–695.

Johnson, J. G., Cohen, P., Gould, M. S., Kasen, S., Brown, J., & Brook, J. S. (2002). Childhood adversities, interpersonal difficulties, and risk for suicide attempts during late adolescence and early adulthood. *Archives of General Psychiatry, 59*, 741–749.

Kann, L., Kinchen, S. A., Williams, B. I., & Ross, J. G. (2000). Youth risk behavior surveillance—United States, 1999. *Journal of School Health, 70*, 271–285.

Kaplan, M. L., Asnis, G. M., Sanderson, W. C., Keswani, L., De Lecuona, J. M., & Joseph, S. (1994). Suicide assessment: Clinical interview versus self-report. *Journal of Clinical Psychology, 50,* 294–298.

Kaufman, J., Birmaher, B., Brent, D., Rao, U., & Ryan, N. (1996). *Kiddie-SADS-Present and Lifetime Version.* Pittsburgh, PA: Department of Psychiatry, University of Pittsburgh.

Kendall, P. C., & Sugarman, A. (1997). Attrition in the treatment of childhood anxiety disorders. *Journal of Consulting and Clinical Psychology, 65,* 883–888.

Kessler, R. C., Borges, G., & Walters, E. E. (1999). Prevalence of and risk factors for lifetime suicide attempts in the National Comorbidity Study. *Archives of General Psychiatry, 36,* 617–626.

King, C. A. (1997). Suicidal behavior in adolescence. In E. W. Maris, M. W. Silverman, & S. S. Canetto (Eds.), *Review of suicidology* (pp. 61–95). New York: Guilford Press.

King, C. A., Segal, H., Kaminski, K., Naylor, M., Ghaziuddin, N., & Radpour, L. (1995). A prospective study of adolescent suicidal behavior following hospitalization. *Suicide and Life-Threatening Behavior, 25,* 327–338.

Kochanek, K. D., Murphy, S. L., Anderson, R. N., & Scott, C. (2004). Deaths: Final data for 2002. *National Vital Statistics Reports, 53*(5). Hyattsville, MD: National Center for Health Statistics.

Kotila, L. (1992). The outcome of attempted suicide in adolescence. *Journal of Adolescent Health, 13,* 415–417.

Kovacs, M., Goldston, D., & Gatsonis, C. (1993). Suicidal behaviors and childhood-onset depressive disorders: A longitudinal investigation. *Journal of the American Academy of Child & Adolescent Psychiatry, 32,* 8–20.

Lewinsohn, P. M., Rohde, P., & Seeley, J. R. (1996). Adolescent suicidal ideation and attempts: Prevalence, risk factors, and clinical implications. *Clinical Psychology: Science and Practice, 3,* 25–46.

Lewinsohn, P. M., Rohde, P., Seeley, J. R., & Baldwin, C. L. (2001). Gender differences in suicide attempts from adolescence to young adulthood. *Journal of the American Academy of Child & Adolescent Psychiatry, 40,* 427–434.

Lewinsohn, P. M., Rohde, P., Seeley, J. R., & Klein, D. N. (1997). Axis II psychopathology as a function of Axis I disorders in childhood and adolescence. *Journal of the American Academy of Child & Adolescent Psychiatry, 36,* 1752–1759.

Linehan, M. M. (1993). *Cognitive–behavioral treatment of borderline personality disorder.* New York: Guilford Press.

Linehan, M. M. (1999). Standard protocol for assessing and treating suicidal behaviors. In D. Jacobs (Ed.), *Harvard Medical School guide to suicide assessment and intervention* (pp. 146–187). San Francisco: Jossey-Bass.

Mann, J. J., Waternaux, C., Haas, G. L., & Malone, K. M. (1999). Toward a clinical model of suicidal behavior in psychiatric patients. *American Journal of Psychiatry, 156,* 181–189.

Marttunen, M. J., Aro, H. M., & Lönnqvist, J. K. (1992). Adolescent suicide: Endpoint of long-term difficulties. *Journal of the American Academy of Child & Adolescent Psychiatry, 31,* 649–654.

Marttunen, M. J., Henriksson, M. M., Aro, H. M., Heikkinen, M. E., Isometsä, E. T., & Lönnqvist, J. K. (1995). Suicide among female adolescents: Characteristics and comparison with males in the age group 13 to 22 years. *Journal of the American Academy of Child & Adolescent Psychiatry, 34*, 1297–1307.

Mazza, J. J. (2000). The relationship between posttraumatic stress symptomatology and suicidal behavior in school-based adolescents. *Suicide and Life-Threatening Behavior, 30*, 91–103.

Middlebrook, D. L., LeMaster, P. L., Beals, J., Novins, D. K., & Manson, S. M. (2001). Suicide prevention in American Indian and Alaska Native communities: A critical review of programs. *Suicide and Life-Threatening Behavior, 31*(Suppl. 1), 132–149.

Miller, A. L., & Glinski, J. (2000). Youth suicidal behavior: Assessment and intervention. *Journal of Clinical Psychology, 56*, 1–22.

Miller, A. L., Nathan, J. S., & Wagner, E. E. (in press). Engaging suicidal multiproblem adolescents with DBT. In D. Castro-Blanco (Ed.), *Elusive alliance: Treatment engagement strategies with high-risk adolescents*. Washington, DC: American Psychological Association.

Miller, A. L., Rathus, J. H., & Linehan, M. M. (2007). *Dialectical behavior therapy with suicidal adolescents*. New York: Guilford Press.

Millon, T., Millon, C., & Davis, R. (1993). *Manual for the Millon Clinical Inventory*. Minneapolis, MN: National Computer Systems.

Minino, A. M., Arias, E., Kochanek, K. D., Murphy, S. L., & Smith, B. L. (2002). Deaths: Final data for 2000. *National Vital Statistics Reports, 50*(15). Hyattsville, MD: National Center for Health Statistics.

Nock, M. K., Holmberg, E. B., Photos, V. I., & Michel, B. D. (2007). The self-injurious behaviors interview: Development, reliability, and validity of a new measure. *Psychological Assessment, 19*, 309–317.

Osman, A., Downs, W. R., Kopper, B. A., Barrios, F. X., Baker, M. T., Osman, J. R., et al. (1998). The Reasons for Living Inventory for Adolescents (RFL-A): Development and psychometric properties. *Journal of Clinical Psychology, 54*, 1063–1078.

Pilowsky, D. J., Wu, L. T., & Anthony, J. C. (1999). Panic attacks and suicide attempts in mid-adolescence. *American Journal of Psychiatry, 156*, 1545–1549.

Reynolds, C. R., & Kamphaus, R. W. (2004). *BASC–2: Behavior Assessment System for Children* (2nd ed.). Circle Pines, MN: AGS Publishing.

Reynolds, W. M. (1987). *Suicidal Ideation Questionnaire*. Odessa, FL: Psychological Assessment Resources.

Robbins, D. R., & Alessi, N. E. (1985). Depressive symptoms and suicidal behavior in adolescents. *American Journal of Psychiatry, 142*, 588–592.

Russell, S. T., & Joyner, K. (2001). Adolescent sexual orientation and suicide risk: Evidence from a national study. *American Journal of Public Health, 91*, 1276–1281.

Schmidtke, A., Bille-Brahe, U., DeLeo, D., & Kerkhof, A. (2004). The WHO/EURO multicentre study on suicidal behavior. In A. Schmidtke, U. Bille-Brahe, D.

DeLeo, & A. Kerkhof (Eds.), *Suicidal behavior in Europe* (pp. 11–14). Ashland, OH: Hogrefe & Huber.

Shaffer, D., Gould, M., Fisher, P., Trautman, M. P., Moreau, D., Kleinman, M., & Flory, M. (1996). Psychiatric diagnosis in child and adolescent suicide. *Archives of General Psychiatry, 53,* 339–348.

Shaffer, D., & Piacentini, J. (1994). Suicide and attempted suicide. In M. Rutter & E. Taylor (Eds.), *Child psychiatry: Modern approaches* (3rd ed., pp. 407–424). Oxford, England: Blackwell Science.

Spirito, A., Brown, L., Overholser, J., & Fritz, G. (1989). Attempted suicide in adolescence: A review and critique of the literature. *Clinical Psychology Review, 9,* 335–363.

Tortolero, S. R., & Roberts, R. E. (2001). Differences in nonfatal suicide behaviors among Mexican and European American middle school children. *Suicide and Life-Threatening Behavior, 31,* 214–223.

Trautman, P. D., Stewart, N., & Morishima, A. (1993). Are adolescent suicide attempters noncompliant with outpatient care? *Journal of the American Academy of Child & Adolescent Psychiatry, 32,* 89–94.

Velting, D. M., & Gould, M. S. (1997). Suicide contagion. In R. W. Maris, M. M. Silverman, & S. S. Canetto (Eds.), *Review of suicidology* (pp. 96–137). New York: Guilford Press.

Velting, D. M., Rathus, J. H., & Asnis, G. M. (1998). Asking adolescents to explain discrepancies in self-reported suicidality. *Suicide and Life-Threatening Behavior, 28,* 187–196.

Velting, D. M., Rathus, J. H., & Miller, A. L. (2000). MACI personality scale profiles of depressed, adolescent suicide attempters: A pilot study. *Journal of Clinical Psychology, 56,* 1381–1385.

Volkmar, F. R. & Woolston, J. L. (1997). Comorbidity of psychiatric disorders in children and adolescents. In S. Wetzler & W. C. Sanderson (Eds.), *Treatment of patients with psychiatric comorbidity* (pp. 307–322). New York: Wiley.

Wagner, B. M. (1997). Family risk factors for child and adolescent suicidal behavior. *Psychological Bulletin, 121,* 246–298.

Wichstrom, L. (2000). Predictors of adolescent suicide attempts: A nationally representative longitudinal study of Norwegian adolescents. *Journal of the American Academy of Child & Adolescent Psychiatry, 39,* 603–610.

World Health Organization (2002). *Suicide rates and absolute numbers of suicide by country.* Retrieved September 15, 2006, from http://www.who.int/mental_health

Wunderlich, U., Bronish, T., & Wiichen, H. U. (1998). Comorbidity patterns in adolescents and young adults with suicide attempts. *European Archives of Psychiatry and Clinical Neuroscience, 248,* 87–95.

5

SUICIDE RISK IN PEOPLE WITH MEDICAL AND TERMINAL ILLNESS

PHILLIP M. KLEESPIES, SIGMUND HOUGH, AND ANGELA M. ROMEO

Certain medical illnesses are associated with suicide rates that exceed those of other physical illnesses and those of the general population (Harris & Barraclough, 1994). Thus, when clinicians assess patients for suicide risk, particular medical illnesses can be factors that should be carefully weighed. This statement is especially relevant for psychologists who work in medical settings, that is, those in behavioral medicine or health psychology, on a consultation–liaison team, or in rehabilitation psychology.

It should be stated at the outset that research on the relationship between medical illness and suicide is underdeveloped. Therefore, in this chapter we focus on establishing the medical illnesses for which there is empirical evidence of an increased risk of suicide and informing clinicians about the research that supports these assertions. Our method is to examine the meta-analytic reviews and large record linkage studies on the subject. Further, we examine how the combination of medical illness and clinical depression heightens suicide risk. Because terminal illness has been considered a particular risk factor for suicide (Kleespies, 2004), we conclude the chapter with a review of the data on the prevalence of suicide among individuals who are terminally ill, with a particular focus on the data on assisted suicide after it was legalized in the state of Oregon (Oregon Death With Dignity Act [ODDA], 1995).

MEDICAL ILLNESS AMONG SUICIDE VICTIMS

There are little data on the prevalence of suicide among individuals who are medically ill as a general category. There is information, however, on how many of those who commit suicide have a medical illness. Larger studies and meta-analytic reviews on this topic from a decade or more ago were examined and summarized by Hughes and Kleespies (2001) and Kleespies, Hughes, and Gallacher (2000). This chapter builds on that previous work but focuses primarily on new findings and developments in the ensuing years.

Prevalence of Medical Illness Among Suicides

Whitlock (1986) and Mackenzie and Popkin (1990) cumulatively reviewed more than 25 psychological autopsy studies, most of which consisted of 100 suicides or more. They found, respectively, that 34% and 43% of the suicides had a medical illness at the time of self-inflicted death. These findings may be contrasted with many psychological autopsy studies that have found that more than 90% of suicides (per the official reports of coroners) experienced a major mental or emotional disorder (Kleespies & Dettmer, 2000). It seems clear that although medical illness is present with some frequency among suicides, it is not present with the same frequency as mental illness.

Despite the fact that mental illness is more prevalent than physical illness among suicides, evidence is emerging that physical illness may have an independent association with suicidal behavior. Thus, in a large probability survey with a young adult population (ages 17–39), Druss and Pincus (2000) collected information about lifetime suicidal ideation and suicide attempts as well as data on general medical conditions, depression, and alcohol use. They found that medical and mental illness each contributed independently to risk of suicidality. In addition, having more than one medical illness conferred even greater risk of suicidal ideation and especially of suicide attempts.

Goodwin, Marusic, and Hoven (2003) examined data from a national comorbidity study of late adolescents and adults (ages 15–54) in an effort to determine the relationship between physical illness, mental illness, and the likelihood of suicide attempts. On the basis of a self-report checklist of medical illnesses and a question about lifetime suicide attempts, these investigators found significantly increased odds of a suicide attempt with physical illness, even after controlling for demographic characteristics and mental disorders. They also found a linear, dose–response association between the total number of physical illnesses and the likelihood of a suicide attempt.

Finally, Ruzicka, Choi, and Sadkowsky (2005) reviewed all completed suicides over a 5-year period (1997–2001) following the introduction of multiple-cause-of-death coding in Australia. Deaths by suicide were compared with deaths by accident. The findings confirmed the significant relationship of suicide with mental health problems, but they also indicated that selected physical diseases (most notably HIV and cancer) were significantly associated with suicide. In addition, Harwood, Hawton, Hope, Harriss, and Jacoby (2006) did a psychological autopsy and case control study with 100 older people who took their own lives in England and found that physical illness was considered the most frequent life problem that contributed to death by suicide.

These findings, of course, do not necessarily indicate a direct relationship between physical illness and suicidal behavior. As Goodwin et al. (2003) pointed out, specific physical illnesses could be associated with underlying temperament or personality factors that predispose to self-harm behaviors and suicide risk; or, as Ruzicka et al. (2005) noted, the suicide risk associated with physical illness could be mediated by secondary mood or affective symptoms. Nonetheless, the data presented by Druss and Pincus (2000) and by Goodwin et al. (2003) seem to suggest that, at the least, multiple concurrent physical illnesses (or perhaps the cumulative burden of these illnesses) warrants inclusion as a risk factor for suicidality.

Suicide and Specific Medical Illnesses or Conditions

There are many medical illnesses and conditions. Most of them, as single diseases or injuries, appear to have no associated risk of suicide (Harris & Barraclough, 1994). As noted earlier, however, a few physical illnesses have been thought to have associated suicide risk.

HIV/AIDS

In the past 25 to 30 years, HIV/AIDS has been frequently cited as an illness that may have a heightened risk of suicide. In a review of studies from 1966 to 1992, Harris and Barraclough (1994) concluded that the relative risk of suicide for men with HIV was 7 times higher than the rate for men in the general population. The level of suicide risk, however, may have been modified with the introduction in 1996 of improved treatments such as highly active antiretroviral therapy (HAART). In this vein, Komiti et al. (2001) reported a review of studies which suggest that although suicide risk is still elevated among patients with HIV/AIDS, there has been a decrease in age-adjusted relative risk over the years, coinciding with the introduction of antiretroviral therapies.

Krentz, Kliewer, and Gill (2005) conducted a study in Southern Alberta, Canada, linking patients with HIV/AIDS to cause-of-death data for the 20-year period from 1984 to 2003. They found that deaths from AIDS-related causes decreased significantly, but deaths from non-AIDS-related causes, including suicide and drug overdose, increased across this time span (both in terms of absolute numbers and in the proportion of all deaths of patients infected with HIV). In a similar fashion, Lu et al. (2006) linked national HIV/AIDS registry data in Taiwan with cause of death and health insurance claims data for the period 1994 to 2002. They also found that deaths from AIDS-related causes had decreased, but deaths by suicide had increased three-fold from the 1994 to 1996 period to the 2000 to 2002 period. Their conclusion was that as the duration of survival for patients with HIV/AIDS increased, the likelihood of suicide also increased.

It should be borne in mind that HAART treatment is lifelong and can result in multiple discomforting side effects that are difficult to tolerate. Some of the medications can cause worsening depression and vivid dreams. As noted by physicians who specialize in infectious disease, many patients discontinue treatment because of these problems (S. K. Schmitt, personal communication, February 14, 2007). On the one hand, it is conceivable that some patients feel that longer life under such conditions does not necessarily lead to better quality of life, and this circumstance could contribute to suicidality. On the other hand, the finding of an increased suicide rate reported by Krentz et al. (2005) and Lu et al. (2006) may be a product of cultural or regional differences. Future investigations will be needed to confirm or deny this possibility. A synthesis of the studies previously noted, however, suggests that at the least clinicians should continue to regard a diagnosis of HIV/AIDS as associated with a heightened risk for suicide.

Cancer

Cancer has consistently been shown to have an elevated risk of suicide that is greater than expected in the general population. In the meta-analytic study by Harris and Barraclough (1994), five studies of cancer cohorts totaling nearly 1 million participants collectively were reviewed. All countries that were represented exhibited comparable increased overall risk, ranging from 1.4 to 2.5 times, with an average of 1.8 times greater than expected.

Since that time, large cohort studies that linked national cancer and death registries (in some instances totaling more than a million patients) have examined suicide risk in patients with cancer. These studies, performed in Norway (Hem, Loge, Haldorsen, & Ekeberg, 2004), Sweden (Björkenstam, Edberg, Ayoubi, & Rosén, 2005), and Denmark (Yousaf, Christensen, Engholm, & Storm, 2005), have found elevated risk similar to that reported by Harris and Barraclough (2004). The risk of suicide ranged from 1.55 to 2.5 times greater than expected for men and from 1.35 to 2.9 for women. A multiple decade cohort study of one Japanese hospital also found similar results, despite a smaller sample size, with an overall increased suicide risk of 1.8 times greater than expected at 5 years after cancer diagnosis (Tanaka et al., 1999).

Three of the aforementioned studies reported that the increased risk of suicide was greatest within the 1st year of cancer diagnosis. Hem et al. (2004) noted a standardized mortality ratio (SMR) of 3.09 for male patients and 2.18 for female patients within 5 months of diagnosis. The rate then dropped to 2.4 and 1.68, respectively, at 11 months postdiagnosis. Yousaf et al. (2005) found that the increased risk for male patients was greatest within 3 months of diagnosis, whereas the greatest risk for female patients was at 3 to 12 months. The greatest increased risk of suicide in the study by Tanaka et al. (1999) was at 3 to 5 months following diagnosis. Closer examination found that seven of the eight suicides committed during that time were shortly after discharge from the hospital.

There have been efforts to investigate whether particular cancer sites are associated with a heightened risk of suicide. In Norway, the relative risk of suicide in male patients was highest in cancer of the respiratory organs, defined as the bronchus, trachea, and lungs, with an SMR of 4.08 (Hem et al., 2004). Although there was a significant drop in relative risk, cancers of the brain, lymphatic and hematopoietic tissue, and esophagus and stomach (with SMRs of 2.4, 2.2, and 2.15, respectively) also showed heightened risk of suicide beyond the overall risk of 1.55 SMR for men. For women in Norway, the relative risk was greatest for cancer of the buccal cavity and pharynx, with an SMR of 3.67. Women also showed a relative risk with cancer of the esophagus and stomach. The risk was 2.5 times greater than that expected and was again significantly greater than the overall SMR of 1.35 for women. In their discussion of increased suicide risk in relation to cancer site, Björkenstam et al. (2005) reported suicide rates across gender. They found the greatest rates in pancreatic cancer, followed by cancer of the esophagus, lungs, and biliary passages and liver.

In Norway (Hem et al., 2004) and Sweden (Björkenstam et al., 2005), researchers found that the overall elevated risk of suicide in patients with cancer decreased over the decades since the 1960s. Although the Denmark SMRs did not show the same effect from the 1970s to the 1990s, the researchers (Yousaf et al., 2005) suggest that the SMR increase across decades in Denmark is due to initially elevated general Danish population suicide rates. Across studies, researchers suggest that the decrease in overall suicide rate is likely due to improvements in both medical understanding and treatment of the disease, as well as to mental health awareness, access to resources, and treatment of other risk factors.

Despite a decrease in recent decades, cancer continues to pose an elevated risk of suicide for patients, with some standardized mortality ratios still suggesting a two- to threefold increased risk over that in the general population. Research consistently shows that the greatest risk of suicide is sometime within the 1st year of diagnosis, with preliminary data suggesting that the time following hospital discharge might be a vulnerable period.

End-Stage Renal Disease

Depression is a frequent mental health complication of end-stage renal disease (ESRD). As Levy (2000) pointed out, depression in patients undergoing renal dialysis may be associated with the many losses and stresses that accompany the disease. Most patients with ESRD are unable to return to work. As a result, they may have a loss of income and a loss of the self-esteem that they derived from employment. They are dependent on a machine and tied to a dialysis routine that can become tedious. There can be a loss of a sense of freedom and a loss of sexual function. Their life expectancy is diminished. Under such conditions, it should come as no surprise that suicidality can become an issue.

Kurella, Kimmel, Young, and Chertow (2005) conducted a large study in which all patients who initiated dialysis from 1995 to 2000 and who were registered in the United States Renal Data System (USRDS), a total of 465,563 people, were linked to the ESRD Death Notification Form and to the national suicide data maintained by the Centers for Disease Control and Prevention. The ESRD Death Notification Form allows for a distinction between those who decided to withdraw from dialysis before death and those who committed suicide. Using this distinction, the investigators nonetheless found a Suicide Incidence Ratio of 1.84, indicating that patients with ESRD had a rate of suicide 84% greater than the general U.S. population rate, even after accounting for demographic differences between the ESRD and general populations.

In the study by Kurella et al. (2005), the rates of suicide among patients with ESRD tended to increase with age, with older people (> 60 years of age) having the highest rates. Such was not the case, however, with patients who had received a kidney transplant. In this regard, Ojo et al. (2000) used transplant registration data from the United Network for Organ Sharing and from USRDS from 1988 to 1997. The sample consisted of 86,502 kidney transplant patients who had retained graft functioning. The investigators obtained cause of death information from a transplant recipient follow-up form and from the ESRD Death Notification Form. They found an elevated rate of suicide among transplant patients (15.7 per 100,000 persons a year) relative to the general population rate (9 per 100,000 persons a year); 35% of the suicides, however, occurred in the first 12 months posttransplant, and the median time from transplantation to suicide was 16 months. In a population that had a mean age of 39 years at the time of transplantation, this finding seems to imply a higher risk of suicide at a younger age than that found with patients undergoing dialysis in the Kurella et al. study. The reasons for this apparent age difference between dialysis patients who commit suicide and transplant patients who commit suicide is as yet undetermined.

There is an increased risk of suicide among patients with a number of neurological disorders (Arciniegas & Anderson, 2002). Many factors (e.g., associated depression, anxiety, cognitive impairment, loss of function, pain) are thought to contribute to this increased risk. In this section we present the neurological disorders for which there is evidence of a heightened risk of suicide.

Epilepsy. It has long been recognized that there is a high incidence of depression among patients with epilepsy (Baker, 2006; Schmitz, 2005). Clinical observations and small studies have also suggested that there is a heightened risk of suicide. Recently, a meta-analytic review of 29 studies involving over 50,000 patients with epilepsy seems to have confirmed that there is an elevated risk (Pompili, Girardi, Ruberto, & Tatarelli, 2005; Pompili, Girardi, & Tatarelli, 2006). In this review, most of the 29 cohorts indicated that suicide in patients with epilepsy was more frequent (and in some studies many times more frequent) than suicide in the general population. Only three of the cohorts had lower suicide rates than the general population.

In a case control study by Nilsson, Ahlbom, Farahmand, Asberg, and Tomson (2002), onset of epilepsy at an early age was found to be strongly associated with an increased risk of suicide. The relative risk was 16 times greater for onset at age 18 or younger compared with onset after age 29, and early onset of epilepsy has been associated with depression and perceived stigma.

A meta-analytic review of 11 studies of suicide after surgical treatment to reduce seizure frequency revealed that suicide in surgically treated patients with epilepsy was more frequent than suicide in the general population (Pompili, Girardi, Tatarelli, Angeletti, & Tatarelli, 2006). The study by Blumer et al. (2002) of over 10,000 patients treated at an epilepsy center in Memphis found five suicides, and all had a history of early onset (mean age = 9.5 years) of longstanding complex partial seizures with very high seizure frequency. Ironically, all committed suicide within a range of 3 months to 3 years after they had obtained full control of seizures for the first time by either temporal lobectomy ($n = 3$), medication ($n = 1$), or vagus nerve stimulation ($n = 1$). All also had symptoms of an interictal dysphoria or depression.

Traumatic Brain Injury. Studies have found a heightened risk of psychiatric disorders (e.g., major depression, panic disorder, obsessive–compulsive disorder, substance abuse), as well as an increased risk of suicidal ideation and suicide attempts, following a traumatic brain injury (Silver, Kramer, Greenwald, & Weissman, 2001; Simpson & Tate, 2002, 2005). Although there were occasional patients in these samples who had a preinjury suicide attempt, the vast majority of suicide attempts occurred postinjury. Moreover, in the study by Silver et al. (2001), the risk of suicide attempt remained elevated after adjusting for demographics and alcohol abuse.

In a large study in Denmark, Teasdale and Engberg (2001b) selected patients on a national register of hospital admissions from 1979 to 1993 for three types of traumatic brain injuries: concussion (n = 126,114), cranial fracture (n = 7560), and cerebral contusion or traumatic intracranial hemorrhage (n = 11,766). They then screened these patients in a national register of deaths for the same period. SMRs, stratified by sex and age, showed that the incidence of completed suicide was increased for all three groups relative to the general population (SMRs equaled 3.0, 2.7, and 4.1, respectively). Furthermore, regression analyses for proportional hazards showed a significantly greater risk of suicide among those with more serious brain injury such as cerebral contusions or intracranial hemorrhages, relative to those with concussions or cranial fractures. It is interesting that there was also an increased rate of suicide among patients with no more than a concussion or a cranial fracture with no known cerebral lesion.

The authors suggested that the greater suicide risk among the more serious cases might be attributed to concomitant risk factors such as the development of psychiatric conditions or the physical, psychological, and social consequences of the injuries. The presence of a codiagnosis of substance abuse was associated with increased suicide rates in all three diagnostic groups. Interestingly, the mortality rates were greater for female patients than for male patients, although the reverse is true in the general population.

Stroke. Studies in Denmark have suggested that there is an elevated risk of suicide in patients who have a stroke. Stenager, Madsen, Stenager, and Boldsen (1998) did a linkage study with stroke patients in a single county of Denmark. They found that SMRs were markedly increased for suicide, particularly among relatively younger patients (< 60 years of age), and among women. Likewise, Bronnum-Hansen, Davidsen, and Thorvalsen (2001) studied causes of death after a first stroke in Copenhagen County from 1982 to 1991. Although the major cause of death was cardiovascular disease, there were other causes of death with elevated risk, including suicide.

Teasdale and Engberg (2001a) attempted to replicate the findings of Stenager et al. (1998) using a full national cohort of stroke patients in Denmark. Their sample consisted of 114,098 patients identified in the computerized National Bureau of Health's Register of Hospitalization during the years 1979 to 1993. The overall annual incidence rate of suicide in the cohort was 83 per 100,000 persons a year, compared with an expected figure of 45 per 100,000 persons a year. Across all age groups, the SMR for men was 1.88 and for women, 1.78. SMRs were greatest (2.85) for patients under age 50, and least (1.30) for patients 80 or older. Survival analysis suggested that the suicide risk was greatest during the first 5 years after stroke.

As Teasdale and Engberg (2001a) and L. Williams (2005) pointed out, poststroke depression is widely recognized. As with epilepsy and traumatic brain injury, depression and other neuropsychiatric sequelae of stroke may be contributing to the heightened risk of suicide.

Multiple Sclerosis. According to meta-analytic studies done 12 to 15 years ago (Harris & Barraclough, 1994; Stenager & Stenager, 1992), patients with multiple sclerosis (MS) appeared to have a suicide rate twice that of the general population rate. This finding has been confirmed in more recent record linkage studies in Denmark and Sweden. Thus, Bronnum-Hansen, Stenager, Stenager, and Koch-Henriksen (2005) linked the Danish Multiple Sclerosis Registry, consisting of more than 10,000 patients and the Cause of Death Registry over the period from 1953 to 1996. They found that the SMR for suicide indicated that the risk for patients with MS was more than twice that for the general population (SMR = 2.12). The increased risk was particularly high in the 1st year after diagnosis (SMR = 3.15). Although risk was greatest in the 1st year, it also remained elevated (relative to the general population) more than 20 years after diagnosis.

In the study by Fredrikson, Cheng, Jiang, and Wasserman (2003), the 12,284 cases of MS in the Swedish Hospital Inpatient Register during the period 1969 to 1996 were linked with the Swedish Cause of Death Register. Suicide risk for patients with MS was again found to be more than twice that in the general population (SMR = 2.3). As in the Danish study, suicide risk was found to be particularly high in the 1st year after diagnosis. In this study, however, a gender difference was noted; the elevation in risk seemed to be greatest in young men (below age 40), but for women, the risk was greatest for those between ages 30 and 59.

Studies have repeatedly found high rates of depression in patients with MS, with lifetime prevalence estimated in the range of 40% to 60% (Caine & Schwid, 2002; Goldman Consensus Group, 2005; Siegert & Abernathy, 2005; Wallin, Wilken, Turner, Williams, & Kane, 2006; R. Williams et al., 2005). A number of factors (e.g., negative psychosocial effects of MS disability, direct effect of lesions on brain structures that regulate mood, immune system dysfunction found in MS) may be involved in the increased incidence of depression. It has also been suspected that depression and suicidality might be a side effect of some of the disease modifying treatments (e.g., interferon-B) that have been used in the past decade to delay the progression of the disease. Studies to date, however, have not provided clear evidence to support such a conclusion (Feinstein, 2000; Goeb et al., 2006; Patten & Metz, 2002).

Depression is the mental and emotional disorder with the highest associated rate of suicide, and it frequently goes undetected in patients with MS (Caine & Schwid, 2002; Goldman Consensus Group, 2005). Practitioners need to be alert to depression and potential suicide risk in patients with MS, and they need to treat it adequately. It should be noted, however, that not all suicides among individuals with MS occur in the context of a depressive episode or disorder. Other factors (e.g., decreased quality of life, decreased ability to participate in meaningful activity, loss of self-determination and control) have also been implicated (R. Williams et al., 2005).

Huntington's Disease. Huntington's disease (HD) is a disorder involving degeneration of nerve cells in the brain. There is progressive loss of mental function including personality change, loss of cognitive ability such as speech and judgment, and neuropsychiatric symptoms (Paulsen, Ready, Hamilton, Mega, & Cummings, 2005). Abnormal facial and body movements are experienced, including rapid jerking movements. An association between mental illness and increased risk for suicide with the diagnosis of HD was recognized as early as 1872 (Huntington, 1872).

More recently, suicidal ideation was investigated in 4,171 individuals in the Huntington Study Group database (Paulsen, Nehl, et al., 2005). Similar to previous research, findings highlighted high rates of depressive symptoms in individuals with HD. More than 40% of patients endorsed having current depressive symptoms, and more than 10% had made a suicide attempt. Findings supported the notion that there are two critical periods for increased risk of suicidal behavior in HD. The first critical period is just before receiving a formal diagnosis, and the second is in Stage 2 of the disease, when independent functioning diminishes. Results showed that 19.8% of at-risk persons with soft neurological signs had suicidal ideation, whereas 23.5% of persons with possible HD had suicidal ideation. In persons who had been formally diagnosed with HD, 16.7% had suicidal ideation in Stage 1 (early stage), and 21.6% had suicidal ideation in Stage 2. The proportion of individuals with suicidal ideation diminished in subsequent stages.

The occurrence of completed suicide in HD has been estimated to be 4 to 5 times that of the general population rate (Farrer, 1986). DiMaio et al. (1993) studied suicide risk in the families of 2,793 individuals who were registered with the National Huntington's Disease Roster. On the basis of 205 (7.3%) identified suicide events, it was clear that suicide rates were higher than in the general population. Sorensen and Fenger (1992) reviewed the etiology of death among 395 Danish people with HD and among 282 of their unaffected siblings. They compared the findings with the suicide rate in the general Danish population. Suicide accounted for 5.6% of deaths among the individuals with HD and 5.3% of deaths among their unaffected siblings. Both occurrences of suicide were significantly higher than the general Danish population rate of 2.7%. In two other studies, Saugstad and Odegard (1986) and Schoenfeld et al. (1984) found completed suicide in HD to be rare, but the risk was increased for ages over 50.

Spinal Cord Injury/Disorder. People with spinal cord injury/disorder (SCI/D) are more vulnerable to life-threatening illnesses such as pneumonia, septicemia, cutaneous and bladder cancer, pulmonary emboli, and stroke. According to mortality studies of people with SCI/D (Imai, Kadowaki, & Aizawa, 2004; Soden et al., 2000), over the past 2 decades there has been a reduction in deaths resulting from these life-threatening illnesses. The result has been an increased life expectancy that approaches 70% of normal for those with complete quadriplegia and 86% of normal for those with complete paraplegia. The death rate by suicide among patients with SCI/D, however, has trebled from an SMR of 2.5 before 1980 to an SMR of 8.7 since 1980 (Soden et al., 2000). As noted earlier in regard to HIV/AIDS, as duration of survival has increased, the likelihood of suicide has also increased.

Harris and Barraclough (1994) and Stenager and Stenager (1992) pointed out that a heightened rate of mood disorders and substance abuse disorders in the SCI/D population may, in part, account for the heightened risk of suicide. Thus, alcohol or drug intoxication is often involved in the accidents that result in spinal cord injuries, and suicide attempts by those who are depressed or abusing substances are, at times, the cause of SCI/D. Estimates of the proportion of spinal cord injuries that result from suicide attempts have been modest (i.e., in the range of 1.5%–3.0%; Harris, Barraclough, Grundy, Bamford, & Inskip, 1996; Kennedy, Rogers, Speer, & Frankel, 1999; Pickett, Simpson, Walker, & Brison, 2003). Charlifue and Gerhart (1991) found that approximately 7% of patients with SCI/D who committed suicide had sustained their SCI/D in a prior suicide attempt.

Findings about a relationship between functional levels of impairment (e.g., complete quadriplegia, incomplete quadriplegia, complete paraplegia) and suicide risk have been inconsistent (e.g., see Hartkopp, Bronnum-Hansen, Seidenschnur, & Biering-Sorensen, 1998; Lidal et al., 2007; Soden et al., 2000). Suicide risk among patients with SCI/D in general, however, appears to be greatest in the first 4 to 5 years after the injury (Charlifue & Gerhart, 1991; DeVivo, Black, Richards, & Stover, 1991). Thus, Charlifue and Gerhart (1991), found in a study of 5,200 individuals with SCI/D covering a 30-year period that of those who died by suicide, 50% did so within 3 years of onset of SCI/D and 76% did so within 4 years. These investigators also found that factors that distinguished suicides from matched nonsuicidal people with SCI/D included (a) postinjury despondency; (b) experiences of shame, apathy, and helplessness; and (c) preinjury family fragmentation.

Depression as a Risk Factor for Suicide in Individuals With Medical Illness

As noted earlier, many medical illnesses that have a heightened risk of suicide also have a heightened rate of depression. In fact, a large body of evidence demonstrates that depression is highly comorbid with specific medical illnesses (Cassem, 1995; Harrington, 2002; Iosifescu, 2007). As Harrington (2002) noted, depression is second only to hypertension as the most common diagnosis in primary care populations. Depression and medical comorbidity has been associated with high use of medical services, unexplained symptoms, increased functional disability, diminished quality of life, and increased morbidity and mortality (Harrington, 2002; Iosifescu, 2007).

It is now generally accepted that the great majority of individuals who commit suicide (an estimated 93% of adult cases) have a major psychiatric disorder (Clark & Fawcett, 1992). As noted previously, depression is the mental disorder most frequently associated with suicide. Thus, an estimated 50% of suicides have depression at the time of death (Pokorny, 1983; Rich, Young, & Fowler, 1986). If serious medical illness is frequently associated with depression, it seems highly probable that there is a heightened risk of suicide among those with comorbid depression and physical illness.

Despite findings such as these, medical staff often fail to detect depression in individuals who are medically ill or view it as appropriate to the patient's condition (Cassem, 1995; Harrington, 2002). Therefore, depression, which is an important risk factor for suicide, is frequently underdiagnosed and undertreated in those with medical illness. Part of the problem may be that the diagnosis of depression is made difficult by the fact that the vegetative symptoms of depression (e.g., loss of appetite, decreased energy) may be caused by the physical disease itself. Moreover, there is difficulty in distinguishing depression and demoralization (or the so-called giving-up syndrome) in those with serious medical illness. Mangelli et al. (2005) have proposed criteria for demoralization and have attempted to clarify how it might be differentiated from clinical depression. They have, for example, pointed out that although a depressed person is incapable of experiencing enjoyment of any sort, a demoralized person can still experience pleasure in certain activities.

Just as the symptoms of depression can overlap with the symptoms of a particular medical disease, so too demoralization and depression can overlap, which makes the diagnosis of depression still more difficult. Nonetheless, given the current state of underdiagnosis and undertreatment of depression, Harrington (2002) recommended having a relatively low threshold, or erring on the side of overinclusion, in the diagnosis and treatment of depression in individuals who are medically ill. His point is underscored when one considers the elevated risk of suicide in this population.

Suicide and Patients With Terminal Illness

In terms of medical illnesses, one might think that illnesses that are in a terminal phase would be the most likely to engender despair and would be found frequently among those who commit suicide. To the contrary, the major psychological autopsy studies conducted over the past 40 years indicate that a rather small percentage of suicide victims (approximately 2%–3%) had a terminal illness at the time of death (Clark & Horton-Deutsch, 1992). Some, however, would argue that this estimate is low given that some suicides among the individuals with terminal illness may be reported to the coroner as deaths caused by their physical illness (Quill, 1991). Jamison (1996), in fact, reported that in his investigation of assisted suicides, the great majority of them

(125 of 140) were recorded as deaths due to natural causes. Be this as it may, it seems unlikely that a large percentage of suicides have a terminal illness.

Perhaps the most significant data on suicide among individuals who are terminally ill can be found in the state of Oregon, where the 1995 voter-approved ODDA (1995) permits physician-assisted suicide for competent persons with terminal illness who voluntarily request it.[1] The ODDA was blocked by a court injunction for 3 years, so it has only been in continuous use since 1998. During the first 9 years of Oregon's law (1998–2006), 292 Oregonians used it to die an assisted death (Oregon Department of Human Services, 2007). Thus, on average, 32 patients with terminal illness per year chose to end their lives under the ODDA. Because Oregon has an average of 31,000 deaths annually, these assisted deaths reflect a very small percentage of the total.

Of those who used the law, 97% were European American and 2% were recorded as Asian American. A few more men (54%) than women (46%) have used the act. The median age has been 70, with an age range of 25 to 96; 58% were in the age range of 65 to 84. Of those who used the ODDA, 46% were married, 25% divorced, 22% widowed, and 8% never married. Those who exercised their right under the law tended to be more highly educated (i.e., 41% had baccalaureate degrees or higher) compared with others in Oregon who died of the same diseases and in the same years (i.e., only 15% had baccalaureate degrees or higher).

Participants have been most likely to have cancer (80%), and cancer of the lung and bronchus has been the most frequent location (20% of those with cancer). Another 9% of the patients had breast cancer and 8% had pancreatic cancer. Of the total number of participants, 8% had amyotrophic lateral sclerosis, 4% had chronic lower respiratory disease, and 2% had HIV/AIDS. Ninety-four percent of the patients died at home, with 87% of them enrolled in hospice. Only 2% did not have health insurance. The median duration of their patient–physician relationship was 12 weeks.

The most frequently mentioned end-of-life concerns were loss of autonomy (86%), decreasing ability to participate in activities that made life enjoyable (85%), loss of dignity (82%), and loss of control of bodily functions (57%). Only 22% mentioned inadequate pain control or concern about it. Under the ODDA, if the patient's judgment is considered impaired by a psychiatric or psychological disorder, the patient must be referred for a psychological examination. Only 13% of patients have been referred for a psychiatric or psychological evaluation.

It should be noted that the report of the Oregon Department of Human Services on the ODDA has not been without its critics. Foley and Hendin (1999) contended that because the ODDA does not require a psychiatric

---

[1]Of note, under the Oregon Death with Dignity Act (1995), ending one's life in accordance with the law is not considered to constitute suicide (Oregon Department of Human Services, 2007).

evaluation for all those who request assisted death, it is possible the report does not have accurate information on the degree to which depression might have impaired the judgment of those making requests. They also argued that the report is based solely on information obtained from physicians and provided no data on how thoroughly physicians assessed the reasons for patients' requests.

The arguments for and against assisted death for the competent, patient with terminal illness who requests it have been discussed at length by Kleespies (2004) and by Rosenfeld (2004), and it is beyond the scope of this chapter to repeat them here. One concern of opponents, however, has not been particularly supported by the Oregon data. Thus, it has been argued that the legitimization of assisted death will put us on a slippery slope whereby it will be too easy for the less scrupulous to coerce vulnerable people, who are lacking in resources, to accept it. The Oregon data suggest that those who have sought an assisted death have actually been people who are relatively well educated and who had health insurance and access to hospice services.

CONCLUSION

Depression has been noted to be a likely contributing factor to suicide in many of the higher risk medical illnesses. Practitioners clearly need to be alert to the fact that depression among individuals who are medically ill constitutes a risk factor for suicide. They should also be aware of the emerging evidence that physical illness itself may have an independent association with suicidal behavior and suicide, particularly when the patient has multiple physical illnesses. It is also noteworthy that with certain physical illnesses and conditions (e.g., cancer, kidney transplant, surgically treated epilepsy, stroke, multiple sclerosis, SCI/D), the risk of suicide seems to be greatest early in the course of the disease or condition. Thus, the clinician should regard the first few months and years following the onset of these illnesses or conditions as a higher risk period for suicide. Mental health clinicians who work in medical settings or with consultation–liaison teams are well positioned to heighten awareness of and evaluate for the potential emergence of a suicidal state in these patients.

REFERENCES

Arciniegas, D., & Anderson, C. A., (2002). Suicide in neurologic illness. *Current Treatment Options in Neurology, 4*, 457–468.

Baker, G. (2006). Depression and suicide in adolescents with epilepsy. *Neurology, 66*(Suppl. 3), 5–12.

Björkenstam, C., Edberg, A., Ayoubi, S., & Rosén, M. (2005). Are cancer patients at higher suicide risk than the general population? *Scandinavian Journal of Public Health, 33,* 208–214.

Blumer, D., Montouris, G., Davies, K., Wyler, A., Phillips, B., & Hermann, B. (2002). Suicide in epilepsy: Psychopathology, pathogenesis, and prevention. *Epilepsy & Behavior, 3,* 232–241.

Bronnum-Hansen, H., Davidsen, M., & Thorvaldsen, P. (2001). Long-term survival and causes of death after stroke. *Stroke, 32,* 2131–2136.

Bronnum-Hansen, H., Stenager, E., Stenager, E. N., & Koch-Henriksen, N. (2005). Suicide among Danes with multiple sclerosis. *Journal of Neurology, Neurosurgery, and Psychiatry, 76,* 1457–1459.

Caine, E., & Schwid, S. (2002). Multiple sclerosis, depression, and the risk of suicide. *Neurology, 59,* 662–663.

Cassem, E. (1995). Depressive disorders in the medically ill: An overview. *Psychosomatics, 36,* S2–S10.

Charlifue, S., & Gerhart, K. (1991). Behavioral and demographic predictors of suicide after traumatic spinal cord injury. *Archives of Physical Medicine and Rehabilitation, 72,* 488–492.

Clark, D., & Fawcett, J. (1992). Review of empirical risk factors for evaluation of the suicidal patient. In B. Bongar (Ed.), *Suicide: Guidelines for assessment, management, and treatment* (pp. 16–48). New York: Oxford University Press.

Clark, D., & Horton-Deutsch, S. (1992). Assessment in absentia: The value of the psychological autopsy method for studying antecedents of suicide and predicting future suicide. In R. Maris, A. Berman, J. Maltsberger, & R. Yufit (Eds.), *Assessment and prediction of suicide* (pp. 144–182). New York: Guilford Press.

DeVivo, M., Black, K., Richards, J. S., & Stover, S. (1991). Suicide following spinal cord injury. *Paraplegia, 29,* 620–627.

Di Maio, L., Squitieri, F., Napolitano, G., Campanella, G., Trofatter, J. A., & Conneally, P. M. (1993). Suicide risk in Huntington's disease. *Journal of Medical Genetics, 30,* 293–295.

Druss, B., & Pincus, H. (2000). Suicidal ideation and suicide attempts in general medical illnesses. *Archives of Internal Medicine, 160,* 1522–1526.

Farrer, L. A. (1986). Suicide and attempted suicide in Huntington disease: Implications for preclinical testing of persons at risks. *American Journal of Medical Genetics, 24,* 305–311.

Feinstein, A. (2000). Multiple sclerosis, disease modifying treatments and depression: A critical methodological review. *Multiple sclerosis, 6,* 343–348.

Foley, K., & Hendin, H. (1999). The Oregon report: Don't ask, don't tell. *The Hastings Center Report, 29*(3), 37–42.

Fredrikson, S., Cheng, Q., Jiang, G., & Wasserman, D. (2003). Elevated suicide risk among patients with multiple sclerosis in Sweden. *Neuroepidemiology, 22,* 146–52.

Goeb, J., Even, C., Nicolas, G., Gohier, B., Dubas, F., & Garre, J. (2006). Psychiatric side effects of interferon-B in multiple sclerosis. *Psychiatry, 21,* 186–193.

Goldman Consensus Group. (2005). The Goldman Consensus statement on depression in multiple sclerosis. *Multiple Sclerosis, 11*, 328–337.

Goodwin, R., Marusic, A., & Hoven, C. (2003). Suicide attempts in the United States: The role of physical illness. *Social Science & Medicine, 56*, 1783–1788.

Harrington, C. (2002). Depression in the medically ill. *Medicine & Health Rhode Island, 85*, 273–277.

Harris, E., & Barraclough, B. (1994). Suicide as an outcome for medical disorders. *Medicine Baltimore, 73*, 281–296.

Harris, E., Barraclough, B., Grundy, D., Bamford, E., & Inskip, H. (1996). Attempted suicide and completed suicide in traumatic spinal cord injury: Case reports. *Spinal Cord, 34*, 752–753.

Hartkopp, A., Bronnum-Hansen, H., Seidenschnur, A., & Biering-Sorensen, F. (1998). Suicide in a spinal cord injured population: Its relation to functional status. *Archives of Physical Medicine and Rehabilitation, 79*, 1356–1361.

Harwood, D., Hawton, K., Hope, T., Harriss, L., & Jacoby, R. (2006). Life problems and physical illness as risk factors for suicide in older people: A descriptive and case-control study. *Psychological Medicine, 36*, 1265–1274.

Hem, E., Loge, J. H., Haldorsen, T., & Ekeberg, Ø. (2004). Suicide risk in cancer patients from 1960 to 1999. *Journal of Clinical Oncology, 22*, 4209–4216.

Hughes, D., & Kleespies, P. (2001). Suicide in the medically ill. *Suicide and Life-Threatening Behavior, 31*(Suppl.), 48–59.

Huntington, G. (1872, April 13). On chorea. *The Medical and Surgical Reporter, 26*, 317–321.

Imai, K., Kadowaki, T., & Aizawa, Y. (2004). Standardized indices of mortality among persons with spinal cord injury: Accelerated aging process. *Industrial Health, 42*, 213–218.

Iosifescu, D. (2007). Treating depression in the medically ill. *Psychiatric Clinics of North America, 30*, 77–90.

Jamison, S. (1996). When drugs fail: Assisted deaths and not-so-lethal drugs. *Journal of Pharmaceutical Care and Pain and Symptom Control, 4*, 223–243.

Kennedy, P., Rogers, B., Speer, S., & Frankel, H. (1999). Spinal cord injuries and attempted suicide: A retrospective review. *Spinal Cord, 37*, 847–852.

Kleespies, P. M. (2004). *Life and death decisions: Psychological and ethical considerations in end-of-life care.* Washington, DC: American Psychological Association.

Kleespies, P. M., & Dettmer, E. (2000). An evidence-based approach to evaluating and managing suicidal emergencies. *Journal of Clinical Psychology, 56*, 1109–1130.

Kleespies, P. M., Hughes, D., & Gallacher, F. (2000). Suicide in the medically ill and terminally ill: Psychological and ethical considerations. *Journal of Clinical Psychology, 56*, 1153–1171.

Komiti, A., Judd, F., Grech, P., Mijch, A., Hoy, J., Lloyd, J., & Street, A. (2001). Suicidal behavior in people with HIV/AIDS: A review. *Australian and New Zealand Journal of Psychiatry, 35*, 747–757.

Krentz, H., Kliewer, G., & Gill, M. (2005). Changing mortality rates and causes of death for HIV-infected individuals living in Southern Alberta, Canada, from 1984 to 2003. *HIV Medicine, 6,* 99–106.

Kurella, M., Kimmel, P., Young, B., & Chertow, G. (2005). Suicide in the United States End-Stage Renal Disease Program. *Journal of the American Society of Nephrology, 16,* 774–781.

Levy, N. (2000). Psychiatric considerations in the primary medical care of the patient with renal failure. *Advances in Renal Replacement Therapy, 7,* 231–238.

Lidal, I., Snekkevik, H., Aamodt, G., Hjeltnes, N., Stanghelle, J., & Biering-Sorenson, F. (2007). Mortality after spinal cord injury in Norway. *Journal of Rehabilitation Medicine, 39,* 145–151.

Lu, T., Chang, H., Chen, L., Chu, M., Ou, N., & Jen, I. (2006). Changes in causes of death and associated conditions among persons with HIV/AIDS after the introduction of highly active antiretroviral therapy in Taiwan. *Journal of the Formosan Medical Association, 105,* 604–609.

Mackenzie, T., & Popkin, M. (1990). Medical illness and suicide. In S. Blumenthal & D. Kupfer (Eds.), *Suicide over the life cycle: Risk factors, assessment, and treatment of suicidal patients* (pp. 205–232). Washington, DC: American Psychiatric Press.

Mangelli, L., Fava, G., Grandi, S., Grassi, L., Ottolini, F. Porcelli, P., et al. (2005). Assessing demoralization and depression in the setting of medical disease. *Journal of Clinical Psychiatry, 66,* 391–394.

Nilsson, L., Ahlbom, A., Farahmand, B., Asberg, M., & Tomson, T. (2002). Risk factors for suicide in epilepsy: A case control study. *Epilepsia, 43,* 644–651.

Ojo, A., Hanson, J., Wolfe, R., Leichtman, A., Agodoa, L., & Port, F. (2000). Long-term survival in renal transplant recipients with graft function. *Kidney International, 57,* 307–313.

Oregon Death With Dignity Act of 1995. *Oregon Revised Statute* §§127.800-127.995 (1995).

Oregon Department of Human Services, Health Services. (2007). *Ninth annual report on Oregon's Death With Dignity Act.* Retrieved May 25, 2007, from http://www.oregon.gov/DHS/ph/pas/ar-index.shtml

Patten, S., & Metz, L. (2002). Interferon B1a and depression in secondary progressive MS: Data from the SECTRIMS Trial. *Neurology, 59,* 744–746.

Paulsen, J. S., Nehl, C., Hoth, K. F., Kanz, J. E., Benjamin, M., Conybeare, R., et al. (2005). Depression and stages of Huntington's disease. *The Journal of Neuropsychiatry and Clinical Neuroscience, 17,* 496–502.

Paulsen, J. S., Ready, R. E., Hamilton, J. M., Mega, M. S., & Cummings, J. L. (2005). Neuropsychiatric aspect of Huntington's disease. *Psychiatric News, 40,* 32.

Pickett, W., Simpson, K., Walker, J., & Brison, R. (2003). Traumatic spinal cord injury in Ontario, Canada. *The Journal of Trauma, Injury, Infection, and Critical Care, 55,* 1070–1076.

Pokorny, A. (1983). Prediction of suicide in psychiatric patients. *Archives of General Psychiatry, 40,* 249–259.

Pompili, M., Girardi, P., Ruberto, A., & Tatarelli, R. (2005). Suicide in the epilepsies: A meta-analytic investigation of 29 cohorts. *Epilepsy & Behavior, 7,* 305–310.

Pompili, M., Girardi, P., & Tatarelli, R. (2006). Death from suicide versus mortality from epilepsy in the epilepsies: A meta-analysis. *Epilepsy & Behavior, 9,* 641–648.

Pompili, M., Girardi, P., Tatarelli, G., Angeletti, G., & Tatarelli, R. (2006). Suicide after surgical treatment in patients with epilepsy: A meta-analytic investigation. *Psychological Reports, 98,* 323–338.

Quill, T. (1991). Death and dignity: A case of individualized decision making. *The New England Journal of Medicine, 324,* 691–694.

Rich, C., Young, D., & Fowler, R. (1986). San Diego suicide study: I. Young vs. old subjects. *Archives of General Psychiatry, 43,* 577–582.

Rosenfeld, B. (2004). *Assisted suicide and the right to die: The interface of social science, public policy, and medical ethics.* Washington, DC: American Psychological Association.

Ruzicka, L., Choi, C., & Sadkowsky, K. (2005). Medical disorders of suicides in Australia: Analysis using multiple-cause-of-death approach. *Social Science & Medicine, 61,* 333–341.

Saugstad, L., & Odegard, O. (1986). Huntington's chorea in Norway. *Psychological Medicine, 16,* 39–48.

Schmitz, B. (2005). Depression and mania in patients with epilepsy. *Epilepsia, 46*(Suppl. 4), 45–49.

Schoenfeld, M., Myers, R. H., Cupples, L. A., Berkman, B., Sax, D. S., & Clark, E. (1984). Increased rate of suicide among patients with Huntington's disease. *Journal of Neurology, Neurosurgery, and Psychiatry, 47,* 283–1287.

Siegert, R., & Abernathy, D. (2005). Depression in multiple sclerosis: A review. *Journal of Neurology, Neurosurgery, and Psychiatry, 76,* 469–475.

Silver, J., Kramer, R., Greenwald, S., & Weissman, M. (2001). The association between head injuries and psychiatric disorders: The findings from the New Haven NIMH Epidemiologic Catchment Area Study. *Brain Injury, 15,* 935–945.

Simpson, G., & Tate, R. (2002). Suicidality after traumatic brain injury: Demographic, injury and clinical correlates. *Psychological Medicine, 32,* 687–697.

Simpson, G., & Tate, R. (2005). Clinical features of suicide attempts after traumatic brain injury. *The Journal of Nervous and Mental Disease, 193,* 680–685.

Soden, R., Walsh, J., Middleton, J., Craven, M., Rutkowski, S., & Yeo, J. (2000). Causes of death after spinal cord injury. *Spinal Cord, 38,* 604–610.

Sorensen, S. A., & Fenger, K. (1992). Causes of death in patients with Huntington's disease and in unaffected first degree relatives. *Journal of Medical Genetics, 29,* 911–914.

Stenager, E. N., Madsen, C., Stenager, E., & Boldsen, J. (1998, April 18). Suicide in patients with stroke: Epidemiological study. *BMJ, 316,* 1206.

Stenager, E. N., & Stenager, E. (1992). Suicide and patients with neurologic diseases. *Archives of Neurology, 49,* 1296–1303.

Tanaka, H., Tsukuma, H., Masaoka, T., Ajiki, W., Koyama, T., Knioshita, N., et al. (1999). Suicide risk among cancer patients: Experience at one medical center in Japan, 1978–1994. *Japanese Journal of Cancer Research, 90,* 812–817.

Teasdale, T., & Engberg, A. (2001a). Suicide after a stroke: A population study. *Journal of Epidemiology and Community Health, 55,* 863–866.

Teasdale, T., & Engberg, A. (2001b). Suicide after traumatic brain injury: A population study. *Journal of Neurology, Neurosurgery, and Psychiatry, 71,* 436–440.

Wallin, M., Wilken, J., Turner, A., Williams, R., & Kane, R. (2006). Depression and multiple sclerosis: Review of a lethal combination. *Journal of Rehabilitation Research and Development, 43,* 45–62.

Whitlock, F. (1986). Suicide and physical illness. In A. Roy (Ed.), *Suicide* (pp. 151–170). Baltimore: Lippincott Williams & Wilkins.

Williams, L. (2005). Depression and stroke: Cause or consequence? *Seminars in Neurology, 25,* 396–409.

Williams, R., Turner, A., Hatzakis, M., Jr., Bowen, J., Rodriquez, A., & Haselkorn, J. (2005). Prevalence and correlates of depression among veterans with multiple sclerosis. *Neurology, 64,* 75–80.

Yousaf, U., Christensen, M. L., Engholm, G., & Storm, H. H. (2005). Suicides among Danish cancer patients 1971–1999. *British Journal of Cancer, 92,* 995–1000.

III

EVALUATION AND MANAGEMENT OF RISK OF VIOLENCE

6

ASSESSMENT AND MANAGEMENT OF ACUTE RISK OF VIOLENCE IN ADULT PATIENTS

DALE E. McNIEL

The assessment and management of risk of violence are core issues in behavioral emergencies. In emergencies, clinicians are expected to be able to assess whether intervention is needed to protect third parties from patients' violence, to assess when patients pose a sufficient level of risk to justify involuntary civil commitment, and to determine what interventions will be sufficient to safely treat patients on an outpatient basis. Adverse outcomes associated with carrying out these risk assessments can expose clinicians to malpractice liability. Most past research on assessing violence potential has focused on long-term or chronic risk, from months to years after the assessment. However, research has begun to address the correlates of acute or short-term risk of violence, that is, within the next few hours, days, or weeks. In this chapter I review the implications of this research for clinical assessment and management of acute risk of violence in adult patients. I consider demographic/personal history, clinical, situational, and clinician variables. Then, I discuss strategies for managing acute risk of violence. Finally, I discuss methods of risk analysis that integrate the risk assessment with planning for risk management.

DEMOGRAPHIC AND PERSONAL HISTORY VARIABLES

History of Violence

A history of violent behavior has consistently been shown to be the best single predictor of future violence (McNiel, Binder, & Greenfield, 1988; Monahan, 2006). It is helpful to assess how recently aggressive behavior has occurred because this may provide information about whether the patient is in an ongoing crisis in which violence is a manifestation. Evaluating whether anyone was harmed during past violent events may aid in assessing the severity of risk in the current situation. Assessing the frequency of past violence is useful because a disproportionate amount of violence is perpetrated by a small number of repeatedly violent individuals (Gardner, Lidz, Mulvey, & Shaw, 1996). It also is helpful to assess for patterns of escalation (e.g., in domestic violence situations), which may provide information about whether the individual is repeating a cycle of violence. It is relevant to consider whether particular symptoms were associated with past violence, the context in which previous violence occurred (e.g., in the community, in the home, in the hospital), whether it was planned or impulsive, any precipitants or immediate triggers to the previous violence, and what the patient's attitude is toward past and current violence and provocation. Seeking information both from the patient and from collateral sources is beneficial. An interview of the patient can include questions such as, "Have you ever hurt or harmed anyone?" and "Have you hurt or harmed anyone in the past month or so?" Preceding these questions by first asking whether the patient has been a victim of such behavior can both facilitate self-disclosure of previous violence and provide useful information about victimization. It is helpful to obtain records from previous health care providers and information from other collateral sources such as family, friends, or others who have been involved in the patient's coming to clinical attention.

Violent Threats and Fantasies

A history of violent threats or fantasies can be elicited with questions such as, "Have you ever tried or threatened to hurt or harm someone?"; "Have you tried or threatened to hurt or harm someone during the past month?"; and "Have you felt like hurting someone?" Issues to consider in evaluating the seriousness of the threat include how specific the threat is, the extent of planning, the availability of means to carry it out, and any preparations that have been made. Although the presence of threats or fantasies does increase the risk of violence (Grisso, Davis, Vesselinov, Appelbaum, & Monahan, 2000), some patients who make threats do not pose a risk of violence, and some patients who are at elevated risk of violence do not make threats (McNiel & Binder, 1989).

Age

Numerous studies have found that violence is most common among younger persons (cf. Klassen & O'Connor, 1994). However, violence is not exclusively exhibited by younger people, and associations between diagnosis and risk of violence appear to vary depending on age. Among elderly patients, there is an increased representation of cognitive disorders such as dementia among patients who become violent (Kalunian, Binder, & McNiel, 1990).

Gender

In general, males have been found to be much more likely to be violent than females (Monahan, 2006). Research suggests that gender-related differences in rates of violence are less pronounced among persons with mental disorders. Research with acute inpatients has found similar rates of aggression among male and female patients, although following release to the community, males patients tend to engage in more severe forms of violence than females (Krakowski & Czbor, 2004; Lam, McNiel, & Binder, 2000; Nicholls, Ogloff, & Douglas, 2004). In the community, female patients who become violent are more likely to target family members than are male patients (Robbins, Monahan, & Silver, 2003).

History of Victimization

A history of being a victim of child abuse or growing up in a violent home increases the risk of violent behavior later in life (cf. Rosenberg, Lu, Mueser, Jankowski, & Cournos, 2007). The risk of future violence is also increased by experiencing or witnessing violence after age 16 (Swanson et al., 2002).

Culture

Among persons with mental disorders, race or ethnicity has not been found to be strongly associated with risk of violent behavior when other correlates of violence such as diagnosis, social class, and so forth, are taken into account (Swanson, Holzer, Ganju, & Jono, 1990). However, culture may be relevant given that some subcultural groups (e.g., some gangs) perceive violence as acceptable.

Socioeconomic Status

Lower socioeconomic status is associated with increased risk of violence in the community (Swanson et al., 1990). However, among patients experiencing acute episodes of mental disorder, the predictive significance of socioeconomic status is attenuated (McNiel et al., 1988).

Intelligence

Lower intelligence has been correlated with crime in general (Hodgins, 1992), and mental retardation has been associated with aggressive behavior in institutionalized populations (Volavka, 2002).

CLINICAL VARIABLES

Diagnosis

Although the proportion of violence in society that is attributable to persons with severe mental disorders is small, there is considerable evidence that the presence of a major mental disorder increases the relative risk of violence (Fazel & Grann, 2006). However, data concerning the relationship between specific psychiatric diagnoses and violence are mixed. For example, some researchers have found a diagnosis of schizophrenia to be associated with higher rates of violence (Brennan, Mednick, & Hodgins, 2000; Wallace, Mullen, & Burgess, 2004); others have found the opposite association (Monahan et al., 2001; Quinsey, Harris, Rice, & Cormier, 2006). Multiple methodological and sampling issues likely affect these disparate findings. For example, many studies have included samples containing a mixture of acute and nonacute patients. Because common major mental disorders (e.g., schizophrenia, bipolar disorder) are episodic, their influence on violence risk may vary according to whether the patient is in an exacerbation of the disorder. Another issue concerns the comparison group: Compared with the general population without major mental disorder, persons with schizophrenia have been found to have an elevated risk of violence (Swanson et al., 1990). However, compared with a group of patients with a documented history of serious violence, current criminal charges, and a high rate of personality disorders incarcerated in a maximum security psychiatric hospital, persons with schizophrenia have been found to have a lower risk of violence (Quinsey et al., 2006).

Acute Schizophrenia, Mania, and Cognitive Disorders

Among acutely ill patients seen in a civil (i.e., nonforensic) context, diagnoses of schizophrenia-spectrum disorders, bipolar disorder, manic episode, and cognitive disorders are associated with elevated short-term risk of violence (McNiel, Gregory, Lam, Binder, & Sullivan, 2003; Tardiff, 2003).

Cognitive disorders associated with brain disease can result in violence. Head injuries have been linked to aggressive behavior (Monahan et al., 2001), as have lesions of the brain, particularly in the temporal lobe and orbitomedial part of the frontal lobe (Volavka, 2002). Cognitive disorders such as delirium and dementia have been associated with violence in psychiatric settings and have diverse causes, many of which can be successfully treated. The violence that is associated with impairment of the brain can be related to generalized dyscontrol or psychotic symptoms such as delusions.

Substance Use Disorders

Substance use disorders are associated with an elevated risk of community violence (Monahan et al., 2001), have an increased prevalence among persons with major mental disorders (Rach-Beisel, Scott, & Dixon, 1999), and substantially increase the risk of violence among the persons with severe mental disorders who have them as co-occurring disorders (Wallace et al., 2004). For example, Swanson (1994) analyzed data from a representative sample of 10,000 people and found that (a) 3.5% of the total sample had completed some type of violence during the previous year, (b) mental disorder alone was twice as prevalent in the violent participants as the nonviolent participants, and (c) substance abuse alone and comorbidly was 5 times as prevalent in the violent group as in the nonviolent group.

The mechanism of the association between substance abuse and community violence appears to be multifaceted. For instance, the disinhibiting effect of alcohol intoxication increases the risk of violence. The agitation, grandiosity, suspiciousness, and delusional beliefs that can accompany intoxication with methamphetamine, cocaine, and phenylcyclidine (i.e., PCP) may increase violence potential, as may the disorganization associated with inhalant intoxication and the irritability and disorganization associated with withdrawal delirium (e.g., from alcohol). Substance-related violence is associated with crimes committed to obtain the substance and with the violent subcultures involved with the commerce associated with drug distribution. In addition, substance abuse may indirectly increase the risk of violence by creating instability in social relationships, employment, finances, housing, and health.

Given the association between substance abuse and violence, it is important to inquire about substance abuse when evaluating a patient's risk of violence. In addition, it is important to observe for acute signs of intoxication or withdrawal. Although the specific syndrome varies according to the substance, common indicators of intoxication include incoordination, unsteady gait, slurred speech, flushed face, changes in pupil size, fluctuating level of consciousness, and disorientation. Common features of withdrawal include sweating, tremors, hypervigilance, anxiety, hallucinations, and elevated vital signs including pulse, blood pressure, and heart rate.

Personality Disorders

A variety of personality disorders have been associated with violent behavior, particularly antisocial personality disorder and less consistently, borderline personality disorder (cf. Moran et al., 2003; Widiger & Trull, 1994). Research has shown a strong association between *psychopathy* and risk of violence. Although not included in the *Diagnostic and Statistical Manual of Mental Disorders* (4th ed., text rev.; American Psychiatric Association, 2000), psychopathy refers to a subset of persons generally diagnosed with antisocial personality disorder who manifest traits assessed by the Psychopathy Checklist—Revised (PCL–R) or similar measures (Hare, 2003). These traits include (a) an interpersonal/affective dimension, manifest by *interpersonal* traits such as glibness or superficial charm, grandiose sense of self-worth, pathological lying, and conning or manipulative and *affective* traits such as lack of remorse or guilt, callousness or lack of empathy, shallow affect, and failure to accept responsibility for own actions and (b) a socially deviant lifestyle, manifest by an *impulsive* lifestyle, for example, a need for stimulation or proneness to boredom, parasitic lifestyle, lack of realistic, long-term goals, impulsivity, and irresponsibility, and *antisocial* traits such as early behavioral problems, poor behavioral controls, juvenile delinquency, revocation of conditional release, and criminal versatility.

People who score above the threshold for classification as a psychopath on the basis of the PCL–R are much more likely than others to show violence over the long term (Hare, 2003). In addition, persons who do not meet criteria for classification as psychopathic but have elevated psychopathic traits are more likely to show violent behavior over the next few months to years, in both forensic (i.e., criminal) and civil (i.e., noncriminal) samples.

Personality disorders appear to be more relevant to assessing long-term, chronic risk than short-term, acute risk of violence in emergency settings (McNiel, Gregory, et al., 2003). This is due in part to the difficulty in obtaining a valid personality disorder diagnosis of a patient who is in the midst of an acute symptomatic (i.e., Axis I) mental disorder, and the limited historical information that is often available in emergency settings (Elbogen, Huss, Tomkins, & Scalora, 2005). However, if sufficient information is available to substantiate a personality disorder, evidence of psychopathy is likely pertinent.

Symptoms

Acute Findings in the Mental Status Examination

There is considerable empirical support for the utility of symptoms as indicators of the short-term risk of violence (Doyle & Dolan, 2006; Linaker & Busch-Iversen, 1995; McNiel & Binder, 1994a; Ogloff & Daffern, 2006). In acutely decompensating patients evaluated at the time of hospital admission, mental status findings, including hostile–suspiciousness (i.e., hostility, suspiciousness, and uncooperativeness), agitation–excitement (i.e., tension and excitement), and thinking disturbance (i.e., conceptual disorganization, hallucinations, and unusual thought content) are associated with aggressive behavior during the next few hours or days.

Anger

An individual's propensity to experience anger and difficulty in controlling its expression represent important risk factors for violence (Doyle & Dolan, 2006; Novaco, 2003). For example, Skeem et al. (2006) found that among a group of high-risk outpatients, those with an increase in anger one week were significantly more likely to engage in serious violence the following week.

Aggressive Attributional Style

A cognitive style involving external hostile attributions, in which the individual responds to stressful events with perceptions of threat, suspiciousness, and hostility, has been associated with increased rates of aggression among psychiatric patients (Doyle & Dolan, 2006; McNiel, Eisner, & Binder, 2003). An extreme variant of this pattern has been described by Link and Stueve (1994), who reported that violence was more likely when individuals have "threat/control override" delusions, that is, psychotic symptoms that cause a person to feel personally threatened or involve the intrusion of thoughts that can override self-controls. Recent data from a large sample support that such beliefs predict violent behavior by male patients in the community (Teasdale, Silver, & Monahan, 2006). Clinically, it can be helpful to ask patients who are experiencing such thoughts what they would do if they came into contact with those they perceive as tormenting or persecuting them.

Command Hallucinations

Command hallucinations involving a voice that tells the patient to harm others increase the risk of violence (McNiel, Eisner, & Binder, 2000; Monahan et al., 2001). The co-occurrence of command hallucinations with associated delusions appears to increase the risk of violence (e.g., a patient who hears a voice telling him to kill his sister and who also has the delusional belief that his sister is the devil).

Conclusion

The association between symptoms and acute risk of violence underscores the importance of a thorough mental status examination in evaluating a patient's risk of violence. For instance, a patient may not threaten violence but may still have symptoms that increase the risk of violence (e.g., a patient who is guarded and paranoid). Similarly, symptoms of decreased orientation and memory raise the possibility of a cognitive disorder that may represent a reversible risk factor. More generally, the associations that research has identified between psychopathology and violence support the importance of careful diagnosis, including assessment of the history of present illness, medical and psychiatric history, and mental status examination.

Treatment Adherence

Treatment of psychopathology that is associated with risk of violence can reduce patients' risk of violence, and lack of adherence to treatment can increase the risk of violence in persons with mental disorders (Swartz et al., 1998).

SITUATIONAL VARIABLES

Even very aggressive patients are usually violent for only a small proportion of the time. A person with a propensity for violence is likely to actually display violent behavior in the context of certain situational precipitants.

Relationship With Potential Victims

Research suggests that more than half of the victims of violence by persons with mental disorders are family members (Monahan et al., 2001; Straznickas, McNiel, & Binder, 1993). Within the family, the person at greatest risk is the primary caregiver (e.g., the mother of a young adult patient with a chronic mental disorder or the spouse or adult child of an older adult with dementia and psychotic symptoms). Clinically, it can be useful to assess the extent of family conflict. For example, the identified patient may not be the only violent person in the family. It can be helpful to evaluate the topic of family conflict; for example, the conflict may pertain to caretaking relationships, to a chronic pattern of family communication, or to a repeating sequence of escalating interchanges (e.g., one spouse criticizes the other, who then gets drunk and becomes violent).

Availability of Potential Victims

The risk of violent behavior can be affected by the availability of and accessibility to potential victims. For instance, an individual with the same propensity for violence would have varying degrees of likelihood of carrying out the violence if the aggressive impulses were focused on a public figure, on a spouse with a restraining order who continued to initiate contact with the patient, or on people who wear black clothing.

Social Support

An individual's social network can increase or decrease the potential for violence, depending on the nature of the network. Estroff, Zimmer, Lachicotte, and Benoit (1994) reported that patients who were married made fewer threats than single patients, and that the risk of violence was reduced by having a mental health professional in the patient's social network. However, Steadman (1982) found that some social networks can actually increase an individual's risk of violence and act as instigators.

Availability of Firearms

The presence of a weapon increases the lethality potential in someone with a propensity for violence. Firearms are used in a majority of homicides in the United States (Bureau of Justice Statistics, 2002). Available data suggest that mental health clinicians can be inconsistent in their assessment of weapon possession (Carney, Allen, & Doebbling, 2002). A recent study compared 100 patients consecutively admitted after a hospital had incorporated routine firearms screening in the workup done at admission, with 100 patients consecutively admitted during an earlier interval when firearms screening had been done on an as-needed basis (McNiel, Weaver, & Hall, 2007). Whereas 1% of patients acknowledged having access to a firearm when screening had been done on an as-needed basis, under conditions of routine screening, 9% of patients reported owning or having access to a firearm. The findings suggest that a substantial proportion of hospitalized patients have access to firearms. Unless clinicians directly ask patients about firearms possession, this information may not come to the attention of professionals.

Homelessness

Compared with other people with mental disorders living in the same community, those who are homeless are proportionately more likely to be arrested for violent crimes or to receive psychiatric emergency services after exhibiting violent behavior (Martell, Rosner, & Harmon, 1995; McNiel & Binder, 2005; McNiel, Binder, & Robinson, 2005).

CLINICIAN VARIABLES

Decision Support Tools

Several instruments have been developed to assist clinical decision making by anchoring the risk assessment in data regarding variables shown by research to be associated with long-term or chronic risk of violence (e.g., Monahan et al., 2005; Quinsey et al., 2006). For example, the Classification of Violence Risk (i.e., COVR) is an interactive software program intended to estimate the risk that a patient on a psychiatric inpatient unit will be violent to others during the several months after discharge (Monahan et al.,

2005). Recently, decision support tools have been developed for assessing short-term, acute risk, including those that follow.

Historical, Clinical, Risk Management—20

The Historical, Clinical, Risk Management—20 (HCR–20) is a strategy for coding 20 variables that the authors concluded had support in the research literature as indicators of violence potential (Webster, Douglas, Eaves, & Hart, 1997). The measure includes 10 Historical items (i.e., previous violence, young age at first violent incident, relationship instability, employment problems, substance use problems, major mental illness, psychopathy, early maladjustment, personality disorder, and prior supervision failure), five Clinical items (i.e., lack of insight, negative attitudes, active symptoms of major mental illness, impulsivity, and unresponsive to treatment), and five Risk Management items (i.e., plans lack feasibility, exposure to destabilizers, lack of personal support, noncompliance with remediation attempts, and stress). The HCR–20, particularly the Historical scale, has been found to predict violence over the long term (Douglas, Ogloff, Nicholls, & Grant, 1999). Recent data support the predictive validity of the Clinical scale of the HCR–20 for short-term risk of violence among persons undergoing acute episodes of major mental disorder (McNiel, Gregory, et al., 2003; Ogloff & Daffern, 2006).

Violence Screening Checklist—Revised

The Violence Screening Checklist (VSC) was designed to screen for short-term risk of violence among patients who are acutely mentally ill admitted to short-term inpatient units (McNiel & Binder, 1994b). The current version of the measure, the Violence Screening Checklist—Revised (VSC–R), includes four items: (a) history of physical attacks and/or fear-inducing behavior during the 2 weeks before hospital admission, (b) absence of recent suicidal behavior (the item is checked if the patient has not shown recent suicidal behavior), (c) schizophrenic or manic diagnosis, and (d) male gender. Research has supported the predictive validity of the measure in patients who are acutely mentally ill, particularly within the first few days after hospital admission (McNiel, Gregory, et al., 2003; Nicholls, Ogloff, & Douglas, 2004).

Broset Violence Checklist

The Broset Violence Checklist (Linaker & Busch-Iversen, 1995) measures the presence or absence of six variables that are frequently observed before violent incidents on acute inpatient units: confusion, irritability, boisterousness, physical threats, verbal threats, and attacks on objects. The measure has been found to reliably indicate the risk of violence during the next 24-hour period for patients on acute psychiatric inpatient units (Almik, Woods, & Rasmussen, 2000).

Short-Term Assessment of Risk and Treatability

The Short-Term Assessment of Risk and Treatability (i.e., START) is a 20-item measure designed to guide the assessment and management of short-term risk of violence (as well as suicide, self-harm, self-neglect, substance abuse, unauthorized leave, and victimization; Webster, Martin, Brink, Nicholls, & Middleton, 2004). Items include social skills, relationships, occupational, recreational, self-care, mental state, emotional state, substance use, impulse control, external triggers, social support, material resources, attitudes, medication adherence, rule adherence, conduct, insight, plans, coping, and treatability. Ratings on the measure correlate with subsequent aggressive behavior in forensic psychiatric inpatients (Nicholls, Brink, Desmarais, Webster, & Martin, 2006).

Dynamic Appraisal of Situational Aggression

The Dynamic Appraisal of Situational Aggression (DYAS) was designed both to assess for acute risk of violence (within the next 24 hours) among inpatients and to assist in treatment planning to reduce the risk (Ogloff & Daffern, 2006). The instrument includes seven items: irritability, impulsivity, unwillingness to follow directions, sensitivity to perceived provocation, easily angered when requests denied, negative attitudes, and verbal threats. Ogloff and Daffern (2006) reported that scores on the DYAS predicted later aggression and that when nurses considered DYAS scores, their clinical risk assessments were more accurate than when made on an unstructured basis.

Therapeutic Alliance

The therapeutic alliance refers to the extent to which the patient is actively collaborating with treatment as a resource for change (Beauford, McNiel, & Binder, 1997). A positive therapeutic relationship may strengthen the clinician's ability to ask difficult questions and elicit information that a patient may be otherwise reluctant to disclose, such as active violent thoughts (Green, Pedley, & Whittingham, 2004). A positive therapeutic relationship can both encourage treatment adherence and assess for nonadherence, which can predict relapse of symptoms associated with violence potential. Among patients with a high base rate of violence (e.g., inpatients), those with a poor initial alliance are at elevated risk of violence (Beauford et al., 1997).

Cognitive Biases

Experimental research on human judgment suggests that people are prone to various cognitive biases when making decisions under conditions of uncertainty, such as neglecting base rate information, selectively attending to information that confirms one's initial assumptions, ignoring disconfirming evidence, judging an uncommon event as likely to occur because it is easily recalled, and so forth (Gilovich, Griffin, & Kahnemann, 2002). Research suggests that when evaluating patients' risk of violence, clinicians tend to overestimate the risk among non-Caucasian minority patients and underestimate the risk among female patients (McNiel & Binder, 1995; Skeem et al., 2005). Previous authors have proposed strategies that clinicians can use to counter such cognitive errors (Borum, Otto, & Golding, 1993). For instance, when assessing a female patient, the clinician would do well not to discount the individual's risk of violence solely on the basis of her gender.

Consultation

In clinical situations in which the decisions have a high potential for adverse consequences or the clinician has limited confidence in the accuracy of his or her evaluation of violence risk, consultation with colleagues can be useful. Some research has indicated that risk assessments in which two clinicians concur have higher predictive validity than individual assessments, especially if there are discordant opinions (McNiel, Lam, & Binder, 2000). In addition, consultation has benefits from the standpoint of management of risk of liability. That is, if despite the clinician's best efforts an adverse outcome occurs and litigation ensues, the clinician will be held accountable to community standards of care. Documentation that consultation was obtained at the time of the clinical decision can support that the clinician's assessment is in accord with prevailing practices of other clinicians (for a more detailed discussion of legal issues in treating violent patients, see chap. 18, this volume).

RISK MANAGEMENT

Management of Acute Violence

Clinical issues associated with the evaluation of biological contributions to violence, and legal issues related to interventions to contain acute violence, call for a varied approach. Multidisciplinary teamwork including physician involvement is usually beneficial when managing acutely violent patients.

Precautions Before the Interview

It is desirable to consider safety in selecting the physical location of the interview, as interviewing a potentially violent patient in an office with the door closed may be unsafe. Alternatives include interviewing the patient in an office with the door open while staff waits outside or interviewing the patient with staff present. If the clinician determines that the risk is low enough to interview the patient in an office with the door closed, there should be a prearranged system for the clinician to communicate that he or she is in danger, such as with a panic button or a predetermined message to a receptionist. Similarly, it is desirable to have a person available outside the office to communicate to the clinician whether there is a dangerous situation before the patient enters the office.

In furnishing the office, the clinician needs to consider the types of patients who will be seen there. For example, pictures, chairs, professional equipment, or other small objects can be used as weapons. Similarly, when preparing to interview patients known to be at acutely elevated risk of violence, the clinician will benefit from attending to his or her own dress (e.g., remove neckties, remove jewelry such as necklaces and dangling earrings, remove eyeglasses).

Rapid Differential Diagnosis

It is desirable to immediately form an opinion about whether the patient has a cognitive disorder (e.g., delirium, dementia), a psychotic disorder, or a nonpsychotic, nonorganic disorder. If the patient has a severe cognitive disorder, verbal intervention is unlikely to be effective and diagnosis and treatment of the underlying medical condition are essential. If the patient is in an acute psychotic episode, verbal intervention will have limited benefit and rapid administration of medication is often most effective. If the patient is not psychotic or cognitively impaired, verbal intervention may be effective, although offering the option of medication may enhance the patient's sense of control (cf. Tardiff, 2003).

Verbal Intervention

In the acute setting, verbal intervention primarily involves limit setting. The clinician clearly points out the behavior that is unacceptable and maladaptive and explains why it is not acceptable. The clinician then explains the consequences that will occur if the behavior persists. It can be helpful to offer the patient choices when limits are set (e.g., "You can have a time-out in your room or the seclusion room," "You can take the medication by mouth or injection"). Safety can be enhanced if the clinician retains a calm appearance and speaks softly in a neutral, concrete, nonjudgmental, respectful, and nonprovocative manner. It can be helpful to avoid intense eye contact, to maintain space between the patient and clinician, to encourage the patient to talk, and not make promises that cannot be kept (see chap. 2 for additional discussion of these issues).

Pharmacological Intervention

The management of an emergency in which an agitated, threatening, and possibly psychotic patient poses an imminent risk of harming others may be facilitated by administration of medication, for example, an antipsychotic medication alone or in combination with a benzodiazepine such as lorazepam (Binder & McNiel, 1999; Citrome, 2007).

Seclusion and Restraint

In emergency situations, if less restrictive interventions have been determined to be ineffective seclusion and restraint may be used as a last resort to ensure physical safety (Centers for Medicare and Medicaid Services, 2006). There is widespread recognition of the desirability of minimizing the use of seclusion and restraint (Substance Abuse and Mental Health Administration, 2006).

Psychiatric Hospitalization

If a clinician concludes that a patient represents an imminent danger to others due to a mental disorder, psychiatric hospitalization is frequently needed. This may involve involuntary civil commitment in accordance with local statutes. Hospitalization accomplishes the purpose of containment of the acute risk of violence and can allow for a more thorough diagnostic evaluation and rapid initiation of treatment. If a patient's dangerousness is not due to a mental disorder the clinician may need to consider other dispositions, such as substance abuse treatment or involvement of the criminal justice system.

Increased Intensity of Treatment

Depending on the level of assessed risk and therapeutic alliance, intensification of treatment short of hospitalization may be sufficient. This may involve participation in a partial hospitalization or intensive outpatient treatment program, increasing the frequency of therapy sessions, increasing medication doses, and so on. Increasing the intensity of treatment also permits increased monitoring for signs of decompensation, adherence with medication, deteriorating social relationships, stressors, and relapse of substance abuse.

Substance Abuse Treatment

Given the association between substance use and community violence, for individuals with substance use problems, engagement in substance abuse treatment programs, motivational interventions, and related cognitive behavioral methods are indicated (Reilly & Shopshire, 2002).

Anger Management

For individuals with a chronic risk of violence, cognitive interventions such as anger management, relaxation training, cognitive restructuring directed toward altering suspiciousness and external hostile attributions, and helping patients avoid situations that are high risk for them as individuals may be of benefit (Reilly & Shopshire, 2002).

Strengthening the Therapeutic Alliance

Strengthening the therapeutic alliance may enhance treatment adherence. This may be facilitated by establishing a problem solving focus, clearly stating the clinician's responsibilities, demonstrating to the patient that what he or she says is heard and taken seriously, involving the patient and developing shared goals, discussing interests and acknowledging positive factors, having consistent regular contact and undertaking increased efforts to make contact (e.g., follow-up calls) as needed, and providing education about mental disorder and its treatment (Green et al., 2004).

Family Intervention

Family interventions may help reduce the risk of violence by patients with mental disorders. Family education about early warning signs of psychiatric decompensation may be helpful, as may referral to peer support groups such as the National Alliance for the Mentally Ill to learn coping strategies used by other families in responding to escalation. When a patient's violence potential is affected by difficulty in family communication or problem solving, family therapy may be helpful. The development of impulse delay procedures such as planned time-outs if conflicts escalate may be beneficial. The family can be educated about the safety benefits of removal of weapons from easy accessibility. In addition, the family can be educated about the role of the criminal justice system in managing violence. In domestic violence situations, it can also be helpful to develop individualized safety plans for persons at risk of victimization (e.g., access to support systems, shelters), referral to victim support groups, and education about decision making concerning orders of protection.

Duty-to-Protect

Throughout the treatment, clinicians must remain aware of their legal duty to protect potential identifiable victims. The *Tarasoff* decision (*Tarasoff v. Regents of the University of California*, 1974, 1976) and subsequent court decisions and legislation established in many jurisdictions that when a patient makes a serious threat of physical violence, the psychotherapist has a duty to protect the intended victim (McNiel, Binder, & Fulton, 1998). To determine whether a threat is serious, the clinician needs to undertake a risk assessment for violence. Although specific actions required of the therapist may be affected by jurisdiction, in many locations if a serious threat is present, the therapist may need to warn the potential victim and the police. Clinically, this process can be enhanced by informing the patient of the necessity of the warning prior to carrying it out (Binder & McNiel, 1996). Aside from warnings, interventions such as those previously listed may help protect the victim (see chapter 18, this volume, for a detailed discussion of duty-to-protect and other legal issues associated with managing behavioral emergencies).

INTEGRATION: RISK ANALYSIS

Multiple authors have proposed models for risk analysis concerning violence (e.g., Gutheil & Appelbaum, 2000; McNiel, Chamberlain, et al., 2007; Monahan, 1993; Tardiff, 2003). The process integrates risk assessment and risk management through four main steps:

1. The clinician gathers information about relevant risk factors and rationally weighs this information to form an evaluation of the level of risk.
2. Based on the risk assessment, the clinician develops an intervention plan to reduce the risk.
3. The clinician implements this plan.
4. The clinician documents the process. Although the extent of detail may vary according to the level of risk and complexity of the situation, documentation of the clinical reasoning in which the previous points were covered is beneficial.

In formulating the risk of violence, it is helpful to consider the extent to which the patient represents an acute or chronic risk of violence. Background, static, historical factors are pertinent to chronic, long-term risk of violence. Clinical, dynamic, and situational factors are especially relevant to acute, short-term violence potential. If the risk of violence is determined to be high and imminent, immediate action is required. If the risk is moderate and more chronic, increased supervision, monitoring, and intensification of treatment may suffice. If the risk is low, no special interventions may be needed. It is useful to consider that the risk of violence varies over time. Hence, reassessments are important for individuals determined to be at elevated risk. For example, if a patient is determined to be at elevated risk at the time of hospital admission, it will be important to reassess the patient's level of risk when discharge is considered.

CONCLUSION

Research has identified a variety of demographic/personal history, clinical, situational, and clinician variables that are relevant to assessing the acute risk of violence in adult patients. On the basis of analysis of how these variables influence a patient's risk, the clinician may select from an array of interventions for managing the risk of violence.

REFERENCES

Almik, R., Woods, P., & Rasmussen, K. (2000). The Broset Violence Checklist: Sensitivity, specificity, and interrater reliability. *Journal of Interpersonal Violence, 15,* 1284–1296.

American Psychiatric Association. (2000). *Diagnostic and statistical manual of mental disorders* (4th ed., text rev.). Washington, DC: Author.

Beauford, J. E., McNiel, D. E., & Binder, R. L. (1997). Utility of the therapeutic alliance in evaluating psychiatric patients' risk of violence. *American Journal of Psychiatry, 154,* 1272–1276.

Binder, R. L., & McNiel, D. E. (1996). Application of the *Tarasoff* ruling and its effect on the victim and the therapeutic relationship. *Psychiatric Services, 47,* 186–188.

Binder, R. L., & McNiel, D. E. (1999). Contemporary practices in managing acutely violent patients in 20 psychiatric emergency rooms. *Psychiatric Services, 50,* 1553–1554.

Borum, R., Otto, R., & Golding, S. (1993). Improving clinical judgment and decision making in forensic evaluation. *Journal of Psychiatry and the Law, 21,* 35–76.

Brennan, P. A., Mednick, S. A., & Hodgins, S. (2000). Major mental disorders and criminal violence in a Danish birth cohort. *Archives of General Psychiatry, 57,* 494–500.

Bureau of Justice Statistics. (2002). *Crime characteristics.* Washington, DC: U.S. Department of Justice.

Carney, D. P., Allen, J., & Doebbeling, R. N. (2002). Receipt of clinical preventive medical services among psychiatric patients. *Psychiatric Services, 53,* 1028–1030.

Centers for Medicare and Medicaid Services. (2006, December 8). Revised restraints regulations. *Federal Register, 71*(236, Part IV).

Citrome, L. (2007). The psychopharmacology of violence with emphasis on schizophrenia: I. Acute treatment. *Journal of Clinical Psychiatry, 68,* 163–164.

Douglas, K. S., Ogloff, J. P., Nicholls, T. L., & Grant, I. (1999). Assessing risk for violence among psychiatric patients: The HCR–20 violence risk assessment scheme and the Psychopathy Checklist: Screening Version. *Journal of Consulting and Clinical Psychology, 67,* 917–930.

Doyle, M., & Dolan, M. (2006). Evaluating the validity of anger regulation problems, interpersonal style, and disturbed mental state for predicting inpatient violence. *Behavioral Sciences & the Law, 24,* 783–798.

Elbogen, E. B., Huss, M. T., Tomkins, A. J., & Scalora, M. J. (2005). Clinical decision making about psychopathy and violence risk assessment in public sector mental health settings. *Psychological Services, 2,* 133–141.

Estroff, S. E., Zimmer, C., Lachicotte, W. S., & Benoit, J. (1994). The influence of social networks and social support on violence by persons with serious mental illness. *Hospital and Community Psychiatry, 45*, 669–679.

Fazel, S., & Grann, M. (2006). The population impact of severe mental illness on violent crime. *American Journal of Psychiatry, 163*, 1397–1403.

Gardner, W., Lidz, C., Mulvey, E. P., & Shaw, E. C. (1996). A comparison of actuarial methods for identifying repetitively violent patients with mental illness. *Law and Human Behavior, 20*, 35–48.

Gilovich, T., Griffin, D., & Kahnemann, D. (Eds.). (2002). *Heuristics and biases: The psychology of intuitive judgment.* Cambridge, England: Cambridge University Press.

Grisso, T., Davis, J., Vesselinov, R., Appelbaum, P., & Monahan, J. (2000). Violent thoughts and violent behavior following hospitalization for mental disorder. *Journal of Consulting and Clinical Psychology, 68*, 388–398.

Green, B., Pedley, R., & Whittingham, D. (2004). A structured clinical model for violence risk intervention. *International Journal of Law and Psychiatry, 27*, 349–359.

Gutheil, T. G., & Appelbaum, P. D. (2000). *Clinical handbook of psychiatry and the law* (3rd ed.). Philadelphia: Lippincott Williams & Wilkins.

Hare, R. D. (2003). *Manual for the Revised Psychopathy Checklist* (2nd ed.). Toronto, Ontario, Canada: Multi-Health Systems.

Hodgins, S. (1992). Mental disorder, intellectual deficiency, and crime: Evidence from a birth cohort. *Archives of General Psychiatry, 49*, 476–483.

Kalunian, D. A., Binder, R. L., & McNiel, D. E. (1990). Violence by geriatric patients who need psychiatric hospitalization. *Journal of Clinical Psychiatry, 51*, 340–343.

Klassen, D., & O'Connor, W. A. (1994). Demographic and case history variables in risk assessment. In J. Monahan & H. J. Steadman (Eds.), *Violence and mental disorder: Developments in risk assessment* (pp. 229–257). Chicago: University of Chicago Press.

Krakowski, M., & Czbor, P. (2004). Gender differences in violent behaviors: Relationship to clinical symptoms and psychosocial factors. *American Journal of Psychiatry, 161*, 459–465.

Lam, J. N., McNiel, D. E., & Binder, R. L. (2000). The relationship between patients' gender and violence leading to staff injuries. *Psychiatric Services, 51*, 1167–1170.

Linaker, O. M., & Busch-Iversen, H. (1995). Predictors of imminent violence in psychiatric inpatients. *Acta Psychiatrica Scandinavica, 92*, 250–254.

Link, B., & Stueve, A. (1994). Psychotic symptoms and the violent/illegal behavior of mental patients compared to community controls. In J. Monahan & H. J. Steadman (Eds.), *Violence and mental disorder: Developments in risk assessment* (pp. 137–159). Chicago: University of Chicago Press.

Martell, D. A., Rosner, R., & Harmon, R. B. (1995). Base rate estimates of criminal behavior by homeless mentally ill persons in New York City. *Psychiatric Services, 46*, 596–601.

McNiel, D. E., & Binder, R. L. (1989). Relationship between threats and later violent behavior by acute psychiatric inpatients. *Hospital and Community Psychiatry, 40*, 605–608.

McNiel, D. E., & Binder, R. L. (1994a). The relationship between acute psychiatric symptoms, diagnosis, and short-term risk of violence. *Hospital and Community Psychiatry, 45*, 133–137.

McNiel, D. E., & Binder, R. L. (1994b). Screening for risk of inpatient violence: Validation of an actuarial tool. *Law and Human Behavior, 18*, 579–586.

McNiel, D. E., & Binder, R. L. (1995). Correlates of accuracy in the assessment of psychiatric inpatients' risk of violence. *American Journal of Psychiatry, 152*, 901–906.

McNiel, D. E., & Binder, R. L. (2005). Psychiatric emergency service use associated with homelessness, mental disorder, and violence. *Psychiatric Services, 56*, 699–704.

McNiel, D. E., Binder, R. L., & Fulton, F. M. (1998). Management of threats of violence under California's "duty to protect" statute. *American Journal of Psychiatry, 155*, 1097–1101. (Correction published in 1998, *American Journal of Psychiatry, 155*, p. 1465)

McNiel, D. E., Binder, R. L., & Greenfield, T. K. (1988). Predictors of violence in civilly committed acute psychiatric patients. *American Journal of Psychiatry, 145*, 965–970.

McNiel, D. E., Binder, R. L., & Robinson, J. (2005). Incarceration associated with homelessness, mental disorder, and co-occurring substance abuse. *Psychiatric Services, 56*, 840–846.

McNiel, D. E., Chamberlain, J. R., Weaver, C. M., Hall, S. E., Fordwood, S. R., & Binder, R. L. (2007). Impact of clinical training on violence risk assessment. *American Journal of Psychiatry, 165*, 195–200.

McNiel, D. E., Eisner, J. P., & Binder, R. L. (2000). The relationship between command hallucinations and violence. *Psychiatric Services, 51*, 1288–1292.

McNiel, D. E., Eisner, J., & Binder, R. L. (2003). The relationship between aggressive attributional style and violence by psychiatric patients. *Journal of Consulting and Clinical Psychology, 71*, 399–403.

McNiel, D. E., Gregory, A. L., Lam, J. L., Binder, R. L., & Sullivan, G. R. (2003). Utility of decision support tools for assessing acute risk of violence. *Journal of Consulting and Clinical Psychology, 71*, 945–953.

McNiel, D. E., Lam, J. N., & Binder, R. L. (2000). Relevance of interrater agreement to violence risk assessment. *Journal of Consulting and Clinical Psychology, 68*, 1111–1115.

McNiel, D. E., Weaver, C. M., & Hall, S. E. (2007). Base rates of firearm possession by hospitalized patients. *Psychiatric Services, 58*, 551–553.

Monahan, J. (1993). Limiting therapist exposure to *Tarasoff* liability: Guidelines for risk containment. *American Psychologist, 48*, 242–250.

Monahan, J. (2006). A jurisprudence of risk assessment: Forecasting harm among prisoners, predators, and patients. *Virginia Law Review, 92*, 391–435.

Monahan, J., Steadman, H. J., Appelbaum, P. S., Grisso, T., Mulvey, E. P., Roth, L. H., et al. (2005). *The Classification of Violence Risk (COVR)* [Computer software]. Lutz, Florida: Psychological Assessment Resources.

Monahan, J., Steadman, H. J., Silver, E., Appelbaum, P. S., Robbins, P. C., Mulvey, E. P., et al. (2001). *Rethinking risk assessment: The MacArthur study of mental disorder and violence.* New York: Oxford University Press.

Moran, P., Walsh, E., Tryer, P., Burns, T., Creed, F., & Fahy, T. (2003). Impact of comorbid personality disorder on violence in psychosis: Report from the UK700 trial. *The British Journal of Psychiatry, 182,* 129–124.

Nicholls, T. L., Brink, J., Desmarais, S. L., Webster, C. D., & Martin, M. L. (2006). The Short-Term Assessment of Risk and Treatability (START): A prospective validation study in a forensic psychiatric sample. *Assessment, 13,* 313–327.

Nicholls, T. L., Ogloff, J. R. P., and Douglas, K. S. (2004). Assessing for violence among male and female civil psychiatric patients: The HCR–20, PCL:SV, and VSC. *Behavioral Sciences & the Law, 22,* 127–158.

Novaco, R. W. (2003). *The Novaco Anger Scale and Provocation Inventory (NAS/PI).* Los Angeles: Western Psychological Services.

Ogloff, J. R. P., & Daffern, M. (2006). The Dynamic Appraisal of Situational Aggression: An instrument to assess risk for imminent aggression in psychiatric inpatients. *Behavioral Sciences & the Law, 24,* 799–813.

Quinsey, V. L., Harris, G. T., Rice, M. E., & Cormier, C. A. (2006). *Violent offenders: Appraising and managing risk* (2nd ed.). Washington, DC: American Psychological Association.

Rach-Beisel, J., Scott, J. & Dixon, L. (1999). Co-occurring severe mental illness and substance use disorders: A review of recent research. *Psychiatric Services, 50,* 1427–1434.

Reilly, P. M., & Shopshire, M. S. (2002). *Anger management for substance abuse and mental health patients: A cognitive–behavioral therapy manual* (DHHS Pub. No. SMA 02-3756). Rockville, MD: Substance Abuse and Mental Health Services Administration.

Robbins, P. C., Monahan, J., & Silver, E. (2003). Mental disorder, violence, and gender. *Law and Human Behavior, 27,* 561–571.

Rosenberg, S. D., Lu, W., Mueser, K. T., Jankowski, M. K., & Cournos, F. (2007). Correlates of adverse childhood events among adults with schizophrenia spectrum disorders. *Psychiatric Services, 58,* 245–253.

Skeem, J. L., Schubert, C., Odgers, C., Mulvey, E. P., Gardner, W., & Lidz, C. (2006). Psychiatric symptoms and community violence among high-risk patients: A test of the relationship at the weekly level. *Journal of Consulting and Clinical Psychology, 74,* 967–979.

Skeem, J. L., Schubert C., Stowman, S., Benson, S., Mulvey, E., Gardner, W., & Lidz, C. (2005). Gender and risk assessment accuracy: Underestimating women's violence potential. *Law and Human Behavior, 29,* 173–186.

Steadman, H. J. (1982). A situational approach to violence. *International Journal of Law and Psychiatry, 5,* 171–186.

Straznickas, K. A., McNiel, D. E., & Binder, R. L. (1993). Violence toward family caregivers of the mentally ill. *Hospital and Community Psychiatry, 44,* 385–387.

Substance Abuse and Mental Health Service Administration (SAMSHA). (2006). *Roadmap to seclusion and restraint free mental health services*. Retrieved July 21, 2008, from http://www.mentalhealth.samhsa.gov/publications/allpubs/sma06-4055

Swanson, J. W. (1994). Mental disorder, substance abuse, and community violence: An epidemiological approach. In J. Monahan & H. J. Steadman (Eds.), *Violence and mental disorder: Developments in risk assessment* (pp. 101–136). Chicago: University of Chicago Press.

Swanson. J. W., Holzer, C. E., Ganju, V. K., & Jono, R.T. (1990). Violence and psychiatric disorder in the community: Evidence from the Epidemiologic Catchment Area surveys. *Hospital and Community Psychiatry, 41*, 761–770.

Swanson, J. W., Swartz, M. S., Essock, S. M., Osher, F. C., Wagner, H. R., Goodman, L. A., et al. (2002). The social–environmental context of violent behavior in persons treated for severe mental illness. *American Journal of Public Health, 92*, 1523–1531.

Swartz, M. S., Swanson, J. W., Hiday, V. A., Borum, R., Wagner, H. R., & Burns, B. J. (1998). Violence and severe mental illness: The effects of substance abuse and nonadherence to medication. *American Journal of Psychiatry, 155*, 226–231.

Tarasoff v. Regents of University of California, S29 P. 2d 553, 118 Cal Rptr. 129 (1974).

Tarasoff v. Regents of University of California, 17 Cal. 3d 425, 551 P. 2d 334, 131 Cal Rptr. 14 (1976).

Tardiff, K. (2003). Violence. In R. E. Hales, S. C. Yudofsky, & J. A. Talbott (Eds.), *Textbook of clinical psychiatry* (4th ed., pp. 1485–1509). Washington, DC: American Psychiatric Press.

Teasdale, B., Silver, E., & Monahan, J. (2006). Gender, threat/control override delusions and violence. *Law and Human Behavior, 30*, 649–658.

Volavka, J. (2002). *Neurobiology of violence* (2nd ed.). Washington, DC: American Psychiatric Press.

Wallace, C., Mullen, P. E., & Burgess, P. (2004). Criminal offending in schizophrenia over a 25-year period marked by deinstitutionalization and increasing prevalence of comorbid substance use disorders. *American Journal of Psychiatry, 161*, 716– 727.

Webster, C. D., Douglas, K. S., Eaves, D., & Hart, S. D. (1997). *HCR–20: Assessing risk for violence* (Version 2) [Computer software]. Burnaby, British Columbia, Canada: Simon Fraser University.

Webster, C. D., Martin, M. L., Brink, J., Nicholls, T. L., & Middleton, C. (2004). *Manual for the Short-Term Assessment of Risk and Treatability (START)* (Version 1.0, consultation ed.) [Computer software]. Hamilton, Ontario, Canada: St. Joseph's Healthcare; and Port Coquitlam, British Columbia, Canada; Forensic Psychiatric Services Commission.

Widiger, T. A., & Trull, T. J. (1994). Personality disorders and violence. In J. Monahan & H. J. Steadman (Eds.), *Violence and mental disorder: Developments in risk assessment* (pp. 203–226). Chicago: University of Chicago Press.

7

CHILDREN AND ADOLESCENTS AT RISK OF VIOLENCE

RANDY BORUM

Clinicians and other human services professionals often wrestle with concerns about potentially violent youth (Borum & Verhaagen, 2006; Hoge, Guerra, & Boxer, 2008). It is difficult enough that children and adolescents are in a continuous state of developmental change; the idea that they might harm someone else makes clinical encounters with them all the more complex. A therapist may face the issue when, for example, her teenage client shows up for his weekly appointment and tells the therapist that his girlfriend cheated on him. He says that he is so angry he "could kill them both." A school psychologist may have to deal with a situation in which an English teacher expresses concern about a student who wrote a poem about killing himself and others. Thoughtful and well-meaning professionals need a practical and systematic approach to gathering information, assessing risk, and managing the case. This chapter addresses some of those issues.

From the mid-1980s to the mid-1990s, there was a sharp and unprecedented increase in nearly all forms of youth violence in the United States. Most troubling was the fact that the number of juvenile homicides nearly doubled. Although rates of youth violence are now, in 2008, down considerably from where they were in the early 1990s (the juvenile homicide rate has dropped most dramatically; Borum, 2000; Hoge et al., 2008; U.S. Department of Health and Human Services, 2001), the level of public and professional concern remains high about serious violent behavior committed by juveniles.

The task of assessing the risk of violence in adolescents is different from similar appraisals with adults. Adolescents' developmental status in physical, cognitive, and psychosocial domains is quite fluid (Borum, 2003; Borum & Verhaagen, 2006; Griffin & Torbet, 2002; Grisso, 1998; McCord, Widom, & Crowell, 2001; Rosado, 2000). Changes tend to evolve and develop gradually, rather than appearing as a sudden or discrete shift. In addition, different physical, cognitive, and social developmental markers emerge at very different rates—and one cannot necessarily be inferred from the other (Grisso, 1996, 1998). Personality traits—and behavioral manifestations of those traits—are less stable and less consistent in juveniles than in adults. One is more likely to see a greater range of variability in styles and behaviors across different contexts (Grisso, 1998).

Biologically, young people are navigating the hormonal (and concomitant emotional) vicissitudes of puberty. Cognitively, new reasoning abilities are emerging, and inhibitory brain structures (those that keep one from doing "stupid" things) are still forming (Borum & Grisso, 2006). Psychosocially, teens are developing capacities for responsibility (i.e., making decisions without undue influence from others), perspective taking (i.e., the ability to see and consider both short- and long-term implications of a decision), and temperance (i.e., the ability to exercise self-restraint and to control one's impulses). As young people mature and become increasingly self-reliant, parental influence progressively declines and peers become more influential (Steinberg & Cauffman, 1999).

With the synergy of these changes, perhaps it should not be surprising that delinquent behavior in adolescence is remarkably common and that the teen years are the peak developmental risk period for initiating an act of serious violence. About one in four girls and nearly half of all boys in high school report being in a physical fight one or more times in the prior 12 months (Kann et al., 1998; U.S. Department of Health and Human Services, 2001). This is markedly above the adult norm. Most of these young people, however, stop engaging in violent behavior before they reach adulthood. After age 17, violence participation rates drop dramatically, and about 80% of those who are violent during adolescence will stop engaging in violent behavior by age 21 (Elliott, Huizinga, & Ageton, 1986; U.S. Department of Health and Human Services, 2001).

In this chapter, I examine the biopsychosocial risk factors that are unique to young people at risk of violence. I also suggest procedures for evaluating and managing risk.

BIOPSYCHOSOCIAL RISK FACTORS

Are there differences between teens who are (or who become) violent and those who are (or who will) not? Although nothing predicts with absolute certainty, there are factors about a youth, including his or her history and social situation, that may increase (i.e., risk factors) or decrease (i.e., protective factors) for the likelihood of engaging in violence (Borum & Verhaagen, 2006; Cottle, Lee, & Heilbrun, 2001; Derzon, 2001; Hawkins et al., 1998; Howard & Jenson, 1999; Howell, 1997; Lipsey & Derzon, 1998; Loeber & Stouthamer-Loeber, 1998). The U.S. Surgeon General's report on youth violence (U.S. Department of Health and Human Services, 2001) found that early onset (ages 6–11) of general delinquent offenses and of substance use showed a large effect in predicting adolescent violence. Among later onset (ages 12–14) factors, weak social ties, antisocial or delinquent peers, and gang membership topped the list, reflecting the increasing developmental importance of peer influence.

Other early and late onset risk factors showed only a moderate or small (but significant) effect. They include being male; low socioeconomic status or poverty; antisocial parents; aggression (for males); psychological condition; hyperactivity; poor parent–child relations; harsh, lax, or inconsistent discipline; abusive or neglectful parents; weak social ties; problem (i.e., antisocial) behavior; exposure to television violence; poor attitude toward or poor performance in school; low IQ; broken home or separation for parents; antisocial attitudes and beliefs; risk taking; and antisocial peers (U.S. Department of Health and Human Services, 2001).

Empirically based risk factors may bear some relevance in emergency risk assessments, but the facts and recent behaviors will probably be the most important elements. Base rates, even if they are known, may not be the most critical factor in appraising clinical concern. A clinician could not dismiss a teen's statement that he intended to leave the office and stab his "cheating bitch girlfriend" simply because the base rate of homicide is statistically low. Portentous communication or behavior combined with other indications of intent or planning could—as a matter of legal foreseeability—pose a prima facie suggestion that the clinician should be concerned and take appropriate action.

A common focus in emergency risk assessments is whether the examinee has made any direct threats to an intended target. Threats of violence should be taken seriously; however, threats should not be regarded as a necessary factor for determining risk. Fein and Vossekuil (1998) suggested that in assessing risk of targeted violence, it is important to distinguish between making a threat (i.e., communicating an intent to harm) and posing a threat (i.e., engaging in behavior that indicates furthering a plan or building capacity for a violent act, such as discussing attack plans with others or acquiring weapons). Although some people who make threats ultimately pose threats, many do not. Similarly, a client may pose a threat of harm to an identifiable victim, even if he or she has not made a direct threat. Persons who appear to pose a threat provoke the greatest level of concern.

Evaluating Risk

The first practical decision facing the evaluator concerns what biopsychosocial information to collect and weigh in his or her risk appraisal. If the clinician's judgment is challenged, the question posed will be whether he or she considered information that most similarly trained professionals would (or should) consider, and in light of that information whether the conclusion reached was one that a reasonable professional could have made. The professional literature on violence risk assessment (which exists mainly for adults) tends to focus on the array of historical, clinical, and contextual factors that have demonstrated a robust, empirically based relationship to violence risk recidivism and on the base rates for violent behavior (Borum, 2000; McNiel et al., 2002; Otto, 2000). Most of these recommendations, however, typically pertain to formal risk assessments in which the clinician is on notice of the assessment question prior to contact with the patient and has adequate time to collect relevant information and conduct the evaluation. In many emergency assessment contexts, the assessment must be done relatively quickly and perhaps with limited collateral information.

Consider Safety Issues

Despite other information that may or may not be readily available, most emergency risk assessments will involve a direct interview with the youth. Before and during the examination, it is important that the examinee, evaluator, and staff feel as safe and comfortable as possible. Clinicians should be familiar with all standard safety procedures used in the setting in which they practice. Routine preevaluation measures such as searches of an examinee's belongings and person vary across clinical settings, but evaluators should consider whether potential weapons may be present. If the patient has not been searched for weapons, this should be done. The evaluator should also be aware of the availability of general and security staff in the area the examination is to be conducted (Borum, Swartz, & Swanson, 1996).

If the examinee is particularly hostile and considered volatile, the interview should be conducted in a large room that permits a comfortable distance between the evaluator and the youth. In some circumstances it may be preferable to conduct the examination in an open area within sight of other personnel. Although a public setting decreases privacy, it may also serve to decrease the intensity of potentially hostile interactions. The optimal exam room has two exits, so that neither assessor nor examinee feels pinned down or trapped during the interview. Leaving a door ajar may also enhance feelings of safety. If at any time the evaluator feels uncomfortable with the examinee, additional staff may be called into the interview. When an optimal physical setting is not available, staff presence should be increased to enhance safety and ensure a basic comfort level (Borum et al., 1996).

Throughout the interview the clinician should be open, although reasonably matter of fact, about safety concerns. For example, the evaluator might say to the young person, "You understand that you and I must feel safe for us to do this interview. To be sure that no one gets hurt, we are going to ask a staff member to sit in with us." The need for a safe climate should be addressed directly. One might begin by telling an examinee, "We are here to discuss and understand any problems you might have. This is not a place for either of us to be hurt or afraid of being hit." The tone should be neutral and nonjudgmental, and the evaluator should openly acknowledge that violence is a behavior to be understood but not acted on. The evaluator also should explain all actions being taken, even explaining a hasty exit, if necessary (Borum et al., 1996).

Inquire About a History of Violence

In emergency assessments, just as it is standard practice to inquire about suicidality, evaluators also should routinely ask a set of screening questions about violent behavior. It is important to investigate multiple sources of information, if available, and to inquire about varying forms of violence and criminal behavior such as arrests, convictions, hospitalizations, in-home violence, and other fights and aggressive behaviors (e.g., arson, violence toward animals—at school, in the neighborhood, on the highway). These questions should be asked as neutrally as possible, as though inquiring about other routine historical information.

If the youth has a significant history of violence or presents with threats or concerns about violent behavior, the evaluator should conduct a more detailed exploration that includes inquiry about the nature and precipitants of any episodes of (a) verbal aggression, (b) physical aggression against objects, and (c) physical aggression against persons. This might include, for example, specific inquiry about the nature and extent of the following:

- injury caused to others;
- the youth's access to and use of weapons;
- the context or settings in which the violence occurred;
- the youth's proximate use of drugs or alcohol; and
- the thoughts, feelings, and behaviors that preceded the violent action.

A detailed examination of the youth's history of violence should help the evaluator discern patterns and indicators that may be useful in forecasting the type of harm that might be of most concern, the likelihood of its occurrence (e.g., are present conditions similar to past conditions in which the youth behaved violently?), and potential management strategies that might be most effective.

It is important, of course, to consider the reliability of the youth's self-report when reviewing his or her history of violent behavior. The evaluator should consider whether obtaining information from third parties (e.g., family members, police, others who accompanied the youth to the evaluation) or reasonably available records is feasible, relevant, and necessary.

Inquire About Current Status and Situation

Another distinctive feature of the emergency assessment is the predominant focus on indicators of intent or imminent action. For this reason, the examiner cannot base an appraisal of risk solely on a youth's history and a tally of risk factors. This requires an assessment that focuses more on the individual's pattern of behavior than on aggregated risk factors. Assessing intent is, in essence, a fact-based inquiry about behaviors that might indicate planning and preparation for violent action. The examiner must search for indications that the youth not only has harbored a passing idea but also has nurtured or embraced the idea, perhaps developed a plan and acted in furtherance of that idea. Overt indicators might include acquiring the means or capacity for the violent act, such as a weapon or other means of inflicting harm; selecting a target or targets; and determining the time, place, and manner in which to approach or otherwise gain access to the target, such as discovering the target's daily schedule (Borum, Fein, Vossekuil, & Berglund, 1999; Fein & Vossekuil, 1998; Fein, Vossekuil, & Holden, 1995; Reddy et al., 2001).

A heuristic device based largely on the work of Fein and Vossekuil (1998; Borum et al., 1999; Fein et al., 1995) was developed for navigating the contours of a fact-based risk inquiry (Borum & Reddy, 2001). It includes six factors and can be remembered by the acronym ACTION: A—attitudes that support or facilitate violence, C—capacity, T—thresholds crossed, I—intent, O—other's reactions, and N—noncompliance with risk reduction interventions (Borum & Reddy, 2001). Each is discussed briefly in the sections that follow.

Attitudes That Support or Facilitate Violence. Research in social psychology suggests that a person's intent to engage in a particular behavior is based in part on the nature and strength of his or her attitude toward that behavior (Azjen, 1985; Jemmott, Jemmott, Hines, & Fong, 2001). This may not be a surprising finding, but it does have implications for violence risk assessments. Beyond asking a young person whether he or she has thought about or made a plan for violent action, it is useful to know how he or she assesses the acceptability and likelihood of success in using violence to attain a goal. Specifically, does the client believe that the use of violence is justified under the circumstances? On the basis of social cognitive theory, the youth's appraisal of his or her circumstances is the most critical factor because that perception, not the professional's perception, will most influence whether violence will occur. In general, people are more likely to engage in violence if they have assessed and affirmed its justification, both cognitively and affectively. In addition, it may be useful to assess a youth's general appraisals of provocation or intentionality from others (i.e., his or her hostile attribution bias), violent fantasies, self-statements, and expectations about success of violence and whether the client thinks violent action will accomplish or further his or her goal. In addition to asking a young person how friends and peers usually treat him or her, one might ask, for example, about how the client has handled situations when he or she was mistreated and wanted to get back at someone.

Capacity. Capacity pertains to the ability and means to carry out the type of violent act that the youth has threatened or suggested might occur. This includes physical and intellectual capabilities, access to means (i.e., weapons or materials necessary to effect the violent act), access to the target, and opportunity to commit the act. The youth's history may give general indications of his or her intellectual and volitional capacity (i.e., what he or she might be willing to do). Different kinds of violence or planned attacks may require vastly different levels of capacity. Weapon access and facility become particularly important in cases in which the idea of weapon use has been raised. As of the year 2000, guns were present in approximately 40 million U.S. households (Cook & Ludwig, 2000). Firearms are very often accessible to children and adolescents. In a 2000 national survey, 43% of homes with children younger than 18 years old that had guns in the house were reported to have at least one unlocked firearm (Schuster, Franke, Bastian, Sor, & Halfon, 2000). Teenage students generally report that they have access to or could get a gun if they wanted to (Callahan & Rivara, 1992; Shapiro, Dorman, Welker, & Clough, 1998; Sheley & Wright, 1993; Wellford, Pepper, & Petrie, 2004).

Thresholds Crossed. In evaluating whether a young person simply had a transient idea or is moving along a pathway to action, it may be useful to explore (including through collateral sources, if possible) what behaviors, if any, have already been undertaken in furtherance of a plan, particularly behaviors that require breaking laws and rules. Acts committed in violation of laws are particularly noteworthy because they indicate a willingness and ability to engage in antisocial behavior to accomplish an objective. In conducting a risk inquiry, it is helpful to ask not only about the existence of a plan but also about the steps the client may have taken to further that plan. These may reveal telling indications of a youth's commitment—and proximity—to action.

Intent. Arguably, there exists an important distinction between having entertained an idea of violence and intent to commit the act. It is probably true that most people who entertain thoughts of harming another person never act on them. As noted before, making a threatening statement does not necessarily mean the youth poses a risk. Similarly, having an idea about harming someone does not necessarily mean a youth intends to do it. A youth's level of intent may be inferred indirectly from the specificity of the plan and the access to means to carry it out, or more directly from behaviors that indicate a commitment to action (Fein et al., 2002). An evaluator might ask, "How committed is this youth to violent action?" To gauge his commitment, the evaluator might explore the extent to which the youth has actively considered and weighed the potential consequences, and considered—and possibly rejected—alternative ways of accomplishing his or her objective. Individuals who are considering violence and believe they have no other available options or have nothing to lose would be expected to have more resolute intent and commitment to the violent act. Attitudes, as noted earlier, can also influence intent.

Others' Reactions and Responses. In emergency risk assessments it may not be possible to review external records or obtain collateral information. However, if information from other people who know the client is available, either directly or from the client's report, that data may be useful in appraising the youth's risk. The psychological *theory of planned behavior* posits that a key factor in determining a person's attitude toward a behavior is the reactions he or she anticipates or expects from others (Azjen, 1985; Jemmott et al., 2001). Thus, knowing about the reactions of others can help the assessment in two ways. First, it may help to gauge the direction of the youth's own attitude toward the act. For example, imagine a scenario in which a young man tells his friends that he is so angry with an older bully that he thought of killing him. If those friends respond by saying, "People like that don't deserve to live," the evaluator might infer that the youth might feel more justified in—or at least less discouraged from—committing violence. Second, knowing how others are responding to the youth helps the evaluator understand the social context in which the youth's ideas about violence exist. If the young examinee has talked to anyone about his ideas or plans for violence, it may be helpful to know whether significant others have discouraged or condemned the ideas, offered no judgment, supported or escalated the violent ideas, or even facilitated the development of capacity or movement from idea to action. If other people say they are concerned that the youth might actually follow through with his or her idea or plan (e.g., "I'm scared he might actually do it"), an evaluator might increase his or her index of concern regarding the propensity for violence.

Noncompliance With Risk Reduction. An additional factor to consider in assessing risk is the youth's interest and willingness to participate in interventions to reduce or mitigate risk. In this regard, an evaluator might consider whether the youth is motivated to prevent or avoid a violent act, whether the youth thinks treatment will be effective, whether the youth has trust and alliance with the provider, and whether he or she has a history of adherence and willingness to comply with conditions of supervision or therapeutic regimens. The likelihood of compliance or participation in an intervention may also be related to *insight*—the extent to which the young person understands and appreciates the severity of his or her own need for treatment or potential for violence. If an examinee appreciates that he or she may be at risk of harming someone and is motivated to take action to avoid that outcome, it seems more likely that his or her movement on a path toward violence can be slowed or redirected.

Consider Special Issues Associated With Targeted Violence in Schools

After the tragic and horrific shootings at Columbine High School in 1999, school systems, parents, and students throughout the United States became increasingly anxious to learn how they might prevent such attacks from occurring where they live. Researchers from the U.S. Secret Service (with nearly a century of experience in assessing and responding to threats against specific individuals) partnered with the U.S. Department of Education to study the problem. Their Safe School Initiative (Vossekuil, Fein, Reddy, Borum, & Modzeleski, 2002) was designed to provide a foundation of clear data, guiding principles, and helpful guidelines for understanding, assessing, and responding to targeted violence in school. The findings and lessons from that study have important implications for risk assessments in school settings.

The researchers reviewed 37 incidents involving 41 attackers for this study. Not surprisingly, all the attackers in the study were boys, and guns were nearly always the weapon of choice. The research revealed that the attacks were rarely, if ever, impulsive acts. The majority of the attackers had a plan at least 2 days prior to the incident, and in some cases, the planning had gone on for up to a year. Revenge was often the motive for the attack; more than three fourths of the attackers held a grievance against particular individuals or the school itself at the time of the attack.

When these attacks occurred, some reports indicated that they came without any warning; however, the vast majority of attackers communicated their idea or plan before the incident. In over three fourths of the incidents, attackers told someone about their interest in mounting an attack at the school. Typically, they told friends or other peer acquaintances. In more than half the cases multiple people knew about the attack prior to its occurrence. Although these school attackers typically told others about what was planned ahead of time, they rarely communicated a threat directly to the target of the attack.

Most of the boys who committed deadly violence in the schools showed signs of needing help before the incident. In almost every case, the attacker engaged in behavior that caused others to be concerned about him. In more than three fourths of the incidents, an adult had expressed concern about the attacker. The vast majority of these boys had difficulty coping with a major loss, and this was known to other individuals, peers and adults alike.

Nearly 75% of these adolescents had previously threatened or tried to commit suicide, and more than half had a history of feeling extremely depressed or desperate.

Bullying seemed to play a key role in the motivation for some, but not all, of the attacks. In more than two thirds of the cases, the attackers felt persecuted, bullied, threatened, attacked, or injured by others prior to the incident. In fact, some of these boys had experienced bullying and harassment that was long-standing and severe. When these shooting incidents occurred they were over quickly, and they typically were concluded before police arrived on the scene. Most of the time a faculty member or another student stopped the attacker. In some cases they decided to stop shooting on their own; in some incidents, they committed suicide. Half the incidents lasted 20 minutes or less.

On the basis of these findings, the researchers suggested that a behavior-based, fact-driven inquiry be used for assessing the potential for targeted violence in schools. Ideally, the available information could be evaluated by a multidisciplinary threat assessment team that might be led by a school administrator, with participation by faculty, school police (e.g., a school resource officer) or security, and a school psychologist. Each member potentially brings a different viewpoint and has access to different kinds of information. The study group recommended that the threat assessment inquiry be focused around a series of 11 key questions (see Exhibit 7.1).

The team first determines whether it has sufficient information available to reasonably answer these questions. If not, and if such information is not attainable, the case may be referred to law enforcement for investigation. If the questions can be reasonably answered, the team must determine whether the weight of the evidence suggests that the young person poses a threat of targeted violence at the school. If the evidence suggests the student is not likely on a pathway toward a violent attack, the inquiry may be terminated. If the evidence suggests, however, that the young person does pose a risk of targeted violence, the inquiry may be referred to law enforcement for follow-up investigation and action (Fein et al., 2002).

Both the general model of emergency assessment and the school-based threat assessment model have the central objective of preventing violence. Managing risk becomes as important, if not more important, than merely assessing it.

Managing Risk

After an evaluator determines that some type of intervention is warranted, he or she should consider which strategies are most likely to reduce the risk of harm. In formulating this decision, consider the type of harm possible, the likelihood of harm, and the conditions that may enhance or mitigate risk as indicated from the assessment.

EXHIBIT 7.1
Eleven Key Investigative Questions for Assessing
Threats of Targeted Violence in Schools

Key investigative questions

1. What are the student's motive(s) and goals?
2. Have there been any communications suggesting ideas or intent to attack?
3. Has the student shown inappropriate interest in any of the following?
   a. school attacks or attackers
   b. weapons (including recent acquisition of any relevant weapon)
   c. incidents of mass violence (e.g., terrorism, workplace violence, mass murderers)
4. Has the student engaged in attack-related behaviors?
5. Does the student have the capacity to carry out an act of targeted violence?
6. Is the student experiencing hopelessness, desperation, or despair?
7. Does the student have a trusting relationship with at least one responsible adult?
8. Does the student see violence as an acceptable—or desirable—or the only—way to solve problems?
9. Are the student's conversation and story consistent with his or her actions?
10. Are other people concerned about the student's potential for violence?
11. What circumstances might affect the likelihood of an attack?

Note. Data from Fein et al. (2002).

Risk assessment and risk management—when done properly—should be integrated functions. A number of treatments and interventions have been proven effective for reducing delinquent and violent recidivism in juveniles (Borum, 2003). A thorough discussion of treatment strategies for delinquent and violent juveniles is beyond the scope of this chapter (see Borum, 2003; Borum & Verhaagen, 2006); rather, I focus here on managing the present emergency or crisis.

Monahan and Shaw (1989) identified three broad categories of intervention for addressing dangerous behavior.

1. *Incapacitation* (e.g., hospitalization). Incapacitation refers to efforts to directly reduce a person's risk to others. Direct restraints may include hospital confinement or observation, or if applicable, legal restraints. Although medications sometimes may be used for persons in the community who are in acutely combative states, they often are slow to act, sometimes ineffective, and always require close and ongoing supervision. As a result, physical containment is the cornerstone of incapacitation.

2. *Target hardening.* Target hardening refers to efforts to alert potential victims or law enforcement of an examinee's potential violence so that persons at risk can reduce their vulnerability. Although warning potential victims may be the first intervention that comes to mind, other strategies may be more appropriate. Warnings to potential victims can be frighten-

ing and unhelpful and should be reserved for occasions when other interventions are implausible or ineffective. In speaking with a potential victim, the clinician should review the nature and seriousness of the threat, and if applicable, discuss specific warning signs, measures to take, and resources to turn to; that is, a warning should help potential victims take measures to protect themselves. Routine warnings or warnings falling on deaf ears do little to reduce the likelihood of harm. For a more in-depth discussion of legal risks associated with treating potentially violent patients or clients, see chapter 17.

3. *Intensified treatment.* Treatment interventions should be driven by needs, rather than placements. Hospitalization may be an option for some potentially violent youth, but one should not assume that treatment in a hospital setting is necessarily better or even more intensive than in a community setting. Research generally suggests that with delinquent and violent youth, community-based interventions work better than residential or inpatient treatments (probably because of ecological generalizability; Borum, 2003). A hospital may offer a venue for therapeutic incapacitation when that is necessary, but intensified treatment may also reduce a youth's risk in a variety of other ways. Frequent visits, home visits, increased supervision, and changes in the treatment modality all may be helpful. Removing youth from their current environment to a safer one may also be warranted.

In keeping with the contours of these broad categories of intervention, a basic risk management model typically will involve the following steps:

1. Determine whether there is a need for immediate containment. If a youth is assessed to be escalating to imminent violence, the evaluator should consider containment options. This may include hospitalization, arrest, or—in extreme cases—restraint. In other cases, containment may occur by separating the youth from a provocative situation or otherwise de-escalating the acuity of the aggression. The main objectives here are to ensure immediate safety and to buy time while diminishing acuity. For a more in-depth discussion of having clients or patients physically restrained, see the discussion about physical restraint in chapter 2.

2. Determine whether target protective measures are necessary. If the evaluator believes that there is a proximate risk to an identified or identifiable target (e.g., a specific named person), it would be wise to consider the necessity and appropriateness of various protective measures. These might include

warning or advising the target or notifying law enforcement. Protective measures should be initiated only if they have a reasonable likelihood of preventing harm. The main objective is to reduce the target's vulnerability. Again, see chapter 17 for a more in-depth discussion of legal risks.

3. Identify the youth's needs. On the basis of the foregoing assessment, the evaluator should determine what resources or services are needed to manage the youth's risk and mitigate his or her critical risk factors. Medical, mental health, social service, criminal justice, or victim service resources might all be considered. The objective is to identify need areas for intervention.

4. Mobilize and coordinate resources. After needs are identified, the evaluator should facilitate or coordinate the process of linking the youth to the proper people or agencies to provide those services. Often a simple referral or handing him or her a phone number will not be sufficient to ensure that the connection is made. The evaluator might consider scheduling a follow-up appointment while the youth is present, before he or she leaves the evaluation, or possibly coordinating reminders before the next visit and following up with the referred professional. The objective here is to engage the youth in a risk management plan and to take concrete steps to mobilize that plan during the emergency assessment.

5. Monitor and follow up. Even the best risk management plans can falter over details. With needs and resources identified and mobilized, the evaluator should think through the action steps of implementing the risk management plan. Who has responsibility for each element? How and when will the intervention be done and monitored? It is usually advisable to have objective markers of redirection or of reduced risk, which could include assessing risk factors such as substance use, intervention adherence, or frequency of angry outbursts or markers such as the youth's level of intent or justification for violence action versus his ability to generate effective nonaggressive solutions to conflict. The plan should include some way of concretely determining whether it is or is not working and whether, when, and the extent to which violence risk has been mitigated.

Unfortunately and tragically, violence does sometimes occur despite everyone's best efforts. As a result, documentation becomes a critical element of risk management. Document the source, content, and date for all information relevant to a risk assessment and intervention. It is equally important to document the reasoning that led to the selected intervention, including recording the risk and benefits of interventions considered. It is better to document your reasoning even if it may turn out to be incorrect than to fail to demonstrate any cogent line of reasoning in the record (see chap. 17 for an in-depth discussion of documentation requirements).

In cases involving the release of individuals from an institutional setting, Poythress (1990) suggested that prerelease records should include a specific form or document that addresses the patient's potential for violence. These structured forms, in addition to enhancing the quality of prerelease documentation, also assist evaluators in conducting a more systematic inquiry about and analysis of violence risk, and help to structure and standardize the clinical risk assessment process (Borum, 1996). Although the specific items, questions, or content may vary for different kinds of institutions, the fundamental objective is to record what key risk-related factors were considered in the release decision and how they support the disposition or action taken.

CONCLUSION

Violence by young people cannot always be prevented, but emergency assessments offer a window of opportunity to manage a risky situation and to redirect a youth from a pathway toward imminent violence. The challenge for evaluators is to be direct, inquisitive, engaging, and systematic in asking questions and seeking information to determine whether there is a reasonable basis for professional concern. If that concern exists, the assessor must be equally rigorous in devising (and initiating) a plan to prevent violence and enhance safety. Having explicit criteria for success in risk reduction and a clear strategy for monitoring and follow-up will multiply the odds of success. When dealing with potentially violent youth in an emergency context, assessment and management actions must be thoroughly integrated and accountably executed.

REFERENCES

Azjen, I. (1985). From intentions to actions: A theory of planned behavior. In J. Kuhl & J. Beckman (Eds.), *Action-control: From cognition to behavior* (pp. 11–39). Heidelberg, Germany: Springer-Verlag.

Borum, R. (1996). Improving the clinical practice of violence risk assessment: Technology, guidelines and training. *American Psychologist, 51,* 945–956.

Borum, R. (2000). Assessing violence risk among youth. *Journal of Clinical Psychology, 56,* 1263–1288.

Borum, R. (2003). Managing at risk juvenile offenders in the community: Putting evidence based principles into practice. *Journal of Contemporary Criminal Justice, 19*, 114–137.

Borum, R., Bartel, P., & Forth, A. (2005). Structured assessment of violence risk in youth (SAVRY). In T. Grisso, G. Vincent, & D. Seagrave (Eds.), *Handbook of mental health screening and assessment in juvenile justice* (pp. 311–323). New York: Oxford University Press.

Borum, R., Fein, R., Vossekuil, B., & Berglund, J. (1999). Threat assessment: Defining an approach for evaluating risk of targeted violence. *Behavioral Sciences & the Law, 17*, 323–337.

Borum, R., & Grisso, T. (2006). Forensic assessment from a developmental perspective. In A. Goldstein (Ed.), *Forensic psychology: Emerging topics and expanding roles* (pp. 553–570). New York: Wiley.

Borum, R., & Reddy, M. (2001). Assessing violence risk in *Tarasoff* situations: A fact-based model of inquiry. *Behavioral Sciences & the Law, 19*, 375–385.

Borum, R., Swartz, M., & Swanson, J. (1996). Assessing and managing violence risk in clinical practice. *Journal of Practical Psychiatry and Behavioral Health, 2*, 205–215.

Borum, R., & Verhaagen, D. (2006). *Assessing and managing violence risk in juveniles.* New York: Guilford Press.

Callahan, C., & Rivara, F. (1992). Urban high school youth and handguns: A school-based survey. *The Journal of the American Medical Association, 267*, 3038–3042.

Cook, P. J., & Ludwig, J. (2000). *Gun violence: The real costs.* New York: Oxford University Press.

Cottle C., Lee R., & Heilbrun, K. (2001). The prediction of criminal recidivism in juveniles: A meta-analysis. *Criminal Justice and Behavior, 28*, 367–394.

Derzon, J. H. (2001). Antisocial behavior and the prediction of violence: A meta-analysis. *Psychology in the Schools, 38*, 93–106.

Elliott, D., Huizinga, D., & Ageton, S. (1986). Self-reported violent offending. *Journal of Interpersonal Violence, 1*, 472–514.

Fein, R., & Vossekuil, B. (1998). *Protective intelligence and threat assessment investigations: A guide for state and local law enforcement officials* (NIJ/OJP/DOJ Publication No. 170612). Washington, DC: U.S. Department of Justice.

Fein, R., Vossekuil, B., & Holden, G. (1995, July). Threat assessment: An approach to prevent targeted violence. *National Institute of Justice: Research in Action.* Washington, DC: U.S. Department of Justice.

Fein R., Vossekuil B., Pollack, W., Borum R., Modzeleski, W., & Reddy M. (2002). *Threat assessment in schools: A guide to managing threatening situations and creating safe school climates.* Washington, DC: U.S. Department of Education and U.S. Secret Service.

Griffin, P., & Torbet, P. (2002). *Desktop guide to good juvenile probation practice.* Washington, DC: Office of Juvenile Justice and Delinquency Prevention.

Grisso, T. (1996). Society's retributive response to juvenile violence: A developmental perspective. *Law and Human Behavior, 20,* 229–247.

Grisso, T. (1998). *Forensic evaluation of juveniles.* Sarasota, FL: Professional Resource Press.

Hawkins, J., Herrenkohl, T., Farrington, D., Brewer, D., Catalano, R., & Harachi, T. (1998). A review of predictors of youth violence. In R. Loeber & D. Farrington (Eds.), *Serious and violent juvenile offenders: Risk factors and successful interventions* (pp. 106–146). Thousand Oaks, CA: Sage.

Hoge, R. D., Guerra, N., & Boxer, P. (Eds.). (2008). *Treating the juvenile offender.* New York: Guilford Press.

Howard, M. O., & Jenson, J. M. (1999). Inhalant use among antisocial youth: Prevalence and correlates. *Addictive Behavior, 41,* 59–74.

Howell, J. (1997). *Juvenile justice and youth violence.* Thousand Oaks, CA: Sage.

Jemmott, J. B., III, Jemmott, L. S., Hines, P. M., & Fong, G. T. (2001). Testing the theory of planned behavior as a model of involvement in violence among African American and Latino adolescents. *Maternal Child Health Journal, 5,* 253–263.

Kann, L., Kinchen, S. A., Williams, B.I., Ross, J. G., Lowry, R., Hill C. V., et al. (1998). Youth risk behavior surveillance—United States, 1997. *MMWR, 47*(3), 1–89.

Lipsey, M., & Derzon, J. (1998). Predictors of violent or serious delinquency in adolescence and early adulthood: A synthesis of longitudinal research. In R. Loeber & D. Farrington (Eds.), *Serious & violent juvenile offenders: Risk factors and successful interventions* (pp. 86–105). Thousand Oaks, CA: Sage.

Loeber, R., & Stouthamer-Loeber, M. (1998). Development of juvenile aggression and violence: Some common misperceptions and controversies. *American Psychologist, 53,* 242–259.

McCord, J., Widom, C. S., & Crowell, N. A. (Eds.) (2001). *Juvenile crime, juvenile justice.* Washington, DC: National Academies Press.

McNiel, D., Borum, R., Douglas, K., Hart, S., Lyon, D., Sullivan, L., & Hemphill, J. (2002). Risk assessment. In J. Ogloff (Ed.), *Taking psychology and law into the 21st century* (pp. 147–170). New York: Kluwer Academic.

Monahan, J., & Shaw, S. (1989). Dangerousness and commitment of the mentally disordered in the United States. *Schizophrenia Bulletin, 15,* 541–53.

Otto, R. (2000). Assessing and managing violence risk in outpatient settings. *Journal of Clinical Psychology, 56,* 1239–1262.

Poythress, N. (1990). Avoiding negligent release: Contemporary clinical and risk management strategies. *American Journal of Psychiatry, 147,* 994–997.

Reddy, M., Borum, R., Vossekuil, B., Fein, R., Berglund, J., & Modzeleski, W. (2001). Evaluating risk for targeted violence in schools: Comparing risk assessment, threat assessment, and other approaches. *Psychology in the Schools, 38,* 157–172.

Rosado. L. (Ed.). (2000). *Kids are different: How knowledge of adolescent development theory can aid decision-making in court.* Washington, DC: American Bar Association Juvenile Justice Center.

Schuster, M., Franke, T., Bastian, A., Sor, S., & Halfon, N. (2000). Firearm storage patterns in US homes with children. *American Journal of Public Health*, 90, 588–594.

Shapiro, J. P., Dorman, R. D., Welker, C. J., & Clough, J. B. (1998). Youth attitudes toward guns and violence: Relations with sex, age, ethnic group, and exposure. *Journal of Clinical Child Psychology*, 27, 98–108.

Sheley, J., & Wright, J. (1993, December). *Gun acquisition and possession in selected juvenile samples* (Publication No. NCJ145326). Washington, DC: National Institute of Justice.

Steinberg, L., & Cauffman, E. (1999, December). A developmental perspective on serious juvenile crime: When should juveniles be treated as adults? *Federal Probation*, 52–57.

U.S. Department of Health and Human Services. (2001). *Youth violence: A report of the Surgeon General*. Rockville, MD: Author.

Vossekuil, B., Fein, R., Reddy, M., Borum, R., & Modzeleski, W. (2002). *The final report and findings of the safe school initiative: Implications for the prevention of school attacks in the United States*. Washington, DC: U.S. Department of Education and U.S. Secret Service.

Wellford, C., Pepper, J., & Petrie, C. (2004). *Firearms and violence: A critical review*. Washington, DC: National Academies Press.

IV

EVALUATION AND MANAGEMENT OF INTERPERSONAL VICTIMIZATION

8

EVALUATION AND ACUTE INTERVENTION WITH VICTIMS OF VIOLENCE

MICHAEL R. McCART, MONICA M. FITZGERALD, RON E. ACIERNO, HEIDI S. RESNICK, AND DEAN G. KILPATRICK

Despite declines in the rates of violent and nonviolent crime in the United States over the past decade, adults continue to experience high levels of criminal victimization. Epidemiological data from the National Crime Victimization Survey (NCVS) indicate that more than 5 million violent crimes (including incidents of rape, robbery, and physical assault) were committed against individuals age 12 and older in 2005 (Catalano, 2006). There are a number of potential psychosocial outcome trajectories among individuals exposed to violent events. Fortunately, the most common is resilience, which is characterized by healthy and relatively stable levels of functioning in the aftermath of a traumatic stressor (Bonanno, 2004). For example, although studies have estimated that between 50% and 70% of individuals in the United States have experienced at least one violent or life-threatening event during their lifetime, most of these people maintain a relatively healthy symptom profile. Estimates suggest that only about 5% to 20% go on to develop posttraumatic stress disorder (PTSD) or other forms of psychological distress (Ozer, Best, Lipsey, & Weiss, 2003; Resnick, Kilpatrick, Dansky,

Saunders, & Best, 1993). Another common trajectory is gradual recovery, in which crime victims experience threshold or sub-threshold levels of psychopathology that subside within several weeks or months of the traumatic event. A third potential trajectory following exposure to criminal victimization is the development of chronic psychopathology (Kessler, Sonnega, Bromet, Hughes, & Nelson, 1995; Kilpatrick et al., 2003). For these individuals, formal treatment may be needed to facilitate recovery to healthy levels of functioning.

As Callahan pointed out in chapter 1 of this volume, many clinicians once believed that it was appropriate to provide psychological treatment to virtually all victims of trauma. This view led to the development of various debriefing interventions that could be applied universally in the acute aftermath of a traumatic event. As mentioned, the data now indicate that a majority of individuals exposed to traumatic stressors do not experience psychological distress at a level that warrants formal clinical intervention (Bonanno, 2004). Furthermore, data suggest that when debriefing interventions are universally applied, they are not universally helpful and may produce iatrogenic effects (Wessley, Rose, & Bisson, 2000). In light of these findings, researchers recently developed a series of preliminary practice guidelines for delivering psychological care to adults immediately following a trauma (Gray & Litz, 2005; McNally, Bryant, & Ehlers, 2003). Drawing heavily from the empirical literature, these guidelines advise against the use of debriefing procedures and advocate for the provision of psychological first aid to adults who request help in the aftermath of a traumatic event. Furthermore, they emphasize the importance of timely assessment to identify at-risk individuals who may benefit from more formal psychological intervention. In this chapter, we discuss how these guidelines can help inform clinical practice with adults who have recently experienced a violent crime. First, however, we provide a brief overview of the prevalence of criminal victimization among adults, and we discuss the difficulties that are commonly faced by individuals following exposure to a violent event.

PREVALENCE OF VIOLENT VICTIMIZATION

Several epidemiological studies document high rates of criminal victimization among adults in the United States. For example, Basile, Chen, Black, and Saltzman (2007) noted that among a nationally representative sample of 9,684 adults participating in the Second Injury Control and Risk Survey, 11% of women and 2% of men reported that they had been raped at some point during their lifetime. Kessler et al. (1995) assessed traumatic events in a sample of 5,877 adults and found that 7% of women and 11% of men reported a history of physical assault. When Resnick et al. (1993) interviewed a nationally representative sample of 4,008 women to assess their lifetime exposure to different violent events, they found that 14% had experienced sexual molestation or attempted rape, 13% had experienced a completed rape, and 10% had a history of physical assault. In addition, research indicates that rape usually occurs more than once to a victim. Tjaden and Thoennes (2000b) reported that in their sample of adult rape victims, the female victims had experienced an average of 2.9 rapes and the male victims had experienced an average of 1.2 rapes in the previous year.

The prevalence of criminal victimization varies by age, sex, and race. According to data from the NCVS, the risk of victimization by violent crime decreases steadily after age 24 (Catalano, 2006). Thus, younger individuals are at increased risk of victimization. For example, although individuals ages 12 to 24 composed 22% of the general population in 2005, they composed 47% of those victimized by rape, robbery, aggravated assault, simple assault, or personal theft. Young women and children are more likely to experience rape and other forms of sexual assault, and incidents of robbery and physical assault are more common among men (Breslau et al., 1998; Hapke, Schumann, Rumpf, John, & Meyer, 2006). In addition, men are more likely to be physically assaulted by strangers and women are more likely to be physically or sexually assaulted by an intimate partner, friend, or acquaintance (Catalano, 2006).

Data related to race from the Centers for Disease Control and Prevention (CDC) indicate that although African American men and women made up about 12% of the population in 2003, they composed 28% of all nonfatal crime victims and 47% of all homicide victims (CDC, 2003). Among the total population, African American and Hispanic men and women are at least 60% more likely to be victims of violent crime than European American men and women across all age categories. A separate report by the Bureau of Justice Statistics (Greenfield & Smith, 1999) indicated that although rates of murder among American Indian men and women are similar to the rates in the general population, rates of violent crime for this ethnic group are higher than those reported by other ethnic groups.

According to several excellent literature reviews (Arrata, 2002; Classen, Palesh, & Aggarwal, 2005), one of the strongest predictors of future victimization is past victimization. Data from the National Violence Against Women Survey (NVAWS) show male and female victims of childhood physical or sexual abuse are 2 to 5 times more likely to experience a subsequent physical or sexual assault in adulthood (Desai, Arias, Thompson, & Basile, 2002). Risk of repeat victimization among women appears to increase at a linear rate. That is, Kilpatrick, Acierno, Resnick, Saunders, and Best (1997) noted that compared with women who had never been physically or sexually assaulted, the odds of experiencing a new assault over a 2-year period doubled for women with one assault, increased about 400% for women with two assaults, and increased about 1,000% for women with three or more prior victimizations. Considering these data, one must be careful not to "blame the victim." As Hanson, Kilpatrick, Falsetti, and Resnick (1995) pointed out, having to remain in violent neighborhoods or being continually accessible to perpetrators (e.g., because of financial hardship, domestic violence) will increase risk of revictimization.

Impact of Victimization

Individuals exposed to interpersonal violence are at risk of experiencing a range of negative outcomes. Examples of common medical and psychological consequences of victimization are described in the sections that follow.

Acute Medical Problems

Interpersonal violence is a common cause of injury and emergency department visits among adult men and women. The NVAWS estimated that about 42% of women and 20% of men who had been physically assaulted sustained injuries during their most recent victimization. Most injuries were minor involving scratches, bruises, or welts (Tjaden & Thoennes, 2000b). More severe physical injuries often occur in the context of intimate partner violence (IPV), which is defined as physical, sexual, or psychological harm perpetrated by a current or former romantic partner or spouse. The NVAWS estimated that about 29% of women and 22% of men had experienced IPV at some point during their lifetime (Coker et al., 2002). IPV results in nearly 2 million emergency department visits and 1,300 deaths each year (CDC, 2003). Common IPV-related injuries include broken bones, contusions, vaginal tearing, knife wounds, and back pain (Campbell et al., 2002; Plichta, 2004; Tjaden & Thoennes, 2000a).

Women who experience rape are also at increased risk of developing a variety of gynecological problems. The prevalence of sexually transmitted diseases in sexual assault populations has been estimated to range between 2% and 30% (Goodman, Koss, & Russo, 1993; Reynolds, Peipert, & Collins, 2000). Other medical problems commonly experienced by female rape victims include vaginal infections, urinary tract infections, and pelvic pain (Campbell et al., 2002).

Acute Psychological Reactions

It is common for adults to experience symptoms of psychological distress in the acute aftermath of a violent event. As described by Bryant (2004), the literature reports high rates of intrusive thoughts, dissociative symptoms (e.g., emotional numbing, derealization, depersonalization, dissociative amnesia), avoidant behaviors, hyperarousal, insomnia, concentration difficulties, irritability, and depressed affect among adults in the initial weeks of a trauma. As mentioned, most individuals will show a decrease in symptoms within a few weeks or months of the traumatic event (Bonanno, 2004). A minority of trauma victims, however, may go on to develop chronic mental health problems, such as PTSD, depression, or substance abuse or dependence.

Chronic Mental Health Problems

PTSD is one of the most commonly observed mental health outcomes associated with interpersonal victimization. As defined in the *Diagnostic and Statistical Manual of Mental Disorders* (*DSM–IV–TR*; 4th ed., text rev.; American Psychiatric Association, 2000), the essential features of PTSD include reexperiencing the event visually through dreams and intrusive thoughts, avoiding reminders of the event, and hyperarousal symptoms that persist for more than 1 month following a traumatic stressor. Criminal victimization tends to be associated with higher rates of PTSD than other traumatic events such as motor vehicle accidents and natural disasters (Breslau et al., 1998; Hapke et al., 2006; Resnick et al., 1993). Women experience higher rates of PTSD than men, and the primary index events differ by gender. For example, whereas combat exposure and witnessed violence are the most common causes of PTSD for men, physical and sexual assault represent the most common precipitating events for women (Kilpatrick & Resnick, 1993). When left untreated, PTSD tends to follow a chronic, unremitting course. Breslau et al. (1998) reported that in a large sample of adults who met criteria for PTSD, the median duration of the disorder was 25 months. Moreover, Kessler et al. (1995) found that although 50% of adults who met criteria for PTSD recovered within 2 years, almost 33% did not experience full remission of symptoms, even after several years.

Major depression is also frequently observed among victims of crime and is highly comorbid with PTSD (Boudreaux, Kilpatrick, Resnick, Best, & Saunders, 1998). In the National Women's Study (NWS; Kilpatrick, Edmunds, & Seymour, 1992), a lifetime occurrence of physical assault increased the odds of current depression by a factor of 3. Data from the NVAWS also reveal strong associations between a history of IPV and current depressive symptoms among both men and women (Coker et al., 2002). In addition, results from a few clinical studies have documented elevated rates of panic attack symptoms and panic disorder among women who experienced rape (Falsetti & Resnick, 1997).

Numerous clinical and epidemiological studies also document high rates of comorbidity between PTSD and substance use disorders (Dansky, Saladin, Brady, Kilpatrick, & Resnick, 1995). In a nationally representative sample of adults, over 50% of men and 28% of women with PTSD also had comorbid problems with alcohol abuse or dependence (Kessler et al., 1995). Data from the NWS (Kilpatrick et al., 1997) suggest that rape and physical assault may lead to substance use and abuse in previously nonusing women. Other data indicate that the risk of victimization by assault is increased among individuals who are already abusing substances (Cottler, Helzer, & Tripp, 1990). Although directionality of the assault–substance abuse relationship remains somewhat ambiguous, the data clearly indicate that victims use substances at significantly elevated rates relative to nonvictims, and this substance use appears to facilitate additional violence (Classen et al., 2005; Cottler, Compton, Mager, Spitznagel, & Janca, 1992).

Risk Factors for Posttraumatic Stress Disorder

Considerable effort has been expended to identify factors that distinguish individuals who will experience transient distress from those who develop longer-term psychopathology (particularly PTSD) following exposure to a traumatic stressor. As noted by Bryant (2003), acutely traumatized individuals who are at risk of developing poor outcomes may be good candidates for early intervention. The diagnosis of acute stress disorder (ASD) was first introduced in the *DSM–IV* (American Psychiatric Association, 1994) as a way to identify individuals who may be at greater risk of eventually developing PTSD. The diagnostic criteria for ASD include three or more dissociative symptoms, one reexperiencing symptom, marked avoidance of stimuli that arouse recollections of the trauma, and symptoms of anxiety or increased arousal that occur within 4 weeks of a traumatic event. The validity of the ASD diagnosis has been called into question by a number of researchers (see Bryant, 2003; Keane, Kaufman, & Kimble, 2001). Furthermore, the disorder has been shown to have limited predictive utility. In a recent review of the literature, Bryant (2006) summarized the findings from 12 prospective studies that assessed the relationship between ASD and subsequent PTSD among traumatized adults. The data indicate that although a majority of individuals with ASD (75%) go on to develop PTSD, less than half of those who eventually develop PTSD initially meet criteria for ASD. Bryant concluded that there are likely to be multiple trajectories along which an individual will develop PTSD, and a diagnosis of ASD in the initial weeks of a trauma appears to represent only one of these paths.

There is also inconsistent evidence for a relationship between acute psychological symptoms (e.g., dissociation, hyperarousal, insomnia) and the development of PTSD (Bryant, 2003). For example, although some studies suggest that initial distress is associated with later psychopathology (Denson, Marshall, Schell, & Jaycox, 2007; King et al., 2000; Koopman, Classen, & Spiegel, 1994), others suggest that acute distress levels do not predict subsequent mental health problems (Harvey & Bryant, 1998; Yehuda, 2002). There is evidence indicating that early biological mechanisms and cognitive responses may represent more powerful predictors of long-term psychological functioning among traumatized adults. For example, trauma survivors who evidence lower cortisol levels, elevated resting heart rates, and panic attack symptoms shortly following a trauma appear to be at higher risk of developing PTSD (Bryant, Harvey, Guthrie, & Moulds, 2000; McFarlane, Atchison, & Yehuda, 1997). Regarding acute cognitive responses, researchers have also noted strong relations between negative cognitive appraisals of the trauma or its sequelae and chronic PTSD (Andrews, Brewin, Rose, & Kirk, 2000; Engelhard, van den Hout, Arntz, & McNally, 2002).

Certain incident characteristics may also increase the probability of a negative outcome among adults exposed to violent events. For example, data from the traumatic stress literature suggest that adults are more likely to develop PTSD if the violent event elicits extreme fear and results in physical injury (Jaycox, Marshall, & Orlando, 2003; Kilpatrick et al., 1989; Weaver & Clum, 1995). Individuals who endure multiple traumas are also more likely to develop PTSD than those who experience fewer than two traumas (Kimerling, Alvarez, Pavao, Kaminski, & Baumrind, 2007). Considering NWS data, Kilpatrick et al. (1997) found that 3% of nonassaulted women had current PTSD, compared with 19% of women with one prior assault and 53% of women with two prior assaults.

Finally, the presence of prior psychiatric problems may increase one's risk of developing PTSD (Ozer et al., 2003). Kessler et al. (1995) reported that the incidence of preexisting psychiatric problems was high in individuals with PTSD. Cottler et al. (1992) specifically studied the risk of PTSD in drug users and found that cocaine abuse was associated with increased risk of PTSD among trauma victims (most often assaultive violence), even after controlling for the effects of depression, age, race, and gender. By contrast, stable sources of social support appear to buffer against development of posttraumatic problems in psychological functioning (Norris et al., 2002).

Acute Interventions for Victims of Violence

Acute interventions are those that are implemented shortly following a traumatic event (i.e., within 4 weeks; National Institute of Mental Health, 2002) with the ultimate aim of reducing risk of the development of chronic mental health problems such as PTSD. As mentioned earlier, a variety of interventions have been developed in recent years to deal with reactions to trauma in the acute phase. However, relatively few of these early interventions have been rigorously evaluated. On the basis of the available evidence, experts have developed a series of preliminary practice guidelines for clinicians working with victims of a recent trauma (Gray & Litz, 2005; McNally et al., 2003). First, clinicians are advised against prescribing formal interventions, particularly psychological debriefing procedures, to all victims in the acute aftermath of a traumatic stressor. Second, although formal interventions are not typically recommended in the acute phase, the provision of psychological first aid is considered reasonable and appropriate. Third, given the transient nature of acute stress reactions, clinicians are advised to wait at least 1 week before conducting symptom-based psychological assessment with trauma-exposed adults. Fourth, for individuals who continue to experience distress symptoms several weeks following the traumatic event, early interventions anchored in cognitive and behavioral principles may be indicated. Each of these practice recommendations is described in more detail in the sections that follow.

Psychological Debriefing

Critical Incident Stress Debriefing (CISD; Mitchell & Everly, 1996) represents one of the most widely used acute interventions for victims of trauma. CISD was originally developed for emergency response personnel (e.g., police, firefighters, paramedics) whose work involves frequent exposure to potentially traumatic events. Over time, this intervention has been applied to a broader range of trauma-exposed adults, including members of the military and victims of disasters (Everly & Mitchell, 1999). CISD is typically conducted in the context of a single group meeting held within a few days of a traumatic event. All exposed individuals are invited to attend the meeting to discuss their emotional reactions to the trauma. A group facilitator normalizes group members' reactions and provides psychoeducation regarding adaptive coping techniques. The main goals of CISD are to reduce immediate distress, prevent the development of PTSD, and identify individuals who are in need of more formal treatment.

Despite its widespread use, CISD has been criticized on a number of grounds. One criticism pertains to the timing of the intervention. For example, researchers have questioned whether individuals can truly benefit from an intervention that is delivered so soon after a traumatic event, before their basic needs (e.g., safety, medical concerns) are addressed (Gray & Litz, 2005). Furthermore, given data indicating that a majority of individuals maintain resilient functioning in the aftermath of a traumatic stressor, the blanket application of CISD to all victims is regarded as unnecessary and potentially misguided (Bonanno, 2004; Litz, Gray, Bryant, & Adler, 2002). Finally, it has been argued that by delivering CISD in a group format, individuals may feel pressured to disclose personal information, which may inadvertently lead to higher, as opposed to lower, levels of distress (Gray & Litz, 2005).

Although a number of early studies documented the effectiveness of CISD (e.g., see Amir, Weil, Kaplan, Tocker, & Witztum, 1998; Chemtob, Tomas, Law, & Cremniter, 1997; Yule, 1992), these studies suffered from a number of significant methodological limitations, including the absence of a control group or the lack of random assignment to the different study conditions. More recent randomized controlled trials of CISD have shown that this intervention is not beneficial (Deahl et al., 2000; Mayou, Ehlers, & Hobbs, 2000; Rose, Brewin, Andrews, & Kirk, 1999) and may even be harmful (Bisson, Jenkins, Alexander, & Bannister, 1997; Hobbs, Mayou, Harrison, & Worlock, 1996). In light of these findings and the mounting criticisms discussed earlier, experts have ultimately concluded that CISD is contraindicated for victims of trauma.

Psychological First Aid

Psychological first aid is currently the most advocated approach for intervening with victims of a recent trauma (Litz et al., 2002; National Institute of Mental Health, 2002). This intervention was developed by researchers at the National Child Traumatic Stress Network and the National Center for PTSD as an evidence-informed approach for supporting individuals exposed to disasters, terrorism, and other potentially traumatic events. The techniques that constitute psychological first aid are in line with empirical research on risk and resilience following trauma, applicable and practical in the field, developmentally appropriate, and culturally informed (National Child Traumatic Stress Network & National Center for PTSD, 2006). Unlike CISD, psychological first aid does not assume that all trauma survivors will develop chronic mental health problems, and it is limited to those who request professional support in the aftermath of a traumatic stressor. The intervention aims to enhance the immediate and ongoing safety of victims, and it assists trauma survivors in addressing current or anticipated problems in a compassionate, nonintrusive manner. A more thorough description of psychological first aid is beyond the scope of this chapter. However, we do provide a brief overview of four intervention components that have particular relevance for victims of violent crime. These include information gathering, safety planning, practical assistance, and offering information on coping.

Information Gathering. An important form of early intervention with the victim of a violent crime involves screening and assessment. The purpose of this assessment should be to identify the victim's immediate needs (e.g., shelter, safety, medical concerns) and to screen for trauma-specific incident characteristics and psychological factors that might place the trauma survivor at increased risk of developing longer-term mental health problems.

Clinicians are advised to follow the crime victim's lead when assessing the trauma, in that trauma survivors should always be given the choice whether to discuss distressing aspects of their assault (McNally, Bryant, & Ehlers, 2003). When a victim expresses a willingness to talk about the incident, initial questions should cover basic areas such as when and where the assault occurred and the relationship of the perpetrator to the victim. The powerful effects exerted by several of the aforementioned incident characteristics on posttrauma functioning also argue for their inclusion in this initial assessment. Inclusion of these factors in assessment increases the precision with which predictions about long-term functioning can be made. For example, repeated physical assault by a spouse involving high-perceived life threat and multiple contusions would be expected to produce different results from a single assault without perceived life threat or physical injury.

When conducting this type of assessment, it is important both clinically and ethically to create an environment in which self-disclosure is met with acceptance, empathy, and encouragement. To maximize sensitivity, assessment questions should include (a) empathetic preface statements that provide appropriate context for answers and (b) behavioral descriptions of index events that elicit closed-ended responses. Victims will disclose extremely personal and frequently humiliating information only when they feel that such disclosure is worthwhile and relevant. Simply asking a woman to describe a rape without appropriate preface statements fails to demonstrate concern for the respondent's welfare and fails to prompt her to think of all potential assault events. Rather, a preface statement should provide a simple context within which interviewees can comfortably respond. Resnick, Falsetti, Kilpatrick, and Freedy (1996) suggested brief prefacing statements that demonstrate concern on the part of interviewer and understanding of the nonrare nature of traumatic events.

Use of behaviorally specific closed-ended questions increases the likelihood that traumatic events will be reported and operationally definable. For example, instead of asking a woman whether she has ever been the victim of a sexual assault, it may be more informative to ask whether she has ever experienced forced unwanted vaginal, oral, or anal penetration by a person's penis, fingers, tongue, or some other object. This is because behavior-based queries are less affected by cultural and individual differences of respondents. In addition, it may be less aversive for some victims to answer *yes* or *no* to questions about particular behavioral events than to generate descriptive information about their assault. As such, sources of error produced by personal definitions of assault, or respondent inability or hesitancy to disclose information relating to victimization, are minimized.

In contrast to epidemiological researchers, clinicians will frequently consider only the trauma that brought the adult in for treatment. However, studies indicate that between 35% and 50% of physically and sexually assaulted individuals have been victimized more than once (Basile et al., 2007; Kilpatrick, 1990). Given these data, adults should be queried about their experiences with multiple types of trauma across the life span. This point is particularly important because the psychological responses and treatment needs of individuals who have been previously assaulted may differ significantly from those who have not experienced such victimization. In addition to these assault parameters, it is also important to screen for other contextual factors that influence posttraumatic outcome, including prior history of psychopathology or suicide attempts, acute emotional reactions such as anxiety or panic, cognitive responses to the traumatic event (e.g., catastrophic thinking), and level of perceived social support.

Suicidality and homicidality should also be assessed among victims of a recent crime. Individuals who present with symptoms of depression may express thoughts of self-harm. Furthermore, crime victims who fear being harmed again or those experiencing intense anger may report a desire to retaliate against the perpetrator of their assault. When screening for suicide and homicide, clinicians are encouraged to pay particular attention to factors that increase the likelihood of these events (e.g., ideation, threats, active preparation, past history of attempts; Linehan, 1993). If an individual is deemed to be at elevated risk of suicide or homicide, efforts should be taken on the part of the clinician to reduce this risk (described in the next section).

Safety Planning. Another important form of early intervention involves safety planning. The crime victim and clinician should work together to evaluate current safety and to determine situations with high risk of future victimization (e.g., frequent contact with the perpetrator at work or in the home). After potentially dangerous situations are identified, the clinician should assist the victim in developing an appropriate action plan. Action plans should be tailored to the different situations the patient is likely to encounter (e.g., when faced with imminent violence, when alcohol and drugs are involved; Dutton, Mitchell, & Haywood, 1996). The clinician should orally review the action plan and provide visual reminders (e.g., reminder card to place in purse or wallet) as a way to increase the probability that the plan will be implemented at the appropriate time. It is also critical to verify that recent crime victims have a safe place to reside in the immediate aftermath of an assault and to refer them to social service agencies (e.g., domestic violence shelters, other emergency housing facilities) if needed.

When indicated, safety planning should also include strategies to prevent suicidality and homicidality. If it is determined that an individual is at high risk of suicide and verbalizes this risk, hospitalization may be necessary to ensure safety. Crime victims who acknowledge thoughts of self-harm but deny intent may still benefit from specific information regarding suicide hotlines, 24-hour crisis lines, social service referrals, and support groups.

If clients express thoughts about retaliating against the perpetrator of their assault, it can be helpful to normalize their anger and to distinguish appropriate actions from thoughts and feelings. However, if the clinician believes that the client is at high risk of committing an act of violence (i.e., he or she has the means and a plan for committing such an act), steps must be taken to ensure the safety of the potential victim (these might include notifying local authorities).

Practical Assistance. It is common for individuals to experience feelings of hopelessness in the aftermath of a violent event. Providing victims with practical assistance to meet their immediate needs may help foster a sense of empowerment and optimism. The victim of a violent crime will likely benefit from information regarding legal advocacy and involvement in the criminal justice system. Clinicians can also provide individuals with contact information for social service agencies that provide short-term housing, financial assistance, or mental health provision. Many victims have a limited understanding of the role of legal-system advocates and the steps involved in prosecuting a case. Furthermore, victims may be eligible for crime victim's compensation, which can help offset financial costs related to medical and mental health treatment directly related to a crime. Whenever possible, clinicians should provide crime victims the telephone numbers of relevant emergency and victims' service agencies so they are able to access needed services such as domestic violence hotlines or shelters, rape crisis advocacy programs, or information about legal system issues. Victims of sexual assault should also be encouraged to seek a medical exam to assess for internal injuries, potential pregnancy, or sexually transmitted infection. If victims present within 72 hours of a sexual assault, forensic evidence can also be collected. These types of protective action are recommended regardless of whether the victim chooses to report the crime.

Information on Coping. Crime victims who are experiencing extreme psychological distress may benefit from psychoeducation about common stress reactions and adaptive coping techniques. Information about symptoms that are common in the aftermath of a traumatic stressor can help validate the crime victim's experience, normalize reactions, and dispel faulty beliefs (McFarlane, 2001). In addition, information about strategies for coping may help reduce immediate distress and promote a sense of personal control. Examples of coping methods that may be helpful for the victim of a recent trauma include spending time with others, scheduling pleasant activities throughout the day, getting adequate rest, and engaging in relaxation techniques. Two commonly used relaxation techniques are diaphragmatic breathing and progressive muscle relaxation. Individuals in acute distress often show signs of hyperventilation, or overbreathing (Holt & Andrews, 1989). Diaphragmatic breathing exercises aim to reduce hyperventilation by teaching clients to engage in slow, regular, rhythmic abdominal breathing whenever they experience elevated levels of tension or stress. During progressive muscle relaxation, the trauma victim learns to distinguish between feelings of tension and relaxation in the body by engaging in different tension–relaxation exercises for each major muscle group. Individuals are also taught to pair cue words (e.g., *relax, calm*) or a pleasant image with feelings of relaxation, and they are encouraged to focus on these cues whenever they experience anxiety or distress. In addition to these relaxation techniques, individuals should be discouraged from engaging in potentially harmful coping methods such as the use of drugs or alcohol, withdrawal from family and friends, or engagement in self-harm behaviors.

Symptom-Based Assessment

Experts typically recommend waiting at least 1 week (Gray & Litz, 2005) or as long as 1 month (Brewin, 2003) before conducting symptom-based psychological assessment with the victim of a recent trauma. Assessments conducted earlier will have limited clinical utility because the level of distress experienced immediately posttrauma is not a strong predictor of risk of later psychological problems (Bryant, 2003; Rothbaum & Foa, 1993). Indeed, it is common for many victims of crime to experience extreme distress in the acute aftermath of a traumatic event. Most of these individuals will go through a process of gradual recovery involving a steady decrease in symptoms over time. When symptoms persist for several weeks or months following a traumatic event, however, this should be viewed as a marker of risk for poor outcomes. By monitoring crime victims' symptom levels from week to week, clinicians may be better able to identify individuals who will benefit from formal intervention.

Symptom-based assessment with the victim of a recent trauma should include measures of ASD (if the assessment occurs within 1 month of the event), as well as more general measures of anxiety, depression, and panic. Two self-report measures that correspond directly to DSM–IV–TR symptom criteria for ASD include the Stanford Acute Stress Reaction Questionnaire (Cardena, Koopman, Classen, Waelde, & Spiegel, 2000) and the Acute Stress Disorder Scale (Bryant, Moulds, & Guthrie, 2000). The Acute Stress Disorder Interview (Bryant, Harvey, Dang, & Sackville, 1998) is a structured clinical interview that is frequently used to assess ASD among adults. An example of a commonly used self-report measure of anxiety severity is the Beck Anxiety Inventory (Beck & Steer, 1991). The Beck Depression Inventory (Beck, Ward, Mendelsohn, Mock, & Erbaugh, 1961) is also frequently used in clinical and research settings to assess depressive symptomatology among adults. A self-report inventory that can be used to assess symptoms of panic is the Physical Reactions Scale (Falsetti & Resnick, 1992). Many of these scales have strong psychometric properties, and they can be administered to adults in a relatively short period of time (5–10 minutes each). Detailed papers have been dedicated to the topic of symptom-based assessment with victims of a recent trauma (e.g., see Bryant, 2004; Orsillo, 2001), and the reader is referred to such sources for more in-depth reviews of available measures.

Formal Treatment for Victims of Acute Trauma

Formal treatment may be indicated for crime victims who continue to report distress symptoms several weeks following the trauma. Bryant, Harvey, Dang, Sackville, and Basten (1998) developed a brief, five-session, cognitive–behavioral intervention for trauma victims with ASD. This individually administered intervention includes psychoeducation, relaxation training, cognitive restructuring, and exposure-based elements. Treatment is usually delivered 2 to 4 weeks posttrauma. During the psychoeducation phase, the therapist provides the client with accurate information about the prevalence of interpersonal victimization and common psychological responses to traumatic events. During the relaxation training phase, clients are taught various anxiety management techniques (e.g., diaphragmatic breathing, progressive muscle relaxation) they can use to cope with trauma-related distress.

Cognitive techniques are also used to reduce anxiety and distress by teaching clients to become aware of their negative thoughts and dysfunctional beliefs (e.g., that the world is unsafe) and to modify them through cognitive restructuring techniques. Imaginal exposure represents a critical component of the intervention. During imaginal exposure, the client is instructed to describe the traumatic event in as much detail as possible, focusing on the environmental stimuli, behavior, cognitions, and emotions that they experienced and observed during the traumatic event. Repeated imaginal exposure is thought to facilitate fear extinction, which refers to the gradual reduction in anxiety over time (see chap. 17, this volume, for a detailed description of these intervention components). The short- and long-term effectiveness of Bryant's intervention has been established in a number of randomized controlled trials with survivors of motor vehicle accidents and physical assaults (e.g., see Bryant et al., 2006; Bryant, Harvey, Dang, Sackville, & Basten, 1998; Bryant, Moulds, Guthrie, & Nixon, 2005; Bryant, Moulds, & Nixon, 2003; Bryant, Sackville, Dang, Moulds, & Guthrie, 1999). This intervention appears to accelerate mental health recovery following a traumatic event, which is important to increasing quality of life and minimizing periods of functional impairment.

Foa, Hearst-Ikeda, and Perry (1995) also developed a brief prevention program for adults who had recently experienced a violent assault. This cognitive–behavioral intervention is delivered in an individual therapy format. It consists of four sessions that are initiated 2 weeks following a traumatic event. The components of the intervention are similar to those used by Bryant, Harvey, Dang, Sackville, and Basten (1998). Foa et al. conducted a pilot study of their program with a small sample of female sexual assault survivors. Adults who received the intervention experienced greater reductions in trauma-related symptoms relative to an assessment-only control condition at posttreatment. Although this is a promising result, it should be mentioned that participants were not randomly assigned to the different study conditions. Thus, randomized controlled trials are needed to increase confidence in conclusions about the efficacy of this program for victims of a recent crime.

RESOURCES FOR CLINICIANS

The following professional organizations and Web sites provide useful and up-to-date information regarding acute psychological interventions for victims of crime and can serve as useful resources for clinicians. The International Society for Trauma Stress Studies is a multidisciplinary organization that works to promote the advancement and exchange of information about trauma and its effects. The organization's Web site (http://www.istss.org) provides valuable information regarding empirically supported interventions for PTSD, fact sheets on the prevalence of different traumatic stressors, and information on training opportunities for clinicians. The National Center for PTSD's Web site (http://www.ncptsd.va.gov) is another helpful educational resource for mental health providers. This Web site provides a link to the complete psychological first aid manual, as well as links to various measures for assessing trauma exposure and PTSD.

The National Child Traumatic Stress Network represents a collaboration among several trauma treatment and research centers in the United States. The network is funded by the Substance Abuse and Mental Health Services Administration. Its mission is to improve the quality, effectiveness, and availability of therapeutic services for children and adolescents experiencing traumatic events. The network's Web site (http://www.nctsnet.org) includes a review of available assessment measures as well as a list of empirically supported treatments for traumatic stress among youth. Finally, the Medical University of South Carolina's National Crime Victims Research and Treatment Center (NCVC) has conducted considerable research over the years aimed at improving the quality of mental health services for victims of crime, abuse, and trauma. Clinicians are referred to the NCVC's Web site (http://www.musc.edu/ncvc) for detailed reviews of this research. It is important to note that several of these Web sites also provide links to handouts for the general public on the prevalence of different traumatic stressors, common psychological reactions, and empirically supported intervention techniques. Many of these handouts are available in both English and Spanish.

CONCLUSION

In sum, the literature indicates that a substantial number of adults are exposed to interpersonal violence. Although many individuals experience psychological distress in the acute aftermath of a traumatic stressor, only a minority go on to develop more chronic mental health problems. Given this, clinicians are advised against delivering formal debriefing interventions to all victims in the acute phase and to instead focus on the provision of psychological first aid to those who request help following a violent event. Furthermore, appropriately timed assessments should be used to monitor changes in the victim's symptom presentation. For adults who continue to experience distress symptoms several weeks following a traumatic event, evidence-based cognitive–behavioral interventions may be indicated.

REFERENCES

American Psychiatric Association. (1994). *Diagnostic and statistical manual of mental disorders* (4th ed.). Washington, DC: Author.

American Psychiatric Association. (2000). *Diagnostic and statistical manual of mental disorders* (4th ed., text rev.). Washington, DC: Author.

Amir, M., Weil, G., Kaplan, Z., Tocker, T., & Witztum, E. (1998). Debriefing with brief group therapy in a homogenous group of non-injured victims of a terrorist attack: A prospective study. *Acta Psychiatrica Scandinavica, 98*, 237–242.

Andrews, B., Brewin, C. R., Rose, S., & Kirk, M. (2000). Predicting PTSD in victims of violent crime: The role of shame, anger, and blame. *Journal of Abnormal Psychology, 109*, 69–73.

Arrata, C. M. (2002). Child sexual abuse and sexual revictimization. *Clinical Psychology: Science and Practice, 9*, 135–164.

Basile, K. C., Chen, J., Black, M. C., & Saltzman, L. E. (2007). Prevalence and characteristics of sexual violence victimization among U.S. adults, 2001–2003. *Violence and Victims, 22*, 437–448.

Beck, A. T., & Steer, R. A. (1991). Relationship between the Beck Anxiety Inventory and the Hamilton Anxiety Rating Scale with anxious outpatients. *Journal of Anxiety Disorders, 5*, 213–223.

Beck, A. T., Ward, C. H., Mendelsohn, M., Mock, J., & Erbaugh, J. (1961). An inventory for measuring depression. *Archives of General Psychiatry, 4*, 561–571.

Bisson, J. L., Jenkins, P. L., Alexander, J., & Bannister, C. (1997). Randomised controlled trial of psychological debriefing for victims of acute burn trauma. *The British Journal of Psychiatry, 171*, 78–81.

Bonanno, G. A. (2004). Loss, trauma, and human resilience: Have we underestimated the human capacity to thrive after extremely aversive events? *American Psychologist, 59*, 20–28.

Boudreaux, E., Kilpatrick, D. G., Resnick, H. S., Best, C. L., & Saunders, B. E. (1998). Criminal victimization, posttraumatic stress disorder, and comorbid psychopathology among a community sample of women. *Journal of Traumatic Stress, 11*, 665–678.

Breslau, N., Kessler, R. C., Chilcoat, H. D., Schultz, L. R., Davis, G. C., & Andreski, P. (1998). Trauma and posttraumatic stress disorder in the community. *Archives of General Psychiatry, 55*, 626–632.

Brewin, C. R. (2003). *Post-traumatic stress disorder: Malady or myth?* New Haven, CT: Yale University Press.

Bryant, R. A. (2003). Early predictors of posttraumatic stress disorder. *Biological Psychiatry, 53*, 789–795.

Bryant, R. A. (2004). Assessing acute stress disorder. In J. P. Wilson & T. M. Keane (Eds.), *Assessing psychological trauma and PTSD* (2nd ed., pp. 45–60). New York: Guilford Press.

Bryant, R. A. (2006). Cognitive–behavioral therapy for acute stress disorder. In V. M. Follette & J. I. Ruzek (Eds.), *Cognitive–behavioral therapies for trauma* (pp. 201–227). New York: Guilford Press.

Bryant, R. A., Harvey, A. G., Dang, S. T., & Sackville, T. (1998). Assessing acute stress disorder: Psychometric properties of a structured clinical interview. *Psychological Assessment, 10*, 215–220.

Bryant, R. A., Harvey, A. G., Dang, S. T., Sackville, T., & Basten, C. (1998). Treatment of acute stress disorder: A comparison of cognitive–behavior therapy and supportive counseling. *Journal of Consulting and Clinical Psychology, 66*, 862–866.

Bryant, R. A., Harvey, A. G., Guthrie, R. M., & Moulds, M. L. (2000). A prospective study of acute psychophysiological arousal, acute stress disorder, and posttraumatic stress disorder. *Journal of Abnormal Psychology, 109*, 341–344.

Bryant, R. A., Moulds, M. L., & Guthrie, R. (2000). Acute Stress Disorder Scale: A self-report measure of acute stress disorder. *Psychological Assessment, 12*, 61–68.

Bryant, R. A., Moulds, M. L., Guthrie, R. M., & Nixon, R. D. V. (2005). The additive benefit of hypnotherapy and cognitive–behavior therapy in treating acute stress disorder. *Journal of Consulting and Clinical Psychology, 73*, 334–340.

Bryant, R. A., Moulds, M. L., & Nixon, R. D. V. (2003). Cognitive–behavior therapy of acute stress disorder: A four-year follow-up. *Behaviour Research and Therapy, 41*, 489–494.

Bryant, R. A., Moulds, M. L., Nixon, R. D. V., Mastrodomenico, J., Felmingham, K., & Hopwood, S. (2006). Hypnotherapy and cognitive–behaviour therapy of acute stress disorder: A 3-year follow-up. *Behaviour Research and Therapy, 44*, 1331–1335.

Bryant, R. A., Sackville, T., Dang, S. T., Moulds, M. L., & Guthrie, R. M. (1999). Treating acute stress disorder: An evaluation of cognitive–behavior therapy and counseling techniques. *American Journal of Psychiatry, 156*, 1780–1786.

Campbell, J. C., Jones, A. S., Dienemann, J., Kub, J., Schollenberger, J., O'Campo, P., et al. (2002). Intimate partner violence and physical health consequences. *Archives of Internal Medicine, 162*, 1157–63.

Cardena, E., Koopman, C., Classen, C., Waelde, L. C., & Spiegel, D. (2000). Psychometric properties of the Stanford Acute Stress Reaction Questionnaire (SASRQ): A valid and reliable measure of acute stress. *Journal of Traumatic Stress, 13*, 719–734.

Catalano, S. M. (2006). *Criminal victimization, 2005* (Publication No. NCJ 214644). Washington, DC: Office of Justice Programs.

Centers for Disease Control and Prevention. (2003). *Costs of intimate partner violence against women in the United States*. Retrieved November 15, 2006, from http://www.cdc.gov/ncipc/pubres/ipv_cost/ipv.htm

Chemtob, C. M., Tomas, S., Law, W., & Cremniter, D. (1997). Postdisaster psychosocial intervention: A field study of the impact of debriefing on psychological distress. *American Journal of Psychiatry, 154*, 415–417.

Classen, C. C., Palesh, O. G., & Aggarwal, R. (2005). Sexual revictimization: A review of the empirical literature. *Trauma, Violence, and Abuse, 6*, 103–129.

Coker, A. L., Davis, K. E., Arias, I., Desai, S., Sanderson, M., Brandt, H. M., & Smith, P. (2002). Physical and mental health effects of intimate partner violence for men and women. *American Journal of Preventive Medicine, 23*, 260–268.

Cottler, L. B., Compton, W. M., Mager, D., Spitznagel, E. L., & Janca, A. (1992). Posttraumatic stress disorder among substance users from the general population. *American Journal of Psychiatry, 149*, 664–670.

Cottler, L. B., Helzer, J. E., & Tripp, J. E. (1990). Lifetime patterns of substance use among general population subjects engaging in high risk sexual behavior: Implications for HIV risk. *American Journal of Drug and Alcohol Abuse*, 16, 207–222.

Dansky, B. S., Saladin, M. E., Brady, K. T., Kilpatrick, D. G., & Resnick, H. S. (1995). Prevalence of victimization and posttraumatic stress disorder among women with substance use disorders: Comparison of telephone and in-person assessment samples. *International Journal of Addictions*, 30, 1079–1099.

Deahl, M., Srinivasan, M., Jones, N., Thomas, J., Neblett, C., & Jolly, A. (2000). Preventing psychological trauma in soldiers: The role of operational stress training and psychological debriefing. *British Journal of Medical Psychology*, 73, 77–85.

Denson, T. F., Marshall, G. N., Schell, T. L., & Jaycox, L. H. (2007). Predictors of posttraumatic distress 1 year after exposure to community violence: The importance of acute symptom severity. *Journal of Consulting and Clinical Psychology*, 75, 683–692.

Desai, S., Arias, I., Thompson, M. P., & Basile, K. C. (2002). Childhood victimization and subsequent adult revictimization assessed in a nationally representative sample of women and men. *Violence and Victims*, 17, 639–653.

Dutton, M. A., Mitchell, B., & Haywood, Y. (1996). The emergency department as a violence prevention center. *Journal of the American Medical Women's Association*, 51, 92–95.

Engelhard, I. M., van den Hout, M. A., Arntz, A., & McNally, R. J. (2002). A longitudinal study of "intrusion-based reasoning" and posttraumatic stress disorder after exposure to a train disaster. *Behaviour Research and Therapy*, 40, 1415–1424.

Everly, G. S., & Mitchell, J. T. (1999). *Critical incident stress management (CISM): A new era and standard of care in crisis intervention* (2nd ed.). Ellicott City, MD: Chevron.

Falsetti, S. A., & Resnick, H. S. (1992). *The Physical Reactions Scale*. Charleston, SC: National Crime Victims Research and Treatment Center, Medical University of South Carolina.

Falsetti, S. A., & Resnick, H. S. (1997). Trauma, posttraumatic stress disorder, and panic attacks: Frequency, severity, and implications for treatment. *Journal of Traumatic Stress*, 10, 683–689.

Foa, E. B., Hearst-Ikeda, D., & Perry, K. J. (1995). Evaluation of a brief cognitive–behavioral program for the prevention of chronic PTSD in recurrent assault victims. *Journal of Consulting and Clinical Psychology*, 63, 948–955.

Goodman, L. A., Koss, M. P., & Russo, N. F. (1993). Violence against women: Physical and mental health effects: Part I. Research findings. *Applied and Preventive Psychology*, 2, 79–89.

Gray, M. J., & Litz, B. T. (2005). Behavioral interventions for recent trauma: Empirically informed practice guidelines. *Behavior Modification*, 29, 189–215.

Greenfield, L. A., & Smith, S. K. (1999). *American Indians and crime* (Publication No. NCJ 173386). Washington, DC: Office of Justice Programs.

Hanson, R. F., Kilpatrick, D. G., Falsetti, S. A., & Resnick, H. S. (1995). Violent crime and mental health. In J. R. Freedy & S. E. Hobfoll (Eds.), *Traumatic stress: From theory to practice* (pp. 129–161). New York: Plenum Press.

Hapke, U., Schumann, A., Rumpf, H. J., John, U., & Meyer, C. (2006). Posttraumatic stress disorder: The role of trauma, pre-existing psychiatric disorder, and gender. *European Archives of Psychiatry & Clinical Neuroscience, 256*, 299–306.

Harvey, A. G., & Bryant, R. A. (1998). Relationship of acute stress disorder and posttraumatic stress disorder following motor vehicle accidents. *Journal of Consulting and Clinical Psychology, 66*, 507–512.

Hobbs, M., Mayou, R., Harrison, B., & Worlock, P. (1996, December 7). A randomised controlled trial of psychological debriefing for victims of road traffic accidents. *BMJ, 313*, 1438–1439.

Holt, P. E., & Andrews, G. (1989). Hyperventilation and anxiety in panic disorder, social phobia, GAD and normal controls. *Behaviour Research and Therapy, 27*, 453–460.

Jaycox, L. H., Marshall, G. N., & Orlando, M. (2003). Predictors of acute distress among young adults injured by community violence. *Journal of Traumatic Stress, 16*, 237–245.

Keane, T. M., Kaufman, M., & Kimble, M. O. (2001). Peritraumatic dissociative symptoms, acute stress disorder, and the development of posttraumatic stress disorder: Causation, correlation or epiphenomena. In L. Sanchez-Planell & C. Diez-Quevedo (Eds.), *Dissociative states* (pp. 21–43). Barcelona, Spain: Springer-Verlag.

Kessler, R. C., Sonnega, A., Bromet, E., Hughes, M., & Nelson, C. B. (1995). Posttraumatic stress disorder in the National Comorbidity Survey. *Archives of General Psychiatry, 52*, 1048–1060.

Kilpatrick, D. G. (1990, August). *Violence as a precursor of women's substance abuse: The rest of the drug-violence story.* Paper presented at the 98th Annual Convention of the American Psychological Association, Boston, MA.

Kilpatrick, D. G., Acierno, R., Resnick, H. S., Saunders, B. E., & Best, C. L. (1997). A 2-year longitudinal analysis of the relationship between violent assault and alcohol and drug use in women. *Journal of Consulting and Clinical Psychology, 65*, 834–847.

Kilpatrick, D. G., Edmunds, C. N., & Seymour, A. K. (1992). *Rape in America: A report to the nation.* Arlington, VA: National Victim Center and Medical University of South Carolina.

Kilpatrick, D. G., & Resnick, H. S. (1993). PTSD associated with exposure to criminal victimization in clinical and community populations. In J. R. Davidson & E. B. Foa (Eds.), *Post-traumatic stress disorder in review: Recent research and future directions* (pp. 113–143). Washington, DC: American Psychiatric Press.

Kilpatrick, D. G, Ruggiero, K. J., Acierno, R., Saunders, B. E., Resnick, H. S., & Best, C. L. (2003). Violence and risk of PTSD, major depression, substance abuse/dependence, and comorbidity: Results from the National Survey of Adolescents. *Journal of Consulting and Clinical Psychology, 71*, 692–700.

Kilpatrick, D. G., Saunders, B. E., Amick-McMullan, A., Best, C. L., Veronen, L. J., & Resnick, H. S. (1989). Victim and crime factors associated with the development of crime-related posttraumatic stress disorder. *Behavior Therapy, 20*, 199–214.

Kimerling, R., Alvarez, J., Pavao, J., Kaminski, A., & Baumrind, N. (2007). Epidemiology and consequences of women's revictimization. *Women's Health Issues, 17*, 101–106.

King, D. W., King, L. A., Erickson, D. J., Huang, M. T., Sharkansky, E. J., & Wolfe, J. (2000). Posttraumatic stress disorder and retrospectively reported stressor exposure: A longitudinal prediction model. *Journal of Abnormal Psychology, 109*, 624–633.

Koopman, C., Classen, C., & Spiegel, D. (1994). Predictors of posttraumatic stress symptoms among survivors of the Oakland/Berkeley, California firestorm. *American Journal of Psychiatry, 151*, 888–894.

Linehan, M. M. (1993). *Cognitive–behavioral treatment of borderline personality disorder*. New York: Guilford Press.

Litz, B. T., Gray, M. J., Bryant, R. A., & Adler, A. B. (2002). Early intervention for trauma: Current status and future directions. *Clinical Psychology: Science and Practice, 9*, 112–134.

Mayou, R., Ehlers, A., & Hobbs, M. (2000). Psychological debriefing for road traffic accident victims: Three-year follow-up of a randomised controlled trial. *The British Journal of Psychiatry, 176*, 589–593.

McFarlane, A. C. (2001). Dual diagnosis and treatment of PTSD. In J. P. Wilson, M. J. Friedman, & J. D. Lindy (Eds.), *Treating psychological trauma and PTSD* (pp. 237–254). New York: Guilford Press.

McFarlane, A. C., Atchison, M., & Yehuda, R. (1997). The acute stress response following motor vehicle accidents and its relation to PTSD. In R. Yehuda & A. C. McFarlane (Eds.), *Psychobiology of posttraumatic stress disorder* (pp. 433–436). New York: New York Academy of Sciences.

McNally, R. J., Bryant, R. A., & Ehlers, A. (2003). Does early psychological intervention promote recovery from posttraumatic stress? *Psychological Science in the Public Interest, 4*, 45–79.

Mitchell, J. T., & Everly, G. S. (1996). *Critical incident stress debriefing: An operations manual for the prevention of traumatic stress among emergency services and disaster workers* (2nd ed.). Ellicott City, MD: Chevron.

National Child Traumatic Stress Network & National Center for PTSD. (2006). *Psychological first aid: Field operations guide* (2nd ed.). Retrieved November 15, 2006, from http://www.ncptsd.va.gov/ncmain/ncdocs/manuals/nc_manual_psyfirstaid.html

National Institute of Mental Health. (2002). *Mental health and mass violence: Evidence-based early psychological intervention for victims/survivors of mass violence: A workshop to reach consensus on best practices* (NIH Publication No. 02-5138). Washington, DC: U.S. Government Printing Office.

Norris, F. H., Friedman, M. J., Watson, P. J., Byrne, C. M., Diaz, E., & Kaniasty, K. (2002). 60,000 disaster victims speak: Part I. An empirical review of the empirical literature, 1981–2001. *Psychiatry, 65*, 207–239.

Orsillo, S. (2001). Measures of acute stress disorder and posttraumatic stress disorder. In M. M. Antony, S. Orsillo, & L. Roemer (Eds.), *Practitioner's guide to empirically based measures of anxiety* (pp. 255–307). New York: Kluwer Academic/ Plenum Publishers.

Ozer, E. J., Best, S. R., Lipsey, T. L., & Weiss, D. S. (2003). Predictors of posttraumatic stress disorder and symptoms in adults: A meta-analysis. *Psychological Bulletin, 129*, 52–73.

Plichta, S. B. (2004). Intimate partner violence and physical health consequences: Policy and practice implications. *Journal of Interpersonal Violence, 19*, 1296–323.

Resnick, H. S., Falsetti, S. A., Kilpatrick, D. G., & Freedy, J. R. (1996). Assessment of rape and other civilian trauma-related PTSD: Emphasis on assessment of potentially traumatic events. In T. W. Miller (Ed.), *Theory and assessment of stressful life events* (pp. 235–271). Madison, CT: International Universities Press.

Resnick, H. S., Kilpatrick, D. G., Dansky, B. S., Saunders, B. E., & Best, C. L. (1993). Prevalence of civilian trauma and PTSD in a representative national sample of women. *Journal of Consulting and Clinical Psychology, 61*, 984–991.

Reynolds, M. W., Peipert, J. F., & Collins, B. (2000). Epidemiological issues of sexually transmitted diseases in sexual assault victims. *Obstetrical and Gynecological Survey, 55*, 51–57.

Rose, S., Brewin, C. R., Andrews, B., & Kirk, M. (1999). A randomized controlled trial of individual psychological debriefing for victims of violent crime. *Psychological Medicine, 29*, 793–799.

Rothbaum, B. O., & Foa, E. B. (1993). Subtypes of posttraumatic stress disorder and duration of symptoms. In J. R. T. Davidson & E. B. Foa (Eds.), *Posttraumatic stress disorder: DSM–IV and beyond* (pp. 23–35). Washington, DC: American Psychiatric Press.

Tjaden, P., & Thoennes, N. (2000a). *Extent, nature, and consequences of intimate partner violence: Findings from the national violence against women survey* (Publication No. NCJ 181867). Washington, DC: U.S. Department of Justice.

Tjaden P., & Thoennes N. (2000b). *Full report of the prevalence, incidence, and consequences of violence against women: Findings from the national violence against women survey* (Publication No. NCJ 183781). Washington, DC: U.S. Department of Justice.

Weaver, T. L., & Clum, G. A. (1995). Psychological distress associated with interpersonal violence: A meta-analysis. *Clinical Psychology Review, 15*, 115–140.

Wessley, S., Rose, S., & Bisson, J. (2000). Brief psychological interventions ("debriefing") for trauma-related symptoms and the prevention of posttraumatic stress disorder. *Cochrane Database of Systematic Reviews, 4*. Available from http:// www.cochrane.org

Yehuda, R. (2002). Posttraumatic stress disorder. *The New England Journal of Medicine, 346*, 108–114.

Yule, W. (1992). Post-traumatic stress disorder in child survivors of shipping disasters: The sinking of the "Jupiter." *Psychotherapy and Psychosomatics, 57*, 200–205.

9

RISK OF INTIMATE PARTNER VIOLENCE: FACTORS ASSOCIATED WITH PERPETRATION AND VICTIMIZATION

DAVID S. RIGGS, MARIE B. CAULFIELD, AND KATHRYN FAIR

Intimate partner violence (IPV) encompasses behaviors ranging from slaps or pushes during an argument through the severe physical violence and coercion identified as abuse or battering to the extreme of femicide or homicide. Determining risk of such violence is difficult and complex because of the variety of definitions for IPV. Risk factors may be different if we are concerned about risk of any violence, risk of severe violence, risk of injury, or risk of death. The problem is further complicated by other issues. Are we interested in risk of perpetration or risk of victimization? Is the issue imminent risk (i.e., Is this person safe to go home today?) or risk over time (i.e., Is this person likely to experience violence some time in the future?)? Clearly, these questions must be answered in the context in which the clinician is operating and the specifics of the case. In this chapter we do not try to answer these questions per se but rather provide a summary of important issues a clinician faces when evaluating risk of domestic violence.

We begin this chapter by exploring how IPV has been defined and then discuss the prevalence and consequences of such violence. We proceed to summarize research on proposed correlates of intimate violence perpetration, intimate violence victimization, and specific incidents of IPV, for the purpose of identifying factors that may be considered clinical markers of risk of either perpetration or victimization. Finally, we provide an overview of the recent development of structured assessment tools to quantify risk of violence.

WHAT IS INTIMATE PARTNER VIOLENCE?

Three forms of behavior have been defined as violent in the context of IPV: (a) emotional or verbal abuse, (b) physical violence, and (c) sexual assault. Each of these is subject to multiple definitions, and not all authors include all forms of violence in their discussions, making it more difficult to clearly summarize the literature. One must also consider the definition of *intimate relationship*. Historically, most IPV research has focused on violence within marital relationships. As the field grew, studies examined violence between unmarried partners (i.e., dating, cohabitating, separated, and divorced). More recently, researchers have begun to look at violence within same-sex couples. Another factor that complicates summaries of the existing literature involves the sampling and data collection strategies used in the research. Studies vary as to whether they use nationally representative samples, convenience samples, or samples drawn from identified cases.

Most IPV research and almost all the risk-related IPV research focuses on physical forms of violence. Furthermore, much of the existing research has examined heterosexual relationships and identified the man as the perpetrator and the woman as the victim, although some studies have included male victims of IPV. Acknowledging that the conclusions drawn from the existing literature are limited by the definitions, sampling procedures, and assessment techniques used, there are some conclusions that may be drawn about IPV.

SCOPE OF THE PROBLEM

Data from the National Crime Victimization Survey conducted by the United States Department of Justice indicate that about 0.38% of women (approximately 476,000) and 0.13% of men (approximately 151,000) were assaulted by a spouse, intimate partner, or ex-partner in 2004. Estimates based on other national surveys provide somewhat higher prevalence estimates. For example, data from the National Violence Against Women Survey indicate that about 1.5% of women and almost 1% of men had been physically or sexually assaulted by an intimate partner in the prior 12 months (Tjaden & Thoennes, 2000). Discrepancies may be due to differences in methodology or actual changes in violence rates over time as suggested by the data from the National Crime Victimization Survey, which show a decrease in the number of IPV incidents reported from 1993 to 2004.

Lifelong rates of IPV are even more dramatic. Data from the National Violence Against Women Survey indicate that almost one fourth of women (24.8%) and 1 of every 12 men (7.6%) were victims of IPV at some point in their lifetimes (Tjaden & Thoennes, 2000). Other results provide somewhat higher rates of IPV. For example, in three samples of young adults and adolescents, Moffitt and Caspi (1999) found 25% to 40% of women and 36% to 50% of men had been victims of IPV. It should be noted that most of these estimates include behaviors ranging from pushing and slapping to more severe forms of violence such as beating up and choking. On the basis of an extensive literature review, Wilt and Olson (1996) reported lifetime rates for severe IPV (e.g., hitting with a fist or hard object, beating up, threatening or assaulting with a weapon) as 9% and 1-year estimates of 0.3% to 0.4%. Their lifetime estimate of total physical violence (including behaviors such as slapping and pushing) was 22%, with the 1-year estimate of 8% to 17%.

IPV is a significant problem across cultures. For example, a review of studies conducted prior to 1999 found that across different countries, between 10% and 50% of women had been victims of physical IPV and between 10% and 30% had experienced sexual IPV at least once (World Health Organization, 2002). In a study that surveyed over 24,000 women across 10 different countries, lifetime rates of IPV (i.e., physical or sexual violence) ranged from 15% (in Japan) to 71% (in Ethiopia). Rates of severe physical violence (e.g., hit with a fist, kicked, beat up) ranged from 4% to 49%, with most countries falling between 13% and 26% (World Health Organization, 2005).

The consequences of IPV can be quite serious, including injuries resulting from the IPV as well as broader physical and mental health problems. It is estimated that more than 40% of women and about 20% of men victims of IPV are injured as a result (Tjaden & Thoennes, 2000), although rates of injury may be considerably higher in samples selected for severe or persistent IPV (e.g., see Campbell et al., 2003). In heterosexual couples, women are more likely than men to be injured and require medical attention (Archer, 2000). IPV is one of the most common causes of injuries among women presenting for treatment in emergency departments (Abbott, 1997), and almost 30% of female homicide victims are killed by intimate partners (Greenfield et al., 1998).

IPV contributes to significant emotional and mental health problems. The rate of posttraumatic stress disorder (PTSD) in women victims of IPV is extremely high. In a meta-analysis of 11 studies that largely sampled shelter and domestic violence treatment populations, the average rate of PTSD was

63.8% (Golding, 1999). This is dramatically higher than the lifetime prevalence estimates of 10% to 12% in the female population (Helzer, Robins, & McEvoy, 1987; Kessler, Sonnega, Bromet, Hughes, & Nelson, 1995). Golding (1999) also found that almost 48% of abused women are depressed (compared with general population prevalence rates of between 10% and 20%).

The high rate of IPV and the significance of the associated consequences make it a significant clinical issue that should be addressed by health care providers. In the balance of this chapter, we present a review of the literature pertaining to the assessment of risk of IPV. Research into the problem of IPV and the recent development and testing of risk assessments provide a growing literature on which to base risk assessments. However, it is important to remember that no risk assessment will provide absolute and completely accurate predictions of IPV.

Assessment of Risk of Intimate Partner Violence

Risk of IPV has been examined in three ways: (a) identification of correlates of violent behavior, (b) structured risk assessments comprising rationally derived items, and (c) actuarial risk assessments based on statistical analysis (Hilton & Harris, 2005). Much of the literature examining correlates of IPV is cross-sectional, with a focus on differentiating individuals with any exposure to IPV from those who have never experienced IPV. In contrast, attempts to develop focused risk assessment tools (whether rationally based or empirically derived) have tended to focus on recidivism (i.e., future violence) among individuals who have already experienced IPV.

The assessment of risk as it pertains to IPV depends to a great degree on what aspect of IPV one is trying to predict. Different variables may be important for identifying perpetrators or victims of IPV. Similarly, risk of any physical violence will differ from risk of battering, which may also differ from risk of femicide or homicide. Studies of severe IPV tend to use samples drawn from clinical, shelter, or legal settings. These data are important, but it is not clear how well the results generalize to individuals who are not seeking help or who have not come to the attention of the legal system. In contrast, many studies that attempt to identify risk factors for any IPV use representative samples or convenience samples. Data obtained using these approaches may be of limited clinical utility. Because each of the approaches used to identify individuals at risk of IPV is limited, we tried to draw on results from all the approaches in this review.

An overwhelming majority of the studies examining correlates of IPV, particularly severe forms of violence, have focused on male perpetrators of violence toward women. Violence by women against male partners can also be a problem, as can IPV in gay and lesbian couples (Lockhart, White, Causby, & Isaac, 1994; Waldner-Haugrud, Gratch, & Magruder, 1997), but there are few data available to identify risk factors in these couples. In the absence of good empirical data on risk of female-to-male violence or violence in same sex relationships, clinicians will probably want to consider the risk markers identified for male-to-female IPV with the awareness that they may not function in the same way in these other populations.

Correlates of Intimate Partner Violence Perpetration

The research attempting to relate personal and psychological factors to IPV largely has compared individuals who have perpetrated IPV with those who have not to better understand the phenomenology of such violence. Research has not focused on trying to determine whether a particular individual will perpetrate IPV. We summarize in the next section the major findings in this area and their limitation in aiding such clinical predictions.

Demographic Characteristics

IPV can and does occur in all demographic groups, but many demographic characteristics such as socioeconomic status (SES), age, and race have been related to IPV perpetration or severity. Indeed, one recent review concluded that "almost all demographic variables assessed show some relation to male to female physical aggression" (Schumacher, Slep, & Heyman, 2001, p. 324). In general, younger men with less education and lower incomes are at greater risk of IPV perpetration than are older men with better educations and greater income. Men who self-identify as African American or Hispanic appear at increased risk of IPV (Leonard & Blane, 1992; Straus & Smith, 1990), although this may arise from racial differences in SES. It is important to note that the associations between demographic characteristics and IPV perpetration tend to be quite weak (Schumacher et al., 2001; Stith, Smith, Penn, Ward, & Tritt, 2004) and therefore of limited clinical utility as risk markers.

Relationship Characteristics

Certain relationship characteristics have been identified as risk markers for IPV perpetration. Among the most consistent is that relationships with IPV are more distressed and experience more conflict than relationships without IPV. In a meta-analysis of 25 studies, only 2 failed to find a significant association between relationship satisfaction and IPV, and the composite effect size computed across the studies was in the large range (Stith et al., 2004). Similarly, all of the studies reviewed by Schumacher et al. (2001) show a significant association between satisfaction and IPV with effect sizes ranging from small/medium to large.

Relationship distress may serve as an effective risk marker for IPV. For example, the proportion of couples (approximately 60%) entering marital therapy that report some level of violence or severe violence (O'Leary, Vivian, & Malone, 1992; Vivian & Malone, 1997) is several times higher than in the general population (e.g., see Straus, Gelles, & Steinmetz, 1980). These findings underscore how important it is for clinicians working with distressed couples to routinely assess for the presence of IPV. However, a large number of IPV couples are generally satisfied with their relationships (Bauserman & Arias, 1992; Brinkerhoff & Lupri, 1988). This may be particularly true for young couples in which IPV is likely to be less severe and bidirectional (O'Leary, Barling, Arias, Rosenbaum, Malone, & Tyree, 1989).

Couple communication styles and the presence of verbal or emotional abuse have been associated with physical IPV. Although findings differ depending on the specific measures used, it appears that couples who have experienced IPV exhibit more negative and less positive behaviors while talking with one another (Schumacher et al., 2001). Similarly, verbal or emotional aggression has been consistently related to the perpetration of IPV (Schumacher et al., 2001). In fact, all 15 studies included in a recent meta-analysis revealed significant associations between verbal aggression and physical IPV, and the composite effect size calculated for this variable was the largest of all those reported (Stith et al., 2004).

Reported aggression by the partner can serve as a risk marker for male-to-female IPV. Regardless of whether the partner's aggression represents self-defense or if the partner initiates the violence, the presence of aggression by the female partner is strongly indicative of IPV by the man. Stith et al. (2004) found that in four of the five studies examined, there was a significant and large effect of the women's aggression on their risk of male-to-female IPV. Women's aggression appears to indicate a risk of future male-perpetrated IPV, particularly more severe IPV (Feld & Straus, 1989).

Psychological Characteristics

Men who perpetrate IPV have been found to differ from those who do not on several psychological factors. Some of these factors reflect pathological processes such as depression and substance abuse, whereas others represent characteristics such as attitudes and cognitions.

Psychopathology. Researchers have identified four distinct psychological syndromes that appear to differentiate men who perpetrate IPV from those who do not: (a) depression, (b) PTSD, (c) substance abuse, and (d) borderline personality disorder. Men who perpetrate IPV tend to be more depressed than those who do not (e.g., see Hanson, Cadsky, Harris, & Lalonde, 1997; Rankin, Saunders, & Williams, 2000) and they may also be more likely to be clinically depressed (Maiuro, Cahn, Vitaliano, Wagner, & Zegree, 1988). All five studies reviewed by Schumacher et al. (2001) and 11 of 14 studies reviewed by Stith et al. (2004) showed significant associations between depression and IPV. However, the strength of the relation can vary greatly depending on the sample, severity of IPV, and the measure used (Schumacher et al., 2001; Stith et al., 2004).

Several studies identified an increased risk of IPV related to PTSD or posttraumatic symptoms. Data from the National Vietnam Veterans Readjustment Survey collected from a nationally representative sample of Vietnam veterans in the late 1980s found 2 to 3 times more IPV in veterans with PTSD than those without (Jordan et al., 1992; Kulka et al., 1990). Two additional studies also found increased risk of IPV among Vietnam veterans with PTSD, and the severity of IPV positively correlated with the severity of PTSD symptoms (Beckham, Feldman, Kirby, Hertzberf, & Moore, 1997; Byrne & Riggs, 1996; Riggs, Byrne, Weathers, & Litz, 1995). The use or abuse of alcohol and drugs has been associated with IPV perpetration across studies (e.g., see Heyman, O'Leary, & Jouriles, 1995; Kyriacou et al., 1999; Leonard & Blane, 1992; O'Farrell, van Hutton, & Murphy, 1999). All the studies reviewed by Schumacher et al. (2001) showed an association between substance use and IPV, and 18 of 23 alcohol studies and 4 of the 5 drug studies included in the Stith et al. (2004) meta-analysis revealed a significant effect. The magnitude of effect sizes varied greatly (Schumacher et al., 2001; Stith et al., 2004), possibly because IPV is more strongly related to patterns of substance use (e.g., binge drinking) than to amount of substances used (Schumacher et al., 2001). Overall, Stith et al. found a medium effect for alcohol abuse and a large effect for illicit drug use. The successful treatment of alcohol problems reduces the likelihood of IPV in the future (O'Farrell, Fals-Stewart, Murphy, & Murphy, 2003; O'Farrell, Murphy, Stephan, Fals-Stewart, & Murphy, 2004; Stuart et al., 2003).

Available data suggest a range of personality disruption among men who perpetrate IPV (see Schumacher et al., 2001), and several studies found characteristics of borderline personality disorder among IPV perpetrators (Beasley & Stoltenberg, 1992; D. G. Dutton, Starzomski, & Ryan, 1996; Murphy, Meyer, & O'Leary, 1993). IPV perpetration has also been related to elevations on personality dimensions including narcissism, aggression, and avoidance (Beasley & Stoltenberg, 1992; Hamberger & Hastings, 1991; Hastings & Hamberger, 1988; Murphy et al., 1993), but these differences may reflect perpetrators' tendency to overendorse negative characteristics (Murphy et al., 1993). These studies do not provide sufficient information to develop specific profiles or cut-scores to enable clinicians to quantify the risk of IPV for a particular individual.

Other Psychological Risk Factors. A number of psychological factors that do not typically constitute pathologies have been related to IPV perpetration. These include personality characteristics (e.g., hostility), attitudes (e.g., accepting aggression as a means of solving problems), and cognitive processes (e.g., problem-solving skills). In general, IPV perpetrators are more angry and hostile than nonviolent groups (e.g., see D. G. Dutton, Saunders, Starzomski, & Bartholomew, 1994; Hanson et al., 1997; Leonard & Senchak, 1993) with effect sizes ranging from medium to large (Schumacher et al.,

2001; Stith et al., 2004). IPV perpetration has been related to authoritarianism (Hastings, 1997; Neidig, Friedman, & Collins, 1986) and lack of assertiveness (Rosenbaum & O'Leary, 1981), but few studies have examined these factors and results are inconsistent (Schumacher et al., 2001).

Perpetrators exhibit lower self-esteem and more jealousy than nonviolent men (D. G. Dutton et al., 1994; Holtzworth-Munroe, Stuart, & Hutchinson, 1997; Neidig et al., 1986). However, low self-esteem may be more strongly related to relationship distress than to IPV (e.g., see Russell et al., 1989; Telch & Lindquist, 1984). Jealousy was associated with IPV in three of four studies reviewed by Stith et al. (2004), with moderate effect sizes. Acceptance of aggression (e.g., see Hanson et al., 1997; Smith, 1990) and traditional sex-role attitudes (e.g., see Hurlbert, Whittaker, & Munoz, 1991; Smith, 1990) have been associated with IPV. Stith et al. found that four of five studies found a significant association between attitudes condoning violence and perpetration of IPV with a large composite effect size, and significant associations between traditional sex-role attitudes and IPV in five of seven studies with a medium composite effect size. These studies provide a profile of characteristics that may be related to IPV. However, these variables have not been shown to predict an individual's propensity for violence.

Family of Origin Violence

IPV perpetration is associated with the perpetrators' childhood experiences of family violence, both violence perpetrated against the child (e.g., see D. G. Dutton et al., 1996; Sugarman & Hotaling, 1989) and violence between parents (e.g., see Beasley & Stoltenberg, 1992; O'Leary, Malone, & Tyree, 1994; Sugarman & Hotaling, 1989). This association is found across studies, but the effect sizes tend to be small to medium in magnitude (Schumacher et al., 2001). Thus, although family of origin violence may identify individuals at somewhat higher risk of IPV, many people grow up in violent families and do not perpetrate violence against their own partners.

Conclusion

Many factors have been associated with IPV perpetration. However, despite the moderate to large associations found in research samples, no single factor or small set of factors has been identified to accurately identify all or even most individuals who will eventually perpetrate IPV. Further, little work has been attempted to translate the identified correlations into clinically useful risk assessments, so it is difficult to determine the relative risk for any given individual. It is also not clear whether the correlates of IPV are useful for determining the risk of IPV during a particular period of time (e.g., Is it safe for this person to return to his family this week?). Rather, this approach allows one to identify individuals, namely those presenting with a number of the risk factors, who should be evaluated more carefully.

Correlates of IPV Victimization

Research to identify correlates of IPV victimization has been less extensive than that focused on perpetration, and the results are less consistent. However, as with perpetration, it is clear that no single variable distinguishes individuals who are at risk of IPV victimization from those who are not.

Demographic Characteristics

In general, the associations between demographic characteristics and IPV victimization are weak or inconsistent (Schumacher et al., 2001; Stith et al., 2004). Indeed, two recent review articles concluded that there is little support for a link between age, race, religion, unemployment, education, or prior marriages and IPV victimization.

Psychological Factors

Two aspects of psychopathology have been related to IPV victimization: PTSD and depression. Depression has been related to IPV victimization in a number of studies (e.g., see Cascardi & O'Leary, 1992; Dienemann et al., 2000; Vivian & Malone, 1997). Stith et al. (2004) found that 5 of 6 studies of IPV victimization and depression revealed significant associations with a medium composite effect size. Golding (1999), in a review of 18 studies, found that almost half of the victims (weighted average = 47.6%) were depressed. Studies have found PTSD symptoms to be elevated in victims of IPV (e.g., see Astin, Lawrence, & Foy, 1993; Saunders, 1994; Vitanza, Vogel, & Marshall, 1995). Golding (1999) reported that in 11 studies, almost two thirds of the women (weighted average = 63.7%) met criteria for PTSD.

It is generally thought that psychological symptoms arise as a result of the violence (and associated experiences), rather than serving as a cause. Because most of these studies are cross-sectional in design and obtain reports of psychological issues concurrent with the IPV or as retrospective reports, it is not possible to draw strong conclusions about the direction of causality. In an attempt to address this question, Schumacher et al. (2001) reviewed only studies in which past psychological diagnoses were related to male-to-female IPV; they concluded that no Axis I or Axis II disorders were strongly associated with IPV victimization. Several studies did indicate that symptoms of depression, psychosis, eating disorders, and antisocial personality disorder had weak associations with IPV victimization.

Three different reviews of the IPV literature concluded that the studies linking IPV victimization to substance use or abuse provide only weak support (Hotaling & Sugarman, 1986; Schumacher et al., 2001; Stith et al., 2004). When significant effects do emerge, they are generally small, and numerous studies have failed to find an association (e.g., see Danielson, Moffitt, Caspi, & Silva, 1998; Russell et al., 1989). Stith et al. (2004) calculated a small composite effect size for alcohol use. The results of the few studies examining drug use and abuse are also mixed, with a few finding a correlation and others suggesting no association (Schumacher et al., 2001).

Family of Origin Violence

Two aspects of family of origin violence have been examined: (a) witnessing violence between parents and (b) experiencing violence by a parent. Numerous studies have concluded that women victims of IPV are more likely to report witnessing parental violence. Indeed, one review concluded that witnessing interparental violence was the only consistent correlate of IPV victimization (Hotaling & Sugarman, 1986). However, other reviews did not find this consistently (Pagelow, 1984; Sedlak, 1988). Most recently, Schumacher et al. (2001) concluded that at most, witnessing violence between parents had only a small effect on the risk of IPV victimization.

Results of studies examining the potential link between childhood victimization and later IPV victimization are also inconsistent. Reviews of the literature on IPV reach strikingly different conclusions, with two concluding that being victimized as a child or adolescent is related to later IPV victimization (Hotaling & Sugarman, 1984; Sedlak, 1988) and two concluding that childhood victimization does not constitute a risk factor for IPV (Hotaling & Sugarman, 1986; Pagelow, 1984). More recently, Schumacher et al. (2001) concluded that physical victimization as a child is only weakly related to IPV victimization but that emotional or verbal victimization may have a more significant effect.

Conclusion

Identification of correlates of IPV victimization has lagged behind that of IPV perpetration; however, although several factors have been associated with the experience of violence at the hands of an intimate partner, none has extremely strong associations with IPV. Experience of violence in the family of origin and demographic characteristics appear largely unhelpful in identifying individuals at risk of IPV victimization. However, the presence of marital distress and symptoms of depression or PTSD should alert professionals to assess for IPV.

Risk Markers for Specific Incidents of Intimate Partner Violence

Most of the correlates previously discussed have differentiated individuals who have experienced IPV from those who have not. It is not clear whether these same variables may be useful in identifying when or if violence will occur. In fact, many of the risk markers have not been tested to see whether they predict future, as opposed to past, IPV. However, some factors that have been examined might best be understood as situational determinants of IPV (Wilkinson & Hamerschlag, 2005). Conclusions must be drawn cautiously because we lack the prospective studies necessary to clearly identify risk factors for IPV incidents, but the following section describes some factors that are thought to set the stage for IPV events.

Relationship Conflict

Research on IPV generally assumes that some conflict or argument precedes the violence. Although this may not be true in cases of long-standing violence or when the couple is separated, results of several studies suggest this assumption is largely correct. Hyden (1995) found that 90% of couples indicated that the violence occurred in the context of a verbal altercation. Similarly, verbal arguments often precede violent interactions in couples seeking relationship therapy (Cascardi & Vivian, 1995). Data from the U.S. Department of Justice indicate that more than 80% of IPV incidents are preceded by arguments and another 14% occur in the context of a lovers' quarrel (Greenfield et al., 1998). In addition, several cross-sectional studies found that violent couples reported more conflict and arguing than nonviolent couples (see earlier discussion). Also, one longitudinal study suggests that there is an increase in arguments and verbal aggression prior to the initial occurrence of physical IPV in that relationship (Murphy & O'Leary, 1994).

Alcohol Use

Alcohol use has been related to some incidents of violence. For example, alcohol use was present in about one fourth of reported IPV incidents (Greenfield et al., 1998; Kantor & Straus, 1987). Two studies examining IPV and alcohol found that physically violent conflicts are more likely than nonviolent arguments to involve alcohol consumption by the male partner (Leonard & Quigley, 1999; Murphy, Winters, O'Farrell, Fals-Stewart, & Murphy, 2005). Incidents of IPV in which the male partner is drinking, compared with those in which he is not, are also more likely to involve severe violence (Martin & Bachman, 1997; Testa, Quigley, & Leonard, 2003).

In sum, although alcohol use is present during some violent episodes, the majority of incidents of IPV likely occur in the absence of alcohol. However, problematic levels of drinking do appear to increase the risk of IPV during a conflict. Again, although no combination of variables will specifically predict IPV, problematic levels of drinking may alert the professional to assess for IPV.

Relationship Termination

It is commonly believed that women who leave a violent relationship may be at increased risk of violence. Although limited, the available data generally support this conclusion with regard to severe violence. Estranged wives are at substantially higher risk than wives in intact couples of being killed by their partner (Wilson & Daly, 1993; Wilson, Daly, & Wright, 1993). Campbell et al. (2003) found that incidents of IPV that resulted in a woman's being killed were roughly 3 times as likely as nonfatal assaults to be triggered by the woman's leaving or attempting to leave the relationship.

Perceived Danger

Some authors have suggested that women who have experienced IPV may be in a better position than anyone to evaluate their risk of future violence (de Becker, 1997; Hart, 1994); others have suggested that abused women systematically underestimate future danger (Campbell, 1995; M. A. Dutton & Dionne, 1991). In a sample of women whose partners had been arrested for IPV, Weisz, Tolman, and Saunders (2000) found that the women's risk ratings were better than a group of risk markers identified in the existing literature for predicting severe violence during a period of 4 months.

Assessment Tools for Intimate Partner Violence Risk

The factors described in the previous section can help identify individuals at risk of IPV, but because we lack prospective studies we know little about how well they work to identify future risk and we cannot quantify the risk associated with one or more of these risk factors (Hilton & Harris, 2005). Indeed, one study found that a set of 25 risk markers accounted for only 15% of the variance in IPV over a 4-month period (Weisz et al., 2000).

Researchers have attempted to develop instruments to assess future risk and, in some cases, quantify the risk for a particular individual. Some approaches involve checklists of rationally derived items (often including the risk markers identified earlier) and provide the user with guidelines to determine risk. Other instruments consist of items empirically shown to differentiate individuals who perpetrate IPV in the future and those who do not. In their review of these approaches, Hilton and Harris (2005) concluded that the empirically derived scales tend to be more accurate than other methods.

We briefly review the literature on IPV risk assessment tools, but this literature is relatively new and somewhat limited. Much of the research examines risk of severe IPV or femicide in men who have already perpetrated IPV. Although this is one of the most important questions regarding IPV risk, this focus limits the conclusions we can draw and the ability to generalize the results to other forms of IPV.

Structured Risk Assessments

A number of risk screening assessments have been developed, and several have been subjected to empirical testing. The Danger Assessment (DA; Campbell, 1986) includes a 15-item checklist (ideally completed in the context of an abuse interview) administered to women who have been victims of IPV. DA items include perpetrator's substance abuse, threats, and escalation of IPV. Goodman, Dutton, and Bennett (2000) found that DA scores were related to the recurrence of IPV in women whose partners had been arrested for IPV. Weisz et al. (2000) found that a 12-item version of the DA had only a weak association with the future occurrence of severe violence. A third study found the DA related to recidivism in a sample of almost 600 IPV perpetrators, but in a smaller sample in this same study, DA scores were not significantly related to IPV reports (Hilton et al., 2004).

Hilton et al. (2004) also examined two other measures, the Spousal Assault Risk Assessment (SARA; Kropp, Hart, Webster, & Eaves, 1999) and the Domestic Violence Supplementary Report (DVSR; Ministry of the Solicitor General, Policing Services Division, 2000). The SARA is a 20-item instrument with items that evaluate the perpetrator's criminal and psychological history, the history of IPV, and the current incident. Scores on the SARA were related to recidivism over 4 years in the large sample but not in the smaller validation sample (Hilton et al., 2004). Other studies of the SARA offer similar mixed results. Kropp and Hart (2000) found that the IPV items, but not the overall score, were related to recidivism. Grann and Wedin (2002) found that total SARA scores were related to new incidents over periods of 2 and 5 years but not over shorter time periods. However, Williams and Houghton (2004) found that the SARA score was significantly related to violence in the 18 months following an arrest for IPV.

The DVSR is somewhat unique in that it is designed to be used by police officers, and the 20 items can be completed with information available when officers are investigating an IPV incident. The single study to investigate the DVSR produced mixed results (Hilton et al., 2004). As with the DA and the SARA, the DVSR was significantly related to recidivism in the large sample examined initially but not in the smaller validation sample.

Actuarial Risk Assessment

The Violence Risk Appraisal Guide (VRAG; Rice & Harris, 1995) was developed to assess risk of recidivism of generally violent perpetrators (Harris, Rice, & Cormier, 2002). However, more recent studies suggest that it may be effective at identifying individuals at risk of IPV (Hilton & Harris, 2005). The VRAG assesses demographic characteristics, childhood history variables, psychological adjustment scores, and criminal history factors found to identify violent offenders who were reconvicted of a violent crime (Rice & Harris, 1995). Among men convicted of wife assault or murder, VRAG scores were related to IPV during the year following their release (Grann & Wedin, 2002).

The Ontario Domestic Assault Risk Assessment (ODARA; Hilton et al., 2004) consists of 13 items that include the perpetrator's history of criminal and domestic violence, substance abuse, and characteristics of the most recent assault. The ODARA was related to the presence, number, and severity of IPV incidents over 5 years in a large sample of men accused of IPV and in a smaller validation sample (Hilton et al., 2004).

Assessing Risk of Femicide

Some effort has been made to identify risk factors for femicide and to evaluate the potential utility of the DA (Campbell, 1986) as a risk assessment. Campbell et al. (2003) found that items from the DA differentiated 220 cases of femicide and 343 victims of nonlethal IPV. Although the Campbell et al. study did not examine the DA in isolation from other risk factors, many of the DA items were retained in the final multivariate model that correctly identified 81% of the femicide cases and 95% of the nonlethal assault survivors.

CONCLUSION

IPV is an unfortunately common and potentially dangerous problem with multiple causes. Researchers are beginning to identify factors that serve to increase or decrease the likelihood that particular individuals will perpetrate or become victims of IPV. However, inconsistencies across studies in methodology, sampling, and definitions of basic concepts make this effort difficult. The recent development of actuarial assessment tools is moving the field in the direction of being better able to quantify risk, but these efforts have focused on predicting risk for men who have already had contact with the legal system as a result of IPV. Because the vast majority of IPV incidents are not reported, it is not clear how well these findings will contribute to the quantification of risk for most IPV cases. Therefore, it is important for clinicians to remain alert to the variety of factors that place their patients at risk of IPV, particularly because a number of these factors may lead individuals to seek care—even if the violence does not.

Clearly, many questions about how to evaluate risk of IPV remain unanswered. For example, little is known about how risk factors interact with one another to affect the likelihood of violence. Data from some studies (e.g., see Hilton et al., 2004) suggest that risk factors can function additively (i.e., the more risk markers present, the more likely the violence). However, some risk markers may account for largely overlapping variance. For example, Murphy and O'Farrell (1994) found that marital satisfaction was not related to risk of IPV perpetration in an alcohol dependent sample. Still other risk factors may work synergistically to increase risk. Thus, binge drinking combined with access to a firearm may increase the likelihood of fatal IPV more than simply adding together the relative risk association with each factor in isolation. Additional research is needed to develop a more complete understanding of the ways in which factors function in combination to increase risk of IPV. Until such research is available, it seems prudent for clinicians to inquire about IPV as part of their standard evaluation and it may be critical to do so when multiple risk markers are present.

REFERENCES

Abbott, J. (1997). Injuries and illnesses of domestic violence. *Annals of Emergency Medicine, 29*, 781–785.

Archer, J. (2000). Sex differences in aggression between heterosexual partners: A meta-analytic review. *Psychological Bulletin, 126*, 651–680.

Astin, M. C., Lawrence, K. J., & Foy, D. W. (1993). Posttraumatic stress disorder among battered women: Risk and resiliency factors. *Violence and Victims, 8*, 17–28.

Bauserman, S. K., & Arias, I. (1992). Relationships among marital investment, marital satisfaction, and marital commitment in domestically victimized and nonvictimized wives. *Violence and Victims, 7*, 287–296.

Beasley, R., & Stoltenberg, C. D. (1992). Personality characteristics of male spouse abusers. *Professional Psychology: Research and Practice, 23*, 310–317.

Beckham, J. C., Feldman, M. E., Kirby, A. C., Hertzberf, M. A., & Moore, S. D. (1997). Interpersonal violence as it correlates in Vietnam veterans with chronic posttraumatic stress disorder. *Journal of Clinical Psychology, 53*, 859–869.

Brinkerhoff, M. B., & Lupri, E. (1988). Interspousal violence. *Canadian Journal of Sociology, 13*, 407–434.

Byrne, C. A., & Riggs, D. S. (1996). The cycle of trauma: Relationship aggression in male Vietnam veterans with symptoms of posttraumatic stress disorder. *Violence and Victims, 11*, 213–225.

Campbell, J. C. (1986). Nursing assessment for risk of homicide with battered women. *Advances in Nursing Science, 8*, 36–51.

Campbell, J. C. (1995). Prediction of homicide of and by battered women. In J. C. Campbell (Ed.), *Assessing dangerousness: Violence by sexual offenders, batterers, and child abusers* (pp. 96–113). Thousand Oaks, CA: Sage.

Campbell, J. C., Webster, D., Koziol-McLain, J., Block, C., Campbell, D., Curry, M. A., et al. (2003). Risk factors for femicide in abusive relationships: Results from a multisite case control study. *American Journal of Public Health, 93*, 1089–1097.

Cascardi, M. A., & O'Leary, K. D. (1992). Depressive symptomatology, self-esteem, and self-blame in battered women. *Journal of Family Violence, 7*, 249–259.

Cascardi, M. A., & Vivian, D. (1995). Context for specific episodes of marital aggression. *Journal of Family Violence, 10*, 265–293.

Danielson, K. K., Moffitt, T. E., Caspi, A., & Silva, P. A. (1998). Comorbidity between abuse of an adult and *DSM–III–R* mental disorders: Evidence from an epidemiological study. *American Journal of Psychiatry, 155*, 131–133.

de Becker, G. (1997). *The gift of fear: Survival signals that protect from violence*. Boston: Little, Brown.

Dienemann, J., Boyle, E., Baker, D., Resnick, W., Weiderhorn, N., & Campbell, J. (2000). Intimate partner abuse among women diagnosed with depression. *Issues in Mental Health Nursing, 21*, 499–513.

Dutton, D. G., Saunders, K., Starzomski, A., & Bartholomew, K. (1994). Intimacy anger and insecure attachment as precursors of abuse in intimate relationships. *Journal of Applied Social Psychology*, *24*, 1367–1386.

Dutton, D. G., Starzomski, A., & Ryan, L. (1996). Antecedents of abusive personality and abusive behavior in wife assaulters. *Journal of Family Violence*, *11*, 113–132.

Dutton, M. A., & Dionne, D. (1991). Counseling and shelter for battered women. In M. Steinman (Ed.), *Women battering: Policy responses* (pp. 113–130). Cincinnati, OH: Anderson.

Feld, S. L., & Straus, M. A. (1989). Escalation and desistance of wife assault in marriage. *Criminology*, *27*, 141–161.

Golding, J. M. (1999). Intimate partner violence as a risk factor for mental disorders: A meta-analysis. *Journal of Family Violence*, *14*, 99–131.

Goodman, L. A., Dutton, M. A., & Bennett, L. (2000). Predicting repeat abuse among arrested batterers: Use of the Danger Assessment Scale in the criminal justice system. *Journal of Interpersonal Violence*, *15*, 63–74.

Grann, M., & Wedin, I. (2002). Risk factors for recidivism among spousal assault and spousal homicide offenders. *Psychology, Crime, and Law*, *8*, 5–23.

Greenfeld, L. A., Rand, M. R., Craven, D., Klaus, P. A., Perkins, C. A., Ringel, C., et al., (1998). *Violence by intimates: Analysis of data on crimes by current or former spouses, boyfriends, and girlfriends*. Washington, DC: U.S. Department of Justice.

Hamberger, L. K., & Hastings, J. E. (1991). Personality correlates of men who batter and nonviolent men: Some continuities and discontinuities. *Journal of Family Violence*, *6*, 131–147.

Hanson, R. K., Cadsky, O., Harris, A., & Lalonde, C. (1997). Correlates of battering among 997 men: Family history, adjustment and attitudinal differences. *Violence and Victims*, *12*, 191–209.

Harris, G. T., Rice, M. E., & Cormier, C. A. (2002). Prospective replication of the *Violence Risk Appraisal Guide* in predicting violent recidivism among forensic patients. *Law and Human Behavior*, *26*, 377–394.

Hart, B. J. (1994). Lethality and dangerousness assessments. *Violence Update*, *4*, 7–8, 10.

Hastings, J. E. (1997). Association of right-wing authoritarianism and income with wife abuse. *Psychological Reports*, *80*, 667–670.

Hastings, J. E., & Hamberger, L. K. (1988). Personality characteristics of spouse abusers: A controlled comparison. *Violence and Victims*, *3*, 31–48.

Helzer, J. E., Robins, L. N., & McEvoy, L. (1987). Post-traumatic stress disorder in the general population: Findings from the Epidemiologic Catchment Area Survey. *The New England Journal of Medicine*, *317*, 1630–1634.

Heyman, R. E., O'Leary, K. D., & Jouriles, E. N. (1995) Alcohol and aggressive personality styles: Potentiators of serious physical aggression against wives? *Journal of Family Psychology*, *9*, 44–57.

Hilton, N. Z., & Harris, G. T. (2005). Predicting wife assault: A critical review and implications for public policy. *Trauma, Violence, and Abuse, 6*, 3–23.

Hilton, N. Z., Harris, G. T., Rice, M. E., Lang, C., Cormier, C. A., & Lines, K. (2004). A brief accurate actuarial assessment for the prediction of wife assault recidivism: The Ontario Domestic Assault Risk Assessment. *Psychological Assessment, 16*, 267–275.

Holtzworth-Munroe, A., Stuart, G. L., & Hutchinson, G. (1997). Violent versus nonviolent husbands: Differences in attachment patterns, dependency, and jealousy. *Journal of Family Psychology, 11*, 314–331.

Hotaling, G. T., & Sugarman, D. B. (1984). An identification of risk factors. In G. L. Bowen, M. A. Straus, A. J. Sedlak, G. T. Hotaling, & D. B. Sugarman (Eds.), *Domestic violence surveillance system feasibility study: Phase I report. Identification of outcome and risk factors* (pp. 3-1–3-66). Rockville, MD: Westat.

Hotaling, G. T., & Sugarman, D. B. (1986). An analysis of risk markers in husband to wife violence: The current state of knowledge. *Violence and Victims, 1*, 101–124.

Hurlbert, D. F., Whittaker, K. E., & Munoz, C. J. (1991). Etiological characteristics of abusive husbands. *Military Medicine, 156*, 670–675.

Hyden, H. (1995). Verbal aggression as prehistory of woman battering. *Journal of Family Violence, 10*, 55–71.

Jordan, B. K., Marmar, C. R., Fairbank, J. A., Schlenger, W. E., Kulka, R. A., Hough, R. L., & Weiss, D. S. (1992). Problems in families of male Vietnam veterans with posttraumatic stress disorder. *Journal of Consulting and Clinical Psychology, 60*, 916–926.

Kantor, G. K., & Straus, M. A. (1987). The "drunken bum" theory of wife beating. *Social Problems, 34*, 213–230.

Kessler, R. C., Sonnega, A., Bromet, E., Hughes, M., & Nelson, C. B. (1995). Posttraumatic stress disorder in the National Comorbidity Survey. *Archives of General Psychiatry, 52*, 1048–1060.

Kropp, P. R., & Hart, S. D. (2000). The Spousal Assault Risk Assessment (SARA) guide: Reliability and validity in adult male offenders. *Law and Human Behavior, 24*, 101–118.

Kropp, P. R., Hart, S. C., Webster, C. D., & Eaves, D. (1999). *Spousal Assault Risk Assessment Guide: Users guide*. North Tonawanda, NY: Multi-Health Systems.

Kulka, R. A., Schlenger, W. E., Fairbank, J. A., Hough, R. L., Jordan, B. K., Marmar, C. R., & Weiss, D. S. (1990). *The National Vietnam Veterans Readjustment Study table of findings and technical appendices*. New York: Brunner/Mazel.

Kyriacou, D. N., Anglin, D., Taliaferro, E., Stone, S., Tubb, T., Linden, J. A., et al. (1999). Risk factors for injury to women from domestic violence. *The New England Journal of Medicine, 341*, 1892–1898.

Leonard, K. E., & Blane, H. T. (1992). Alcohol and marital aggression in a national sample of young men. *Journal of Interpersonal Violence, 7*, 19–30.

Leonard, K. E., & Quigley, B. M. (1999). Drinking and marital aggression in newlyweds: An event-based analysis of drinking and the occurrence of husband marital aggression. *Journal of Studies on Alcoholism, 60*, 537–545.

Leonard, K. E., & Senchak, M. (1993). Alcohol and premarital aggression among newlywed couples. *Journal of Studies in Alcohol, 11*, 96–108.

Lockhart, L. L., White, B. W., Causby, V., & Isaac, A. (1994). Letting out the secret: Violence in lesbian relationships. *Journal of Interpersonal Violence, 9*, 469–492.

Maiuro, R. D., Cahn, T. S., Vitaliano, P. P., Wagner, B. C., & Zegree, J. B. (1988). Anger, hostility, and depression in domestically violent versus generally assaultive men and nonviolent control subjects. *Journal of Consulting and Clinical Psychology, 56*, 17–23.

Martin, S. E., & Bachman, R. (1997). The relationship of alcohol to injury in assault cases. In M. Gatner (Ed.), *Recent developments in alcoholism: Vol. 13. Alcoholism and violence* (pp. 41–56). New York: Plenum Press.

Ministry of the Solicitor General, Policing Services Division. (2000). *A guide to the Domestic Violence Supplementary Report Form*. Toronto, Ontario, Canada: Author.

Moffitt, T. E., & Caspi, A. (1999). *Findings about partner violence from Dunedin Multidisciplinary Health and Development Study* (Publication No. NCJ 170018). Washington, DC: U.S. Department of Justice.

Murphy, C. M., Meyer, S. L., & O'Leary, K. D. (1993). Family of origin violence and MCMI–II psychopathology among partner assaultive men. *Violence and Victims, 8*, 165–176.

Murphy C. M., & O'Farrell, T. J. (1994). Factors associated with marital aggression in male alcoholics. *Journal of Family Psychology, 8*, 321–335.

Murphy, C. M., & O'Leary, K. D. (1994). Research paradigms, values, and spouse abuse. *Journal of Interpersonal Violence, 9*, 207–223.

Murphy, C. M., Winters, J., O'Farrell, T. J., Fals-Stewart, W., & Murphy, M. (2005). Alcohol consumption and intimate partner violence by alcoholic men: Comparing violent and nonviolent conflicts. *Psychology of Addictive Behaviors, 19*, 35–42.

Neidig, P. H., Friedman, D. H., & Collins, B. S. (1986). Attitudinal characteristics of males who have engaged in spouse abuse. *Journal of Family Violence, 1*, 223–233.

O'Farrell, T. J., Fals-Stewart, W., Murphy, M., & Murphy, C. M. (2003). Partner violence before and after individually based alcoholism treatment for male alcoholic patients. *Journal of Consulting and Clinical Psychology, 71*, 92–102.

O'Farrell, T. J., Murphy, C. M., Stephan, S. H., Fals-Stewart, W., & Murphy, M. (2004). Partner violence before and after couples-based alcoholism treatment for male alcoholic patients: The role of treatment involvement and abstinence. *Journal of Consulting and Clinical Psychology, 72*, 202–217.

O'Farrell, T. J., van Hutton, V., & Murphy, C. M. (1999). Domestic violence before and after alcoholism treatment: A two-year longitudinal study. *Journal of Studies on Alcohol, 60*, 317–321.

O'Leary, K. D., Barling, J., Arias, I., Rosenbaum, A., Malone, J., & Tyree, A. (1989). Prevalence and stability of physical aggression between spouses: A longitudinal analysis. *Journal of Consulting and Clinical Psychology, 57*, 263–268.

O'Leary, K. D., Malone, J., & Tyree, A. (1994). Physical aggression in early marriage: Prerelationship and relationship effects. *Journal of Consulting and Psychology, 62,* 594–602.

O'Leary, K. D., Vivian, D., & Malone, J. (1992). Assessment of physical aggression in marriage: The need for a multimodal method. *Behavioral Assessment, 14,* 5–14.

Pagelow, M. D. (1984). *Family violence.* New York: Praeger Publishers.

Rankin, L. B., Saunders, D. G., & Williams, R. A. (2000). Mediators of attachment style, social support, and sense of belonging in predicting women abuse by African American men. *Journal of Interpersonal Violence, 15,* 1060–1080.

Rice, M. E., & Harris, G. T. (1995). Violent recidivism: Assessing predictive validity. *Journal of Consulting and Clinical Psychology, 63,* 737–748.

Riggs, D. S., Byrne, C. A., Weathers, F. W., & Litz, B. T. (1995, July). The cycle of trauma: Marital violence in Vietnam veterans with PTSD. Paper presented in D. Saunders (Chair), *Issues in batterer treatment.* Symposium conducted at the Fourth International Family Violence Research Conference, Durham, NH.

Rosenbaum, A., & O'Leary, K. D. (1981). Marital violence: Characteristics of abusive couple. *Journal of Clinical and Consulting Psychology, 41,* 63–71.

Russell, M. N., Lipov, E., Phillips, N., & White, B. (1989). Psychological profiles of violent and nonviolent maritally distressed couples. *Psychotherapy, 26,* 81–87.

Saunders, D. G. (1994). Posttraumatic stress symptom profiles of battered women: A comparison of survivors in two settings. *Violence and Victims, 9,* 31–44.

Schumacher, J. A., Slep, A. M. S., & Heyman, R. E. (2001). Risk factors for male-to-female partner physical abuse. *Aggression and Violent Behavior, 6,* 281–352.

Sedlak, A. J. (1988). Prevention of wife abuse. In V. B. Van Hasselt, R. L. Morrison, A. S. Bellack, & M. Hersen (Eds.), *Handbook of family violence* (pp. 319–358). New York: Plenum Press.

Smith, M. D. (1990). Patriarchal ideology and wife beating: A test of a feminist hypothesis. *Violence and Victims, 5,* 257–273.

Stith, S. M., Smith, D. B., Penn, C. E., Ward, D. B., & Tritt, D. (2004). Intimate partner physical abuse perpetration and victimization risk factors: A meta-analytic review. *Aggression and Violent Behavior, 10,* 65–98.

Straus, M. A., Gelles, R. J., & Steinmetz, S. K. (1980). *Behind closed doors: Violence in the American family.* New York: Doubleday/Anchor.

Straus, M. A., & Smith, C. (1990). Violence in Hispanic families in the United States: Incidence rates and structural interpretations. In M. A. Straus & R. J. Gelles (Eds.), *Physical violence in American families* (pp. 95–131). New Brunswick, NJ: Transaction.

Stuart, G. L., Ramsey, S. E., Moore, T. M., Kahler, C. W., Farrell, L. E., Recuperon, P. R., & Brown, R. A. (2003). Reductions in marital violence following treatment for alcohol dependence. *Journal of Interpersonal Violence, 18,* 1113–1131.

Sugarman, D. B., & Hotaling, G. T. (1989). Violent men in intimate relationships: An analysis of risk markers. *Journal of Applied Social Psychology, 19,* 1034–1048.

Telch, C., & Lindquist, C. (1984). Violent versus nonviolent couples: A comparison of patterns. *Psychotherapy, 21,* 242–248.

Testa, M., Quigley, B. M., & Leonard, K. E. (2003). Does alcohol make a difference? Within-participants comparison of incidents of partner violence. *Journal of Interpersonal Violence, 18,* 163–180.

Tjaden, P., & Thoennes, N. (2000). *Prevalence, incidence, and consequences of violence against women: Findings from the national violence against women survey.* Washington, DC: U.S. Department of Justice.

Vitanza, S., Vogel, L. C. M., & Marshall, L. L. (1995). Distress and symptoms of posttraumatic stress disorder in abused women. *Violence and Victims, 10,* 23–24.

Vivian, D., & Malone, J. (1997). Relationship factors and depressive symptomatology associated with mild and severe husband-to-wife physical aggression. *Violence and Victims, 12,* 3–18.

Waldner-Haugrud, L. K., Gratch, L. V., & Magruder, B. (1997). Victimization and perpetration rates of violence in gay and lesbian relationships: Gender issues explored. *Violence and Victims, 12,* 173–184.

Weisz, A. N., Tolman, R. M., & Saunders, D. G. (2000). Assessing the risk of severe domestic violence: The importance of survivors' predictions. *Journal of Interpersonal Violence, 15,* 75–90.

Wilkinson, D. L., & Hamerschlag, S. J. (2005). Situational determinants in intimate partner violence. *Aggression and Violent Behavior, 10,* 333–361.

Williams, K. R., & Houghton, A. B. (2004). Assessing the risk of domestic violence reoffending. *Law and Human Behavior, 28,* 437–455.

Wilson, M., & Daly, M. (1993). Spousal homicide risk and estrangement. *Violence and Victims, 8,* 3–16.

Wilson, M., Daly, M., & Wright, C. (1993). Uxoricide in Canada: Demographic risk patterns. *Canadian Journal of Criminology, 35,* 263–291.

Wilt, S., & Olson, S. (1996). Prevalence of domestic violence in the United States. *Journal of the American Medical Women's Association, 51,* 77–88.

World Health Organization. (2002). *World report on violence and health.* Geneva, Switzerland: Author.

World Health Organization. (2005). *WHO multi-country study on women's health and domestic violence against women.* Geneva, Switzerland: Author.

V

EMERGENCY-RELATED
CRISES AND CONDITIONS

10

SELF-INJURY: TREATMENT OF A COMPLEX ADAPTATION

PAMELA J. DEITER-SANDS AND LAURIE ANNE PEARLMAN

Self-injury often derives from traumatic experiences. It differs from suicidal behavior because it is essentially an adaptive strategy, intended to allow the individual to endure and carry on. It therefore does not always call for the interventions described in Part II of this volume. Nonetheless, for those who work with patient emergencies, it is important to be able to distinguish those who injure themselves as an adaptation from those who injure themselves with intent to die; of course, emergency intervention may be required for the physical effects of self-injury. If an adaptation that is more constructive than self-injury is to develop, however, long-term treatment, rather than emergency or crisis intervention, is typically required.

The behavior of self-injury is an adaptive strategy to manage intense physiological arousal and emotional suffering. For many people, self-injury begins as a response to unbearable circumstances in which response choices are restricted. It is adaptive because it allows these overwhelming states and unbearable circumstances to be managed so the individual survives, and therefore has the opportunity to change and grow. There are physiological mechanisms through which self-injury may serve to adapt to trauma, including self-injury's effect of quieting an oversensitized alarm system in the brain, and self-injury's effect of stimulating hormones that reduce distress. Thus, treatment and intervention needs for self-injury differ greatly from those for suicidality. In this chapter, we first provide a conceptualization of self-injury as an adaptive strategy and then explains the physiological mechanisms through which self-injury may help individuals adapt to trauma. Next, we offer a constructivist self-development theory (CSDT) as a framework for treatment. We then discuss clinical applications of the theory for self-injury, as well as clinical implications of how trauma affects the body. Finally, we warn against possible negative effects of treatment on the provider and remind the provider to attend to his or her own personal and professional needs.

CONCEPTUALIZATION

Definitions

In this chapter, we use the terms *self-injury* and *direct self-injury* to refer to deliberate acts resulting in damage to one's own body tissues, when these acts have psychological significance and are not intended to bring about death. By specifying psychological significance, we mean the behaviors that typically come to the attention of mental health professionals, not the casual, normative self-injury (e.g., mild cuticle picking or biting) that reflects no particular distress, nor the comparatively rare, stereotypic self-injury seen with some severe developmental disabilities. The most familiar forms of self-injury are cutting, burning, or scratching at one's skin, especially on wrists and forearms and most frontal surfaces of the body (e.g., arms, chest, thighs), along with hair pulling, head-banging, and self-hitting. Direct self-injury may take many other forms, including destruction of tissues through biting, self-hitting, swallowing and insertion of objects into the body, injurious masturbation, scalding, and aggravation of wounds. This class of behavior is often identified by other names, including parasuicidal behavior, self-mutilation (i.e., repetitive or episodic), and deliberate self-harm.

Authors and researchers express varying opinions about whether another class of behaviors constitute self-injury; we classify these behaviors as *indirect self-harm*. For example, drug abuse, alcohol abuse, eating and evacuation practices (e.g., starvation, vomiting, enemas), excessive exercise, unprotected or overtly risky sex, and frequent elective surgeries have been excluded from most, although not all, self-injury research (Favazza, 1992; Pattison & Kahan, 1983). Similarly, behaviors such as neglecting a medical condition; withholding medication, warm clothing, or other necessities; spending time in dangerous places or with dangerous people; and provoking injury by others may serve self-injurious purposes and place individuals at risk of serious harm. Indirect self-harm is frequently reported by people who practice direct self-injury.

Behaviors that injure or modify the body have a variety of meanings and purposes in human society (Favazza, 1998). Piercing, branding and tattoos, and ritualized self-injuries such as adolescent rites of passage are usually decorative and socially accepted in a way that pathological self-injurious behavior is not (Yates, 2004). The main difference between culturally acceptable body modification and pathological self-injury is the sociocultural and intrapsychic context, as noted by Gasperoni: "One is a shared act of pride [or defiance]; the other a secretive act steeped in shame" (as cited in Yates, 2004, p. 36).

Trautmann and Connors (1994) cautioned that "behavior alone does not constitute self-injury . . . any particular behavior can be viewed in different lights, depending on the social and personal context within which it occurs" (p. 59). Categorization of behaviors is ultimately an empirical question about behavior, and one of considerable importance for research, as ongoing definitional issues are evident in the literature and continue to interfere with developing knowledge about self-injury. However, individuals often defy categorization. Clinically, it is the internal meaning and purpose of self-injury for each person that guides intervention.

Prevalence

Rather than viewing it as deviant, clinicians have good reason to see self-injury as a natural outcome of particular distress. Self-injury is not rare or bizarre; it is a behavior reported by many distressed people and observed among animals. Rates in the nonclinical adult population are estimated to be about 4% (Briere & Gil, 1998; Klonsky, Oltmanns, & Turkheimer, 2003). Self-injury occurs among 4% to 20% of adult psychiatric patients, according to estimates by Briere and Gil (1998) and Favazza (1998). These estimates are quite likely modest. The authors surveyed 233 adults in outpatient psychiatric care and found 58% reported a history of direct self-injury (Deiter, Nicholls, & Pearlman, 2000). In an inpatient adolescent sample researched by Clery (2000), 21% reported self-injury. According to Yates (2004), "other researchers have observed rates as high as 40–60% among adolescent populations" (p. 40). High school students report self-injury at a rate of 14% (Ross & Heath, 2002) to 21% (Zoroglu, Tuzun, Sar, Tutkun, Savas, & Ozturk, 2003). Among college students, reports range from 14% (Favazza, DeRosear, & Conterio, 1989) to 35% (Gratz, 2001). Some researchers and authors have observed that self-injury is becoming increasingly common (Klonsky et al., 2003; Ross & Heath, 2002; Walsh & Rosen, 1988; Whitlock, Powers, & Eckenrode, 2006).

Self-injury has been observed in many primates other than humans, including rhesus monkeys, squirrel monkeys, chimpanzees, and gorillas. However, "self-injurious behavior is by no means limited to primates" (Dellinger-Ness & Handler, 2006, p. 506) and has been observed in other types of animals. Social isolation (particularly at an early age), abnormal rearing, and repeated use in animal experiments were associated with animal self-injurious behavior by Dellinger-Ness and Handler (2006), who concluded that self-injurious behavior served as a form of affect regulation for the captive animals. Allen (2001) reported that animal research has "construed self-injury as 'self-aggression' that often has its origins in a history of social isolation and is prompted by threat or frustration" (p. 218).

Self-Injury and Suicide

Nonsuicidal self-injury is essentially a survival technique. It is a reaction to almost unendurable physiological and emotional distress. It is intended to allow the individual to endure and to carry on.

In general, self-injury is distinct from suicide attempts. Self-injury and suicidality differ in many ways, and the treatment and intervention needs for self-injury differ greatly from treatment and intervention needs for a suicide attempt. Most authors and researchers working in the area of self-injury agree that the behaviors of self-injury are, by definition, not suicidal (cf. Gratz, 2006; Muehlenkamp, 2005). The intentions are different, and the behaviors of suicide attempts are distinct from the rituals of self-injury (Allen, 1995; Gratz, 2006).

However, it has been reported that individuals who self-injure are at heightened risk of later suicide (Muehlenkamp, 2005). It is important to note that the distinct behaviors of self-injury and suicide can exist in the same individual at different times. Sansone, Songer, and Sellbom (2006, p. 148) reported that in their sample "individuals with histories of suicide attempts . . . were significantly more likely to report a greater number of low-lethal self-harm behaviors" (e.g., cutting, scratching, hitting oneself) in addition to suicidal behaviors. Finally, self-injury can be unintentionally life threatening. Harm from direct self-injury (such as deep cutting) could lead to accidental death.

For adolescents, suicide attempts peak between 16 and 18 years of age in the U.S. population. Completed suicide is most frequent among those ages 15 to 24, with risk leveling out for several decades after the mid-20s (after which risk gradually rises to peak among the elderly; Gould, Shaffer, & Greenberg, 2003). Ross and Heath (2002) found that teens who self-injured reported higher levels of anxiety and depression than their peers. There is little research to guide clinicians in the area of self-injury and adolescence. The generally heightened risk of suicide in this age group and the awareness that self-injury indicates intense distress suggest that adolescents who self-injure should be considered at increased risk of suicide.

Assessment and corresponding decisions about protection and treatment should take place in dialogue with the person who self-injures. Straightforward discussion of suicide risk is often possible and necessary in the context of assessing self-injury. A standard suicide assessment interview is called for (i.e., assessing level of depression, perceived helplessness and hopelessness, suicidal intent, plan, preparations, access to means, previous attempts, social supports, history of suicide in family members, recent bereavement, relationship loss, job loss, age, gender, etc.). Special attention should be paid to subjective experiences of depression and hopelessness and to signs of aggression and impulsivity, which may elevate suicide risk (Mann, Waternaux, Haas, & Malone, 1999). Guidance can be found in the description of a sensitive emergency assessment by Kleespies and Richmond in chapter 2 of this volume. Walsh (2006) outlined a cognitive–behavioral assessment for self-injury, including attention to place and pattern of wounds, which he suggested provide clues to the individual's level of organization, intention, self-control, and to the content and process of thought at the time of the injury.

Meaning in Self-Injury

Rituals, methods, reasons, and meanings for self-injury vary among people who self-injure and may change with time. In general, though, a consensus seems to be emerging in the literature that people who self-injure frequently describe increasing tension, anger, anxiety, and depersonalization or other dissociative phenomena, with a rising focus on the upcoming act of self-injury to provide rapid relief (cf. Allen, 2001; Connors, 2000). Immediate precipitants "tend to share a theme of real or perceived rejection or abandonment and include a stressful situation" (Muehlenkamp, 2005, p. 325). Commonly reported reasons for self-injury include (a) to regulate affect, (b) to express affect, (c) to relieve tension, (d) to manage dissociation, (e) to feel a sense of control, and (f) to influence others (Muehlenkamp, 2005).

The meanings of self-injury are often complex and may be related to past or present experiences that are difficult to communicate. Calof (1995) noted that much of the logic that governs self-injury is *trance logic*, which may include elements of primary process, magical thinking, and affect-driven problem solving. It may be marked by dissociated memories and related functions of self-injury. Miller (1994) viewed individuals who persistently injure or abuse their bodies as unconsciously reenacting elements of past abuses they have endured—specifically, unconsciously enacting the object relational dynamic among victim, perpetrator, and nonprotective bystander, all internalized as aspects of the self. Walsh and Rosen (1998) illuminated the experience of self-injury by identifying a series of events, feelings, and behaviors that individuals experience both in an episode of child abuse and in an episode of self-injury. Bearing in mind the idiosyncratic and unarticulated meanings possible in trance logic and reenactments can help clinicians and clients together come to an understanding of self-injury. A perspective of curiosity, openness, patience, and respect can help the client and the treatment provider when the meaning of self-injury is not yet clear.

HOW SELF-INJURY MAY PHYSIOLOGICALLY HELP INDIVIDUALS ADAPT TO TRAUMA

The link between trauma and self-injury has grown clear in recent research. The past decade has seen a much deeper appreciation for the neurophysiology of trauma, the effect of trauma on the brain and on the subsequent health of the mind and body. The effect of trauma on the brain is especially clear and compelling in the lives of abused children. Childhood abuse has profound and lasting physiological effects, leading to depression, hyperarousal, and other highly aversive physical and affective states (Briere, 1995; Davies & Frawley, 1994; van der Kolk, 2006) that individuals may attempt to manage in many ways, including through self-injury.

The self-injury literature has identified several predisposing factors for self-injury. These include childhood physical and/or sexual abuse, chaotic and neglectful homes in childhood, childhood separation from caregivers, parental alcoholism, early surgical or medical trauma, and childhood and adolescent residence in an institutional setting. Histories of abuse are common among people who self-injure, and research evidence for the association between abuse and self-injury is ample (cf. Briere & Gil, 1998; Gratz, Conrad, & Roemer, 2002; Klonsky et al., 2003).

The literature offers compelling information on the frequency of abuse. "Abuse and neglect of children are extremely common in our society, and their effects are well-documented to persist over time" (van der Kolk, Roth, Pelcovitz, Sunday, & Spinazzola, 2005, p. 390).

> In the United States approximately 3 million children are reported for abuse or neglect each year; at least 15 out of every 1,000 children in the United States have substantiated histories of abuse. In a survey of 16,000 adults who belonged to an HMO in California, 22% reported having been sexually abused and 30% were physically abused as children. (van der Kolk, 2003, p. 295)

These rates are similar to those found in other large samples of the general population, but they are lower than childhood abuse rates reported in clinical samples. However, rates can vary; for example, Deiter et al. (2000) found that 69% of a sample of adult psychiatric outpatients reported childhood abuse.

"In adult survivors of childhood sexual abuse, severe self-injury shows a positive correlation to greater frequency, severity, and sadism of early abuse" (Calof, 1995, p. 11). It appears that earlier abuse leads to more self-directed aggression. Van der Kolk, McFarlane, and Weisaeth (1996) reported that in one sample, "Abuse during early childhood and latency was strongly correlated with suicide attempts, self-mutilation, and other self-injurious behavior" (p. 190), with sexual abuse, separation, and neglect predicting increased severity and chronicity over a 4-year follow-up period.

Brain Development and Attachment

The human brain at birth is unfinished in that it is incompletely developed and has many more neurons (i.e., brain cells) than it will contain in adulthood. The first several years of life involve the maturation of brain structures and the development of elaborate connections among brain structures, allowing increasingly complex mental and physical functions while pruning away less-used neurons. The unfinished brain allows each of us to customize ourselves, as we are sculpted by experience to fit the demands of our unique early life circumstances and advance our likelihood of survival in those circumstances (Sunderland, 2006). It is important that as we develop, we use and reuse particular structures and pathways. They become more efficient and more likely to be activated through subsequent experience (van der Kolk, 2006).

The early years of life are significant for forging pathways between the limbic system and the neocortex (Schore, 2003). The limbic system takes in emotionally charged information and activates strong reactions such as rage, fear, separation distress, pleasure, social bonding, and nurturing. The neocortex is responsible for reasoning, self-control, awareness, and empathy (Sunderland, 2006). With normal development, the neocortex responds to and inhibits action of the limbic system. Thus, human beings develop more emotional insight, self-control, reasoning ability, social judgment, and ability to soothe their own distress over time, as these structures cooperate and mature (cf. Ford, 2005b; Schore, 2003; Sunderland, 2006; van der Kolk, 2006).

The brain structures described here do not work alone, of course. They control hormone systems, they are activated by and inhibit neurotransmitters, and they send and receive information from other parts of the brain, muscles, and vital organs, interacting at all times with the larger nervous system. Essentially, they create and maintain the neurophysiobiological environment of the individual (Allen, 2001; Marvasti, 2004; Schore, 2003; van der Kolk, 2003).

Much of the development of the brain and body system takes place through relationships with other human beings, especially primary caregivers. Thus, rational, comforting, well-controlled parents stimulate the pathways, structures, and chemical systems important to the functioning of rational, comforting, well-controlled children (Fonagy, Gergely, Jurist, & Target, 2004; Sunderland, 2006).

On defining *attachment*, Kinniburgh, Blaustein, and Spinazzola (2005) wrote,

> Attachment describes the interactions between children and their caregivers that have a longstanding impact on the development of identity and personal agency, early working models of self and other, and the capacity to regulate emotions. Nurturing and consistent caregiving pro-

motes skill development and a safety net for coping with difficult experiences. Secure attachment in childhood has been linked to numerous positive outcomes and is a significant predictor of resilience. (p. 426)

It is through secure attachment, in part, that caregivers positively shape the neurophysiology of children. This is achieved through modeling and encouraging behaviors that create internal balance and stability. As caregivers repeat attuned responses to distress over thousands of occasions (e.g., the caregiver calmly comforts an upset child), the child internalizes the regulated state of the caregiver (i.e., the child calms), partly by replicating the responses of the caregiver (i.e., by acting like the calm and comforting caregiver; Fonagy et al., 2004; Sunderland, 2006). Gradually, this internalized response becomes the regulated state of the child (i.e., the child is generally calm and can be comforted when distressed). As the child grows, the many brain and body structures and systems developed to maintain a calm, easily comforted state are further reinforced, elaborated, and refined through practice, and the child becomes an adult who is capable of remaining generally calm and easily comforted and training his or her own children in the same manner.

Approximately 90% of all child abuse occurs at the hands of parents or other relatives (van der Kolk, 2003); children are overwhelmingly likely to be abused by a primary caregiver or another loved one. Eighty percent of traumatized children have disorganized attachment patterns (van der Kolk, 2003). Disorganized attachment resulting from caregiver abuse is associated with chronic heightened physiological arousal and inability to self-soothe, leading to overwhelming emotional and physical distress. Heightened arousal, inability to self-soothe, and resulting overwhelming emotional and physical distress set the stage for self-injury (cf. Pearlman, 1998; van der Kolk, Perry, & Herman, 1991; Walsh, 2006; Yates, 2004).

The Physiology of Trauma and Self-Injury

Researchers have suggested various biological mechanisms through which trauma relates to self-injury, asserting that "we therapists must appreciate the biological basis of trauma to empathize with our clients who so try to 'get over it,' but cannot" (Allen, 2001, p. 139).

Research has suggested that trauma sensitizes the amygdala, which is intended to act as an alarm system for the body (Ford et al., 2005; Marvasti, 2004; Walsh, 2006). It signals danger. In addition, the brain is equipped with "a filing cabinet of previous experiences (hippocampus) and a problem-solving center (frontal cortex). . . . When extreme stress or trauma occurs, the alarm signal in the brain becomes so highly activated that . . . it interferes with the ability to access the other parts of the brain" so one cannot use the "filing cabinet" (i.e., the hippocampus) and the "problem-solving center" (i.e., the frontal cortex) to consider past experience and make a decision about how to act. Furthermore,

> During normal stress the alarm shuts off automatically when the danger is over. After . . . trauma the alarm center in the brain can become greatly sensitized . . . people find that anything that reminds them of trauma will set off the alarm . . . and it does NOT turn off automatically. It is this constant alarm that leads people to extreme behaviors . . . in an attempt to shut it off. (Ford, 2005a, p. 18)

Additional hypotheses linking stress and trauma-related changes to self-injury include changes in the opiate system and reduced serotonin levels. Stress and trauma-related changes in the (endogenous) opiate system may lead to a subjective sense of numbing, as well as the physical pain insensitivity often notable with self-injury (Allen, 2001; Walsh, 2006). It has been speculated that self-injury serves to stimulate the system, creating a mood change in the self-injurer (van der Kolk, 1988): "Stated in lay person's terms, when an individual harms his or her body, the brain may release naturally occurring opiate-like chemicals (e.g., endorphins) that are experienced as pleasurable and/or as relief from emotional distress" (Walsh, 2006, p. 64). Grossman and Siever (2001) suggested that self-injury takes place in people with lower than normal serotonin levels and cited research using selective serotonin reuptake inhibitors to diminish depression and self-injury. Other medications used to address self-injury include antianxiety medications, opiate antagonists, mood stabilizers, alpha-agonists, and antipsychotics. Walsh (2006) reported that most of these medications appear useful in case reports, but few have been empirically tested.

As Muehlenkamp (2005) noted, "Research into the neurobiological processes that may underlie impulsive self-injurious behavior has been very limited. Therefore, much of what we know or hypothesize is extrapolated from studies of related entities, such as impulsive aggression or suicide" (p. 69). Because of the link between trauma and self-injury, the trauma literature and its recent discoveries are the source for the most useful inferences about self-injury and provide insight into clinical treatment.

When considering research that confirms the dire effects of abuse on the brain and the functioning of related systems, clinicians must be aware of the hopeful implications, as well. The brain is most of all an adaptive organ. Particularly in the cortex, new associations and pathways are constantly added by experience (Doidge, 2007; Sunderland, 2006). Humans continue to learn, especially through social means in relationship, throughout their lives. It appears that the brain changes itself through experience, particularly in response to emotional and social stimulation (Begley, 2007; Doidge, 2007; Johnson, 2004). Psychotherapy may provide conditions in which healing change can take place.

Working with self-injury, which is a complex adaptation to unbearable states arising often from past abuse, requires a theory and therapeutic approach that takes into account a lifetime of experience with attachment, as well as the effects of trauma on physiology and the development of the self.

CONSTRUCTIVIST SELF-DEVELOPMENT THEORY

CSDT (McCann & Pearlman, 1990; Pearlman & Saakvitne, 1995) can provide a framework for treatment providers and survivors in their work together, making self-injury understandable and guiding treatment of survivors who self-injure. CSDT integrates psychoanalytic theories, particularly object relations, interpersonal psychiatry, and self-psychology, with theories of constructivism, social learning, and cognitive development. It recognizes that the physiological experiences of survivors can be shaped by trauma, especially trauma in childhood. It views the impact of traumatic experiences as unique to every individual, determined by an interaction of psychological aspects of the event with aspects of the individual, including psychological and physical resources, defenses, and needs. The impact of trauma is further shaped by the cultural and social context within which it occurs. Different aspects of the self that are impacted by trauma include frame of reference (including identity, worldview, and spirituality), psychological needs, ego resources, the memory system, and self-capacities. The last of these aspects—self-capacities—is particularly important because of their connection to self-injurious behaviors.

CSDT describes three self-capacities, or inner abilities, people require to maintain a state of internal balance and sense of self (Brock, Pearlman, & Varra, 2006; Pearlman, 1998). They are (a) the ability to maintain a sense of inner connection with benign others; (b) the ability to experience, tolerate, and integrate strong affect; and (c) the ability to maintain a sense of self as viable, benign, and positive. As suggested, states of inadequate self-capacities are both emotional and physiological, related to the activities of a brain and nervous system that has developed and practiced particular responses to extreme stress, possibly including abuse, and a psychological self that has developed without the reliable influence of accurately attuned caregiving. They should not be confused with simple attitudes, beliefs, or even behaviors. Self-capacities describe essential regulatory functions of the self. The development of self-capacities is central to work with self-injurers who are trauma survivors. In emergency interventions, considering self-capacities allows the treatment provider to identify areas of need and strength. In addition, the provider and client can develop temporary measures to shore up or increase self-capacities to help the client through a crisis. Self-capacity development is the work of long-term psychotherapy. Pearlman et al. (Pearlman, 1998; Saakvitne, Gamble, Pearlman, & Lev, 2000) have written elsewhere in detail about clinical work to help develop self-capacities. The following description of self-capacities is based on more elaborate explanations elsewhere (e.g., see Pearlman, 1998; Pearlman & Saakvitne, 1995; Saakvitne et al., 2000).

Inner Connection

The capacity to maintain a sense of connection with benign others is the basis from which affect regulation and self-worth develop. The adult survivor with impaired self-capacities may live in alienation instead of connection, experience terrible affects that he or she cannot soothe, and experience him- or herself as toxic, unworthy of living, or unable to live.

The ability to maintain a sense of connection cannot fully develop when empathic attunement, affection, and nurturance are lacking. Ideally, connection to others is fostered by early, empathic, and consistent care from loved ones, that is, in the context of secure attachment. When children experience shaming and punitive rhetoric or physical torment rather than responsive words, there can be no effective internalization of loving others. Instead, the images and voices the individual internalizes are challenging, harsh, and mocking. When the physical emergencies of separation, pain, hunger, and other physical states are not corrected and soothed away by the physical care of a parent, the child is left in a neurochemical "stew" of panic, arousal, and unmet need. When this is the repeated experience of childhood it becomes the most efficient pathway for future experience to travel, and one involuntarily becomes expert at panic, arousal, and unmet need, alienation, and the management of harsh and mocking introjects.

When the capacity to maintain an inner sense of connection with others is impaired, self-injury can help manage the work of connection. Self-injury can be a way to manage conflict internally because interpersonal conflict has in the past been dangerous. Self-injury might demonstrate loyalty to perpetrators and symbolize identification with the aggressor. Self-injury can also be a way of taking control of victimization—being the one to decide when, how, and how much one will be injured. Self-injury may at times be an effort to obtain recognition, attention, or other forms of interpersonal connection that are sometimes identified as secondary gain. Such efforts demonstrate the degree of an individual's desperation to connect and the nature of past objectification of self and other. Self-injury also offers the benefits of private experience; when connection is too risky, the self meets its own complex needs, in part through a relationship to the body.

Strong Affect

The ability to experience, tolerate, and integrate strong affect cannot fully develop when strong feelings are met with punishment or derision and need and longing are met with neglect or humiliation. The child learns not to want and not to need. To accomplish this, he or she must also learn not to feel. Thus, numbing, dissociation, or self-punishment (through words of criticism or through actions of self-harm) may become natural responses to or protection from feelings. Through repetition of this, one involuntarily becomes expert at numbing and dissociation and self-punishment. Thus, numbing, dissociation, or self-punishment occurs in response to all kinds of triggers, many of which call for self-protective judgment or sensitivity to the self. Revictimization is one outcome; loss of felt experience and internal coherence are others.

If the capacity to experience and tolerate strong affect is impaired, self-injury may present a solution. The rituals and sensations around it are generally experienced as reducing unbearable tension. This can be self-soothing for individuals who never had the opportunity to internalize a soothing other. Self-injury can serve as punishment for affect that is forbidden or split off. It can be a way to deal with sexual feelings, especially if sexual abuse has served to link terror, pain, and sexual feeling together (Davies & Frawley, 1994). Self-injury is also commonly used to manage depersonalization and extreme levels of dissociation. Some people report that it is useful to induce dissociation or trance; others that it brings them back to their bodies and to physical sensation, reducing the dysphoria or the terror of prolonged dissociation. Finally, self-injury can be used to invoke a sense of safety and relief. If abuse is inevitable, its occurrence removes dread and terror. If the safest times of a child's life are the hours following an abusive episode, the aftermath of abuse may feel comforting and safe (Calof, 1994; Sakheim, 1996).

Expression or externalizing of affective states is a primary function of self-injury, and developing new ways of expressing, especially in connection with others, is central to treatment. Calof (1996) wrote in detail about the difficulty childhood abuse survivors experience in feeling, naming, and comprehending anger. The ability to feel and name affects is impaired. This was termed *alexythymia* by Krystal (1978) and was linked to self-injury in one study (Zlotnik et al., 1996). The individual moves from arousal to action without mediating stages of feeling awareness, feeling identification, feeling expression, and self-soothing. This rapid and unmediated movement from arousal to action is demonstrated in the rising sense of tension that self-injurers describe, the preoccupation with achieving self-injury, and the sense of relief that accompanies or follows the act. This is a good example of overuse of parts of the limbic system without the full aid of the neocortex. Brain imaging research suggests that people having traumatic memories are in a physical state of speechless terror, during which they reexperience the trauma but are prevented from translating the experience to language (van der Kolk, 2006).

Self-Worth

Finally, the ability to maintain a sense of self as viable, benign, and positive cannot fully develop when a child's existence and accomplishments are met with silence or abusive words or actions. The child does not learn that he or she is a person of value. Rather, the lesson is existential self-doubt and self-loathing. Experience does not teach the child that relational experiences can reassure and cheer the child. The child's brain does not sculpt pathways of easy access to a sense of resilient self-worth. Instead, states of low stimulation, boredom, emptiness, and self-disgust dominate.

When the capacity to maintain a sense of self as viable, benign, and positive is impaired, self-injury serves a host of functions. It may be used for purification, transcendence, or penance, as in many mystical practices. It may provide punishment and degradation of the unworthy self. It may serve to reassure the survivor that he or she is a human being—flesh and blood. It may serve to threaten or remind the individual of his or her unworthiness, intrinsic vileness, and fragile hold on the world of other people. It may also serve to reassure the individual that he or she is indeed tough, resilient, and able to take abuse and carry on.

Without strong self-capacities and stable external supports, a self-injurer cannot afford to let go of the adaptations that have helped her or him survive the original abusive environment or the current inner emotional and physical life that has resulted. When self-capacities are undeveloped, self-injury can act as a substitute for their essential regulatory functions. Self-injurious behavior, then, may be viewed as a complex adaptation to powerful psychological and physiological circumstances rooted in otherwise impossible developmental conditions and personal suffering.

CLINICAL APPLICATION OF CONSTRUCTIVIST SELF-DEVELOPMENT THEORY FOR SELF-INJURY

Short-Term Goals

CSDT provides a way to understand self-injury and a framework for action. This is particularly important in crisis and emergency settings in which contact may be brief and clinical information minimal. CSDT allows the treatment provider to move with respect and purpose to assist the self-injuring individual in a crisis. Within this framework, three organizing principles guide short-term intervention: (a) return control to the individual in crisis, (b) develop short-term strategies to shore up self-capacities, and (c) link self-injury to an external or internal antecedent event. The treatment provider should first assess how this encounter has come about, how the individual is reacting to the setting, and the possibility that the self-injuring individual may have a history of childhood abuse. The intervention process has been described in previous publications (e.g., see Deiter & Pearlman, 1998; Saakvitne et al., 2000). It applies to all persons who present with self-inflicted injuries, including those who are not childhood trauma survivors.

Under the stress of emergency situations, an acronym can help clinicians maintain focus and simplify interpersonal communication. The acronym reminds clinicians to make therapeutic contacts RICH, by focusing on respect, information, connection, and hope (Saakvitne et al., 2000). This approach is applied here to self-injury intervention.

Respect

Attention to the interpersonal context is an essential beginning in responding respectfully to the self-injuring person. Childhood abuse survivors are exquisitely attuned to manipulation and deception, and the encounter cannot succeed if the provider is behaving in an authoritarian, indirect, or otherwise disrespectful manner. The circumstances of an individual's presentation to an emergency service or urgent care clinic are significant to the process of addressing his or her safety, and unfavorable circumstances may set a negative tone if the provider does not address them directly. Someone who is dragged against his or her will to an emergency service will respond differently than someone who has entered the treatment setting independently. It is respectful to acknowledge the circumstances and help the client be in a position of control.

In the rushed and impersonal climate of emergency or crisis settings, respectful attention to circumstances and the interpersonal context can feel time-consuming and therefore stressful for the provider. It may be useful to remember Kluft's (1993) maxim, "The slower you go, the faster you get there" (p. 42).

The goal is to help the individual regain control and dignity and create safety. To do this, the provider asks the client's opinion about what level and type of assistance will help and initiates a collaborative discussion about treatment decisions. This approach minimizes the possibility of retraumatizing events in the crisis setting, including affect-driven escalation on the part of the client or provider and reenactments of past abuses such as restraint, labeling, rejection, or abandonment.

Information

The provider should ensure that the client has information about the current situation. For example, the real limits, procedures, and risks of the setting should be reviewed to enable the client to make informed decisions about behavior. Clients in a hospital emergency department need to be informed of the gross criteria for release and for admission, so both parties can operate in an above-board and respectful fashion with reduced fears of being manipulated, trapped, or abandoned. The provider can help the client regain control and move toward safety through compassionate understanding of self-injury and by discussing the client's experience in a sensitive, nondramatic, and accepting manner. Offering education about the effects of trauma and about living in a sensitized body can be helpful for some clients. It is important that clients know their behavior is an outcome of understandable human distress, not a sure sign of being "crazy" or otherwise "bad." The provider can offer assistance by answering questions about specific symptoms, crisis services, trauma treatment, and by sharing information about resources for self-injuring people. Educational and support resources for self-injury are listed in the appendix at the end of this chapter.

Connection

By sharing information about resources, clinicians also offer the self-injuring person the possibility of connection. Encouraging the client to call a local crisis service when distressed, sharing knowledge about Internet sites for self-injuring people, referring to a book or workbook, and offering information about therapy groups or therapists who are sensitive to the client's issues reassure the client that he or she is not alone in the world, that other people self-injure, and that others understand the distress and isolation he or she may be feeling.

Connection can also refer to connecting past and present affect states; connecting bodily sensations, emotions, and beliefs about self and others; and connecting psychological needs to feeling states. In a crisis setting, clinicians can help by acknowledging these connections as they emerge.

Most important may be the connection that is offered in the person of the provider. A RICH encounter with a kind and well-prepared person in a position of benevolent authority can challenge and counter many of a self-injuring person's past relational experiences. It may open the door to risking connection with other providers. If the encounter goes well, referrals to other resources are much more likely to be accepted.

Hope

People can and do stop self-injuring. Self-injury arises out of extreme need and lack of options. When it is no longer needed and a client finds other useful strategies for surviving, self-injury can end. This is likely to happen over time, through psychotherapy that is sensitive to trauma and self-injury. More immediate hope may emerge as the client and therapist determine together the immediate precipitant to this episode of self-injury. When a sequence of events is understood, the self-injuring person may feel understood and more in control. In addition, it may be possible to think together about the points at which another decision could be made and other choices considered and to make a plan for the next time the desire to self-injure arises. Gently determining what was needed to change the events that led to self-injury and making plans to meet the need differently can be enormously useful.

Long-Term Goals

The long-term goals for treatment of self-injury are to explicate the adaptive function of the behavior, support the individual in living without self-injury, and help the individual develop self-capacities.

Explicate the Adaptive Function of Self-Injury

In longer-term therapy with survivors of childhood trauma, the client and therapist work to grasp the adaptive functions of symptoms, including self-injury. How did the symptom serve the goal of survival? How has the symptom changed with time? Is the adaptation still useful? Can it be replaced with something else, reduced or transformed? What will be lost to the survivor if this adaptation is challenged, altered, or transcended? What could be gained? What resources will be needed to make the loss bearable and to make useful that which is gained?

In the treatment of individuals with self-injury, there should not be an early focus on elimination of symptoms as the measure of treatment success. Symptoms have original contexts that made them adaptive; to ignore or reject the functional quality of symptoms is to empathically fail the individual, encourage self-loathing and confusion, and discourage an important survival strategy. Managing self-injury until it is no longer needed is one reasonable goal. This is a highly collaborative task and requires work on using alternative strategies and minimizing physical harm.

Support the Individual in Living Without Self-Injury

Early work on self-capacities and concrete, planful work on self-care and alternatives to self-injury help the client and the therapist track self-injury and address safety. Escalating or dangerous forms of self-injury should be evaluated clinically and interpreted in light of affective challenges, external stressors, current memory content and nature, and the therapeutic relationship. Escalation suggests the need for more structure (including inpatient care), careful pacing, and continuing work on self-capacities through the development of the therapeutic relationship. Returning again to work on self-care, self-capacities, and moment-to-moment survival strategies is necessary.

The therapist must be clear from the outset about his or her own position on self-injury. If the therapist cannot tolerate any injury in the course of therapy, it is important to state that at the consultation stage. The pair can then consider carefully whether they should go forward as a therapy dyad and if so, how urges to self-injury will be handled.

Help the Individual Develop Self-Capacities

The development of self-capacities takes place within the context of therapeutic relationships (McCann & Pearlman, 1990; Pearlman, 1998;

Saakvitne et al., 2000). Connection to benign others is likely the most feared, the most longed-for, and often the most needed experience of survivors. Patient work on the development of trust and esteem between the therapist and client is required. It is within this relationship that the client has an opportunity to work from a secure base, to use the relationship to fill missing ego functions, and to develop self-capacities. It is within this context that the client has a new opportunity to develop in relationship with a person who can teach self-soothing and managing behavior in times of distress.

The therapist and client can work together to consider episodes of self-injury relationally (Saakvitne et al., 2000). Could self-injury be serving a function that is like the original functions (Deiter et al., 2000)? Is it serving to reassure the client of the therapist's concern? To overwhelm the therapist? To make the therapist serve as a helpless witness to abuse? To express an untold story of suffering? Is the therapist being asked to express horror, outrage, fear, hope, or compassion? Is self-injury the only way to achieve these goals, tell the story, survive the feelings, or elicit the reactions? Can the client imagine ever having another way?

Self-injury can be seen as an expression of a pressing need. The need may well be related to affect, memory, relational patterns, hyperresponsiveness of the nervous system, lack of ability to soothe, or other vestiges of abuse. The therapy relationship can be used to identify the pressing need and find other ways of meeting and expressing it.

Clinical Applications of Knowledge About the Effects of Trauma on the Body

Trauma's effect on the body and speculations about the link to self-injury have implications for treatment. It is increasingly clear that trauma-related disorders involve not simply conditioned responses, not simply psychological effects, not even just personality-level impacts but also neuropsychophysiological effects on the body and many of its systems, including the nervous system and brain. "The entire organism is affected" (van der Kolk, 2006, p. 310). Indeed, "traditional therapies have relied either on words and meaning-making or on medications to help modulate these neurobiologic systems" (van der Kolk, 2006, p. 309). Van der Kolk (2006) called for the addition of therapies that teach through felt experience. The teaching relies on safety and supportive relationships. It involves use of the body and is aimed at increased regulation, increased tolerance of the effects of trauma, and *interoception*, or perception of the self and the state of the self.

Survivors can benefit from education about living with sensitized nervous systems and other outcomes of trauma exposure. Allen (2001) encouraged education of clients, careful attention to new and ongoing sources of stress, self-care for health maintenance, and the practice of responding to reexperiencing trauma as a medical emergency because of its extremely harmful physical and neurological effects on the sensitized systems of trauma survivors.

Self-injury is one of the "extreme behaviors" Ford (2005a) identified as helping calm the "alarm system in the brain." In fact, most of the extreme behaviors he identifies are forms of indirect or direct self-injury. Ford developed a group education and training program called Trauma Adaptive Recovery Group Education and Therapy (TARGET). TARGET teaches voluntary, practiced activities for shutting down or resetting the alarm by creating access to the frontal cortex. This allows people to think clearly and respond in ways that meet the needs of the moment. Ford's techniques involve psychoeducation and careful rehearsal of cognitive–behavioral strategies. They are highly adaptable for individual therapy (Ford, 2005a; Marvasti, 2004).

Adjunct therapies may be helpful in treatment. For example, psychodrama, art therapy, eye movement desensitization and reprocessing, and other treatment approaches that use the body and mind together may offer potentially healing experiences. Yoga, meditation, and self-defense may offer opportunities for clients to develop control and understanding of the body. Building specific skills for managing physical effects of trauma may relieve trauma-induced changes. Ford (2005a) taught techniques to decrease hyperarousal. Rothschild (2000) was careful to address the physical basis and outcome of trauma as well as the emotional dimensions through eclectic strategies. Dialectical behavior therapy (Linehan, 1993) focuses in part on increasing distress tolerance skills. Levine (1997) drew attention to the body's response to the original emergency experience. Intrapsychic and physical resources can be strengthened and matched with a stable, supportive interpersonal network and adequate therapeutic care before deeper therapy work is approached (McCann & Pearlman, 1990; Miller, 1994). Therapy with a self-injuring trauma survivor requires resources for both the client and the therapist. A skilled psychiatrist or other prescribing provider may be important. Nonpsychiatric medical care may be needed but may be feared, creating the need for a careful alliance with a medical provider. In addition, the therapist will need supervision, and the client can benefit from relationships with peers.

Seeking such resources together over time and experimenting with adding more people and experiences to the recovery strategy are important for both the therapist and the client. The combination of internal and external resources and emotional and physical resources sets the stage for psychotherapeutic work on the meaning, purpose, and interpersonal and dynamic functions of self-injury and other complex adaptations.

The Self of the Provider

Clinicians encountering self-injury can be surprised by the complexity and depth of personal feeling they confront. Each provider must work to understand and monitor reactions to this kind of work, protect his or her internal resources, and make him- or herself available to clients without harmful judgment, panic, blaming, exhaustion, or other common reactions to self-injury. *Vicarious trauma* is the negative transformation in the helper that results from empathic engagement with trauma survivors and their trauma material, combined with a commitment or responsibility to help. Its hallmark is disrupted spirituality; as with direct trauma, the signature loss is that of meaning and hope (McCann & Pearlman, 1990; Pearlman & Caringi, in press; Pearlman & Saakvitne, 1995). It is a natural outcome of this type of work and must be addressed through ongoing attention to one's professional and personal needs and the personal work we all have of making meaning in our lives. Only through these means can we clinicians hope to remain vital, alert, and attuned to the complex needs of self-injuring trauma survivors.

CONCLUSION

By acknowledging the importance of childhood trauma in the life of the self-injuring survivor and working toward collaboration in the goal of increased safety, treatment providers offer clients an opportunity to explore self-injury in a compassionate, respectful, and nonjudgmental way. Understanding the forces that underlie self-injury, including the physiology of trauma and impairments of self-capacities, allows the provider to greet the relational challenge and invitation of self-injury in emergency settings and longer-term therapy. This kind of work requires access to internal and external resources for both the client and the provider and should be guided by theory. CSDT teaches that clients can heal from trauma and evolve from self-injury to other strategies for living. This takes place most effectively in a carefully developed therapeutic relationship characterized by respect, information, connection, and hope.

APPENDIX 10.1: EDUCATIONAL AND SUPPORT RESOURCES FOR SELF-INJURY

Treatment providers can find guidelines for educating clients about trauma and related issues at the end of every chapter in Jon Allen's (2001) book *Traumatic Relationships and Serious Mental Disorders*, and self-injuring adults might consider Kristy Trautmann and Robin Connors's (1994) *Understanding Self-Injury: A Workbook for Adults*. Other books and workbooks are listed, described, or reviewed on the Self-Harm and Self-Injury Booklets page of the Web site for Self-Injury and Related Issues (SIARI; http://www.siari.co.uk), which also offers discussion boards and additional resources. Self-help books and booklets for families of young people and information for professionals can also be accessed through http://www.selfharm.org.uk/default.aspa. In addition, the Sidran Institute offers educational resources for professionals (http://www.sidran.org/index.cfm). Sidran also has a telephone information line to help direct people to resources around trauma and related issues (for Help Desk instructions, go to http://www.sidran.org/sub.cfm?sectionID=5), and Sidran Press publishes the quarterly newsletter *The Cutting Edge* (also accessible through Sidran's Web site) for self-injuring people. Other informative Web sites include that of Focus Adolescent Services (FocusAS; www.focusas.com/SelfInjury.html) and that of Self Mutilators Anonymous (http://selfmutilatorsanonymous.org), which provides information on local and telephone meetings. Finally, S.A.F.E. Alternatives advertises a hotline (1-800-DONTCUT [366-8288]) on its Web site (http://www.selfinjury.com).

REFERENCES

Allen, J. G. (1995). *Coping with trauma.* Washington, DC: American Psychiatric Press.

Allen, J. G. (2001). *Traumatic relationships and serious mental disorders.* New York: Wiley.

Begley, S. (2007). *Train your mind change your brain.* New York: Random House.

Briere, J. (1995, November). *Attacks on the body: Meaning and management of self-mutilation in trauma therapy.* Clinical symposium presented at the XI Annual Meeting of the International Society for Traumatic Stress Studies, Boston, Massachusetts.

Briere, J., & Gil, E. (1998). Self-mutilation in clinical and general population samples: Prevalence, correlates, and functions. *American Journal of Orthopsychiatry, 68,* 609–620.

Brock, K., Pearlman, L., & Varra, E. (2006). Child maltreatment, self-capacities and trauma symptoms. *Journal of Emotional Abuse, 6,* 103–125.

Calof, D. L. (1994, November). *Self-injury and self-mutilation in trauma survivors*. Paper presented at the Healing the Heart–sponsored seminar, Madison, CT.

Calof, D. L. (1995). Chronic self-injury in adult survivors of childhood abuse. *Treating Abuse Today, 5–4/5,* 31–36.

Calof, D. L. (1996). Chronic self-injury in adult survivors of childhood abuse. *Treating Abuse Today, 5*(4/5), 31–36.

Clery, C. (2000). Self-directed violence in adolescence: A psychotherapeutic approach. In G. Boswell (Ed.), *Violent children and adolescents: Asking the question why* (pp. 91–103). London: Whurr.

Connors, R. E. (2000). *Self-injury psychotherapy with people who engage in self-inflicted violence*. New Jersey: Jason Aronson.

Davies, J. M., & Frawley, M. G. (1994). *Treating the adult survivor of childhood sexual abuse: A psychoanalytic perspective*. New York: Basic Books.

Deiter, P. J., Nicholls, S., & Pearlman, L. A. (2000). Self-injury and self-capacities: Assisting and individual in crisis. *Journal of Clinical Psychology, 56,* 1173–1193.

Deiter, P. J., & Pearlman, L. A. (1998). Responding to self-injurious behavior. In P. M. Kleespies (Ed.), *Emergencies in mental health practice: Evaluation and management* (pp. 235–257). New York: Guilford Press.

Dellinger-Ness, L. A., & Handler, L. (2006). Self-injurious behavior in human and non-human primates. *Clinical Psychology Review, 26,* 503–514.

Doidge, N. (2007). *The brain that changes itself*. New York: James H. Silberman Books.

Favazza, A. R. (1992). Repetitive self-mutilation. *Psychiatric Annals, 22,* 60–63.

Favazza, A. R. (1998). The coming of age of self-mutilation. *The Journal of Nervous and Mental Disease, 186,* 259–268.

Favazza, A. R., DeRosear, L., & Conterio, K. (1989). Self-mutilation and eating disorders. *Suicide and Life-Threatening Behavior, 19,* 352–361.

Favazza, A. R., & Rosenthal, R. J. (1993). Diagnostic issues in self-mutilation. *Hospital and Community Psychiatry, 44,* 134–140.

Fonagy, P., Gergely, G., Jurist, E., & Target, M. (2004). *Affect regulation, mentalization, and the development of the self*. New York: Other Press.

Ford, J. D. (2005a, March). *Trauma adaptive recovery group education and therapy (TARGET)*. Paper presented at University of Connecticut Health Center, Farmington, CT.

Ford, J. D. (2005b). Treatment implications of altered neurobiology, affect regulation and information processing following child maltreatment. *Psychiatric Annals, 35,* 410–419.

Ford, J. D., Courtois, C., Steele, K., van der Hart, O., & Nijenhuis, E. R. (2005). Treatment of complex posttraumatic self-dysregulation. *Journal of Traumatic Stress, 18,* 437–447.

Gould, M. S., Shaffer, D., & Greenberg, T. (2003). The epidemiology of youth suicide. In R. King & A. Apter (Eds.), *Suicide in children and adolescents* (pp. 1–40). Cambridge, England: Cambridge University Press.

Gratz, K. L. (2001). Measurement of deliberate self-harm: Preliminary data on the deliberate self-harm inventory. *Journal of Psychopathology and Behavioral Assessment, 23*, 253–263.

Gratz, K. L. (2006). Risk factors for deliberate self-harm among female college students: The role and interaction of childhood treatment, emotional inexpressivity, and affect intensity/reactivity. *American Journal of Orthopsychiatry, 76*, 238–250.

Gratz, K. L., Conrad, S. D., & Roemer, L. (2002). Risk factors for deliberate self-harm among college students. *American Journal of Orthopsychiatry, 72*, 128–140.

Grossman, R., & Siever, L. (2001). Impulsive self-injurious behaviors: Neurobiology and psychopharmacology. In D. Simeon & E. Hollander (Eds.), *Self-injurious behaviors: Assessment and treatment* (pp. 117–148). Washington, DC: American Psychiatric Press.

Johnson, S. (2004). *Mind wide open*. New York: Scribner.

Kinniburgh, K. J., Blaustein, M., & Spinazzola, J. (2005). Attachment, self-regulation, and competency. *Psychiatric Annals, 35*, 424–430.

Kleespies, P. M., Deleppo, J. D., Mori, D. L., & Niles, B. L. (1998). The emergency interview. In P. M. Kleespies (Ed.), *Emergencies in mental health practice: Evaluation and management* (pp. 41–72). New York: Guilford Press.

Klonsky, E. D., Oltmanns, T. F., & Turkheimer, E. (2003). Deliberate self-harm in a nonclinical population: Prevalence and psychological correlates. *American Journal of Psychiatry, 160*, 1501–1508.

Kluft, R. P. (1993). Basic principles in conducting the psychotherapy of multiple personality disorder. In R. P. Kluft & C. G. Fin (Eds.), *Current perspectives in multiple personality disorder* (pp. 19–50). Washington, DC: American Psychiatric Press.

Krystal, H. (1978). Trauma and affects. *Psychoanalytic Study of the Child, 33*, 81–117.

Levine, P. A. (1997). *Waking the tiger: Healing trauma*. Berkeley, CA: North Atlantic Books.

Linehan, M. (1993). *Cognitive–behavioral treatment of borderline personality disorder*. New York: Guilford Press.

Mann, J. J., Waternaux, C., Haas, G. L., & Malone, K. M. (1999). Toward a clinical model of suicidal behavior in psychiatric patients. *American Journal of Psychiatry, 156*, 181–189.

Marvasti, J. A. (2004). *Psychiatric treatment of victims and survivors of sexual trauma: A neurobiopsychological approach*. Springfield, IL: Charles C Thomas.

McCann, I. L., & Pearlman, L. A. (1990). *Psychological trauma and the adult survivor: Theory, therapy, and transformation*. New York: Brunner/Mazel.

Miller, D. (1994). *Women who hurt themselves: A book of hope and understanding*. New York: Basic Books.

Muehlenkamp, J. J. (2005). Self-injurious behavior and as a separate clinical syndrome. *American Journal of Orthopsychiatry, 75*, 324–333.

Muehlenkamp, J. J. (2006). Empirically supported treatment and general therapy guidelines for nonsuicidal self-injury. *Journal of Mental Health Counseling, 28*, 166–185.

Pattison, E. M., & Kahan, J. (1983). The deliberate self-harm syndrome. *American Journal of Psychiatry, 140,* 867–872.

Pearlman, L. A. (1998). Trauma and the self: A theoretical and clinical perspective. *Journal of Emotional Abuse, 1,* 7–25.

Pearlman, L. A., & Caringi, J. (in press). Vicarious traumatization and complex trauma. In C. A. Courtois & J. D. Ford (Eds.), *Complex traumatic stress disorders: An evidence-based clinician's guide.* New York: Guilford Press.

Pearlman, L. A., & Saakvitne, K. W. (1995). *Trauma and the therapist: Countertransference and vicarious traumatization in psychotherapy with incest survivors.* New York: Norton.

Ross, S., & Heath, N. (2002). A study of the frequency of self-mutilation in a community sample of adolescents. *Journal of Youth and Adolescence, 31,* 67–77.

Rothschild, B. (2000). *The body remembers: The psychophysiology of trauma and trauma treatment.* New York: Norton.

Saakvitne, K., Gamble, S., Pearlman, L. A., & Lev, B. T. (2000). *Risking connection: A training curriculum for working with survivors of childhood abuse.* Baltimore: Sidran Press.

Sakheim, D. K. (1996). Clinical aspects of sadistic ritual abuse. In L. Michelson & W. J. Ray (Eds.), *Handbook of dissociation: Theoretical, empirical, and clinical perspectives* (pp. 569–594). New York: Plenum Press.

Sansone, R. A., Songer, D. A., & Sellbom, M. (2006). The relationship between suicide attempts and low-lethal self-harm behavior among psychiatric patients. *Journal of Psychiatric Practice, 12,* 148–152.

Schore, A. N. (2003). *Affect regulation and the repair of the self.* New York: Norton.

Sunderland, M. (2006). *The science of parenting.* New York: DK Publishing.

Trautmann, K., & Connors, R. (1994). *Understanding self-injury: A workbook for adults.* Pittsburgh, PA: Pittsburgh Action Against Rape.

van der Kolk, B. A. (1988). The trauma spectrum: The interaction of biological and social events in the genesis of the trauma response. *Journal of Traumatic Stress, 1,* 273–290.

van der Kolk, B. A. (2003). The neurobiology of childhood trauma and abuse. *Child and Adolescent Psychiatric Clinics of North America, 12,* 293–317.

van der Kolk, B. A. (2006). Clinical implications of neuroscience research in PTSD. *Annals of the Academy of Science, 1071,* 277–293.

van der Kolk, B. A., McFarlane, A. C., & Weisaeth, L. (Eds.). (1996). *Traumatic stress: The effects of overwhelming experience on mind, body, and society.* New York: Guilford Press.

van der Kolk, B. A., Perry, C., & Herman, J. L. (1991). Childhood origins of self-destructive behavior. *American Journal of Psychiatry, 148,* 1665–1671.

van der Kolk, B., Roth, S., Pelcovitz, D., Sunday, S., & Spinazzola, J. (2005). Disorders of extreme stress: The empirical foundation of complex adaptation to trauma. *Journal of Traumatic Stress, 18,* 389–399.

Walsh, B. W. (2006). *Treating self-injury: A practical guide*. New York: Guilford Press.

Walsh, B. W., & Rosen, P. (1988). *Self-mutilation: Theory, research, and treatment*. New York: Guilford Press.

Whitlock, J. L., Powers, J. L., & Eckenrode, J. (2006). The virtual cutting edge: The Internet and adolescent self-injury. *Developmental Psychology, 42*, 407–417.

Yates, T. M. (2004). The developmental psychopathology of self-injurious behavior: Compensatory regulation in posttraumatic adaptation. *Clinical Psychology Review, 24*, 35–74.

Zlotnick, C., Shea, M. T., Pearlstein, T., Simpson, E., Costello, E., & Begin, A. (1996). The relationship between dissociative symptoms, alexithymia, impulsivity, sexual abuse, and self-mutilation. *Comprehensive Psychiatry, 37*, 12–16.

Zoroglu, S. S., Tuzun, U., Sar, V., Tutkun, H., Savas, H. A., & Ozturk, M. (2003). Suicide attempt and self-mutilation among Turkish high school students in relation with abuse, neglect, and dissociation. *Psychiatry and Clinical Neurosciences, 57*, 119–126.

11

CONTEMPORARY ISSUES IN THE EVALUATION AND MANAGEMENT OF ALCOHOL- AND DRUG-RELATED CRISES

GLENN R. TREZZA AND HARRIET SCHEFT

Trezza and Popp (1998) sought to delineate the key substance-induced emergency situations a clinician might face and to detail appropriate interventions, both medical and behavioral. A subsequent article (Trezza & Popp, 2000) examined the potential for violence and self-harm in the patient using substances. The purposes of this chapter are to update those reviews with new evidence-based information on the management of alcohol- and drug-induced emergency situations and to call attention to new issues in the field of substance abuse triage.

Substance abuse is an issue in a large number of emergency department (ED) presentations. For instance, Rockett, Putnam, Jia, and Smith (2006) found that overall use of eight targeted substances was 56% for women and

We, the chapter authors, thank our colleague Susan Vickory, RN, for helpful assistance with the literature review of this chapter and for help with training in the clinical use of the Clinical Institute Withdrawal Assessment Scale for Alcohol instruments.

69% for men among 1,502 admissions to seven registered acute care, adult nonpsychiatric hospitals in Tennessee. Such presentation is not limited to the young or to alcohol. Schlaerth, Splawn, Ong, and Smith (2004) found that of 107 adults with positive urine toxicology screens presenting to an ED in Los Angeles, 63% (ages 50 years and older) were using cocaine and another 16% were using opiates. Substance use may present in a manner similar to a variety of psychiatric disorders and in base rates that approach the base rates of these psychiatric disorders. For instance, Caton et al. (2005) found that of 400 patients seen in New York City psychiatric EDs, 217 (54%) were diagnosed as having a primary psychosis, but another 169 (44%) were diagnosed with a substance-induced psychosis. Substance-induced psychosis was better predicted by a history of parental substance abuse, a diagnosis of any drug dependence, and any presence of visual hallucinations than was primary psychosis.

The principal simple substance use–related crises and emergencies that clinicians encounter remain substance intoxication, substance withdrawal, and substance overdose. More complicated substance use emergency situations occur in the presence of comorbid addiction and psychiatric disorder, comorbid addiction and medical problems, and substance use–enhanced risks for violence and self-harm. In covering the psychiatric ED and in teaching, we find that the principal clinical mistake made by many emergency clinicians is neglecting to assess for the role of substance use in emergency situations. A second mistake appears to be a lack of up-to-date knowledge about newer assessment technologies. These newer technologies include, for instance, the Clinical Institute Withdrawal Assessment Scale for Alcohol (CIWA; Sullivan, Sykora, Schneiderman, Naranjo, & Sellers, 1989), and the Clinician Administered Opiate Withdrawal Scale (COWS; Wesson & Ling, 2003) for measuring need for withdrawal interventions. A third mistake has to do with a lack of information about the clinical presentation of "new" substances, principally designer drugs, in both emergency and nonemergency situations. Finally, a lack of familiarity with the current literature on dangerousness may complicate adequate and safe assessment and treatment of the substance-using individual. This chapter attempts to address some of these gaps in knowledge to help clinicians better prepare themselves to handle alcohol- and drug-use emergency situations.

We begin this chapter with a brief discussion of key strategies for clinicians to consider in evaluating all types of substance use–related crises and with a table designed for quick reference about evaluating and managing intoxication and withdrawal states. We then examine how clinicians can work with patients with withdrawal syndromes and present information about standardized, empirically validated assessment instruments for managing withdrawal from alcohol, sedatives, and opiates. Next, we examine the management of intoxication states, with particular attention on what is known in the literature about dealing with the possibility of dangerous behaviors in an intoxicated patient. Finally, we discuss the management of substance over-dose situations and, in particular, detail some of what is known about the overdose potential of designer, or "club," drugs. We discuss designer drugs at some length as part of our attempt to educate and sensitize clinicians to the risks presented by the growing use of this not well-known but highly prob-lematic group of substances.

KEY STRATEGIES FOR CLINICIANS

Regardless of the type of crisis or emergency that arises and the types of substances involved in such situations, there are several key strategies for providers. First, clinicians must make decisions within a limited amount of time, both because of the pace of the ED or urgent care clinic (UCC) and because of medical problems or problems with violence that can arise quickly in a substance use situation. The behavioral clinician must therefore do a thorough assessment of the triage situation quickly, using available assess-ment technologies and making decisions on when to call for a physician evaluation. In conducting triage evaluation and making diagnostic decisions, the behavioral ED or UCC clinician should always consider the possibility of a substance use diagnosis to account for a large variety of presenting psychi-atric or medical symptoms.

Evaluation of potential substance use situations should always include toxic screening (i.e., urine screens and Breathalyzer tests for alcohol) and as complete an interview as possible of both the substance-using patient and any available collateral relatives or friends. The interviewer should make sure to include detailed questions about the type, frequency, and amount of substance use and withdrawal symptom history as well as standard questions about medical and psychiatric status and also conduct an adequate mental status exam. In making diagnostic decisions, it remains important to con-sider the possibility of a substance use diagnosis to account for a variety of psychiatric or medical symptoms.

The importance of physiological screens remains paramount, however. Although clinical identification of substance use often occurs correctly, toxic screens can pick up substance use missed by clinicians. For instance, Bjornaas et al. (2006) found that toxic screens identified an additional 143 cases of substance use among patients admitted for self-poisoning in an acute medi-cal hospital in Oslo, Norway. Cherpitel, Bond, et al. (2005) found that Breathalyzer tests more accurately measured alcohol intoxication than did clinical assessment among 4,798 patients admitted for injuries to EDs in 12 countries. Serum alcohol levels, in turn, are better predictors of alcohol tox-icity than Breathalyzers. The latter can underestimate the degree of alcohol toxicity (Currier, Trenton, & Walsh, 2006). Thus, behavioral clinicians working in the ED or UCC should always be careful to order or have medical clinicians order urine or serum toxic screens whenever possible to determine correctly the presence of substances. With the one exception of serum collection to quantify blood alcohol level, the urine specimen is most sensitive for purposes of detection of substances of abuse in the toxicology lab. Certain hospitals package various screens together, but often not all drugs are included in any one screening panel. Particularly in the presence of possible multiple drug use, clinicians should be prepared to obtain multiple urine or blood samples to run the various tests that will ensure that substances have not been missed. Multiple screens may also be critical if a patient has overdosed and if no confirmed collateral report is available as to which substances the patient had been using.

Information to help clinicians in the ED and UCC evaluate signs and symptoms of intoxication and withdrawal and determine treatments for withdrawal from a number of key substances is included in Table 11.1.

Withdrawal Syndromes

Withdrawal syndromes remain one of the principal substance use–related triage situations the behavioral clinician may confront. Of various withdrawal syndromes, alcohol and sedative withdrawal present with the most medical risks to the patient, and opiate withdrawal remains one of the most subjectively uncomfortable for the patient in terms of feeling ill and out of sorts. Alcohol and sedative withdrawal is also the type of withdrawal that may elicit some of the most difficult behavioral problems in the patient.

Alcohol and Sedative Withdrawal

Patients experiencing substance withdrawal present a number of challenges for the ED or UCC behavioral clinician. Some withdrawal states (e.g., associated with nicotine and caffeine) have primarily behavioral manifestations that include irritability, paranoia (most prominent in stimulant withdrawal), restlessness, insomnia, fatigue, and increased appetite. In the most problematic cases, these may require some form of destimulating environment or psychiatric medication. Other withdrawal states such as alcohol, benzodiazepines, and barbiturates may present with more problematic medical symptoms that require intensive medical intervention.

Uncomplicated withdrawal from alcohol, benzodiazepines, or barbiturates may include agitation, increased pulse and blood pressure, diaphoresis, flushing, fever, anorexia, and sleep disturbance. Complicated withdrawal can become a significant medical emergency, as the patient may begin to present with seizures, hallucinations, confusion, disorientation, and/or delusional thinking. Typically, these symptoms set in about 48 to 96 hours after cessation or significant reduction of alcohol or sedative use. However, they can sometimes occur much sooner, depending on the overall psychiatric and medical health of the patient and on the other substances the patient might

TABLE 11.1

Clinical Presentation of Intoxication and Withdrawal States and Treatment of Withdrawal

Drug	Clinical presentation of intoxication	Clinical presentation of withdrawal	Treatment of withdrawal
Alcohol Benzodiazepines	Slurred speech and dysarthria, incoordination, ataxia, nausea, vomiting, mood changes	Mild to moderate: tremor, tachycardia, anxiety, diaphoresis, insomnia, elevated blood pressure	Benzodiazepines, p.o. fluids, rest
	Severe: obtundation, coma	Severe: seizure, delirium, agitation, incontinence, psychosis	Benzodiazepines, IV access, Haloperidol, medical monitoring
Opioids	Euphoria, myosis, pruritis, sedation	Restlessness, muscle and joint pain, abdominal cramps, mydriasis, piloerection, yawning, rhinorrhea, insomnia, lacrimation, nausea, vomiting, diarrhea, irritability	Full agonist or partial agonist opioids, antispasmodics, antidiarrheals, antiemetics, nsaids/acetaminophen
	Severe: respiratory depression		
Sympathomim- etics	Hyperfocus, anxiety, bruxism, headache, mydriasis, tachycardia, hypertension, chest pain, arrhythmia, hyperthermia, agitation, hyperreflexia, psychosis, paranoia	Hypersomnolence, fatigue, depressed mood, anxiety, increased appetite, anhedonia, decreased concentration	Benzodiazepines prn, p.o. fluids
Cocaine Amphetamines Designer drugs			
MDMA	Agitation, confusion, anxiety, tachycardia, elevated blood pressure and temperature, nystagmus, bruxism	Comparable to mild stimulant withdrawal	
GHB	Lethargy, bradycardia, somnolence, agitation, myoclonic jerks, vomiting, seizures, vertical nystagmus, amnesia, respiratory depression	HTN, tachycardia, tremor, nausea, vomiting, diaphorsis, insomnia, anxiety, delirium, auditory and visual hallucinations	Cardiovascular and respiratory support, fluid maintenance and electrolyte balance, benzodiazepines
			Severe: propofol
Ketamine	Tachycardia, elevated blood pressure, agitation, psychosis	No recognized withdrawal syndrome	

Note. nsaids = nonsteroidal anti-inflammatory drugs; p.o. = per os (i.e., by mouth); IV = intavenous; prn = as needed; MDMA = 3,4-methylenedioxymethamphetamine; GHB = gammahydroxybutyrate; HTN = hypertension.

also have been using. Traditionally, symptoms from complicated withdrawal from alcohol, benzodiazepines, or barbiturates have been treated with benzodiazepines along with behavioral monitoring and, at times, treatment for delirium (Trezza & Popp, 1998).

The determination of degree of alcohol or sedative withdrawal, however, was for a long time not terribly well regulated, and concerns have been reported about overmedication of the patient withdrawing from alcohol (Mayo-Smith, 1997). We, the chapter authors, have on a number of occasions had to deal with a patient entering our substance abuse rehabilitation unit still somnolent or disorganized from iatrogenic benzodiazepine intoxication. In the absence of concrete medical information, a clinician should probably always treat alcohol or sedative withdrawal conservatively. This is particularly true for patients who present with increased risks for withdrawal seizures. Patients at relatively higher risk of withdrawal seizures include the elderly, the homeless (who may be malnourished or harboring covert infection), those living with HIV, and those with any history of head injury, seizure disorders, or withdrawal seizures (Morton, Laird, Crane, Partovi, & Frye, 1994; Trezza & Popp, 1998). Such elevated risk of withdrawal seizures is also the case for patients with increased risk for psychotic spectrum symptomatology (i.e., patients with known psychotic disorders, with stimulant-use or withdrawal-related paranoia, or with prior histories of hallucinations or delusions in the presence of alcohol withdrawal).

In the past decade, scales have been developed to standardize clinical assessment and improve diagnosis and treatment for those patients undergoing alcohol withdrawal syndrome (AWS). The principal assessment scale currently used in the United States is the revised Clinical Institute Withdrawal Assessment Scale for Alcohol (CIWA-Ar; Sullivan, Sykora, Schneiderman, Naranjo, & Sellers, 1989). The CIWA-Ar is a 10-item scale that rates a number of withdrawal symptoms (including nausea/vomiting, paroxysmal sweats, agitation, headache/head fullness, anxiety, tremor, visual disturbances, tactile disturbances, auditory disturbances, and orientation/sensorium clouding) on Likert-type scales.

The Addiction Research Foundation Clinical Institute Withdrawal Assessment Scale for Alcohol (CIWA-AD; Sellers, Sullivan, Somer, & Sykora, 1991), which is based on the *Diagnostic and Statistical Manual of Mental Disorders* (*DSM–III–R*; 3rd ed., rev.; American Psychiatric Association, 1987), is a version of the CIWA-Ar that condenses perceptual disturbances into one question, formally includes autonomic hyperactivity (pulse rate), and maps more closely than the CIWA-Ar on the *DSM* symptoms of alcohol withdrawal. The CIWA-AD has been found to generate slightly higher withdrawal severity scores than the CIWA-Ar (Reoux & Oreskovich, 2006). The authors, however, did not believe the statistically significant difference between the two scales to be of great clinical significance.

An initial CIWA-Ar total score greater than or equal to 10 was found to be a significant predictor of severe AWS in a retrospective study of 284 inpatients admitted for alcohol withdrawal at the Manchester VA Medical Center in New Hampshire. Other significant predictors of severe AWS included (a) use of a morning eye-opener, (b) past benzodiazepine use, (c) self-reported history of delirium tremens, and (d) prior participation in two or more alcohol treatment programs (Kraemer, Mayo-Smith, & Calkins, 2003). The authors found a significantly higher risk of severe AWS in the presence of three or more identified risk factors. Use of the CIWA to individualize therapy for AWS has resulted in administration of significantly less medication and shorter treatment stays (Mayo-Smith, 1997).

CIWA-Ar and CIWA-AD scores, therefore, seem to have real clinical utility in predicting severe alcohol withdrawal and providing guidance about the need for benzodiazepine medication. In recent literature, however, there has been some debate on what scores constitute a flag for treating alcohol or sedative withdrawal with benzodiazepines, with scores from 10 or higher (Kraemer et al., 2003) or from 20 or higher (McMullin & Queen, 2004) being cited as a threshold for withdrawal medication.

The CIWA-Ar pointedly does not include hypertension or tachycardia as symptoms for evaluating alcohol withdrawal. These symptoms can be absent in mild alcohol withdrawal and are generally poor predictors of worsening AWS. Absence of these symptoms can be particularly true in patients who have been using other substances (McMullin & Queen, 2004). As such, a degree of clinical judgment supported by good interview data and toxic screen information should still be used in managing alcohol or sedative withdrawal syndromes. Other medical conditions and other substance use may affect CIWA scores, for example, use of opiates and withdrawal from same may artificially inflate CIWA-Ar and CIWA-AD scores (Reoux & Oreskovich, 2006).

The CIWA scales have empirical support for their utility in determining the need for medication treatment for AWS. Use of the scales can help prevent overmedication and track the course of a patient's withdrawal if changes in CIWA scale scores are observed over time. Although highly recommended by the research literature and by converted clinicians, the scales are not always used routinely in triage settings. One concrete recommendation we offer is that behavioral clinicians should be trained in the use of the instrument by clinicians experienced in administering it. When a patient presents with alcohol or sedative withdrawal, therefore, the behavioral clinician should conduct a clinical interview, use vital sign data taken by the UCC or triage nurse, and compute an initial CIWA-Ar or CIWA-AD scale score. The nurse can then consult with available physicians about the advisability of instituting benzodiazepine therapy.

For less complicated cases of alcohol or sedative withdrawal, behavioral clinicians may become engaged in providing a destimulating environment for potentially agitated patients; however, more complicated AWS may necessitate physical or further chemical restraints. Very mild cases of alcohol or sedative withdrawal may require some time in the ED or UCC under observation, some outpatient prescriptions, and outpatient medical and addiction treatment follow-up. Complicated cases of AWS almost always result in some form of inpatient admission, although lengths of stay appear to be decreasing with appropriate detoxification protocols being guided by CIWA scales and by American Society of Addiction Medicine substance withdrawal criteria (American Society of Addiction Medicine, 2003; Mayo-Smith, 1997, 2003; Myrick, Anton, & Kasser, 2003).

Whereas assessment of alcohol and sedative withdrawal has become more systematized in the past 10 years, treatment (if needed as indicated by CIWA assessment) has remained relatively constant. Reviews of treatment episodes of patients who are in withdrawal continue to indicate that benzodiazepines, in preference to beta-blockers, clonidine, carbamazepine, or neuroleptics, do the best job in preventing severe alcohol- and sedative-associated withdrawal symptoms such as delirium, seizures (Jaeger, Lohr, & Pankratz, 2001; Kosten & O'Connor, 2003; Mayo-Smith, 1997; O'Brien, 2005), and autonomic hyperactivity (e.g., perspiration, tremor, palpitation; Berglund et al., 2003). This last review notes that although other medications do have benefits in terms of nonspecific withdrawal features, only benzodiazepines have demonstrated utility in preventing seizures and delirium tremens; thus, we as yet have no other form of monotherapy that can be strongly recommended to treat complicated AWS.

Opiate Withdrawal

Even though patients in opiate withdrawal will report that their subjective sense of distress is life threatening, opiate withdrawal is rarely life threatening. The two exceptions in terms of medical emergency are (a) untreated, intractable vomiting, which could lead to Mallory-Weiss syndrome (i.e., esophageal tears caused by retching and vomiting), and (b) untreated, intractable diarrhea, which in combination with vomiting could lead to dehydration, hypotension, and electrolyte imbalance. However, such severe opiate withdrawal reactions are relatively infrequent. The bulk of patients undergoing opiate withdrawal will generally experience some combination of flu-like symptoms, such as diaphoresis, rhinorrhea, non-life-threatening nausea, vomiting, abdominal cramps, diarrhea, increased heart rate and blood pressure, muscle spasms, weakness, and periods of irritability (O'Connor, Kosten, & Stine, 2003).

A number of scales have been developed to measure opiate withdrawal, including the Himmelsbach's Point System for Measuring Opioid Abstinence Syndrome Intensity by the Day or Hour (Himmelsbach, 1941), the Subjective and Objective Opiate Withdrawal Scales (Handelsman et al., 1987; Turkington & Drummond, 1989), the Short Opiate Withdrawal Scale (Gossop, 1990), and the Subjective Opiate Withdrawal Questionnaire (Loimer, Linzmayer, & Grunberger, 1991). The scale receiving the most attention currently, however, is the empirically supported COWS, as detailed by Wesson and Ling (2003).

The COWS is an 11-item, clinician-administered pencil-and-paper questionnaire that rates resting pulse rate, sweating, restlessness, pupil size, bone/joint aches, runny nose/tearing, gastrointestinal (GI) upset, tremor, yawning, anxiety/irritability, and gooseflesh skin on Likert-type scales. Wesson and Ling (2003, p. 257) noted that the scale, modified from the CIWA-Ar, can be administered in about 2 minutes and that the COWS can be serially administered to track changes in severity of opiate withdrawal symptoms over time or in response to treatment.

Wesson and Ling (2003) also noted that severe COWS scores can be an indicator of the advisability of using buprenorphine or other opiate replacement therapy in the treatment of severe opiate withdrawal. The scale is also a validated, objective way of determining how intense an uncomfortable opiate-dependent person's symptoms actually are. Wesson and Ling indicated that the various items on the COWS were all drawn from previously validated assessment instruments, but in general, less clinical research on the COWS (as compared with the CIWA-Ar) has appeared in the literature.

Medical complications of opiate withdrawal are most closely associated with dehydration. Treatment of opiate withdrawal may consist of rehydration, monitoring of vital signs, and initiation of opiate full agonists such as methadone or partial agonists such as buprenorphine. The behavioral clinician often has to engage in behavioral management strategies to deal with patient complaints, help a patient remain calm and hydrate properly, and provide accurate information about recent substance use.

INTOXICATION AND DANGEROUSNESS ISSUES

Intoxication is a difficult management issue for the behavioral clinician. Patients who are intoxicated frequently present with the most disinhibition of all patients with substance abuse problems who come to the ED or UCC. Often referred by concerned relatives or friends or by other treatment providers, patients who are intoxicated frequently require a destimulating environment, possible rehydration, monitoring of vital signs, and regular monitoring for signs and symptoms of substance withdrawal.

Common symptoms of alcohol and sedative intoxication include (a) disinhibition and labile affect; (b) slurred speech; (c) unsteady gait; (d) concentration, memory, and attentional difficulties; (e) GI distress; (f) an odor of alcohol; and in severe cases (g) respiratory depression and coma. Symptoms of opiate intoxication include (a) sedation; (b) euphoria or apathy; (c) increased pain tolerance; (d) pinpoint pupils; (e) pruritus (i.e., itching); (f) decreased pulse, blood pressure, and respiratory rate; and (g) inattention or memory problems.

Stimulant intoxication may depend on dosing. At lower doses, the cocaine- or amphetamine-intoxicated patient may have dry mouth; dilated pupils; elevated temperature and respiration; elevated pulse and blood pressure; increased energy, rate of speech, and motor activity; grandiosity; hypersexual behavior; and diaphoresis. At higher levels, stimulants may cause paranoia, irritability, labile affect, impulsivity, hallucinations, delusions, cardiac symptoms, and seizures (Trezza & Popp, 1998). Amphetamine intoxication, as detailed in the section on designer drugs in this chapter, is becoming a common concern, and intoxication states of other "designer," or "club," drugs are discussed below. Hallucinogens and inhalants are also classified as having intoxication states. Intoxication with hallucinogens is characterized by hallucinations, derealization, synesthesias, paranoid ideation and ideas of reference, loss of appetite, and insomnia. The latter is characterized by apathy, belligerence, euphoria, dizziness, blurred vision, impaired gait and coordination, lethargy, and in severe cases, tremor, muscle weakness, stupor, or coma.

Intoxication states certainly increase clinician concerns about harm to others and especially harm to self. Patients frequently fall, accidentally burn themselves, or get assaulted by others whom they have irked in their disinhibited, intoxicated state. Whether being intoxicated increases a patient's potential for being actively suicidal or homicidal, however, remains uncertain. Trezza and Popp (2000) examined literature on dangerousness and substance use and noted that (a) research studies seemed to support a relationship between heavy alcohol use and completed suicides, but the existing data were based on samples of Anglo-Caucasian men and did not speak to the issues of drug use or comorbid drug–alcohol use; (b) clinicians must assess history of recent losses, prior suicide attempts, psychiatric comorbidity, and recent hospitalizations in addition to substance abuse parameters in evaluating and treating suicide risk in substance-using persons; (c) alcohol use on the part of victims appeared to have been a factor more often in stranger-rape situations than in acquaintance-rape events; (d) alcohol use did appear to have a role in domestic violence; and (e) there remained a number of problems with definitions, frequency and accuracy of reporting of violence, and identification of clear causal pathways between substance use and violence (especially with other drugs besides the most-often-studied alcohol).

Conversely and more definitively, the MacArthur Violence Risk Assessment Study, which sampled admissions at acute civil inpatient facilities in one small and two mid-size American cities, found that of many hundreds of violence incidents studied, 54.1% were preceded by drinking just before the incident and 23.0% were preceded by use of illegal drugs just before the incident. The MacArthur study indicated clearly that alcohol use was a major predictor of violent assaults on the part of patients studied, that more men than women in their sample had histories of violent acts along with concomitant alcohol dependence issues, and that men were more likely than women to have used alcohol and drugs prior to committing a violent act (Monahan et al., 2001).

More recent research has also indicated that aggression by men against women is 8 to 11 times more likely on days when men have been drinking (Fals-Stewart, 2003) and that partner violence decreased significantly after alcohol-dependent veterans underwent behavioral couples treatment for alcohol dependence (O'Farrell, Fals-Stewart, Murphy, & Murphy, 2003).

Other studies have attempted to quantify a number of variables associated with substance use and dangerousness to self and others. Cherpitel, Ye, and Bond (2005) did a meta-analysis of studies that involved 17,708 persons presenting to EDs in seven countries. They found that violence-related injuries were more associated with drinking right before an injury rather than with patterns of drinking (such as chronic vs. sporadic) and that this effect was stronger for men than for women, with no age-specific differences. Cherpitel et al. noted that their observed effect sizes were small and that sociocultural factors (including typical amounts of consumption by nation and varying levels of stigmatization about drinking) contributed strongly to the heterogeneity of their results.

Tiett, Ilgen, Byrnes, and Moos (2006) examined suicide attempts among patients who are substance use disordered in 150 Veterans Affairs medical centers. Using clinical diagnostic and Addiction Severity Index data to identify the 30-day risk of suicide attempt among veterans who reported suicidal ideation in the 30 days prior to intake assessment, the investigators found that current drinking to intoxication and current cocaine use were both factors in a decision tree about suicide risk for these veterans. Other factors were a history of prior suicide attempts, first occasion of suicidal ideation, and difficulty controlling violent behavior. Doshi, Boudreaux, Wan, Pelletier, and Camargo (2005) studied 412,000 annual ED visits for a 5-year period from 1997 to 2001 that involved suicide attempt and self-inflicted injury. The researchers found that such ED visits were more frequent for teenagers, for female rather than male patients, and among African American rather than Anglo-Caucasian patients. They also found that such ED visits did not vary by metropolitan status or region, and that self-poisoning (68%) and cutting/piercing (20%) were the most frequent methods of self-injury. Depressive disorder was recorded for 34% of such ED visits for suicide attempt, and alcohol abuse was recorded in 16% of cases. Other drug use was apparently not assessed.

Borges, Walters, and Kessler (2000) reviewed data from the 1990–1992 U.S. National Comorbidity Survey. The authors found that current alcohol and drug use predicted subsequent suicide attempts after controlling for sociodemographics and comorbid mental disorders but that previous substance use was not a predictor of suicide among current nonusers. They further noted that the number of substances used is more important than the types of substances used in predicting suicidal behavior. They concluded with a take-home message for clinicians to be aware that current substance use, even in the absence of abuse or dependence, is a significant risk of unplanned suicide attempts among ideators.

Thus, the state of the literature about substance use and violence to self and others remains somewhat diverse, with continuing variability in what substances are studied, what violence is reported and assessed, and how much of an etiological role substance use is actually playing in harm to self and to others. The literature does indicate, however, that recent substance use does appear to be a risk factor for increased chances of violence, particularly when prior substance use has been associated with prior violent acting out.

The literature suggests that the behavioral clinician working in the ED must think complexly in looking at violence and self-harm in the substance-using patient. In terms of assessment and treatment strategies, the clinician should be concerned about increased potential for violence and self-harm in patients who are intoxicated or in withdrawal, because of issues of disinhibition, physical anesthesia, increased irritability and libido, and distress over physical discomfort. However, the clinician should evaluate this potential in terms of other factors, including history of harm to self and others (in an intoxicated state or otherwise), presence of psychotic symptoms, history of past or current depression, history of recent losses, and presenting picture of medical comorbidity.

OVERDOSE

Today, the growing presence of designer drugs threatens to make overdose a regular occurrence in EDs nationwide. In this section, we first discuss the general management of overdose situations (which clinically require medical involvement). We then give concentrated attention to the reality of designer and club drugs and the issues they present in critical overdose situations and, more generally, in terms of intoxication and withdrawal states. We make a point of highlighting these drugs together because they represent a potential tidal wave of ED presentations nationally (and are already a frequent issue on the West Coast of the United States) and because despite many calls to arms, many clinicians are still unfamiliar with the particulars of these substances.

General Management of Overdose

Overdose may be defined as a potentially life-threatening condition secondary to drug ingestion that can present on a continuum of altered mental status from agitation to delirium to coma to respiratory and cardiac arrest. This situation represents a medical emergency that requires immediate intervention by ED or UCC medical staff. Although the mental health clinician may be called on to help parse the purposeful versus accidental overdose, until the patient is medically stable this distinction must remain a secondary concern.

The workup of the overdosed patient requires a meticulous physical and mental status examination, along with collection of drug ingestion history with corroboration of information from witnesses whenever possible. Although supportive medical treatment to stabilize airway/breathing, circulation, and temperature is initiated on the basis of clinical presentation, urine and blood toxicology analyses are of particular importance for confirmation of diagnosis because patients may misrepresent their ingestion intentionally or by mistake. The medical staff will often have no drug ingestion data, for example, when the patient arrives comatose. Certain substances have specific antidotes (e.g., full agonist opioids, naloxone), which underscores the need for accurate identification of the substances ingested (Dickinson, Mayo-Smith, & Eickelberg, 2003; Taylor, Cohan, & White, 1985).

The importance of comprehensive toxicology screening in the ED is further highlighted by the Drug Abuse Warning Network data from 2005 (also supported in previous work; Taylor, Cohan, & White, 1985). These data indicated that of an estimated 598,542 ED visits for nonmedical use of prescription or over-the-counter pharmaceuticals, 55% of these visits involved multiple drugs, 20% implicated pharmaceuticals in combination with illicit drugs, and 6% involved pharmaceuticals in combination with both alcohol and illicit drugs (see http://www.DAWNinfo.samhsa.gov). Polydrug ingestion will affect clinical presentation. For example, rapid onset and brief duration symptoms of gamma hydroxybutyrate (GHB) ingested alone contrast strongly with the sustained manifestation of symptoms plus increased agitation and aggression observed when alcohol is combined with GHB (Gonzalez & Nutt, 2005; Liechti, Kunz, Greminger, Speich, & Kupferschmidt, 2006). Thus, a patient who presents as ataxic, agitated, and smelling strongly of alcohol should not necessarily be presumed to have ingested only alcohol on board because he or she may need treatment for GHB ingestion also.

In general, a frequent danger in overdose situations is that unidentified multiple drug ingestion may result in the inadvertent withholding of a specific treatment. The ED or UCC clinicians treating patients who have overdosed must therefore be knowledgeable about the testing capabilities of their hospital's toxicology laboratory. The triage team should be aware of which drugs are included in standard urine screens and which drugs need to be ordered specially. For example, certain designer drugs such as GHB and ketamine will be detected by gas chromatography/mass spectrometry but not by routine immunoassay urine screen. Mental health clinicians may be engaged in an evaluation during the evolution of an overdose as the patient proceeds from an intoxicated state to coma. The clinician needs to be cognizant of the range of clinical symptoms and signs of overdose of a wide range of substances.

Alcohol, Drugs of Abuse, and Overdose States

Alcohol will cause marked motor and mental dysfunction at a wide range of blood alcohol concentrations, depending on the individual's tolerance. Loss of consciousness is common when blood alcohol concentration reaches 400 mg/dl to 600 mg/dl and is accompanied by respiratory depression, hypotension, and hypothermia. Mortality may be the endpoint of profound central nervous system (CNS) shutdown (Mayo-Smith, 2003). Sedative–hypnotic agents, specifically benzodiazepines, generally do not cause mortality secondary to overdose unless combined with other CNS depressants, such as alcohol. Although medical management of overdose is beyond the scope of this chapter, it is worthwhile to note that benzodiazepine-induced respiratory depression and coma can be reversed, albeit for a brief duration, by the antagonist flumazenil, which carries its own potentially adverse effect of precipitating seizures in the benzodiazepine-dependent patient.

Opioids in overdose will cause sedation and respiratory depression that may progress to coma and respiratory arrest. Intravenous injection of naloxone, a mu opioid receptor antagonist, will reverse full agonist opioid-induced coma. The caveat for naloxone administration is awareness of its short duration of action, particularly when used to reverse the effects of a long-acting opioid agonist such as methadone. The experience of finding a hastily transferred patient comatose in his bed after naloxone's effects have dissipated, a patient who arrived minutes before awake and alert from the ED to the floor of the general medical ward, is not soon forgotten.

Signs of amphetamine and cocaine overdose, perhaps more accurately described as the extreme effects of intoxication, are the cardiovascular complications of myocardial infarction or arrhythmia and neurological dysregulation resulting in agitation and psychosis. In addition, patients may present with sympathomimetic-induced seizures—single seizures or status epilepticus, hypothermia, and rhabdomyolysis (Smets et al., 2005).

In summary, drug overdose is a medical emergency that requires a rapid response of comprehensive assessment, supportive intervention to stabilize the patient medically, and when relevant, administration of a specific antidote.

Designer Drugs

Ingestion of designer drugs (also known as club drugs) should be suspected in a healthy young person who presents to the ED with an acute onset of altered mental status. Systematic workup and management should include vital sign measurement; airway protection; IV access with complete blood count, serum chemistries, creatine kinase, myoglobin, and lactic acid tests sent to the lab; urine specimen for osmolality, sodium, and creatine kinase sent to the lab; EKG monitoring; toxicology screening; administration of glucose, thiamine, or naloxone; and brain imaging to rule out lesions or bleeds (Ricaurte & McCann, 2005). One particular designer drug worth noting is GHB, which may cause bradycardia, agitation, incontinence, somnolence, confusion, seizures, respiratory arrest, and coma in overdose (Gonzalez & Nutt, 2005; Miro, Nogue, Espinosa, To-Figueras, & Sanchez, 2002). Large doses will precipitate overdose, and frequent users have a high probability of having experienced overdose more than once (Gonzalez & Nutt, 2005). There is no specific medication that will reverse the effects of GHB overdose, and mortality may be the consequence.

GHB, which originally was sold as a bodybuilding and fat burning compound, is now abused by bodybuilders, partying high school "ravers," and gay men, particularly those attending "circuit parties" (i.e., large-scale dance parties happening in a planned circuit across a variety of American and Canadian cities). Most often found in liquid form, GHB is also available in powder or capsule formats and is often mixed in drinks for ingestion. The drug initially produces euphoria, increased sociability, and increased libido, then leads to ataxia, somnolence, vomiting, aggression, headaches, nausea, confusion, and incontinence. The drug presents sexual risks to users. GHB has been implicated in a number of sexual assaults and appears to raise the risk of HIV transmission because of its disinhibiting and libido-enhancing effects (Gonzalez & Nutt, 2005; Shoptaw, 2006). In doses over 30 mg per kilogram, GHB can cause hallucinations, myoclonic jerks, and anesthesia; in doses over 60 mg per kilogram, the drug can induce coma (Gonzalez & Nutt, 2005).

Often used to enhance the high of other drugs such as Ecstasy, cocaine, crystal meth, and alcohol, GHB can have fatal overdose potential, particularly when combined with alcohol. Management of such overdose may include blood pressure and fluid support, endotracheal intubation, and in severe cases, mechanical ventilation (Liechti et al., 2006). GHB overdose can also present with a withdrawal syndrome that can look similar to alcohol withdrawal, including symptoms of insomnia, tremulousness, anxiety, chills, sweating, and increased heart rate and blood pressure. Withdrawal management recommendations include emotional support and possible benzodiazepine administration, particularly as patients in GHB withdrawal often are presenting with alcohol withdrawal as well (Ricaurte & McCann, 2005). Gamma butyrolactone and 1,4-butanediol, both precursors to GHB, are sometimes abused in themselves and have similar overdose and withdrawal profiles (Ricaurte & McCann, 2005).

In addition to GHB use, an epidemic of use of the stimulant methamphetamine, or crystal meth, has been expanding in the Midwest and on the West Coast (but has not yet fully hit the East Coast; Parsons, 2007). The crystal meth epidemic is affecting a number of target populations, including high school age youth and adult gay and bisexual men (Hopfer, Mendelson, Van Leeuwen, Kelly, & Hooks, 2006; Jones, 2005; Shoptaw, 2006; Wu, Schlenger, & Galvin, 2006). Moreover, other club, party, or designer drugs (along with OxyContin) have been playing a larger role in the presentations of chemically dependent individuals, including a large number of young veterans of the Afghanistan and Iraq wars. These drugs, in addition to crystal meth, include Ecstasy (i.e., X, MDMA, 3,4-methulenedioxy-methamphetamine), ketamine (i.e., K, "special K," N-methyl-D-aspartate), flunitrazepam (i.e., flumazenil, the "date rape" drug), the previously discussed GHB (i.e., G or "liquid X"), and although somewhat less often, Viagra and resurgently popular club inhalants such as amyl and butyl nitrate and nitrous oxide (Britt & McCance-Katz, 2005; Romanelli, Smith, & Pomeroy, 2003). These club drugs are often used in combination with more traditional substances including alcohol, cocaine, and opiates.

For a number of behavioral and medical clinicians, even those experienced with substance abuse, designer drugs remain a large hole in knowledge and clinical acumen, with a number of providers not knowing all the names and street names of current drugs. Clinicians are often unaware of the current epidemiology of these substances and unfamiliar with clinical manifestations of such drugs. Moreover, many clinicians lack access to toxic screens that routinely test for the presence of them. Although most of the designer drugs can be found through laboratory testing, screens for virtually all designer drugs are omitted from otherwise routine serum and urine toxic screens, which is a serious limitation to adequate screening at a time such drugs are becoming more commonly used among the young.

Most serious among current designer drugs is methamphetamine. Known also as "crystal meth," "crystal," "tina," "meth," and "speed," methamphetamine may be smoked, snorted, injected, taken orally, or "booty bumped" (i.e., taken by inserting a solution of water and methamphetamine rectally through a syringe). Subjective symptoms of intoxication include euphoria, increased alertness, reduction of fatigue and appetite, increased libido, increased confidence, and decreased fears about living with or about acquiring HIV or other sexually transmitted diseases. Physiologically, crystal meth can cause acute increases in heart rate, blood pressure, pupil size, respiration, and sensory acuity, and eventually can cause chronic tremor, weakness, dry mouth, weight loss, cough, sinus infection, skin damage, headaches, and anorexia, along with marked dental damage (e.g., bruxism, rotting of teeth near the gums, multiple caries). Evidence suggests a connection between crystal meth use and increased risk of acquiring HIV and other sexually transmitted diseases (Jones, 2005; Shoptaw, 2006). After a weekend of intense methamphetamine use, users may present to an ED in a "crash" state, with depression and anxiety from work and relationship problems, paranoia such as that seen in the presence of other stimulants, and possible violent acting out. Shoptaw

(2006) noted the alarming epidemiology of crystal meth use. He cited (a) 2004 statistics from the United Nations that more than 35 million people worldwide use amphetamines, making them the second most popular global drug of abuse after cannabis (United Nations Office on Drugs and Crime, 2004) and (b) domestic treatment admission data showing that over 50% of substance abuse treatment admissions in California are for methamphetamine use and methamphetamine admission outpaced cocaine and heroin treatment admissions in 14 U.S. states in the West, Midwest, and South. In many parts of the United States, however, toxic screens for methamphetamine use are not routinely collected (and they are available.) Moreover, many ED and UCC staff are still unfamiliar with the presentation of methamphetamine intoxication or withdrawal and are unfamiliar with the presenting high risk groups for crystal meth use.

Lack of familiarity with other designer drugs is also a concern. Of crystal meth's fellow club drugs, many also have serious side effects. Smets et al. (2005) reported on several cases of serious amphetamine toxicity induced by MDMA (i.e., 3,4-methylenedioxymethamphetamine, Ecstasy) use. One patient suffered severe hepatic toxicity and coma, requiring liver transplant; a second had prolonged seizures, psychotic symptoms, and marked aggressiveness; and a third died of MDMA-induced central hyperthermia and pulmonary edema. Smets et al. noted that MDMA can also cause disseminated intravascular coagulation and rhabdomyolysis, which can lead to renal failure. Management of MDMA overdose is similar to that for most overdose states, that is, monitoring of vital signs, EKG, urine and serum toxicology screens, routine blood analyses, intubation as necessary, and adequate nutrition and hydration to stabilize the patient (Wilkins, Mellott, Markvitsa, & Gorelick, 2003).

Ketamine, or special K, is an animal tranquilizer that can be injected, snorted, or smoked. Introduced in the 1960s and a derivate of phenylcyclidine hydrochloride, ketamine is a dissociative anesthetic that in social settings is most commonly snorted. Analgesic in lower doses, ketamine causes amnestic effects in higher doses, including a prolonged dissociative state referred to by users as "being in a K-hole." Ketamine can also cause visual hallucinations and decreases in coordination (Romanelli, Smith, & Pomeroy, 2003; Shoptaw, 2006). Although death from ketamine use is rare, the drug can cause hypertension, tachycardia, and arrhythmias, and overdose hazards are compounded by combination with alcohol. Thus, a patient should be monitored carefully if any ketamine use is reported or detected. A ketamine-intoxicated patient may need a destimulating environment, behavioral monitoring, and vital sign monitoring to manage any hallucinations that are manifested and to manage marked uncoordinated, dissociative states.

Because it is colorless, odorless, and tasteless, ketamine is also used as one of several date-rape drugs; the other common drug used in this way is flunitrazepam. Similar in effect to benzodiazepines, to which it is chemically related, flunitrazepam causes a number of CNS-depressing toxic effects similar to those seen in benzodiazepine intoxication. Patients need to be monitored for such possible effects. Overdose on flunitrazepam is rare, unless the drug is combined with alcohol or with other CNS-depressants such as benzodiazepines. Gradual taper with a long-acting benzodiazepine, such as diazepam, is the treatment of choice for possible flunitrazepam withdrawal (Ricuarte & McCann, 2005).

In addition to designer drugs, current trends in drug use also lead to concern about the intoxication and withdrawal effects of certain over-the-counter medications, including diphenhydramine (or Benadryl, an antihistamine and sleeping aid), Flexeril (i.e., an antispasm muscle relaxant), and dextromorphan (i.e., a synthetic opiate commonly used in a number of over-the-counter cough suppressants). Miller (2005) noted that dextromorphan, for instance, has dependence and withdrawal risks, can cause dissociative and psychotic states and may lead to dissociation-induced accidents.

CONCLUSION

We tried in this chapter to include useful reference information on the empirically supported clinical management of intoxication, withdrawal, and overdose states for ED and UCC clinicians and for a general mental health professional audience. In addition, we attempted to highlight key new areas with which the behavioral clinician dealing with substance use issues should become familiar. In particular, in this chapter we strove to (a) make clinicians more familiar with contemporary scales for managing alcohol–sedative and opiate withdrawal, (b) briefly survey recent literature on the relationship of substance abuse to acts of self- and other-harm, and (c) detail pointedly the presentation of designer drugs and the ways in which these drugs may present in ED and UCC settings. For the behavioral clinician to successfully manage a range of alcohol- and drug-related crises, he or she must combine longstanding methods of intervention with attention to developing substance use patterns and newer methods of assessment and intervention.

REFERENCES

American Psychiatric Association. (1987). *Diagnostic and statistical manual of mental disorders* (3rd ed., rev.). Washington, DC: Author.

American Society of Addiction Medicine. (2003). Summary of the ASAM patient placement criteria for adult patients in need of detoxification services. In A. Graham, T. K. Schultz, M. F. Mayo-Smith, R. K. Ries, & B. B. Wilford (Eds.), *Principles of addiction medicine* (3rd ed., pp. 619–620). Chevy Chase, MD: Author.

Berglund, M., Thelander, S., Salaspuro, M., Franck, J., Andreasson, S., & Ojehagen, A. (2003). Treatment of alcohol abuse: An evidence-based review. *Alcoholism: Clinical and experimental research, 27,* 1645–1656.

Bjornaas, M. A., Hovda, K. E., Mikalsen, H., Andrew, E., Rudberg, N., Ekeberg, Ø., & Jacobsen, D. (2006). Clinical vs. laboratory identification of drugs of abuse in patients admitted for acute poisoning. *Clinical Toxicology, 44,* 127–134.

Borges, G., Walters, E. E., & Kessler, R. C. (2000). Associations of substance use, abuse, and dependence with subsequent suicidal behavior. *American Journal of Epidemiology, 151,* 781–789.

Britt, G. C., & McCance-Katz, E. F. (2005). A brief overview of the clinical pharmacology of "club drugs." *Substance Use & Misuse, 40,* 1189–1201.

Caton, C. L. M., Drake, R. E., Hasin, D. S., Dominguez, B., Shrout, P. E., Samet, S., & Schanzer, W. B. (2005). Differences between early-phase primary psychotic disorders with concurrent substance use and substance-induced psychoses. *Archives of General Psychiatry, 62,* 137–145.

Cherpitel, C., Bond, J., Ye, Y., Room, R., Poznyak, V., Rehm, J., & Peden, M. (2005). Clinical assessment compared with Breathalyzer readings in the emergency room: Concordance of ICD-10 Y90 and Y91 codes. *Emergency Medicine Journal, 22,* 689–695.

Cherpitel, C., Ye, Y., & Bond, J. (2005). Attributable risk of injury associated with alcohol use: Cross-national data from the Emergency Room Collaborative Alcohol Analysis Project. *American Journal of Public Health, 95,* 266–272.

Currier, G. W., Trenton, A. J., & Walsh, P. G. (2006). Relative accuracy of breath and serum alcohol readings in the psychiatric emergency service. *Psychiatric Services, 57,* 34–36.

Dickinson, W. E., Mayo-Smith, M. F., & Eickelberg, S. J. (2003). Management of sedative-hypnotic intoxication and withdrawal. In A. Graham, T. K. Schultz, M. F. Mayo-Smith, R. K. Ries, & B. B. Wilford (Eds.), *Principles of addiction medicine* (3rd ed., pp. 633–650). Chevy Chase, MD: American Society of Addiction Medicine.

Doshi, A., Boudreaux, E. D., Wan, N., Pelletier, A. J., & Camargo, C. A., Jr. (2005). National study of U.S. emergency department visits for attempted suicide and self-inflicted injury, 1997–2001. *Annals of Emergency Medicine, 46,* 369–375.

Fals-Stewart, W. (2003). The occurrence of partner physical aggression on days of alcohol consumption: A longitudinal diary study. *Journal of Consulting and Clinical Psychology, 71,* 41–52.

Gonzalez, A., & Nutt, D. J. (2005). Gamma hydroxy butyrate abuse and dependency. *Journal of Psychopharmacology, 19,* 195–204.

Gossop, M. (1990). The development of a short opiate withdrawal scale (SOWS). *Addictive Behaviors, 15,* 487–490.

Handelsman, L., Cochrane, K. J., Aronson, M. J., Ness, R., Rubinstein, K. J., & Kanof, P. D. (1987). Two new rating scales for opiate withdrawal. *American Journal of Drug and Alcohol Abuse, 13,* 293–308.

Himmelsbach, C. K. (1941). The morphine abstinence syndrome, its nature and treatment. *Annals of Internal Medicine, 15,* 829–839.

Hopfer, C., Mendelson, B., Van Leeuwen, J. M., Kelly, S., & Hooks, S. (2006). Club drug use among youths in treatment for substance abuse. *The American Journal on Addictions, 15*, 94–99.

Jaeger, T. M., Lohr, R. H., & Pankratz, V. S. (2001). Symptom-triggered therapy for alcohol withdrawal syndrome in medical inpatients. *Mayo Clinical Procedure, 76*, 695–701.

Jones, K. (2005). Methamphetamine, the brain, HIV, and mental health. *Focus: A Guide to AIDS Research and Counseling, 20*(6), 1–4.

Kosten, T. R., & O'Connor, P. G. (2003). Management of drug and alcohol withdrawal. *The New England Journal of Medicine, 348*, 1786–1795.

Kraemer, K. L., Mayo-Smith, M. F., & Calkins, D. R. (2003). Independent clinical correlates of severe alcohol withdrawal. *Substance Abuse, 24*, 197–209.

Liechti, M. E., Kunz, I., Greminger, P., Speich, R., & Kupferschmidt, H. (2006). Clinical features of gamma-hydroxybutyrate and gamma-butyrolactone toxicity and concomitant drug and alcohol use. *Drug and Alcohol Dependence, 81*, 323–326.

Loimer, N., Linzmayer, L., & Grunberger, J. (1991). Comparison between observer assessment and self-rating of withdrawal distress during opiate detoxification. *Drug and Alcohol Dependence, 28*, 265–268.

Mayo-Smith, M. F. (1997). Pharmacological management of alcohol withdrawal: A meta-analysis and evidence-based practice guideline. *The Journal of the American Medical Association, 278*, 144–151.

Mayo-Smith, M. F. (2003). Management of alcohol intoxication and withdrawal. In A. Graham, T. K. Schultz, M. F. Mayo-Smith, R. K. Ries, & B. B. Wilford (Eds.), *Principles of addiction medicine* (3rd ed., pp. 621–633). Chevy Chase, MD: American Society of Addiction Medicine.

McMullin, N., & Queen, J. (2004). A construction worker with recent confusion, disorientation, and somnolence. *Cleveland Clinic Journal of Medicine, 71*, 809–814.

Miller, S. C. (2005). Dextromethorphan psychosis, dependence, and physical withdrawal. *Addiction Biology, 10*, 325–327.

Miro, O., Nogue, S., Espinosa, G., To-Figueras, J., & Sanchez, M. (2002). Trends in illicit drug emergencies: The emerging role of gamma-hydroxybutyrate. *Clinical Toxicology, 40*, 129–135.

Monahan, J., Steadman, H. J., Silver, E., Appelbaum, P. A., Robbins, P. C., Mulvey, E. P., et al. (2001). *Rethinking risk assessment: The MacArthur Study of Mental Disorder and Violence.* New York: Oxford University Press.

Morton, W. A., Laird, L. K., Crane, D. F., Partovi, N., & Frye, L. H. (1994). A prediction model for identifying alcohol withdrawal seizures. *American Journal of Drug and Alcohol Abuse, 20*, 75–86.

Myrick, H., Anton, R., & Kasser, C. L. (2003). Management of intoxication and withdrawal: General principles. In A. Graham, T. K. Schultz, M. F. Mayo-Smith, R. K. Ries, & B. B. Wilford (Eds.), *Principles of addiction medicine* (3rd ed., pp. 611–618). Chevy Chase, MD: American Society of Addiction Medicine.

O'Brien, C. P. (2005). Benzodiazepine use, abuse, and dependence. *Journal of Clinical Psychiatry, 66*(Suppl. 2), 28–33.

O'Connor, P. G., Kosteon, T. R., & Stine, S. M. (2003). Management of opioid intoxication and withdrawal. In A. Graham, T. K. Schultz, M. F. Mayo-Smith, R. K. Ries, & B. B. Wilford (Eds.), *Principles of addiction medicine* (3rd ed., pp. 651–667). Chevy Chase, MD: American Society of Addiction Medicine.

O'Farrell, T., Fals-Stewart, W., Murphy, M., & Murphy, C. (2003). Partner violence before and after individually based alcoholism treatment for male alcoholic patients. *Journal of Clinical and Consulting Psychology, 71*, 92–102.

Parsons, J. T. (2007, March). *Methamphetamine use among young gay and bisexual men in New York City.* Paper presented at the 10th Annual CHAPS Conference, London, England.

Reoux, J. P., & Oreskovich, M. R. (2006). A comparison of two versions of the Clinical Institute Withdrawal Assessment for Alcohol: The CIWA-Ar and CIWA-AD. *The American Journal on Addictions, 15*, 85–93.

Ricaurte, G. A., & McCann, U. D. (2005, June 18). Recognition and management of complications of new recreational drug use. *The Lancet, 365*, 2137–2145.

Rockett, I. R. H., Putnam, S. L., Jia, H., & Smith, G. S. (2006). Declared and undeclared substance use among emergency department patients: A population-based study. *Addiction, 101*, 706–712.

Romanelli, F., Smith, K. M., & Pomeroy, C. (2003). Use of club drugs by HIV-seropositive and HIV-seronegative gay and bisexual men. *International AIDS Society—USA: Topics in HIV Medicine, 11*, 25–32.

Schlaerth, K. R., Splawn, R. G., Ong, J., & Smith, S. D. (2004). Change in the pattern of illegal drug use in an inner city population over 50: An observational study. *Journal of Addictive Diseases, 23*, 95–107.

Sellers, E. M., Sullivan, J. T., Somer, G., & Sykora, K. (1991). Characterization of *DSM–III–R* criteria for uncomplicated alcohol withdrawal provides an empirical basis for *DSM–IV. Archives of General Psychiatry, 48*, 442–447.

Shoptaw, S. (2006, January). *Men who have sex with men, club drugs, and HIV.* Paper presented at the HIV Office for Psychology Education (HOPE) National Training Conference, Memphis, TN.

Smets, G., Bronselaer, K., De Munnynck, K., De Feyter, K., Van de Voorde, W., & Sabbe, M. (2005). Amphetamine toxicity in the emergency department. *Emergency Medicine, 12*, 193–197.

Sullivan, J. T., Sykora, K., Schneiderman, J., Naranjo, C. A., & Sellers, E. M. (1989). Assessment of alcohol withdrawal: The Revised Clinical Institute Withdrawal Assessment for Alcohol Scale (CIWA-Ar). *British Journal of Addiction, 84*, 1353–1357.

Taylor, R. L., Cohan, S. L., & White, J. D. (1985). Comprehensive toxicology screening in the emergency department. *The American Journal of Emergency Medicine, 3*, 507–511.

Tiett, Q. Q., Ilgen, M. A., Byrnes, H. F., & Moos, R. H. (2006). Suicide attempts among substance-use disorder patients: An initial step toward a decision tree for suicide management. *Alcoholism: Clinical and Experimental Research, 30,* 998–1005.

Trezza, G. R., & Popp, S. M. (1998). The evaluation and management of alcohol- and drug-related crises. In P. M. Kleespies (Ed.), *Emergencies in mental health practice* (pp. 258–276). New York: Guilford Press.

Trezza, G. R., & Popp, S. M. (2000). The substance user at risk of harm to self or others: Assessment and treatment issues. *Journal of Clinical Psychology, 56,* 1193–1205.

Turkington, D., & Drummond, D. C. (1989). How should opiate withdrawal be measured? *Drug and Alcohol Dependence, 24,* 151–153.

United Nations Office on Drugs and Crime. (2004). *Amphetamines: A global survey 2003.* Available at www.unodc.org/pdf/research/wdr07/WDR_2006_1.5_ats.pdf

Wesson, D. R., & Ling, W. (2003). The Clinical Opiate Withdrawal Scale (COWS). *Journal of Psychoactive Drugs, 35,* 253–259.

Wilkins, J. N., Mellott, K. G., Markvitsa, R., & Gorelick, D. A. (2003). Management of stimulant, hallucinogen, marijuana, phencyclidine, and club drug intoxication and withdrawal. In A. Graham, T. K. Schultz, M. F. Mayo-Smith, R. K. Ries, & B. B. Wilford (Eds.), *Principles of addiction medicine* (3rd ed., pp. 671–695). Chevy Chase, MD: American Society of Addiction Medicine.

Wu, L. T., Schlenger, W. E., & Galvin, D. M. (2006). Concurrent use of methamphetamine, MDMA, LSD, ketamine, GHB, and flunitrazepam among American youths. *Drug and Alcohol Dependence, 84,* 102–113.

12

SUICIDE RISK IN PERSONALITY DISORDERS: AN ARGUMENT FOR A PUBLIC HEALTH PERSPECTIVE

PAUL DUBERSTEIN AND TRACY K. WITTE

Only recently has suicide emerged from the shadows of religion and the law as a topic of legitimate inquiry in clinical science. Research initiated in the early to mid-20th century established that many people who died by suicide were in considerable emotional distress at the time of death. As diagnostic nomenclature and postmortem research methods became more refined, it seemed clear that most people who died by suicide in industrialized countries had a diagnosable, but frequently undiagnosed, mental disorder when they took their lives (Cavanagh, Carson, Sharpe, & Lawrie, 2003). Postmortem studies revealed that mood disorders, schizophrenia, or substance use disorders were common. With the advent of biomedical understanding, mental disorders became the lingua franca of contemporary Western suicidology. Treatments for mood disorders, schizophrenia, or substance use disorders are now considered vital components of suicide prevention efforts.

Work on this chapter was supported by U.S. Public Health Service Grants K24MH072712 and F31MH077386. Nikki Mason and Kelly McCollumn provided technical and editorial assistance.

Despite these advances, we now must contend with the danger of ascribing too much explanatory power to the mental disorders that are present in the days, weeks, or months prior to death. Doing so may lead researchers, clinicians, and policymakers to underestimate the role of nonproximal, distal risk markers and misdirect treatment and prevention efforts. Risk markers exist at multiple levels of analysis (Cacioppo & Bernston, 1992). At the *individual* level, *temporally distal* risk markers include longstanding personality traits, processes, and disorders that precede the onset of the suicidal crisis. At the *macro* or *societal* level of analysis, *structurally distal* markers include economic indicators such as the unemployment rate, or health service indicators such as the availability of mental health services in a particular geographic region, as well as indicators of culturally mediated attitudes such as stigma and self-reliance.

Recognizing that suicide risk is a product of individual processes interacting with macro level forces, the focus here is on an individual level variable, personality disorders, defined in terms of the criteria appearing in the *Diagnostic and Statistical Manual of Mental Disorders* (DSM; American Psychiatric Association, 1980, 1987, 1994, 2000) or the *International Classification of Diseases* (ICD; World Health Organization, 1992). Our premise is that progress in suicide prevention will be advanced by identifying personality disorders that could be targeted (a) prior to the development of potentially malignant disorders of mood, cognition, or substance use and (b) alongside the treatment of these disorders. A public health perspective (Kaplan, 2000; Knox, Conwell, & Caine, 2004) points to the potential value of both macro level interventions designed to mitigate risk prior to the development of a frank crisis such as attempted suicide and individual treatments designed to ensure that risk is contained after the crisis has emerged. Risk conferred by personality disorders ought to be addressed both at the macro as well as the individual level.

PERSONALITY DISORDERS AND SUICIDE RISK

Which personality disorders confer risk? To answer this question, many clinicians and patients might turn to authoritative guides such as the DSM. They would be misled, however, as the information on suicide risk contained in that manual is not based on scientifically meaningful contemporary evidence. In their review of all English language publications reporting data on the contributions of personality disorders to suicide, Duberstein and Conwell (1997) concluded that a substantial proportion of people who died by suicide met criteria for *avoidant* or *schizoid* personality disorder. Yet the DSM fails to mention suicide risk in either of these disorders. Consistent with nearly a century of psychological theorizing on the role of aggression in suicide (Freud, 1917/1957; Hendin, 1991; Zilboorg, 1937), that review also revealed that *antisocial* and *borderline* personality disorders both confer risk. Here, too, the *DSM* provides misleading information in its assertion that 8% to 10% of patients with borderline personality disorder take their own lives (American Psychiatric Association, 1994, 2000).

Covering the years 1986 to 1996, Duberstein and Conwell's (1997) review included six retrospective studies reporting data on 731 suicides and eight cohort studies yielding data on 48 suicides. Given the significant conceptual and methodological weaknesses in the available research, Duberstein and Conwell cautioned that knowledge concerning the relationship between personality disorders and suicide may change markedly as more rigorous studies are conducted in more diverse contexts. Among the most notable weakness was the absence of data on suicide risk in community samples: All cohort studies had been conducted on treatment-seeking individuals with personality disorders. However, a significant proportion of people who die by suicide were never in mental health treatment (Luoma, Martin, & Pearson, 2002), and this is particularly true of elderly people (Conwell, Duberstein, & Caine, 2002; Salib & Green, 2003) and in countries with rapidly evolving health care delivery systems (Yang et al., 2005). Even more problematic was the evidence for sample bias. For example, the IQ scores of patients in two studies (McGlashan, 1986; Stone, Stone, & Hurt, 1987) were close to 2 standard deviations above the population mean. These studies accounted for more than 40% of the suicides reported in the literature by 1996 (Duberstein & Conwell, 1997).

In the ensuing 10 years (1997–2006), 11 retrospective studies (see Table 12.1) containing data on personality disorders in 1,288 suicides have been published, along with 10 cohort studies containing data on 109 suicides among 4,251 participants. The pace of research increased, as has its geographic breadth: Between 1997 and 2006, the first studies on suicide and personality disorders were conducted in Germany (Schneider et al., 2006), Taiwan (Cheng, Mann, & Chan, 1997), France (Bioulac et al., 2000), Turkey (Senol et al., 1997), and India (Vijayakumar & Rajkumar, 1999). The significance of this enhanced geographic diversity should not be underestimated, as suicide risk is contingent on numerous circumstances, such as population density and access to firearms and health care, that vary across geographic and political regions (Neeleman, 2002). Research on the interaction of macro and individual level variables is new and rapidly evolving, and firm conclusions have not yet been reached. Still, macro level issues must be considered in clinical risk formulations.

Definition of Suicide

Any review of the suicide literature must begin with a clear operational definition of *suicide*. We use the term to refer to a self-inflicted act that leads to death; we are not concerned here with attempted suicide, nonlethal self-

TABLE 12.1
Axis II Assessments in Case Control Studies: 1997–2006

Location	Publications reporting Axis II data	Study period	Age range: M, SD	N (% suicides recruited); sex	Comparison group	Diagnostic nomenclature; assessment instrument	Reliability of Axis II diagnoses	% with Axis II diagnosis	No. (%) Axis II Cases with Axis I comorbidity	Control for informant status	Control for Axis I
Hualien and Taitung counties, Taiwan	Cheng, Mann, and Chan (1997)	July 1989 to December 1991	Ages 15 and older	116 (99%); 71M, 45F	Living comparison group matched for ethnicity, age (± 5 yrs), sex, and area of residence during the year before death	ICD-10[a]; Standardized Assessment of Personality[b]	κ values range from 0.89 to 1.0	61.9% cases, 23.5% comparison group	70 (62%)	NR—relatives, significant others	NR
Northern Ireland	Foster, Gillespie, and McClelland (1997); Foster, Gillespie, McClelland, and Patterson (1999)	July 1992 to July 1993	Ages 16–79	118 (77%); 93M, 25F	Living comparison group matched for age, sex, and marital status	DSM-III-R[c]; Standardized Assessment of Personality[b]	NR	44.0% cases, 8.5% comparison group	48 (41%)	NR—relatives, significant others	Yes
Manchester, England	Appleby, Cooper, Amos, and Faragher (1999)	January 1995 to June 1996	Ages 13–34; M = 26.8	84 (60%); 68M, 16F	Living comparison group matched for age (=/- 5 yrs) and sex	ICD-10[a]; Personality Assessment Schedule[d]	NR	32.0% cases, 6% comparison group	NR	NR—nonprofessional informants	NR
Staffordshire, England	Boardman, Grimbaldeston, Handley, Jones, and Willmott (1999)	January 1991 to December 1995	Ages 14–89; under age 45 = 58.1%M and 44.4%F	212 (100%); 167M, 45F	Individuals dying from unnatural causes other than suicide matched for age (± 5 yrs) and sex; matched year of death for 172 pairs (81%)	ICD-10[a]; review of medical records	NR	13.2% cases, 7.5% comparison group	NR	NR—no related informants (coroner, general practitioner)	NR

Location	Study	Dates	Age	Sample	Comparison group	Diagnostic instrument	Reliability	Prevalence	Number	Informant	
Southeast Scotland	Cavanagh, Owens, and Johnstone (1999)	1996 to 1998	M = 35.0, SD = 13.6	45 (46%); 71% M, 29% F	Living comparison group matched for age (± 5yrs), sex, and Axis I disorders	ICD-10[a] Personality Assessment Schedule[d]	NR	2.2% cases, 0% comparison group	NR	NR—all relatives	NR
Chennai, India	Vijayakumar and Rajkumar (1999)	January 1994 to Feb. 1995	Ages 15 and older	100 (83%); 55M, 45F	Living comparison group matched for age (± 2 yrs), sex, area of residence, and socioeconomic status	DSM-III-R[c] Standardized Assessment of Personality[b]	NR	20.0% cases, 3% comparison group	30 (30%)	NR—close relative	NR
Oxford, England	Harwood, Hawton, Hope, and Jacoby (2001)	January 1995 to May 1998	Ages 60–91, M = 72.2, SD = 8.42	100 (51%); 132M, 63F in original sample of 195 suicides	Individuals dying by natural causes in a hospital during the same time period matched for age (± 30 mo) and sex	ICD-10[a] Personality Assessment Schedule[d]	NR	16.0% cases, 3.7% comparison group	15 (93.8%)	NR—person in closest contact w/ informant year before death	yes
Canterbury, New Zealand	Conner, Beautrais, and Conwell (2003)	September 1991 to May 1994	Ages 18 and older, M = 37.7, SD = 15.9	193 (94%); 149M, 44F	Living community comparison group matched for age and sex stratified proportional to know distribution of population ages 18 and over	DSM-III-R[c] SCID-III-R[e]	κ values > 0.94	14% cases and 4.3% comparison group had either conduct disorder as a child or antisocial personality disorder as an adult	NR	NR—next-of-kin	NR

(continues)

TABLE 12.1
Axis II Assessments in Case Control Studies: 1997–2006 (Continued)

Location	Publications reporting Axis II data	Study period	Age range; M, SD	N (% suicides: recruited); sex	Comparison group	Diagnostic nomenclature; assessment instrument	Reliability of Axis II diagnoses	% with Axis II diagnosis	No. (%) Axis II Cases with Axis I comorbidity	Control for informant status	Control for Axis I
Montreal, Canada	Kim et al. (2003)	Not reported	Ages 18–65, M = 28.9, SD = 8.4	115[f] (56%) 115M	Living comparison group matched for residential area, marital status, occupation, and age	DSM-IV;[g] Interview Schedule for Children	Kappas not reported for this group of participants.[f]	BPD: 27.0% cases, 3.7% comparison group. AnPD: 15.7% cases, 4.9% comparison group. UnPD: 19.1% cases, 11.0% comparison group	NR	NR—relatives, significant others	NR
England and Wales, United Kingdom	Hawton et al. (2002)	January 1994 to December 1997	Ages 20–59	42 (39.6%); 42F	Living comparison group matched for age (±10 years), specialty, seniority	ICD-10;[c] Personality Assessment Schedule[d]	NR	38.1% vs. 1.2%	16 (100%)	NR—reative or friend; offered a Bereavement Information Pack (Hill, Hawton, Malmberg, & Simkin, 1997)	NR
Frankfurt/Main Germany	Schneider et al. (2006)	January 1999 to December 2000	M = 49.8%, SD = 19.3	163 (62.0%)	Living comparison group matched by age, gender, residential area	DSM-IV;[f] SCID-II[e]	κ values above 0.79 for most Axis I and above 0.65 for most personality disorder diagnoses	72.3% male cases, 27.0% male comparison group. 66.7% female cases, 24.4% female comparison group	68.9%	NR—relatives	yes

Note. M = male, F = female; NR = not reported; *DSM* = *Diagnostic and Statistical Manual of Mental Disorders; ICD* = *International Classification of Diseases;* SCID = Structured Clinical Interview for *DSM* Disorders; BPD = borderline personality disorder; AnPD = antisocial personality disorder; UnPD = unspecified personality disorder. [a]World Health Organization (1992). [b]Mann, Jenkins, Cutting, and Cowen (1991). [c]American Psychiatric Association (3rd ed., rev.; 1987). [d]Tyrer and Alexander (1979). [e]Spitzer, Williams, Gibbon, and First (1988). [f]Kappa coefficients were calculated for a previously studied subgroup of subjects. The kappa coefficients for key diagnoses were as follows: major depression (0.98), alcohol dependence (0.94), schizophrenia (0.98), and borderline personality disorder (0.81). [g]American Psychiatric Association (4th ed.; 1994).

harm, or parasuicide, although each present considerable management and treatment challenges to the practitioner. These issues are covered in other chapters in this book. We focus exclusively on death by suicide. In reviewing the literature, it is important to draw a sharp distinction between studies of suicide and studies of nonlethal self-harm. Important differences have been observed in the demographic and psychological characteristics of those who engage in lethal and nonlethal self-harm (Tsoh et al., 2005; Useda et al., 2007). By definition, a public health perspective affords an aerial view of the field. It allows us to identify areas of neglect in the clinical literature, in which fires are burning and first responders have not yet appeared. People are dying in part because mental health providers have not known where to deliver services. In this chapter, we aim to inform mental health practitioners of the risk conferred by certain personality disorders that have not yet been subject to treatment research. We also argue that patients with these disorders are reluctant to seek help in standard mental health delivery settings (Tyrer, Mitchard, Methuen, & Ranger, 2003). New treatments in novel venues are needed. Given the significant influence of research design on the interpretation of findings in the suicide literature (Duberstein & Conwell, 1997), we organize our review by study design. After reviewing postmortem studies of personality disorders and suicide, we review cohort studies. We then consider the implications of the data on suicide risk in personality disorders for the conceptualization of prevention.

Postmortem Studies

Postmortem studies typically rely on a technique known as the *psychological autopsy*, which involves a review of all available records (e.g., school, criminal, medical) and interviews with informants, most frequently relatives, friends, and health care professionals (Cavanagh et al., 2003). Studies conducted prior to the publication of the *DSM–III* (3rd ed.; American Psychiatric Association, 1987) provided data on the proportion of suicide deaths in a given region with nonspecific personality disturbances (Barraclough, Bunch, Nelson, & Sainsbury, 1974; Dorpat & Ripley, 1960). Estimates derived from psychological autopsy studies published from 1986 to 1996 indicate that 30% to 40% of suicides met criteria for a personality disorder (Duberstein & Conwell, 1997). However, other researchers concluded that 16.2% of the suicides in the postmortem studies they reviewed met criteria for a personality disorder (Arsenault-Lapierre, Kim, & Turecki, 2004). This is an underestimate because postmortem studies that based their diagnoses solely on record review were included, as opposed to psychological autopsy interviews. Yet many people who take their own lives never seek mental health treatment and thus will have no mental health records.

The first-generation psychological autopsy studies of suicide in patients with Axis II disorders all used *DSM* criteria (Apter et al., 1993; Henriksson et al., 1993; Rich et al., 1986; Runeson, 1989), and all reported data on antisocial personality disorder and borderline personality disorder. These groundbreaking studies were methodologically limited. All were uncontrolled and only one reported data on the reliability of their Axis II assessments (Henriksson et al., 1993). None attempted to determine whether informant characteristics affected the quality or quantity of the data provided on personality, a potentially important issue (Riso, Klein, Anderson, Ouimette, & Lizardi, 1994).

The first controlled studies on Axis II and suicide were published in 1994 (Brent et al., 1994; Lesage et al., 1994). Table 12.1 shows all controlled retrospective studies of Axis II disorders in completed suicide that have been published from 1997 through 2006. Controlled retrospective studies without data on personality disorders (e.g., see Chen et al., 2006) and uncontrolled studies (e.g., see Hawton, Malmberg, & Simkin, 2004) are not shown. Table 12.2 shows the findings from the two studies that have attempted to calculate a prevalence rate of all personality disorders listed in the *DSM*.

Although the use of control groups and the routine use of established structured interviews represent clear advances over prior research, the methodological rigor in this area of research is still quite poor. Table 12.1 shows that no studies have attempted to examine the effect of informant mental status on the data. Diagnostic reliability ratings have rarely been reported, and only three attempts have been made to determine whether Axis II disorders conferred risk independent of the presence of Axis I disorders (Foster, Gillespie, McClelland, & Patterson, 1999; Harwood, Hawton, Hope, & Jacoby, 2001; Schneider et al., 2006).

The median rate of Axis II disorders in postmortem samples is 32%, consistent with Duberstein and Conwell's (1997) estimate. Although this consistency with prior research is encouraging, the range of reported rates is striking and warrants further scrutiny and study. How can one investigation yield a rate of 2.2% (Cavanagh, Owens, & Johnstone, 1999) and another 72.3% (Schneider et al., 2006)?

Duberstein and Conwell (1997) also observed interstudy variability, though not quite as dramatic. They ascribed the variability to differences in sample demographics, diagnostic assessment tools, and diagnostic manuals. These methodological explanations are not satisfactory, however. In their review, Arsenault-Lapierre et al. (2004) similarly concluded that the observed cross-study geographic difference is not merely a methodological artifact but an interesting issue that warrants further exploration. Isometsä et al. (1997) reported rural versus urban differences in rates of personality disorders that cannot be explained by methodological artifacts. If indeed risk factors and markers for suicide differ in their relative potency across geographic regions, interventions targeting these factors will be differentially effective in different geographic contexts (Kraemer et al., 1997).

TABLE 12.2

Rates of Axis II Disorders in Foster, Gillespie, McClelland, and Patterson (1999) and Schneider et al. (2006)

Publication		Personality disorder										
	AnPD	BPD	NPD	HPD	PPD	SzPD	StPD	AvPD	DPD	P-APD	CPD
Foster, Gillespie, McClelland, and Patterson (1999)	8.5	9.3	0.8	4.2	14.4	5.9	0.0	19.5	8.5	1.7	0.8
Schneider et al. (2006)											
Men	7.9	28.1	27.7	10.8	20.0	10.8	6.5	23.1	6.2	26.2	23.1
Women	2.6	25.6	20.5	17.9	17.9	12.8	5.1	15.4	5.1	12.8	17.9

Note. Data are all percentages. AnPD = antisocial personality disorder; BPD = borderline personality disorder; NPD = narcissistic personality disorder; HPD = histrionic personality disorder; PPD = paranoid personality disorder; SzPD = schizoid personality disorder; StPD = schizotypal personality disorder; AvPD = avoidant personality disorder; DPD = dependent personality disorder; P-APD = passive–aggressive personality disorder; CPD = compulsive personality disorder.

Table 12.2 lists postmortem studies of suicide that have reported prevalence rates of all *DSM*-defined personality disorders. In addition, Cheng et al. (1997) reported prevalence rates of all personality disorders using *ICD* criteria. For the sake of comparison, we also review recent studies of the prevalence of personality disorders in community settings (Coid, Yang, Tyrer, Roberts, & Ullrich, 2006; Grant et al., 2004; Jackson & Burgess, 2000; Samuels et al., 2002; Torgersen, Kringlen, & Cramer, 2001).

Consistent with the earlier studies (Duberstein & Conwell, 1997), research conducted throughout the past decade has revealed that people with *DSM*-defined borderline personality disorder and antisocial personality disorder are at elevated risk (Foster et al., 1999; Schneider et al., 2006). Moreover, Cheng et al. (1997) reported that 46.0 % of suicides in Taiwan met *ICD-10* (World Health Organization, 1992) criteria for borderline personality disorder, 40.7% of whom met criteria for the *impulsive type*, characterized primarily by emotional instability and lack of impulse control. The remaining 5.3% were thought to have the *borderline type*, which includes disturbances in self-image and identity in addition to emotional instability. The rates of borderline personality disorder in these postmortem studies of suicide are much higher than the rates recorded in recent community studies of living individuals; the highest rate reported in the latter type of study is 1.2% (Samuels et al., 2002). Interestingly, the rate reported by Foster et al. (1999) in their postmortem sample is consistent with the rate reported in a study of treatment-seeking outpatients, 9.3% (Zimmerman, Rothschild, & Chelminski, 2005).

Duberstein and Conwell (1997) tentatively concluded that patients with schizoid and avoidant personality disorder may be at risk. Recent data provide mixed support for this conclusion. In Taiwan, for example, people with these disorders do not appear to be at elevated risk (Cheng et al., 1997). However, rates of avoidant personality disorder in postmortem suicide samples (see Table 12.2) are alarmingly high, especially when viewed in the context of the low prevalence of avoidant personality disorder in community studies, which have ranged from 0.8% (Coid et al., 2006) to 5% (Torgersen et al., 2001). Zimmerman et al. (2005) reported a rate of 14.7% among mental health outpatients, a figure that is slightly lower than the rates shown in Table 12.2. Clearly, there are subgroups of at-risk patients with avoidant personality disorder that are not engaged with the mental health care delivery system. Table 12.2 shows that the rates of schizoid personality disorder reported in postmortem samples are considerably higher than the rates typically reported in community studies of living people, which, with one outlier (Grant et al., 2004), are no higher than 1.9% (Jackson & Burgess, 2000). Ten years ago, data on suicide risk in individuals with *dependent* personality disorder and *paranoid* personality disorder were unavailable or inconsistent (Duberstein & Conwell, 1997). Our review suggests that rates of both disorders are elevated in postmortem samples (see Table 12.2). Rates of dependent personality disorder are no higher than 1.5 % in community samples but range from 3.5% (Cheng et al., 1997) to 8.5% (Foster et al., 1999) in postmortem samples. With the exception of a methodologically limited study (Grant et al., 2004), rates of paranoid personality disorder in community samples are no higher than 1.9% (Jackson & Burgess, 2000), but range from 3.5% to 17.9% in individuals who died by suicide.

Research comparing suicide decedents with personality disorders with those without could inform clinical risk assessments. Using reasonably large postmortem samples, researchers in Finland (Heikkinen, Henriksson, et al., 1997; Heikkinen, Isometsä, et al., 1997; Isometsä et al., 1996, 1997) and Canada (Dumais et al., 2005; Kim et al., 2003, 2004) have pursued this strategy. Heikkinen, Henriksson, et al. (1997) compared 56 suicides with a personality disorder with 56 age- and sex-matched suicides without a personality disorder. Among the former, life events were more common, particularly job problems, family discord, financial trouble, unemployment, and interpersonal loss. Heikkinen, Henriksson, et al. concluded that these events may be explained by the victim's own behavior. Using the same sample, Heikkinen, Isometsä, et al. (1997), showed that suicides with personality disorders were more likely to be unmarried and live alone in an urban area; Isometsä et al. (1997) showed that borderline, antisocial, *histrionic*, and *narcissistic* disorders were also more common in urban regions, as were alcohol disorders, which they speculated could be a function of urbanization. Kim et al. (2003) found that suicides with impulsive and aggressive traits were more likely to have multiple Axis I diagnoses, a finding that is consistent with data from Finland (Isometsa et al., 1996). In summary, postmortem research from 1997 to 2006 continues to document elevated rates of suicide in individuals with borderline and antisocial personality disorders; further evidence for risk in individuals with avoidant and schizoid personality disorders has been provided, and important data have been presented on risk in individuals with dependent and paranoid personality disorders. Interstudy variability in reported prevalence rates is not uncommon and occasionally large in magnitude. Even within the same study, rates of personality disorder are nonrandomly distributed in rural versus urban regions (Heikkinen, Isometsä, et al., 1997; Isometsä et al., 1997). We tentatively conclude that variations in reported rates are only partially attributable to methodological differences. Substantive scientific hypotheses must be developed and tested. Just as alcohol dependence is a more potent risk factor in Sweden than in France (Nortstrom, 1995), some personality disorders might be a more potent driver of risk in some countries or regions and less potent in others.

Cohort Studies

In contrast to postmortem studies, cohort studies examine suicide rates prospectively among a group of individuals; in theory, they are also able to identify risk factors within particular cohorts. Given the rarity of death by suicide, it is common for researchers to focus on at-risk individuals, which makes it more likely that there will be deaths by suicide in a sample. One potential limitation of this design is that the researcher often makes a priori predictions as to which groups are at risk and merit inclusion in the sample. This leaves open the possibility that certain at-risk groups will be excluded from cohort studies. Their suicide risk will be overlooked.

Suicide Rates

Table 12.3 lists the 10 cohort studies of personality disorders and suicide that were published between 1996 and 2006. Cohort studies of personality *traits* and suicide (Angst & Clayton, 1998; Maser et al., 2002; Yen & Siegler, 2003) were excluded. Of the 4,198 individuals with personality disorders who could be traced (98.8%), 109 died by suicide, making the overall suicide rate for personality disorders between 2.56% and 2.60%, depending on whether the denominator is the total number of participants at baseline or the total number who were traced. The geographic differences observed in the postmortem studies are not evident here, with the possible exception of the study by Bioulac et al. (2000), but the small sample size does not permit us to draw any firm conclusions.

Borderline Personality Disorder. Cohort studies have predominantly focused on individuals with borderline personality disorder. Of the 1,131 individuals with borderline personality disorder drawn from five studies (Davies & Campling, 2003; Paris & Zweig-Frank, 2001; Senol et al., 1997; Tidemalm, Elofsson, Stefanson, Waern, & Runeson, 2005; Zanarini et al., 2005), 40 died by suicide (3.54% of the total sample; 3.68% of those who were traced). Davies and Campling (2003) did not specify whether the two suicides in their sample had diagnoses of borderline personality disorder or another emotionally unstable personality disorder. Removing these two suicides leads to a negligible change in the suicide rate (i.e., 3.31% of the total sample and 3.50% of those who were traced). These rates are lower than the rate reported in a previous review (i.e., 5.1%–6.8%; Duberstein & Conwell, 1997). Combining the suicide deaths in the current sample with those in the previous report (Duberstein & Conwell, 1997) yields a total of 86 suicides out of 2,040 people with borderline personality disorder, 1,793 (88%) of whom were traced. Thus, the overall suicide rate ranges from 4.21% to 4.80%. The DSM and many authors have repeatedly asserted that the rate of suicide for individuals with borderline personality disorder is between 8% and 10% (e.g., see Black et al., 2004). Our results suggest that this figure is a considerable overestimate.

Clearly, individuals with borderline personality disorder have a higher likelihood of death by suicide than individuals in the general population. Nevertheless, most patients with borderline personality disorder will not die by their own hand. Thus, there is a need for researchers to identify those at elevated risk. Unfortunately, no cohort study published during the past decade has attempted to differentiate between patients with borderline personality disorder who die by suicide and those who do not. Earlier cohort studies (Paris, Brown, & Nowlis, 1987; Stone et al., 1987) tried but failed to distinguish patients with borderline personality disorder who died by suicide from those who did not, although one group noted the concurrence of "drug abuse, alcoholism, incest, chaotic family life, and impulsivity including promiscuity" in 5 of the 19 suicides in their sample (Stone et al., 1987, p. 191).

Other Personality Disorders. Rates for each of the following personality disorders were reported in only one study: paranoid personality disorder, schizoid personality disorder, schizotypal personality disorder, and antisocial personality disorder. Tidemalm et al. (2005) were able to trace 100% of the original sample. They found that of the 122 individuals in their sample with paranoid personality disorder, 2 died by suicide (1.64%); of the 107 in their sample diagnosed with schizoid personality disorder, 1 died by suicide (0.93%). Given that it is possible that individuals in this sample had additional comorbid Axis II psychopathology, this rate should be viewed with caution. Fenton, McGlashan, Victor, and Blyler (1997) found that out of 33 patients diagnosed with schizotypal personality disorder, 1 died by suicide. Thus, the suicide rate ranged from 3.03% to 3.33%, depending on whether the denominator is baseline participants versus those who were able to be traced ($n = 30$). Black et al. (1996) found that of the 71 men enrolled in the cohort diagnosed with antisocial personality disorder, 1 died by suicide (i.e., 1.41% of total sample and 1.51% of those who were traced).

Methodological Considerations

There have been several notable improvements since Duberstein and Conwell's (1997) review. Recent studies have had remarkably high trace rates of 98.8%. This stands in contrast to the previous review, which found that less than 80% of patients with borderline personality disorder were traced. Furthermore, recent studies used more precise means of determining death by suicide, with four (Baxter & Appleby, 1999; Black, Baumgard, Bell, & Kao, 1996; Kullgren, Tengstrom, & Grann, 1998; Tidemalm et al., 2005) relying on death certificates or national death registers and one (Fenton et al., 1997) relying on informant interviews. The remaining five studies did not clearly state how cause of death was determined, which could potentially be a source of error.

No study has been published on personality disorders and suicide in a random community sample. The generalizability of the available findings to individuals who do not seek treatment in the mental health sector is dubious. Many at-risk individuals are never seen in specialty mental health care (Luoma et al., 2002). Bostwick and Pankratz (2000) described three distinct subgroups of individuals diagnosed with affective disorders: Patients who were hospitalized specifically for suicidal behaviors have the highest risk of death

TABLE 12.3
Cohort Studies of Axis II Disorders and Death by Suicide

Study	Country	Index N	Traced N (%)	Diagnostic method	Reliability rating	Follow-up length	Suicide N (% Index N → Traced N)	Inpatient versus outpatient
Baxter and Appleby (1999)	United Kingdom	779 personality disorders	779 (100%)	Wing et al. (1980) system; ICD-8[a]	No	Up to 18 years	21 (2.7%)	Inpatient and out-patient
Bioulac et al. (2000)[b]	France	7 personality disorders	7 (100%)	DSM–II[c]	No	8	1 (14.3%)	Inpatient
Black, Baumgard, Bell, and Kao (1996)	United States	71 men with AnPD	66 (93%)	DSM–II[c]	No	20–45 years	1 (1.4% → 1.5%)	Inpatient
Davies and Campling (2003)[d]	United Kingdom	52 patients with either BPD or emotionally unstable personality disorders. N = 45 definitely had BPD	52 (100%)	ICD-10[e]; file review	No	Up to 3 years	2 (3.8% of total → 4.4% of BPD)	Inpatient

Study	Country	Sample	Diagnosis (%)	Diagnostic method	Reliability	Follow-up	Suicide rate	Setting
Fenton, McGlashan, Victor, and Blyler (1997)	United States	33 StPD	30 (91%)	DSM–III[c]; positive and negative Syndrome Scale[f]; structured file review	No	Mean = 18.8 years	1 (3.0% → 3.3%)	Inpatient
Kullgren, Tengstrom, and Grann (1998)	Sweden	920 PD	920 (100%)	ICD-9[g]; interviews, psychological tests	No	4–8 years	24 (2.8%) PD	Inpatient
Paris and Zweig-Frank (2001)[h]	Canada	100 BPD	81 BPD (81%)	Retrospective DIB-R[i]	Yes, κ = .74	12 years	3 (3% → 3.7%)	Inpatient
Senol, Dereboy, and Yuksel (1997)	Turkey	75 BPD	61 (81%)	DSM–III[c]; file review by three clinicians who achieved consensus	No formal reliability calculated, but 100% agreement reportedly achieved	4–5 years	2 (3.3% → 2.7%)	Inpatient

(continues)

TABLE 12.3
Cohort Studies of Axis II Disorders and Death by Suicide (Continued)

Study	Country	Index N	Traced N (%)	Diagnostic method	Reliability rating	Follow-up length	Suicide N (% Index N → Traced N)	Inpatient versus outpatient
Tidemalm Elofsson, Stefanson, Waern, and Runeson (2005)[j]	Sweden	122 PaPD 107 SzPD 621 BPD 259 OSPD 815 UnPD	1924 (100%)	ICD-9[g]; chart review	No	1–7 years	PaPD = 2 (1.6%) SzPD = 1 (1%) BPD = 22 (3.5%) OSPD = 9 (3.5%) PD NOS = 21 (2.6%)	Outpatient
Zanarini Frankenburg, Hennen, Reich, and Silk (2005)	United States	290 BPD	278 (96%) of BPD	DIB-R[i] and DSM–III–R[k]; semistructured interview	Yes; interrater κ = .54–.94 (median = .85); test–retest κ = .47–1.0 (median = .87)	2–6 years (mean = 3.5)	BPD = 11 (3.7% → 3.9%)	Inpatient

Note. ICD = International Classification of Diseases; DSM = Diagnostic and Statistical Manual of Mental Disorders; AnPD = antisocial personality disorder; BPD = borderline personality disorder; PD = personality disorder; DIB-R = Revised Diagnostic Interview for Borderlines; PaPD = paranoid personality disorder; SzPD = schizoid personality disorder; StPD = schizotypal personality disorder; OSPD = other specific personality disorder; UnPD = unspecified personality disorder. [a]World Health Organization (1967). [b]In French. [c]American Psychiatric Association (1980). [d]It is possible that neither of these cases were diagnosed with BPD. [e]World Health Organization (1992). [f]Kay, Fiszbein, and Opler (1987). [g]World Health Organization (1977). [h]This is a follow-up study of Paris, Brown, and Nowlis (1987), which was included in Duberstein and Conwell's (1997) review. Paris and Zweig-Frank (2001) conducted a follow-up study of the 100 living patients who had agreed to participate in the earlier study. The rate reported here is based on these 100 to not be redundant with our prior review; Zanarini, Gunderson, Frankenburg, and Chauncey (1989). [i]There may be overlap because some of the suicide cases had comorbid Axis II disorders. Individuals who died by suicide and had comorbid disorders were counted in the rates of each separate personality disorder, although each participant is only counted once in the overall suicide rate for personality disorders. [k]American Psychiatric Association (1987).

by suicide, followed by those hospitalized for symptoms related to their disorder. Outpatients, the third subgroup, have a substantially lower risk of suicide than either of the inpatient groups. Although these subgroups likely exist among patients with personality disorders, detailed information regarding sample selection was rarely provided.

Our review of cohort studies appears most relevant to the subgroup of inpatients who are hospitalized for largely unspecified reasons. Only two studies included outpatients (Baxter & Appleby, 1999; Tidemalm et al., 2005), and none followed individuals who were hospitalized for suicidal behavior. It is possible that the subgroups described by Bostwick and Pankratz (2000) are not at differential risk among patients with personality disorders, however. Baxter and Appleby (1999) and Tildemalm et al. (2005) reported rates that do not deviate markedly from the rates reported in studies of inpatient samples. However, without a larger number of cases than those reported in these two studies, one of which is a combination of inpatients and outpatients (Baxter & Appleby, 1999), no firm conclusion can be drawn. The suicide rates reported here may be an underestimate for those who are hospitalized for suicidal behavior and an overestimate for outpatients with personality disorders. Future cohort studies of patient samples should describe in detail how and where the sample was recruited, make an effort to include outpatients, and provide data on the primary reason for which inpatients are hospitalized (i.e., suicidal behavior vs. other reasons).

None of the cohort studies included in the prior review (Duberstein & Conwell, 1997) contained data on suicide for reliably diagnosed Axis II disorders other than borderline personality disorder. Unfortunately, little progress on this front has been made in the past decade. Only two studies reported reliability ratings for borderline personality disorder (Paris & Zweig-Frank, 2001; Zanarini et al., 2005), and no reliability data were provided for any other personality disorders. Additionally, only two studies used a structured interview to assess personality disorder symptoms (Paris & Zweig-Frank, 2001; Zanarini et al., 2005). Given the difficulty inherent in diagnosing personality disorders accurately, it seems crucial that researchers use well-validated assessment tools.

Another common trend was the propensity to lump personality disorders together into one heterogeneous group. It is probable that there are distinctly different risk levels for suicide amongst the different personality disorders. One would not propose to combine all Axis I disorders into one group to determine risk of suicide; it seems equally imprudent to do so for personality disorders.

None of the studies published between 1996 and 2006 provided information regarding predictors of suicide within diagnostic categories. Although individuals with borderline personality disorder have elevated suicide rates, greater than 90% will not die by suicide. It is critical that researchers identify the characteristics that differentiate patients with borderline personality disorder who take their lives from those who do not. In theory, the cohort design is well suited to provide this type of information because researchers typically collect a wide array of data from participants at baseline, which could then be analyzed postmortem. We recognize, however, that lack of statistical power may make it difficult to identify statistically significant predictors. Duberstein and Conwell (1997) identified two prospective cohort studies that added a postmortem follow-up component (Hagnell & Rorsman, 1980; Rao, Weissman, Martin, & Hammond, 1993); neither focused on personality disorders. Among the studies included in this review, no attempt has been made to add a follow-back component to ongoing prospective cohort studies of personality disorders. At least two cohort studies of personality disorders are currently being conducted (Skodol et al., 2005; Zanarini et al., 2005). It would be useful and cost-effective to add a postmortem surveillance component to these ongoing studies. By interviewing friends, relatives, and clinicians postmortem, researchers could determine the extent to which stressful life events, service utilization, treatment adherence, and other clinical parameters distinguish patients with particular personality disorders who take their lives from those who do not. Still, we acknowledge that cohort designs are not particularly efficient: Suicide and personality disorders occur at low base rates in the general population, and suicide occurs at relatively low base rates among those with personality disorders. Very large sample sizes will be required to examine the effects of mediators (e.g., life events, service utilization). Finally, it is worth noting that not a single cohort study of suicide in patients with avoidant personality disorder has been published, although postmortem studies revealed that the risk of suicide in patients with that disorder is clearly elevated. One would be hard-pressed to find a better illustration of the downside of cohort studies conducted on treatment-seeking patients.

Need for a Public Health Perspective

Rose (1992) divided preventive interventions into high-risk strategies and population (or universal) strategies. Examples of universal strategies include restricting access to lethal means, crafting economic policies that lead to the creation of new jobs, shifting cultural norms concerning the acceptability of suicide, and enhancing mental health literacy. Despite the label, so-called universal programs do not reach everyone. Among other consequences, this could serve to increase the risk of suicide among those not reached (Neeleman, 2002), which might disproportionately include the socioeconomically disenfranchised, racial and ethnic minorities, and of greatest relevance here, those with particular personality traits or disorders. Moreover, some population-based strategies, such as gun control, are vulnerable to political gridlock because they are perceived as restricting a freedom rather than conferring a benefit.

Nonetheless, population-level interventions can potentially save more lives than interventions targeting high-risk groups, because more suicides will be observed in large populations at relatively low risk than in small, high-risk populations. Consider this example: In a population of 10,000,000, the risk of suicide is 0.1%, corresponding to 10,000 suicide deaths annually. If a policy were implemented that reduced the rate by only 5%, 500 lives would be saved. Instead of 10,000 suicides annually, there would be 9,500. Alternatively, one could exclusively target a sample of 1,000 high-risk people, in which the risk of suicide is 50% (which is extraordinarily high but is useful for illustrative purposes). Without intervention, 500 people would die by suicide. Even if one were to implement an intervention with an 80% efficacy rate (again, extraordinarily high), instead of 500 people dying, only 100 would die, which translates to a total of 400 lives saved, a smaller amount than the number saved using a much less potent public health campaign. This illustration points to the tremendous potential of large public health campaigns, which have rarely been used in suicide prevention efforts.

High-risk approaches are less controversial because they typically involve providing a treatment or service to an at-risk population, as opposed to restricting the autonomy of average citizens. High-risk approaches are also thought to be more relevant to clinical care, because the standard model in clinical psychology involves treating people in distress as opposed to preventing morbidity and enhancing wellness (Kaplan, 2000; Levine, 1998; Sarason, 1981). Unfortunately, only 10 treatment studies have examined rates of suicide as an outcome (M. M. Linehan, personal communication, October 6, 2006), few of which have focused on personality disorder. Only one reported a significant reduction in mortality (Motto & Bostrom, 2001). The others did not (Allard, Marshall, & Plante, 1992; Hawton et al., 1987; Linehan, Armstrong, Suarez, Allmari, & Heard, 1991, 1993; Litman & Wold, 1976; Moller, 1989; Motto & Bostrum, 2001; Tyrer, Thompson, et al., 2003; Vaiva et al., 2006; van Heeringen et al., 1995), presumably because of inadequate power. Beyond this inherent difficulty in documenting significant effects, there are other problems with high-risk approaches:

1. Many at-risk patients will not avail themselves of treatment because of their attitudes toward help seeking; this is perhaps especially true of patients with avoidant or schizophrenic tendencies.
2. Few treatments are tailored to patients' needs and preferences, which could lead to poor levels of treatment adherence and high levels of dropout; we are aware of no research on the treatment preferences of patients with avoidant personality disorder, for example.
3. High-risk approaches, although less vulnerable to political problems, are not immune to them, as it can be argued that

there has been an inequitable distribution of clinical and research resources, favoring patients with borderline personality (Coid, 2003).

4. Many patients cannot afford mental health treatment, and
quality services are not available throughout the United States.

Ideally, a public health perspective on suicide would be informed by
systematic studies of the costs of suicide (economic and otherwise) that could
be ascribed to different categories of personality disorder. No consensus has
emerged on the measurement of the cost of suicide, but most would agree
that such a definition would include the number of lives lost, years of life
lost, and economic impact. This is the area in which there is a significant
disconnect between what we need to know about suicide in personality disorders and what is known. Postmortem studies have shown that suicide risk
is elevated for individuals with borderline, antisocial, avoidant, and schizoid
personality disorders and recent data suggest that risk may be elevated for
those with dependent and paranoid personality disorders as well. Yet there is
little data available to inform the work of the practicing clinician, as treatment research has almost exclusively focused on borderline personality disorder, perhaps because those patients have strong treatment-seeking tendencies and are known to burden the health care delivery system (Coid, 2003).
In this regard it might be useful to consider the potentially important conceptual distinction between treatment rejecting and treatment seeking personality disorders (Tyrer, Mitchard, et al., 2003). Although no consensus has
yet emerged in this new literature (Ansell, Sanislow, McGlashan, & Grilo,
2007; Bender et al., 2006), studies of patient samples suggest that individuals
diagnosed with borderline personality disorder have higher rates of treatment utilization than patients with other personality disorders (Ansell et al.,
2007). This is most readily seen in studies of emergency services and hospitalization (Ansell et al., 2007). However, other individuals with personality
disorders who are disengaged from the care delivery system remain at risk.

To be sure, treatment studies of patients with borderline personality
disorder have yielded encouraging results (Bateman & Fonagy, 2001; Linehan
et al., 1991; Linehan, Heard, & Armstrong, 1993). But from a public health
perspective they are limited. First, treatment resources and other mental health
resources (e.g., grant funding, time and attention of clinicians and researchers, policymakers) must be allocated to other personality disorders that confer risk. When Duberstein and Conwell reviewed the literature in 1997, the
risk of suicide for individuals with avoidant personality disorder was unexpected. Ten years later, it is no longer news. What is striking is the absence of
treatment research on this disorder.

Second, developing mechanisms to encourage at-risk individuals to
obtain some form of effective treatment is as pressing a public health need as
developing more potent treatments. Few people who die by suicide had re-

ceived any mental health treatment (Luoma et al., 2002), let alone specialized, evidence-based interventions. No matter how well they are designed, randomized controlled trials conducted on treatment-seeking, or even treatment-referred, populations cannot address this problem. Although good data are not yet available, we suspect that treatment seeking is far more common among patients with borderline personality disorder who take their lives than among patients with avoidant personality disorder who take their lives. Individual practitioners will need to treat people with personality disorders who bristle at the idea of being seen in outpatient mental health care or emergency services to have any impact on suicide mortality. Third, given that personality disorders typically precede the Axis I mental disorders that elevate suicide risk, opportunities to intervene are present long before the development of acute suicide risk. Preventionists can mount interventions targeting individuals who are at risk by virtue of the presence of a personality disorder known to confer suicide risk. But where should these interventions be implemented? Rather than waiting in vain for treatment rejecting individuals with personality disorders to appear in traditional mental health service delivery settings, psychologists must work to actively construct a care delivery system that accommodates these at-risk individuals elsewhere.

A public health perspective requires research aimed at identifying the mediators of suicide risk and gaining a deeper understanding of where, why, and how at-risk patients engage with formal and informal health care providers and services. Such research could be used to identify points of entry for the implementation of prevention programs, such as jails and prisons (which may be particularly relevant for individuals with antisocial personality disorder) and employee assistance programs (for those with avoidant personality disorder).

Fourth, a public health perspective allows clinicians, researchers, and policymakers to consider the possibility that the wide geographic variation in suicide rates could be ascribed to local, not universal, care delivery conditions. Young women in China are at greater risk than young women in industrialized countries because the fundamental transportation infrastructure is inadequate (Yang et al., 2005). The absence of good roads makes it difficult to obtain high quality, timely medical care after the ingestion of pesticide. In contrast, patients with borderline personality disorder in the United States are more likely to survive after an overdose because it is easier for them to be transported to a hospital. The care-delivery infrastructure can be pathogenic, however. To what extent is the care-delivery system in the United States designed to accommodate patients with disorders that compromise one's ability to ask for help, even indirectly? We speculate that the high rates of suicide in patients with avoidant and schizoid disorders can be explained in part by the failure of our health care delivery system to meet their unique help-seeking needs. Although suicide hotlines are widely available throughout the United States and may provide care for those who are housebound or lack transportation, they still require the individual to make an effort to reach out for help.

CONCLUSION

Suicide prevention resources might be misdirected (Sarason, 1981) if clinicians and researchers ascribe too much explanatory power to the mental disorders that are present in the days, weeks, or months prior to death. Clearly, suicide prevention requires researchers and clinicians to focus on the treatment of mood disordered patients with comorbid borderline personality disorder who have been hospitalized for a suicide attempt. However, it is just as important—and potentially more cost-effective—to identify at-risk patients with personality disorders long before they develop a mood disorder, let alone a suicidal crisis.

We focused on an individual level variable, but it is highly likely that the suicide risk conferred by any particular personality disorder is moderated by macro level influences. Suicide rates in the United States vary twofold, with states in the Intermountain West recording rates twice that of the Middle Atlantic States and New England (American Association of Suicidology, 2006). Our review of the literature suggests that there is significant geographic (study site) variability in rates of personality disorder detected postmortem that is unlikely to be attributable to methodological differences between sites. It would not be surprising if some of the regional and national variability in suicide rates were ascribed to interactions between individual level and macro level variables. For example, the risk of suicide for individuals with borderline personality disorder might be greater in regions of the United States where mental health services are less accessible. Suicide in those with avoidant personality disorder might be greater in local cultures characterized by pathological self-reliance in which receipt of mental health service is more stigmatized. Despite the potential need for geographically sensitive risk assessments, the available data offer little guidance to clinicians, public health officials, or policy makers.

Of the six personality disorders that definitely (i.e., borderline, antisocial, avoidant, and schizoid) or probably (i.e., dependent and paranoid) confer risk, only borderline personality disorder has been the subject of intervention research. It has also been studied far more frequently using the prospective cohort design. Much remains to be learned about the mediators of suicide risk in that group. Still, from a public health perspective, it is important to develop novel interventions targeting individuals with other personality disorders that confer suicide risk. Although clinical initiatives might be most effective with patients that are already engaged with the health care delivery system, prevention programs are needed to reach those who are disengaged or treatment rejecting. Ideally, the design and implementation of new treatments and interventions will be informed by the next generation of postmortem and prospective cohort studies.

REFERENCES

Allard, R., Marshall, M., & Plante, M. C. (1992). Intensive follow-up does not decrease the risk of repeat suicide attempts. *Suicide and Life-Threatening Behavior*, 22, 303–314.

American Association of Suicidology. (2006). *Fact sheet*. Retrieved November 22, 2006, from http://www.suicidology.org/associations/1045/files/2003statedatapgc.pdf

American Psychiatric Association. (1980). *Diagnostic and statistical manual of mental disorders* (3rd ed.). Washington, DC: Author.

American Psychiatric Association. (1987). *Diagnostic and statistical manual of mental disorders* (3rd ed., rev.). Washington, DC: Author.

American Psychiatric Association. (1994). *Diagnostic and statistical manual of mental disorders* (4th ed.). Washington, DC: Author.

American Psychiatric Association. (2000). *Diagnostic and statistical manual of mental disorders* (4th ed., text rev.). Washington, DC: Author.

Angst, J., & Clayton, P. C. (1998). Personality, smoking, and suicide: A prospective study. *Journal of Affective Disorders*, 51, 55–62.

Ansell, E. B., Sanislow, C. A., McGlashan, T. H., & Grilo, C. M. (2007). Psychosocial impairment and treatment utilization by patients with borderline personality disorder, other personality disorders, mood and anxiety disorders, and a healthy comparison group. *Comprehensive Psychiatry*, 48, 329–336.

Appleby, L., Cooper, J., Amos T., & Faragher, B. (1999). Psychological autopsy study of suicides by people aged under 35. *The British Journal of Psychiatry*, 175, 168–174.

Apter, A., Bleich, A., King, R., Kron, S., Fluch, A., Kotler, M., & Cohen, D. (1993). Death without warning? A clinical postmortem study of suicide in 43 Israeli adolescent males. *Archives of General Psychiatry*, 50, 138–142.

Arsenault-Lapierre, G., Kim, C., & Turecki, G. (2004). Psychiatric diagnoses in 3275 suicides: A meta-analysis. *BMC Psychiatry*, 4, 37–42.

Barraclough, B. M., Bunch, J., Nelson, B., & Sainsbury, P. (1974). 100 cases of suicide—clinical aspects. *The British Journal of Psychiatry*, 125, 355–373.

Bateman, A., & Fonagy, P. (2001). Treatment of borderline personality disorder with psychoanalytically oriented partial hospitalization. *American Journal of Psychiatry*, 158, 36–42.

Baxter, D., & Appleby, L. (1999). Case register study of suicide risk in mental disorders. *British Journal of Psychiatry*, 175, 322–326.

Bender, D. S., Skodol, A. E., Pagano, M. E., Dyck, I. R., Grilo, C. M., Shea, M. T., et al. (2006). Prospective assessment of treatment use by patients with personality disorders. *Psychiatric Services*, 57, 254–257.

Bioulac, S., Bourgeois, M., Ekouevi, D. K., Bonnin, J. M., Gonzales, B., & Castello, M. F. (2000). Predictive factors of suicide: An 8-year prospective longitudinal study of 200 psychiatric inpatients. *Encephale, 26*, 1–7.

Black, D. W., Baumgard, C. H., Bell, S. E., & Kao, C. (1996). Death rates in 71 men with antisocial personality disorder. *Psychosomatics, 37*, 131–136.

Black, D. W., Blum, N., Pfohl, B., & Hale, N. (2004). Suicidal behavior in borderline personality disorder: Prevalence, risk factors, prediction, and prevention. *Journal of Personality Disorders, 18*, 226–239.

Blair-West, G. W., Cantor, C. H., Mellsop, G. W., & Eyeson-Annan, M. L. (1999). Lifetime suicide risk in major depression: Sex and age determinants. *Journal of Affective Disorders, 55*, 171–178.

Boardman, A. P., Grimbaldeston, A. H., Handley, C., Jones, P. W., & Willmott, S. (1999). The North Staffordshire suicide study: A case-control study of suicide in one health district. *Psychological Medicine, 29*, 27–33.

Bostwick, J. M., & Pankratz, V. S. (2000). Affective disorders and suicide risk: A reexamination. *American Journal of Psychiatry, 157*, 1925–1932.

Brent, D. A., Johnson, B. A., Perper, J. A., Connolly, J., Bridge, J., Bartle, S., & Rather, C. (1994). Personality disorder, personality traits, impulsive violence, and completed suicide in adolescents. *Journal of the American Academy of Child & Adolescent Psychiatry, 33*, 1080–1086.

Brent, D. A., Perper, J. A., Moritz, G., Allman, C., Friend, A., Roth, C., et al. (1993). Psychiatric risk factors for adolescent suicide: A case-control study. *Journal of American Academy of Child & Adolescent Psychiatry, 27*, 362–366.

Cacioppo, J. T., & Bernston, G. G. (1992). Social psychological contributions to the decade of the brain. *American Psychologist, 47*, 1019–1028.

Cavanagh, J. T., Carson, A. J., Sharpe, M., & Lawrie, S. M. (2003). Psychological autopsy studies of suicide: A systematic review. *Psychological Medicine, 33*, 395–405.

Cavanagh, J. T., Owens, D. G. C., & Johnstone, E. C. (1999). Suicide and undetermined death in Southeast Scotland: A case-control study using the psychological autopsy method. *Psychological Medicine, 29*, 1141–1149.

Chen, Y. H., Chan, W. S., Wong, P. W., Chan, S. S., Chan, C. L., & Law, Y. W. (2006). Suicide in Hong Kong: A case-control psychological autopsy study. *Psychological Medicine, 36*, 815–825.

Cheng, A. T. A, Mann, A. H., & Chan, K. A. (1997). Personality disorder and suicide: A case-control study. *The British Journal of Psychiatry, 170*, 441–446.

Coid, J. (2003). Epidemiology, public health, and the problem of personality disorder. *The British Journal of Psychiatry, 182*(Suppl. 44), 3–10.

Coid, J., Yang, M., Tyrer, P., Roberts, A., & Ullrich, S. (2006). Prevalence and correlates of personality disorder in Great Britain. *The British Journal of Psychiatry, 188*, 423–431.

Conner, K. R., Beautrais, A. L., & Conwell, Y. (2003). Moderators of the relationship between alcohol dependence and suicide and medically serious suicide attempts: Analyses of Canterbury suicide project data. *Alcoholism: Clinical and Experimental Research, 27,* 1156–1161.

Conwell, Y., Duberstein, P. R., & Caine, E. D. (2002). Risk factors for suicide in later life. *Biological Psychiatry, 52,* 193–204.

Davies, S., & Campling, P. (2003). Therapeutic community treatment of personality disorder: Service use and mortality over 3 years' follow-up. *The British Journal of Psychiatry, 182*(Suppl. 44), 24–27.

Dorpat, T. L., & Ripley, H. S. (1960). A study of suicide in the Seattle area. *Comprehensive Psychiatry, 1,* 349–359.

Duberstein, P. R., & Conwell, Y. (1997). Personality disorders and completed suicide: A methodological and conceptual review. *Clinical Psychology: Science and Practice, 4,* 359–376.

Dumais, A., Lesage, A. D., Lalovic, A., Seguin, M., Tousignant, M., Chawky, N., & Turecki, G. (2005). Is violent method of suicide a behavioral marker of lifetime aggression? *American Journal of Psychiatry, 162,* 1375–1378.

Fenton, W. S., McGlashan, T. H., Victor, B. J., & Blyler, C. R. (1997). Symptoms, subtype, and suicidality in patients with schizophrenia spectrum disorders. *American Journal of Psychiatry, 154,* 199–204.

Foster, T., Gillespie, K., & McClelland, R. (1997). Mental disorders and suicide in Northern Ireland. *The British Journal of Psychiatry, 170,* 447–452.

Foster, T., Gillespie, K., McClelland, R., & Patterson, C. (1999). Risk factors for suicide independent of DSM–III–R Axis I disorder. *The British Journal of Psychiatry, 175,* 175–179.

Freud, S. (1957). Mourning and melancholia. In J. Strachey (Ed. & Trans.), *The standard edition of the complete psychological works of Sigmund Freud* (Vol. 14, pp. 248–610). London: Hogarth Press. (Original work published 1917)

Grant, B. F., Hasin, D. S., Stinson, F. S., Dawson, D. A., Chou, S. P., Ruan, W. J., & Pickering, R. P. (2004). Prevalence, correlates, and disability of personality disorders in the United States: Results from the National Epidemiologic Survey on Alcohol and Related Conditions. *Journal of Clinical Psychiatry, 65,* 948–958.

Gururaj, G., Isaac, M., Subbakrishna, D., & Ranjani, R. (2004). Risk factors for completed suicides: A case-control study from Bangalore, India. *Injury Control and Safety Promotion, 11,* 183–191.

Hagnell, O., & Rorsman, B. (1980). Suicide in the Lundby Study: A controlled prospective investigation of stressful life events. *Neuropsychobiology, 6,* 319–332.

Harwood, D., Hawton, K., Hope, T., & Jacoby, R. (2001). Psychiatric disorder and personality factors associated with suicide in older people: A descriptive and case-control study. *International Journal of Geriatric Psychiatry, 16,* 155–65.

Hawton, K., Malmberg, A., & Simkin, S. (2004). Suicide in doctors: A psychological autopsy study. *Journal of Psychosomatic Research, 57,* 1–4.

Hawton, K., McKeown, S., Day, A., Martin, P., O'Connor, M., & Yule, J. (1987). Evaluation of outpatient counseling compared with general practitioner care following overdoses. *Psychological Medicine, 17,* 751–761.

Hawton, K., Simkin, S., Rue, J., Haw, C., Barbour, F., Clements, A., et al. (2002). Suicide in female nurses in England and Wales. *Psychological Medicine, 32*, 239–250.

Heikkinen, M. E., Henriksson, M. M., Isometsä, E. T., Marttunen, M. J., Aro, H. M., & Lönnqvist, J. K. (1997). Recent life events and suicide in personality disorders. *Journal of Nervous and Mental Disease, 185*, 373–381.

Heikkinen, M. E., Isometsä, E. T., Henriksson, M. M., Marttunen, M. J., Aro, H. M., & Lönnqvist, J. K. (1997). Psychosocial factors and completed suicide in personality disorders. *Acta Psychiatrica Scandinavica, 95*, 49–57.

Hendin, H. (1991). Psychodynamics of suicide, with particular reference to the young. *American Journal of Psychiatry, 148*, 1150–1158.

Henriksson, M. M., Aro, H. M., Marttunen, M. J., Heikkinen, M. E., Isometsä, E. T., Kuoppasalmi, K. I., & Lönnqvist, J. K. (1993). Mental disorders and comorbidity in suicide. *American Journal of Psychiatry, 150*, 935–940.

Hill, K., Hawton, K., Malmberg, A., & Simkin, S. (1997). *Bereavement Information Pack: For those bereaved by suicide or other sudden death.* Retrieved on August 3, 2008, from http://www.rcpsych.ac.uk/publications/books/rcpp/1901242080.aspx

Houston, K., Hawton, K., & Shepperd, R. (2001). Suicide in young people aged 15–24: A psychological autopsy study. *Journal of Affective Disorders, 63*, 159–170.

Isometsä, E. T., Heikkinen, M., Henriksson, M., Marttunen, M., Aro, H., & Lönnqvist, J. K. (1997). Differences between urban and rural suicides. *Acta Psychiatrica Scandinavia, 95*, 297–305.

Isometsä, E. T., Henriksson, M. M., Heikkinen, M. E., Aro, H. M., Marttunen, M. J., Kuoppasalmi, K. I., & Lönnqvist, J. K. (1996). Completed suicide in personality disorders. *American Journal of Psychiatry, 153*, 667–673.

Jackson, H. J., & Burgess, P. M. (2000). Personality disorders in the community: A report from the Australian national survey of mental health and well-being. *Social Psychiatry & Psychiatric Epidemiology, 35*, 531–538.

Kaplan, R. M. (2000). Two pathways to prevention. *American Psychologist, 55*, 382–396.

Kay, S. R., Fiszbein, A., & Opler, L. A. (1987). The Positive and Negative Syndrome Scale (PANSS) for schizophrenia. *Schizophrenia Bulletin, 13*, 261–276.

Kessler, R. C., Borges, G., & Walters, E. E. (1999). Prevalence of and risk factors for lifetime suicide attempts in the National Comorbidity Survey. *Archives of General Psychiatry, 56*, 617–626.

Kim, C. D., Lesage, A. D., Seguin, M., Chawky, N., Vanier, C., Lipp, O., & Turecki, G. (2003). Patterns of comorbidity in male suicide completers. *Psychological Medicine, 33*, 1299–1309.

Kim, C. D., Lesage, A. D., Seguin, M., Chawky, N., Vanier, C., Lipp, O., & Turecki, G. (2004). Seasonal differences in psychopathology of male suicide completers. *Comprehensive Psychiatry, 45*, 333–339.

Knox, K. L., Conwell, Y., & Caine, E. D. (2004). If suicide is a public health problem, what are we doing to prevent it? *American Journal of Public Health, 94*, 37–45.

Kovacs, M. (1985). The Interview Schedule for Children (ISC). *Psychopharmacology Bulletin, 21*, 991–994.

Kraemer, H. C., Kazdin, A. E., Offord, D. R., Kessler, R. C., Jensen, P. S., & Kupfer, D. J. (1997). Coming to terms with the terms of risk. *Archives of General Psychiatry, 54*, 337–343.

Kullgren, G., Tengstrom, A., & Grann, M. (1998). Suicide among personality-disordered offenders: A follow-up study of 1,943 male criminal offenders. *Social Psychiatry & Psychiatric Epidemiology, 33*(Suppl. 1), 102–106.

Lesage, A. D., Boyer, R., Grunberg, E., Vanier, C., Morisette, R., Menard-Buteau, C., & Loyer, M. (1994). Suicide and mental disorders: A case-control study of young men. *American Journal of Psychiatry, 151*, 1063–1068.

Levine, M. (1998). Prevention and community. *American Journal of Community Psychology, 26*, 189–206.

Linehan, M. M., Armstrong, H. E., Suarez, A., Allmari, D., & Heard, H. L. (1991). Cognitive–behavioral treatment of chronically parasuicidal borderline patients. *Archives of General Psychiatry, 48*, 1060–1064.

Linehan, M. M., Heard, H. L., & Armstrong, H. E. (1993). Naturalistic follow-up of a behavioral treatment for chronically parasuicidal borderline patients. *Archives of General Psychiatry, 50*, 971–974.

Litman, R. E., & Wold, C. I. (1976). Beyond crisis intervention. In E. S. Shneidman (Ed.), *Suicidology: Contemporary developments* (pp. 528–546). New York: Grune & Stratton.

Luoma, J. B., Martin, C. E., & Pearson, J. L. (2002). Contact with mental health and primary care providers before suicide: A review of the evidence. *American Journal of Psychiatry, 159*, 909–916.

Mann, A. H., Jenkins, R., Cutting, J. C., & Cowen, P. J. (1981). The development and use of a standardized assessment of abnormal personality. *Psychological Medicine, 11*, 839–847.

Maser, J. D., Akiskal, H. S., Schettler P., Scheftner, W., Mueller, T., Endicott, J., et al. (2002). Can temperament identify affectively ill patients who engage in lethal or nonlethal suicidal behavior? A 14-year prospective study. *Suicide and Life-Threatening Behavior, 32*, 10–32.

McGlashan, T. H. (1986). The Chestnut Lodge follow-up study: Long-term outcome of borderline personalities. *Archives of General Psychiatry, 43*, 20–30.

Moller, H. J. (1989). Efficacy of different strategies of aftercare for patients who have attempted suicide. *Journal of the Royal Society of Medicine, 82*, 643–647.

Motto, J. A., & Bostrom, A. G. (2001). A randomized controlled trial of postcrisis suicide prevention. *Psychiatric Services, 52*, 828–833.

Neeleman, J. (2002). Beyond risk theory: Suicidal behavior in its social and epidemiological context. *Crisis, 23*, 114–120.

Nortstrom, T. (1995). Alcohol and suicide: A comparative analysis of France and Sweden. *Addiction, 90*, 1463–1490.

Paris, J., Brown, R., & Nowlis, D. (1987). Long-term follow-up of borderline patients in a general hospital. *Comprehensive Psychiatry, 28,* 530–535.

Paris, J., & Zweig-Frank, H. (2001). A 27-year follow-up of patients with borderline personality disorder. *Comprehensive Psychiatry, 42,* 482–487.

Portzky, G., Audenaert, K., & van Heeringen, K. (2005). Suicide among adolescents: A psychological autopsy study of psychiatric, psychosocial, and personality-related risk factors. *Social Psychiatry & Psychiatric Epidemiology, 40,* 922–930.

Rao, U., Weissman, M. M., Martin, J. E., & Hammond, R. W. (1993). Childhood depression and risk of suicide: A preliminary report of a longitudinal study. *Journal of the American Academy of Child & Adolescent Psychiatry, 32,* 21–27.

Rich, C. L., Young, D., & Fowler, R. C. (1986). San Diego suicide study: I. Young vs. old subjects. *Archives of General Psychiatry, 43,* 577–582.

Riso, L. P., Klein, D. N., Anderson, R. L., Ouimette, P. C., & Lizardi, H. (1994). Concordance between patients and informants on the Personality Disorder Examinations. *American Journal of Psychiatry, 151,* 568–573.

Rose, G. (1992). *The strategy of prevention medicine.* Oxford, England: Oxford University Press.

Runeson, B. (1989). Mental disorders in youth suicide. *Acta Psychiatrica Scandinavica, 79,* 490–497.

Salib, E., & Green, L. (2003). Gender in elderly suicide: Analysis of coroners' inquests of 200 cases of elderly suicide in Cheshire 1989–2001. *International Journal of Geriatric Psychiatry, 18,* 1082–1087.

Samuels, J., Eaton, W. W., Bienvenu, O. J., III, Brown, C., Costa, P. T., Jr., & Nestadt, G. (2002). The prevalence of personality disorders in a community sample. *The British Journal of Psychiatry, 180,* 536–542.

Sarason, S. B. (1981). An asocial psychology and a misdirected clinical psychology. *American Psychologist, 36,* 827–836.

Schneider, B., Wetterling, T., Sargk, D., Schneider, F., Schnabel, A., Maurer, K., & Fritze, J. (2006). Axis I disorders and personality disorders as risk factors for suicide. *European Archives of Psychiatry & Clinical Neuroscience, 256,* 17–27.

Senol, S., Dereboy, C., & Yuksel, N. (1997). Borderline disorder in Turkey: A 2- to 4-year follow-up. *Social Psychiatry & Psychiatric Epidemiology, 32,* 109–112.

Skodol, A. E., Gunderson, J. G., Shea, M. T., McGlashan, T. H., Morey, L. C., Sanislow, C. A., et al. (2005). The Collaborative Longitudinal Personality Disorders Study (CLPS): Overview and implications. *Journal of Personality Disorders, 19,* 487–504.

Spitzer, R. L., Williams, J. B. W., Gibbon, M., & First, M. B. (1988). *Structured Clinical Interview for DSM–III–R—Patient version.* Washington, DC: American Psychiatric Association.

Stone, M., Stone, D. K., & Hurt, S. W. (1987). The natural history of borderline patients: I. Global outcome. *Psychiatric Clinics of North America, 10,* 185–205.

Tidemalm, D., Elofsson, S., Stefanson, C. G., Waern, M., & Runeson, B. (2005). Predictors of suicide in a community-based cohort of individuals with severe mental disorder. *Social Psychiatry & Psychiatric Epidemiology, 40,* 595–600.

Torgersen, S., Kringlen, E., & Cramer, V. (2001). The prevalence of personality disorders in a community sample. *Archives of General Psychiatry, 58,* 590–596.

Tsoh, J. M. Y., Chiu, H. F. K., Duberstein, P. R., Chan, S. S. M., Chi, I., Yip, P., & Conwell, Y. (2005). Attempted suicide in the Chinese elderly: A multi-group controlled study. *American Journal of Geriatric Psychiatry, 13,* 562–571.

Tyrer, P., & Alexander, J. (1979). Classification of personality disorder. *The British Journal of Psychiatry, 135,* 163–67.

Tyrer, P., Mitchard, S., Methuen, C., & Ranger, M. (2003). Treatment rejecting and treatment seeking personality disorders: Type R and type S. *Journal of Personality Disorders, 17,* 263–268.

Tyrer, P., Thompson, S., Schmidt, U., Jones, V., Knapp, M., Davidson, J., et al. (2003). Randomized controlled trial of brief cognitive–behavior therapy versus treatment as usual in recurrent deliberate self-harm: The POPMACT study. *Psychological Medicine, 33,* 969–976.

Useda, J. D., Duberstein, P. R., Beckman, A., Franus, N., Tu, X., & Conwell, Y. (2007). Differences in attempted versus completed suicide: Informant report of personality traits in adults 50 years of age and older. *Journal of Consulting and Clinical Psychology, 75,* 126–133.

Vaiva, G., Ducrocq, F., Meyer, D., Mathieu, D., Philippe, A., Libersa, C., & Goudemand, M. (2006, May 27). Effects of telephone contact on further suicide attempts in patients discharged from an emergency department: Randomised controlled study. *BMJ, 332,* 1241–1245.

van Heeringen, C., Jannes, S., Buylaert, W., Henderick, H., de Bacquer, D., & van Remoortel, J. (1995). The management of noncompliance with referral to outpatient after-care among attempted suicide patients: A controlled intervention study. *Psychological Medicine, 25,* 963–970.

Vijayakumar, L., & Rajkumar, S. (1999). Are risk factors for suicide universal? A case-control study in India. *Acta Psychiatrica Scandinavica, 99,* 407–11.

Wing, J. K. (1980). Methodological issues in psychiatric case-identification. *Psychological Medicine, 10,* 5–10.

World Health Organization. (1967). *Manual of the international classification of diseases, injuries, and causes of death* (8th rev.). Geneva: Author.

World Health Organization. (1977). *International classification of diseases and related health problems* (9th rev.). Geneva: Author.

World Health Organization. (1992). *International classification of diseases and related health problems* (10th rev.). Geneva: Author.

Yang, G. H., Phillips, M. R., Zhou, M. G., Wang, L. J., Zhang, Y. P., & Xu, D. (2005). Understanding the unique characteristics of suicide in China: National psychological autopsy study. *Biomedical and Environmental Sciences, 18,* 379–389.

Yen, S., & Siegler, I. C. (2003). Self-blame, social introversion, and male suicides: Prospective data from a longitudinal study. *Archives of Suicide Research, 7,* 17–27.

Zanarini, M. C., Frankenburg, F. R., Hennen, J., Reich, B., & Silk, K. R. (2005). The McLean Study of Adult Development (MSAD): Overview and implications of the first six years of prospective follow-up. *Journal of Personality Disorders, 19,* 505–523.

Zanarini, M. C., Gunderson, J. G., Frankenburg, F. R., & Chauncey, D. L. (1989). The revised Diagnostic Interview for Borderlines: Discriminating BPD from other Axis II disorders. *Journal of Personality Disorder, 3,* 10–18.

Zhang, J., Conwell, Y., Zhou, L., & Jiang, C. (2004). Culture, risk factors, and suicide in rural China: A psychological autopsy case control study. *Acta Psychiatrica Scandinavica, 110,* 430–437.

Zilboorg, G. (1937). Considerations on suicide, with particular reference to the young. *American Journal of Orthopsychiatry, 7,* 15–31.

Zimmerman, M., Rothschild, L., & Chelminski, I. (2005). The prevalence of *DSM– IV* personality disorders in psychiatric outpatients. *American Journal of Psychiatry, 162,* 1911–1918.

VI

MEDICAL CONDITIONS PRESENTING AS BEHAVIORAL EMERGENCIES

13

COMMON NEUROLOGICAL DISORDERS ASSOCIATED WITH PSYCHOLOGICAL–BEHAVIORAL PROBLEMS

ROBERTA F. WHITE, MAXINE H. KRENGEL,
AND TERRI ANN THOMPSON

The purpose of this chapter is to provide an overview of neurological syndromes and neuropsychological or cognitive–behavioral symptoms that either can present in an emergent situation or are present in the medical context and are in need of follow-up evaluation to ensure appropriate treatment. Because neurological syndromes and behavioral symptoms largely coexist and the dichotomy between the two is untenable, it is essential for clinicians to be able to identify the types of symptoms that commonly occur and appreciate the need for medical follow-up when necessary. What is known is that many disorders that historically fell under the purview of the psychiatrist are clearly shown to have a neurological basis, including schizophrenia and bipolar disorder, in addition to disorders involving mood and affect, such as major depression or posttraumatic stress disorder. Even in the case of Axis II diagnoses such as obsessive–compulsive personality disorders, dysfunction may be, at least in part, attributed to specific cerebral structures (Rauch et al., 1994; Saint-Cyr, Taylor,

& Nicholson, 1995). Likewise, patients with such neurological disorders as traumatic brain injury or primary progressive dementias often present initially and receive initial care from mental health practitioners.

In this chapter we provide symptom clarification to determine appropriate diagnostic clarification and treatment recommendations. We review a series of symptoms such as hallucinations, delusions, paranoia, apathy, restlessness, agitation, sadness/depression, anxiety, denial, and regression as they appear in the context of neurological conditions. The types of disorders we discuss include primary progressive dementias such as Alzheimer's disease (AD) and frontal lobe dementias, motor disorders such as Parkinson's disease (PD) and Huntington's disease (HD), diseases involving multiple cerebral lesions such as cerebrovascular diseases (CVD) and multiple sclerosis (MS), traumatic brain injury, and epilepsy. We cannot provide an exhaustive review of all disorders (which would require an entire volume) but focus on common conditions that present frequently in the context of behavioral emergencies.

Because the neurological literature tends to focus on neuropathology and physical findings, the neuropsychological literature on cognitive deficits, and the psychiatric literature on disorders other than those we discuss here, the literature on the co-occurrence of these symptoms is rather sparse. Our discussion here, therefore, largely emanates from our own extensive clinical experience as clinical psychologists with a subspecialty in neuropsychology. We focus our discussion on the systematic expression of behavioral changes in neurological disease that go beyond the traditional cognitive deficits assessed in neuropsychology.

DEVELOPMENTAL, SOCIAL, AND MEDICAL INDICATORS OF POSSIBLE NEUROLOGICAL DISORDERS

Although the psychological interview is well described in chapter 3 of this volume, a few points should be highlighted when evaluating patients in emergent situations who may have neurologic illness. We focus this review on the developmental, social, and medical indicators of possible neurological disease that can be elicited on history when taking a history.

Developmental and Educational History

The need to document pre- and perinatal complications arises because patients who have experienced exposures to neurotoxins in utero or through birth trauma, early head injuries, or encephalitis/meningitis are at greater risk of neurological disorders later in life, including epilepsy. Epilepsy may result in a history of behavioral complications such as daydreaming or "blanking out" episodes in school or at home in addition to personality changes and emotional dyscontrol. School history, including difficulty paying attention, restlessness, hyperactivity, or a tendency to leave tasks incomplete in childhood, can be seen in patients with attention-deficit disorder. In cases such as this, impulsivity and an inability to inhibit may lead one to make inappropriate choices, resulting in emergent psychiatric crises. These same kinds of problems can be seen in patients with below average general intelligence, childhood or adolescent onset of a neurogenetic disorder (such as HD), or childhood exposure to neurotoxins such as lead at unsafe levels. These issues will likely result in varying treatment methodologies, depending on the cause of the behavioral issues.

Social and Occupational History

In a number of patients with primary neurological disorder, initial manifestation of the illness can be seen in the patient's social or occupational life. Undiagnosed brain tumors, strokes, primary progressive dementias, neurotoxin exposures, or MS can result in deterioration of social relationships and an inability to retain a job. In some occupational histories, the patient's job status may decline as an undiagnosed illness progresses. When these patients are questioned closely, it often becomes apparent that they lost jobs because of a decline in cognitive or motor capacity to carry out job demands prior to diagnosis. In other cases, the patient may have insufficient insight at the time of evaluation to note the cause of job status changes. Other patients present as behavioral emergencies because of a social change noted in behavioral control. The patient may have suddenly or gradually become irritable and aggressive, paranoid, sexually disinhibited, unable to follow rules or obey the law or normal codes of behavior, apathetic, or consistently confused. These kinds of changes can be seen in patients with primary progressive dementias but can also occur in patients with slow-growing lesions such as brain tumors.

Medical History

A number of medical conditions predispose patients to the development of neurological disease, which can then present as behavioral emergencies. Chronic heart failure, hypertension, and diabetes are all associated with an increased risk of cerebrovascular disorders or sudden changes in behavioral control. Any patient with a history of stroke or transient ischemic attacks should be considered at risk of behavioral or cognitive changes attributable to the vascular condition.

Physical Symptoms

Physical symptoms that can be seen in many neurological disorders include incontinence, fatigue, dizziness, and headaches. Visual disturbances (e.g., double vision, blindness) are common in MS and may wax and wane or even disappear completely for years. Sensitivity to heat is also often seen in MS, at which time symptoms seem to worsen. Gait disturbance and tremors or abnormal movements may be seen in patients with PD, HD, or other disorders involving the brain's motor system (including strokes in motor areas and in particular, nutritionally related alcoholic neuropathies and exposure to environmental neurotoxins, inhalant abuse, and other causes). Weight loss in the year prior to diagnosis is commonly reported in patients who develop primary progressive dementias, and these patients may also develop sensitivity to cold (e.g., start wearing sweaters or inappropriate clothing). Paresthesias (i.e., numbness or tingly feelings in the skin) may also be seen with peripheral nervous system involvement (e.g., in alcoholic and toxin-induced disorders).

PSYCHOLOGICAL AND BEHAVIORAL SYMPTOMS IN NEUROLOGICAL DISORDERS

In this section we discuss a number of neurological disorders. We begin with a general description of the medical features of a disorder. Next, we summarize the types of psychological symptoms that may herald the onset of a disorder or be prominently featured in a patient with a disease who presents with a behavioral emergency.

Alzheimer's Disease

AD is a neurodegenerative disorder that causes progressive cognitive decline, especially a striking memory impairment in addition to behavioral changes early in the process. The dementia associated with AD has an insidious onset, and there is a progressive decline in almost all areas of cognitive functioning. Neuropathologically, AD is characterized by the development of neuritic plaques and neurofibrillary tangles throughout the brain. It is diagnosed presumptively and confirmed by autopsy or biopsy (see Cummings & Cole, 2002, for a review of the neuropathology of the disease process and the neuropsychological consequences).

In addition to the deterioration in cognitive function that defines the dementia associated with AD (i.e., impairments in memory, attention, executive system functioning, language, and visuospatial abilities identified on neuropsychological testing), profound psychological sequelae and personality changes are associated with the disease process. In the early stages of the disease, patients often show a loss of interest, apathy, lowered energy levels, and depressed mood (Hamdy, 1998). The risk of suicide increases in early-stage compared with later stage AD prior to the loss of insight, although the classic suicide risk factors are not commonly apparent.

Among patients with AD, the frequency of apathy has been reported to range from 25% to 50% (Starkstein, Jorge, Mizrahi, & Robinson, 2006). Apathy is far more frequent in mild AD compared with delusions, irritability, anxiety, agitation, and hallucinations, which tend to occur in later stages (Meguro et al., 2004). Several studies have demonstrated a significant association between apathy and both reduced metabolic activity in prefrontal regions and more severe motor findings such as Parkinsonism, suggesting that neuropathological changes in specific brain areas may underlie the high frequency of apathy in AD, although severity of cognitive deficits is not directly correlated with level of apathy.

The depression associated with AD is qualitatively different from the clinical depression defined in the *Diagnostic and Statistical Manual of Mental Disorders*, (4th ed.; American Psychiatric Association, 1994). Patients with AD are often described as appearing less interested and less willing to engage in activities that they once found pleasurable. However, this change can be best described as reflecting apathy and passivity rather than feelings of sadness, worthlessness, or the anhedonia seen in depression.

As the disease process progresses, common behavioral symptoms may include anxiety, agitation, extreme restlessness, and irritability. It is not uncommon for a patient with AD to present with delusions or hallucinations, which may occur in as many as 40% to 60% of patients (Eror, Lopez, Dekosky, & Sweet, 2005; M. F. Folstein & Bylsma, 1994). The hallucinations are most often visual or auditory but can be olfactory or tactile. Common delusions include the belief that people are stealing from the patient, that there are unwanted people living in their home, or that the house they are living in is not their real home. Although wandering is commonly seen in AD, it may also occur in the context of a delusion in which the patient experiences the need to find his or her "real" house. The wandering, coupled with the severe memory impairments, may lead to patients becoming lost and brought to the emergency department after being found by police. The delusions dissipate as the dementia becomes more severe (M. F. Folstein & Bylsma, 1994). Clinically, psychosis in AD has been associated with more rapid cognitive decline and increased risk of agitated and aggressive behavior.

Although mania is rare in patients with AD, it may be seen in patients who have disturbances in their sleep–wake cycle. These patients may present with symptoms similar to mania, such as irritability, agitation, poor judgment, and sleep disturbances.

Word finding difficulties and impaired confrontational naming evidenced on neuropsychological tests are hallmarks of the language disturbance in AD. These language disturbances are markedly different from the language disturbances seen in schizophrenia and its related disorders. Qualitatively, the language and speech problems observed in patients with AD often include circumlocutions that are reflective of naming problems. The loosening of associations and the speech disorder that is indicative of a thought disorder are not present. However, in the later stages of AD speech may become neologistic and incomprehensible.

Frontal Lobe Dementias

A few primary progressive dementing disorders affect the frontal lobes most extensively (see Moss, Albert, & Kemper, 1992, for a description of the typical pathological features of these disorders). Although these conditions, such as Pick's disease, primary progressive aphasia, and frontotemporal dementia are relatively rare, the initial presentations are frequently behavioral, and patients are often evaluated initially in emergency settings. The cardinal features of the change evident in these disorders are best summarized as a loss of behavioral control or monitoring. The patient may become irritable and aggressive and fail to use self-control to monitor behavior. These patients are unable to inhibit aggressive acts that were previously inhibited, and they have diminished social comportment. Similarly, behavior may become sexually disinhibited, with the patient approaching inappropriate persons, exhibiting an increased sexual drive, or talking about sexual activity inappropriately. Occasionally, patients with no history of criminality or antisocial behavior begin to break the law, stealing objects or money or breaking into buildings. Faulty behavioral monitoring can be seen as a lack of insight into behavioral changes, in which the patient does not notice the inappropriateness of behaviors or even that he or she is acting differently than in the past. Finally, we see patients diagnosed with this type of dementia who appear to have lost the capacity for guilt, failing to ascribe any fault for behaviors considered antisocial. In one case, the patient came to medical attention because he had begun stealing tools from a coworker and was making sexual advances toward female family members besides his wife. He remembered and acknowledged these acts but said that he took advantage of the proximity of tools or women because they were convenient and he needed them. When asked whether other people would consider these acts to be wrong, he acknowledged that this was the case. He also denied personal feelings of guilt.

Cerebrovascular Disease

Cerebrovascular disease (i.e., CVD) is a term referring to the constellation of lesions that occur because of vascular pathology in the brain. It encompasses entities known as multi-infarct dementia (Hachinski, Lassen, & Marshall, 1974), leukoariosis (Hachinski, Potter, & Merskey, 1987), and Binswanger's disease (Binswanger, 1894). Patients with vascular disease may have experienced large clinical strokes, often with other small lesions identifiable by magnetic resonance imaging (MRI), or may have no clinically identified strokes despite showing evidence of lesions on MRI scans and exhibiting cognitive, behavioral, and neurological signs of such lesions. By the time of diagnosis, patients may have a variety of lesions that can involve the cortex, connections between cortical regions or subcortical white matter, basal ganglia, cerebellum, brain stem, or combinations of these areas. Patients with multiple lesions may show behavioral changes that are attributable to lesions occurring in specified brain regions or systems, and they may also show secondary or cumulative effects of having multiple lesion sites (Tatemichi, 1990). The latter generally show up in group studies of these patients as "frontal system" dysfunction observable on neuropsychological tests of attention and executive functioning (Wolfe, Linn, Babikian, Knoefel, & Albert, 1990). Focal deficits are harder to establish in group studies of patients with CVD, presumably because the sites of these lesions vary among patients. CVD is thought to occur rather commonly, perhaps accounting for 57% of dementia diagnoses (Tatemichi, 1990).

From the perspective of behavioral emergencies, CVD is an important disorder because behavioral (especially affective) changes are often the first symptoms that bring a patient in for diagnosis; recent research has shown increased psychiatric symptomatology with increased severity of white matter changes in the brain (Lee et al., 2006).

In our experience, CVD is a diagnostic category that is also common among geriatric patients receiving inpatient psychiatric evaluation and care (especially when the admission is the first psychiatric admission they have experienced). We frequently find that history of strokes, abnormal MRI findings, and evidence of multifocal vascular disease are ignored etiologically in evaluation of the patient's behavioral status.

Symptomatic changes that are behavioral in nature and that occur across the many types of presentations of multiple lesions in patients with CVD are often seen as a new presentation of agitation or agitated depression. The patient is frequently at a loss to explain any precipitants for periods or episodes of agitation or a sense of anxiety and may be quite debilitated because of it. The agitation may also be accompanied by easy tearfulness or irritability. In lesions involving the frontal lobes, aggression, major depression, and generalized anxiety are not uncommon (Chan, Campayo, Moser, Arndt, & Robinson, 2006). Many patients with CVD are apathetic or amotivational when presented with cognitive tasks or life dilemmas, even when the agitation or anxiety is severe enough to produce pronounced restlessness. When patients are apathetic or lethargic, their behavioral changes may be interpreted by others as reflecting a depression, although diagnosis and treatment for clinical depression would be inappropriate. Finally, patients with diffuse lesions may show evidence of behavioral changes attributable to frontal dysfunction and similar to those seen in frontal dementias (see the previous section).

Patients with severe bilateral CVD may exhibit a chronic or episodic confusional state. This state can be accompanied by a number of symptoms, including paranoid delusions. These delusions are often fixed in terms of their central theme (e.g., the belief that the patient's landlord is spying into the patient's home). However, details of the patient's report about incidents that recently occurred in relation to the delusion are often highly variable from one report to another, and the patient may completely forget having reported specific information related to the delusion. For example, the patient may report one afternoon that the landlord spied on him with a television camera and another day say the spying occurred with a tape recorder. Sometimes it may be the landlord who is the culprit; other times it is the next-door neighbor. In addition to delusions, *illusions*, or interpretations of sensory distortions caused by damage to the parietal or occipital lobes, are seen. One patient, for example, thought that a big black raven was sitting on his shoulder. This illusion was also vague and changeable, with the patient sometimes reporting that the bird was always there (other times it was not) and with the bird switching between the right and left shoulders.

A similar phenomenon known as *reduplicative paramnesia* can occur, in which the patient multiplies objects or people in the environment. Common manifestations include the patient's belief that he or she has two or more hospital rooms or homes. However, the belief can extend to the patient's body, so that the patient believes that he or she has many arms or legs. In the most dramatic case of this phenomenon we have seen, the patient believed that he had a double of himself who followed him around. Another behavioral anomaly that may be seen in patients with posterior cortical damage is that of *anosagnosia*, in which the patient expresses a form of denial about medical status or physical functioning. In such cases, he or she may refuse to acknowledge having had a clinical stroke and may refuse to acknowledge hemiparesis, even when it is quite severe. This phenomenon does not seem to represent classic psychoanalytical denial but rather reflects the patient's altered perception of somatic functioning as a result of brain damage.

In addition to these changes, patients may exhibit a wide variety of behavioral symptoms related to focal or lateralized brain damage. Patients with left hemisphere strokes may develop depressive symptoms that are not entirely reactive in nature, and patients with right hemisphere strokes may show an unawareness of deficit or an indifference or lack of emotional comprehension. For example, a patient may begin to cry whenever he hears his father mentioned; on questioning, the patient states that he was very upset about his father's death a year ago, but he did not feel sad when his father was mentioned and did not realize that he was sad until he began to cry. Similarly, a patient may lose the ability to read the emotional states other people reveal in facial expressions or body posture and may be surprised by statements others make about their feelings. Patients with right frontal lesions may develop paranoid delusions. Those with left temporal lesions may report auditory hallucinations, whereas other patients with temporal lesions may become extremely religious. Occipital lesions may be associated with visual hallucinations (often of lights, colors, or spots), and gustatory or olfactory hallucinations are seen in some patients with temporal lesions. Finally, changes in sexual behavior, including hypersexuality, are sometimes seen in these individuals (Chae & Kang, 2006).

Multiple Sclerosis

MS is a neurological disorder in which the myelin sheaths of nerve fibers are damaged, producing lesions called *demyelinating plaques*. These lesions may occur throughout the central nervous system; therefore, there is wide variability in symptom presentation. Symptoms are transient in the early stages of the illness. There is often motor weakness, visual disturbance (partial or total loss of vision that may last several days), numbness, vertigo, seizures, unformed auditory hallucinations, fatigue, and mood changes. Additionally, apathy, irritability, and hypersexuality are not uncommon (Lopez-Meza, Corona-Vazquez, Ruano-Calderon, & Ramirez-Bermudez, 2005). The course of the illness may be rapidly progressive, relapsing and remitting, or chronic progressive, but the disease often persists for many years (Victor & Ropper, 2000).

MS is sometimes confused with hysteria or somatoform disorder. This is because of the fleeting, evanescent nature of the physical symptoms of MS, preoccupation with physical functioning that occurs in some MS patients, and the tendency of MS patients to show profiles similar to those seen in patients with hysteria or somatoform disorders on personality tests.

Affective disorders are commonly seen in MS. In one study (Schiffer, Wineman, & Weitkamp, 1986), the rate of affective disorder was found to be twice as high as expected in the general population on the basis of the individual occurrence rates of the two disorders. Patients may be described as euphoric. In fact, even as early as 1926, Cottrell and Wilson characterized the majority of their patients as "abnormally" optimistic. Manic episodes may occur with restlessness, grandiosity, reduced need for sleep, and indiscriminant spending. We have seen patients whose depression appeared to be the most troubling of their symptoms. In some cases, depression may be the first sign of the disease (Goodstein & Farrell, 1977). White (1990) previously described her experiences with MS patients. For one patient, the initial MS symptom was suicidal ideation. Another's depression intensified as his MS progressed. As the disease progresses, it is not uncommon for patients to experience emotional lability. Patients may present to the emergency department with suicidal ideation, apathy, fatigue, irritability, and recent mood changes. Suicidality in individuals with MS is believed to be twice that in the general population (Turner, Williams, Bowen, Kivlahan, & Haselkorn, 2006).

A smaller subgroup of patients with MS present with delusions and hallucinations. Patients may have fixed persecutory delusions. They may also have symptoms consistent with frontal and temporal dysfunction (see earlier discussion related to CVD), including hyperreligiosity (White, Nyenhuis, & Sax, 1992).

Parkinson's Disease

Idiopathic PD is characterized by motor symptoms such as tremor, rigidity, fatigue, slowness of movements, and an inability to initiate movement. Gait disturbance, slurred speech, and small and tremulous writing are also cardinal features of the disease. It is a progressive illness, with patients in the early stages showing mild motor signs (beginning with unilateral involvement and moving to bilateral involvement) and patients later in the disease process showing more severe motor impairment. Cognitive deficits can be seen at various stages, including visuospatial processing deficits, impaired retrieval of information, and attentional variability. Mood changes are also commonly seen in patients with PD. In addition, psychiatric symptoms such as hallucinations and paranoia are seen in patients with PD, even early in the disease process.

Depression is fairly common in patients with untreated PD, ranging from 40% to 60% (Santamaria, Tolosa, & Balles, 1986). There is controversy about whether mood changes are a result of organic changes or a reaction to having the illness. It is fairly well documented that the mood changes do not correlate reliably with motor signs (Huber, Paulson, & Shuttleworth, 1988), age of onset, or duration of the motor symptoms (Celesia & Wanamaker, 1972). There is some indication that patients who are young at disease onset are more likely to have depressive symptoms predating the motor symptoms. When motor symptoms are treated, the depression may initially improve slightly. However, this change in mood does not appear to hold over time, even with continued improvement in motor symptoms.

Patients with early PD may present with visual hallucinations. These most often involve fuzzy animals, hooded people, or indistinct people (White, Au, Durso, & Moss, 1992). Later in the course of the illness, patients may present with confusion and psychosis. The hallucinations may involve both auditory and visual modalities and are seen during confusional states (White, Au, et al., 1992). Paranoid beliefs or delusions are seen to a lesser extent; however, when they occur they are associated with anxiety and fear (Williams-Gray, Foltynie, Lewis, & Barker, 2006). It is unclear which, if any, of these symptoms are related to medication side effects, although some patients complain of visual hallucinations even before they begin taking medications.

There is some indication that medication treatments for PD may cause vivid and disturbing dreams (Moskovitz, Moses, & Klawans, 1978), visual hallucinations, and paranoid delusions (Celesia & Barr, 1970). Other treatment effects include confusional states with disorientation as to time or place, anxiety, or mania. This is especially true for older patients (Saint-Cyr, Taylor, & Lang, 1993).

Visual hallucinations are the most common side effect of medication (Cummings, 1992), and the frequency of hallucinations ranges from 6% to 38% of patients treated with anti-Parkinsonian medications. Fully formed images of humans or animals are common. They are most often experienced at night and are recurrent nearly every night. Most patients report these as nonthreatening hallucinations. Older patients who are taking anticholinergic drugs and are on medications longer are most likely to have visual hallucinations (Tanner, Bogel, Goetz, & Klawans, 1983).

Delusions are rare in untreated PD. However, they are found in conjunction with a variety of medication treatments (Crow, Johnstone, & McClelland, 1976), ranging from 3% to 30% of patients, and may represent emerging toxicity. Delusions from anti-Parkinsonian treatment tend to be persecutory in nature, involving fears of being harmed or tape-recorded (Moskovitz et al., 1978).

Mood elevation, which varies from euphoria to full-blown manic episodes, has been reported in patients on anti-Parkinsonian medications. Again, these episodes are related to amount of drug use and diminish with decreased drug use. Less common symptoms that have been found to relate to amount of drug use include increased anxiety, irritability, and insomnia.

Delirious states with fluctuating arousal, impaired attention, and incoherent verbal output have been observed in 5% to 25% of treated PD patients, most often later in the disease process after years of medication treatment (Cummings, 1992). Overall, PD patients who are older, with dementia, on higher dosages of medication, and with a history of psychiatric illness predating the PD motor signs are described as more likely to have psychiatric symptoms (Tanner et al., 1983).

Huntington's Disease

Although HD is a relatively rare disorder, the presenting symptoms are often behavioral and psychological in nature and deserve review in this section. HD is an autosomal dominant genetic disease with complete penetrance, meaning that the offspring of an affected individual has a 50% chance of being affected. It is characterized by a combination of symptoms that are described as an example of a subcortical triad (McHugh & Folstein, 1975; Peyser & Folstein, 1990). The triad includes uncontrollable involuntary movements (known as *chorea*), psychiatric disturbances, and progressive dementia. McHugh (1989) described these cardinal features as a triad of Ds: dyskinesia, dementia, and depression. After the initial appearance of the symptoms there is a progressive decline in cognitive and motor functioning.

Patients with HD show considerable variability in the onset of motor symptoms and in emotional and cognitive disturbances (Caine & Shoulson, 1983; Conneally, 1984; White, Vasterling, Koroshetz, & Myers, 1992).

The characteristics of the behavioral and personality changes observed in HD share features with other basal ganglia diseases. For example, depression and apathy are commonly seen in PD as well as in HD (Mayeux, Stern, Rosen, & Leventhal, 1981; McHugh, 1989; Sano, 1991). These mood state or affective changes are not typically a reaction to having a debilitating degenerative disease. Investigators have found evidence of behavioral and mood changes occurring several years before the onset of the motor impairments (Bird, 1980; S. E. Folstein, Abbott, Chase, Jensen, & Folstein, 1983; Hayden, 1981; Mayeux et al., 1981; Webb & Trzepacz, 1987). The finding that HD patients experience manic episodes in addition to depression (S. E. Folstein, 1989; McHugh, 1989; Pflanz, Besson, Ebmeier, & Simpson, 1991) also constitutes evidence suggesting the organic nature of the changes. Peyser and Folstein (1990) reported that approximately 10% of their sample had manic episodes. Neither bipolar disorder nor mania is an expected functional reaction to living with this debilitating disease.

Presently, affective disorders (including depression, mania, and bipolar disorder) are reported as the most common psychiatric syndrome in HD. Up to 40% of HD patients sampled report major affective illness (Caine & Shoulson, 1983; S. E. Folstein & Folstein, 1983). Some studies found that close to 60% of their HD samples were described as irritable (Burns, Folstein, Brandt, & Folstein, 1990; Pflanz et al., 1991). The irritability was at times severe enough to warrant the diagnosis of intermittent explosive disorder (S. E. Folstein, Franz, Jensen, Chase, & Folstein, 1983; Webb & Trzepacz, 1987). Burns et al. (1990) found aggression in 59% of their HD sample. S. E. Folstein and Folstein (1983) hypothesized that the episodes of aggression observed in HD patients are an exacerbation of a premorbid personality trait. They proposed that as a result of the disease process, there may be a dysfunction in the normal regulatory (i.e., dampening) mechanisms and, therefore, there is heightened aggression.

Patients with HD may have difficulty inhibiting impulsive behavior (Caine, Hunt, Weingartner, & Ebert, 1978; Caine & Shoulson, 1983). There is a great deal of evidence of antisocial behavior associated with HD, ranging from criminal assaults and minor crimes to child abuse and neglect (Dewhurst, Oliver, & McKnight, 1970; S. E. Folstein, Franz, et al., 1983; Hayden, 1981; Oliver & Dewhurst, 1969). However, the relationships between development of these symptoms and the social effects of living in an HD family and neuropathology of the disease are controversial (S. E. Folstein, 1989).

Some investigators believe that affected individuals often have a history of alcohol as well as substance abuse (e.g., see Dewhurst et al., 1970; S. E. Folstein, Abbott, et al., 1983; S. E. Folstein & Folstein, 1983). White, Vasterling, et al. (1992) described a significant level of alcohol and drug abuse in some HD patients and their families. White, Vasterling, et al., as well as Webb and Trzepacz (1987), observed that the majority of alcohol use was during earlier stages of the disease and tended to drop as the disease progressed. They raised the possibility that for some, the use of alcohol and other recreational drugs may be a form of self-medication.

Disorders related to schizophrenia were reported to occur in between 5% and 10% of HD patients (Shoulson, 1990), with hallucinations and paranoid delusions frequently reported by HD patients (Caine & Shoulson, 1983; S. E. Folstein & Folstein, 1983; White, Vasterling, et al., 1992). White, Vasterling, et al. (1992) also pointed out that there are significant changes in mood state that do not reach the level of diagnosable affective disorders. Vegetative, biological signs of depression are common in HD, including psychomotor retardation as a result of the disease, insomnia (Shoulson, 1990; White, Vasterling, et al., 1992) often resulting from the patient's chorea and restlessness (White, Vasterling, et al., 1992), and anorexia (Hayden, 1981; White, Nyenhuis, & Sax, 1992). White, Nyenhuis, et al. (1992) noted that some HD patients reported diminished appetites; Hayden (1981) remarked on the dramatic weight loss observed even in patients who reported having excellent appetites. He suggested that the caloric expenditure exceeds what would be expected from the increase in movement alone and may in some way be related to the disease process itself.

The extraordinarily high suicide rate in this population (Dewhurst et al., 1970; Kessler & Block, 1989; Reed & Chandler, 1958; Schoenfeld et al., 1984) was noticed by Huntington, and he remarked on it qualitatively in his seminal paper (Huntington, 1872). A quantitative study by Schoenfeld et al. (1984) found that after statistically adjusting for age and sex, the suicide rate in an HD group was more than 8 times the suicide rate in the Massachusetts population for individuals ages 50 to 69. Further, they concluded that because the preponderance of successful suicides was committed by individuals who had not yet been diagnosed, suicide may occur more frequently in earlier stages of the disease. White, Vasterling, et al. (1992) described patients who experienced command hallucinations regarding suicide, some who reported a compulsive urge to kill themselves, and some for whom suicidal ideation is secondary to their depression and demoralization related to the disease. Kessler (1987; Kessler & Block, 1989) made the provocative suggestion that passive encouragement on the part of the patient's family and professional health care workers is a major factor underlying some of the suicides.

Traumatic Brain Injury

There are two types of head injuries, open and closed. Open head injuries occur when the skull is penetrated. Closed head injuries (CHIs) occur more frequently. Motor vehicle accidents, falls, and sporting accidents resulting in head injuries are most likely to be CHIs. Therefore, CHI is the subject of the following discussion.

Brain damage can result when a person is moving and strikes an obstacle (i.e., the brain accelerates and quickly decelerates) or when a person is struck by an object (i.e., creating pressure gradients from the skull distortion). Contusions and tissue shearing seen with more severe CHI result and may cause losses in consciousness. The duration of the loss of consciousness (or the length of coma) and the duration of the posttraumatic amnesia correlate with the severity of the head injury in terms of mortality and cognitive and emotional functioning (see Lezak, Howieson, & Loring, 2004, for detailed reviews of the neuropathological and neuropsychological consequences of CHIs).

Patients who experience these psychological and personality disturbances are remarkable in that they often appear physically healthy. Often, no physical or neurological consequences of the CHI remain, yet the behavior and personality changes that result from the injury cause significant difficulty and stress. Lezak et al. (2004) reported that for some patients, behavioral and emotional disturbances are more debilitating than residual cognitive and physical disabilities; often, patients who survive severe head injuries are unable to resume their studies or return to their previous level of employment.

The exact nature of the behavioral and cognitive disturbances associated with head injuries is directly dependent on the location of the primary as well as any secondary injuries (see the earlier discussion of the different psychological or psychiatric disturbances commonly associated with the dysfunction of specific areas of the brain in this chapter). In addition to behavioral consequences related to the specific site of injury, diffuse damage (i.e., small lesions and lacerations throughout the brain) often accompanies the injury. Even patients with mild injuries who were never admitted to a hospital, may not have gone to an emergency department at the time of their injury, and whose laboratory findings including computed tomography, MRI, and electroencephalogram are all normal may experience physical (e.g., pain, nausea, dizziness) and emotional symptoms. In addition, multiple mild CHIs may result in significant behavioral disturbance, even in the absence of frank symptoms immediately following any of the injuries alone.

Lezak et al. (2004) depicted the kinds of alterations in the brain-injured patient's character that can cause the most distress and adjustment problems for patients' families and loved ones. These include impaired social perceptiveness and an inability to reflect and monitor behavior. Patients may lose insight and empathy, so that their understanding of and feelings for others are diminished. In addition, brain-injured patients often become impulsive, restless, and impatient; this may lead to legal problems resulting from the commission of criminal acts (Morse & Montgomery, 1992). There is often a lack of drive and an impaired capacity for social learning; although a patient's ability to learn new information may be intact, he or she fails to learn from experience. In addition to impulsivity and heightened emotional experiences, some CHI patients may experience mania and paranoia, leading them to seek psychiatric assistance (Lezak et al., 2004).

Idiopathic Temporal Lobe Epilepsy

Seizures are a common symptom of a wide range of neurological disorders and the hallmark symptom of epilepsy. A seizure results when an overactive group of neurons (i.e., the *seizure focus*) is released from its usual physiological control, resulting in abnormal electrical rhythms in the brain. This transient disturbance is caused by an excessive discharge of cortical neurons. The excitation can spread and excite adjacent regions. Depending on the number of neurons affected, the excitation can lead to widespread electrical dysrhythmias. These generalized seizures are characterized by loss of consciousness and stereotyped motor activity, including convulsions (see Greenberg & Seidman, 1992; Trimble & Thompson, 1986; Victor & Ropper, 2000, for a more comprehensive review of epilepsies).

Seizures can result from infections, head injuries, vascular malformations, strokes, tumors, toxic chemicals, high fevers, and other neurological disorders. Seizures of unknown etiology are referred to as idiopathic seizures. Idiopathic temporal lobe epilepsy (ITLE) has been of particular interest to neuropsychologists, and psychiatric and psychological problems are common in patients with ITLE. Patients with ITLE often experience affective and behavior disturbances, hallucinations, psychosis, and personality changes.

During the seizure itself (i.e., *ictus*) patients can experience a wide variety of sensory, motor, and emotional phenomena, including autonomic sensations (e.g., fullness or "butterflies" in the stomach, blushing), cognitive disturbances (e.g., feelings of déjà vu, hallucinations), alterations in mood (e.g., fear, panic, depression, elation), illusions (i.e., misperception or misinterpretation of real external stimuli), and automatisms (e.g., lip smacking, grimacing, automatic behavior; Greenberg & Seidman, 1992).

ITLE is thought to be the type of epilepsy most frequently associated with the psychiatric changes known as the *interictal behavioral syndrome* (IBS). However, there is considerable controversy in neuropsychology regarding the specificity of this association (Osview, 1989). The personality disturbances commonly described as part of the IBS include changes in sexual behavior (most often hyposexuality), *viscosity* (i.e., social clinging), religiosity, hypergraphia, and experiencing emotions more intensely (Blumer, 1975). Viscosity can be manifested in different ways. Some patients treat new acquaintances with the same degree of intimacy and candor that they extend to a close friend, and they seem to have difficulty ending conversations, even at the conclusion of professional appointments.

They can also show considerable changes in the manner of their interactions and conversations. Their speech is often circumstantial, weighted

down with numerous unnecessary details, overly serious, and perhaps pedan-
tic. An important difference between this type of circumstantial speech and
the disordered (i.e., tangential) speech of schizophrenics is that patients with
ITLE, if given enough time, will eventually reach their point; however, patients with a thought disorder are pulled away from the point and are not
able to return to it.

Patients with ITLE often have trouble controlling their anger. Irritable
and impulsive behavior in the form of angry outbursts is common, and on
rare occasions behavior may be violent or abusive (Lezak et al., 2004). Often, a specific quality of moral indignation or feeling that an injustice has
occurred that accompanies the anger or aggressive outburst. For some patients the IBS can be more debilitating than the seizure disorder itself
(Greenberg & Seidman, 1992).

Psychological and psychiatric attention is often required for patients
who are experiencing not only anger and aggression more intensely but fear
and depression as well. The depression of some patients is so severe that they
are at risk of suicide. Interictal psychosis is less frequently seen than personality and affective changes. In the latter stages of ITLE, a paranoid psychosis
can develop that resembles schizophrenia (Greenberg & Seidman, 1992).

CONCLUSION

In this chapter we provided an update on the behavioral and psychological symptoms often seen in patients who have neurological conditions.
We included examples of psychological emergencies during which affected
patients may come to the attention of mental health care workers. We attempted to illustrate that thinking of disorders as either psychiatric or neurological imposes a false dichotomy and that in the context of what may appear
to be a behavioral emergency, it may be beneficial to consider the patient's
neurological and medical status. It is of the utmost importance to understand
the need for follow-up care when these issues emerge. When an individual
provides knowledge of cardiovascular risk factors, toxic exposures, or history
of traumatic brain injury, the clinician would be wise to refer him or her for
more a extensive medical workup to rule out medical causes of behavioral
limitations. In addition, a family history of neurologic illness may raise concerns about potential causes for behavioral changes and should also be further evaluated.

REFERENCES

American Psychiatric Association. (1994). *Diagnostic and statistical manual of mental
disorders* (4th ed.). Washington, DC: Author.

Binswanger, O. (1894). Die abgrenzung der allgemeinen progressiven paralyse [The definition of general progressive paralysis]. *Beliner Klinische Wochenschrift, 31,* 1103–1186.

Bird, E. D. (1980). Chemical pathology of Huntington's disease. *Annual Review of Pharmacology and Toxicology, 20,* 533–551.

Blumer, D. (1975). Temporal lobe epilepsy and its psychiatric significance. In D. Benson & D. Blumer (Eds.), *Psychiatric aspects of neurological disease* (pp. 171–198). New York: Grune & Stratton.

Burns, A., Folstein, S. E., Brandt, J., & Folstein, M. F. (1990). Clinical assessment of irritability, aggression, and apathy in Huntington's and Alzheimer's disease. *Journal of Nervous and Mental Disease, 178,* 20–26.

Caine, E. D., Hunt, R. D., Weingartner, H., & Ebert, M. H. (1978). Huntington's dementia: Clinical and neuropsychological features. *Archives of General Psychiatry, 35,* 377–384.

Caine, E. D., & Shoulson, I. (1983). Psychiatric syndromes in Huntington's disease. *American Journal of Psychiatry, 140,* 728–733.

Celesia, G. G., & Barr, A. N. (1970). Psychosis and other psychiatric manifestations of levodopa therapy. *Archives of Neurology, 23,* 193–200.

Celesia, G. G., & Wanamaker, W. M. (1972). Psychiatric disturbances in Parkinson's disease. *Diseases of the Nervous System, 33,* 577–583.

Chae, B.-J., & Kang, B.-J. (2006). Quetiapine for hypersexuality and delusional jealousy after stroke. *Journal of Clinical Psychopharmacology, 26,* 331–332.

Chan, K.-L., Campayo, A., Moser, D. J., Arndt, S., & Robinson, R. G. (2006). Aggressive behavior in patients with stroke: Association with psychopathology and results of antidepressant treatment on aggression. *Archives of Physical Medicine and Rehabilitation, 87,* 793–798.

Conneally, P. M. (1984). Huntington's disease: Genetics and epidemiology. *American Journal of Human Genetics, 36,* 506–526.

Cottrell, S. S., & Wilson, S. A. K. (1926). The affective symptomatology of disseminated sclerosis. *Journal of Neurology and Psychopathology, 7,* 1–30.

Crow, T. J., Johnstone, E. C., & McClelland, H. A. (1976). The coincidence of schizophrenia and Parkinsonism: Some neurochemical implications. *Psychology of Medicine, 6,* 227–233.

Cummings, J. L. (1992). Neuropsychiatric complications of drug treatment of Parkinson's disease. In S. J. Huber & J. L. Cummings (Eds.), *Parkinson's disease: Neurobehavioral aspects* (pp. 313–327). New York: Oxford University Press.

Cummings, J. L., & Cole, G. (2002). Alzheimer's disease. *The Journal of the American Medical Association, 287,* 2335–2338.

Dewhurst, K., Oliver, J. E., & McKnight, A. L. (1970). Sociopsychiatric consequences of Huntington's disease. *The British Journal of Psychiatry, 116,* 255–258.

Eror, E. A., Lopez, O. L., Dekosky, S. T., & Sweet, R. A. (2005). Alzheimer disease subjects with psychosis have increased schizotypal symptoms before dementia onset. *Biological Psychiatry, 58,* 325–330.

Folstein, M. F., & Bylsma, F. W. (1994). Noncognitive symptoms of Alzheimer's disease. In R. D. Terry, R. Katzman, & K. L. Bick (Eds.), *Alzheimer's disease* (pp. 27–40). New York: Raven Press.

Folstein, S. E. (1989). *Huntington's disease: A disorder of families.* Baltimore: Johns Hopkins University Press.

Folstein, S. E., Abbott, M. H., Chase, G. A., Jensen, B. A., & Folstein, M. F. (1983). The association of affective disorder with Huntington's disease in a case series and in families. *Psychology of Medicine, 13*, 537–542.

Folstein, S. E., & Folstein, M. F. (1983). Psychiatric features of Huntington's disease: Recent approaches and findings. *Psychological Development, 2*, 193–205.

Folstein, S. E., Franz, M. L., Jensen, B. A., Chase, G. A., & Folstein, M. F. (1983). Conduct disorder and affective disorder among the offspring of patients with Huntington's disease. *Psychology of Medicine, 13*, 45–52.

Goodstein, R. K., & Farrell, R. B. (1977). Multiple sclerosis presenting as a depressive illness. *Disorders of the Nervous System, 38*, 127–131.

Greenberg, M. S., & Seidman, L. J. (1992). Temporal lobe epilepsy. In R. F. White (Ed.), *Clinical syndromes in adult neuropsychology: The practitioner's handbook* (pp. 345–379). Amsterdam: Elsevier.

Hachinski, V. C., Lassen, N. A., & Marshall, J. (1974, July 27). Multi-infarct dementia: A cause of mental deterioration in the elderly. *Lancet, 2*, 207–210.

Hachinski, V. C., Potter, P., & Merskey, H. (1987). Leukoaraiosis. *Archives of Neurology, 44*, 21–23.

Hamdy, R. C. (1998). Clinical presentation. In R. C. Hamdy, J. M. Turnbull, W. Clark, & M. M. Lancaster (Eds.), *Alzheimer's disease: A handbook for caregivers* (3rd ed., pp. 74–86). Saint Louis, MO: Mosby.

Hayden, M. R. (1981). *Huntington's chorea.* New York: Springer-Verlag.

Huber, S. J., Paulson, G. W., & Shuttleworth, E. C. (1988). Relationships of motor symptoms, intellectual impairment, and depression on Parkinson's disease. *Journal of Neurology, Neurosurgery, and Psychiatry, 5*, 855–858.

Huntington, G. W. (1872). On chorea. *Medical Surgical Report, 26*, 317–321.

Kessler, S. (1987). Psychiatric implications of presymptomatic testing for Huntington's disease. *American Journal of Orthopsychiatry, 57*(2), 212–219.

Kessler, S., & Block, M. (1989). Social system responses to Huntington's disease. *Family Process, 28*, 59–68.

Lee, D. Y., Choo, I. H., Kim, K. W., Jhoo, J. H., Youn, J. C., Lee, U. N., & Woo, J. I. (2006). White matter changes associated with psychotic symptoms in Alzheimer's disease patients. *Journal of Neuropsychiatry and Clinical Neurosciences, 18*, 191–198.

Lezak, M. D., Howieson, D. B., & Loring, D. W. (2004). *Neuropsychological assessment* (4th ed.). New York: Oxford University Press.

Lopez-Meza, E., Corona-Vazquez, T., Ruano-Calderon, L. A., & Ramirez-Bermudez, J. (2005). Severe impulsiveness as the primary manifestation of multiple sclerosis in a young female. *Psychiatry and Clinical Neurosciences, 59*, 739–742.

Mayeux, R., Stern, Y., Rosen, J., & Leventhal, J. (1981). Depression, intellectual impairment, and Parkinson's disease. *Neurology, 31,* 659–662.

McHugh, P. R. (1989). The neuropsychiatry of basal ganglia disorders: A triadic syndrome and its explanation. *Neuropsychiatry, Neuropsychology, and Behavioral Neurology, 2,* 239–247.

McHugh, P. R., & Folstein, M. F. (1975). Psychiatric syndromes of Huntington's chorea: A clinical and phenomenological study. In D. Benson & D. Blumer (Eds.), *Psychiatric aspects of neurological disease* (pp. 267–286). New York: Grune & Stratton.

Meguro, K., Meguro, M., Tanaka, Y., Akanuma, K., Yamaguchi K., & Itoh, I. (2004). Risperidone is effective for wandering and disturbed sleep/wake patterns in Alzheimer's disease. *Journal of Geriatric Psychiatry and Neurology, 17,* 61–67.

Morse, P. E., & Montgomery, C. E. (1992). Neuropsychological evaluation of traumatic brain injury. In R. F. White (Ed.), *Clinical syndromes in adult neuropsychology: The practitioner's handbook* (pp. 85–176). New York: Elsevier.

Moskovitz, C., Moses, H., III, & Klawans, H. L. (1978). Levodopa-induced psychosis: A kindling phenomenon. *American Journal of Psychiatry, 135,* 669–675.

Moss, M. B., Albert, M. S., & Kemper, T. L. (1992). Neuropsychology of frontal lobe dementia. In R. F. White (Ed.), *Clinical syndromes in adult neuropsychology: The practitioner's handbook* (pp. 387–303). Amsterdam: Elsevier.

Oliver, J. E., & Dewhurst, K. E. (1969). Six generations of ill-used children in a Huntington's pedigree. *Postgraduate Medical Journal, 45,* 757–760.

Osview, F. (1989). Interictal behavior syndrome in temporal lobe epilepsy: The views of three experts. *Journal of Neuropsychiatry and Clinical Neuroscience, 1,* 308–318.

Peyser, C. E., & Folstein, S. E. (1990). Huntington's disease as a model for mood disorders, clues from neuropathology and neurochemistry. *Molecular and Chemical Neuropathology, 12,* 99–119.

Pflanz, S., Besson, J. A. O., Ebmeier, K. P., & Simpson, S. (1991). The clinical manifestation of mental disorder in Huntington's disease: A retrospective case record study of disease progression. *Acta Psychiatrica Scandinavica, 83,* 53–60.

Rauch, S. L., Jenike, M. A., Alpert, N. M, Baer, L., Breiter, H. C., Savage, C. R., & Fischman, A. J. (1994). Regional cerebral blood flow measured during symptom provocation in obsessive–compulsive disorder using oxygen 15-labeled carbon dioxide and positron emission tomography. *Archives of General Psychiatry, 51,* 62–70.

Reed, E., & Chandler, J. H. (with Hughes, E. M., & Davidson, R. T.). (1958). Huntington's chorea in Michigan: I. Demography and genetics. *American Journal of Human Genetics, 10,* 201–225.

Saint-Cyr, J. A., Taylor, A. E., & Lang, A. E. (1993). Neuropsychological and psychiatric side effects in the treatment of Parkinson's disease. *Neurology, 43*(Suppl. 6), 47–52.

Saint-Cyr, J. A., Taylor, A. E., & Nicholson, K. (1995). Behavior and the basal ganglia. *Advances in Neurology, 65,* 1–28.

Sano, M. (1991). Basal ganglia diseases and depression. *Neuropsychiatry, Neuropsychology, and Behavioral Neurology, 4*, 41–48.

Santamaria, J., Tolosa, E., & Balles, A. (1986). Parkinson's disease with depression: A possible subgroup of idiopathic Parkinsonism. *Neurology, 36*, 1130–1133.

Schiffer, R. B., Wineman, N. M., & Weitkamp, L. R. (1986). Association between bipolar affective disorder and multiple sclerosis. *American Journal of Psychiatry, 143*, 94–95.

Schoenfeld, M., Myers, R. H., Cupples, L. A., Berkman, B., Sax, D. S., & Clark, E. (1984). Increased rate of suicide among patients with Huntington's disease. *Journal of Neurology, Neurosurgery, and Psychiatry, 47*, 1283–1287.

Seidman, L. J., Cassens, G. P., Kremen, W. S., & Pepple, J. R. (1992). Neuropsychology of schizophrenia. In R. F. White (Ed.), *Clinical syndromes in adult neuropsychology: The practitioner's handbook* (pp. 213–251). Amsterdam: Elsevier.

Shoulson, I. (1990). Huntington's disease: Cognitive and psychiatric features. *Neuropsychiatry, Neuropsychology, and Behavioral Neurology, 3*, 15–22.

Starkstein, S. E., Jorge R., Mizrahi R., & Robinson, R. G. (2006). A prospective longitudinal study of apathy in Alzheimer's disease. *Journal of Neurology, Neurosurgery, and Psychiatry, 77*, 8–11.

Tanner, C. M., Bogel, C., Goetz, C. G., & Klawans, H. L. (1983). Hallucinations in Parkinson's disease: A population study. *Annals of Neurology, 14*, 136.

Tatemichi, T. K. (1990). How acute brain failure becomes chronic: A view of the mechanisms of dementia related to stroke. *Neurology, 40*, 1652–1659.

Trimble, M. R., & Thompson, P. J. (1986). Neuropsychological aspects of epilepsy. In I. Grant & K. M. Adams (Eds.), *Neuropsychological assessment of neuropsychiatric disorders* (pp. 321–346). New York: Oxford University Press.

Turner, A. P., Williams, R. M., Bowen, J. D., Kivlahan, D. R., & Haselkorn, J. K. (2006). Suicidal ideation in multiple sclerosis. *Archives of Physical Medicine and Rehabilitation, 87*, 1073–1078.

Victor, M., & Ropper, A. (2000). *Principles of neurology* (7th ed.). New York: McGraw-Hill.

Webb, M., & Trzepacz, P. T. (1987). Huntington's disease: Correlations of mental status with chorea. *Biological Psychiatry, 22*, 751–761.

White, R. F. (1990). Emotional and cognitive correlates of multiple sclerosis. *Journal of Neuropsychiatry, 2*, 422–428.

White, R. F., Au, R., Durso, R., & Moss, M. B. (1992). Neuropsychological function in Parkinson's disease. In R. F. White (Ed.), *Clinical syndromes in adult neuropsychology: The practitioner's handbook* (pp. 213–251). Amsterdam: Elsevier.

White, R. F., Nyenhuis, D. S., & Sax, D. S. (1992). Multiple sclerosis. In R. F. White (Ed.), *Clinical syndromes in adult neuropsychology: The practitioner's handbook* (pp. 177–212). Amsterdam: Elsevier.

White, R. F., Vasterling, J. J., Koroshetz, W., & Myers, R. (1992). Neuropsychology of Huntington's disease. In R. F. White (Ed.), *Clinical syndromes in adult neuropsychology: The practitioner's handbook* (pp. 213–251). Amsterdam: Elsevier.

Williams-Gray, C. H., Foltynie, T., Lewis, S. J. G., & Barker, R. A. (2006). Cognitive deficits and psychosis in Parkinson's disease: A review of pathophysiology and therapeutic options. *CNS Drugs, 20,* 477–506.

Wolfe, N., Linn, R., Babikian, V. L., Knoefel, J. E., & Albert, M. E. (1990). Frontal systems impairment following multiple lacunar infarcts. *Archives of Neurology, 47,* 129–132.

14

PSYCHOLOGICAL AND BEHAVIORAL SYMPTOMS IN ENDOCRINE DISORDERS

KARINA TSATOURIAN AND JACQUELINE A. SAMSON

Accurate diagnosis is essential to the treatment of behavioral emergencies in acute and chronic medical conditions. Among the most difficult of diagnostic discriminations is the differential diagnosis of primary mental disorders versus behavioral manifestations of endocrine disorders. In this chapter, we review the main characteristics of the endocrine system and the behavioral manifestation of endocrine disorders that may appear to represent psychiatric conditions. As we note in this chapter, the *Diagnostic and Statistical Manual of Mental Disorders* (DSM–IV; 4th ed.; American Psychiatric Association, 1994) differential diagnoses that are most typical for patients with endocrine pathology are mostly found in the categories of anxiety and mood disorders. However, in acute or severe chronic conditions, psychotic and other psychopathological manifestations are possible. The psychological, cognitive, and behavioral signs and symptoms that can be found secondary to endocrine dysfunction are somewhat nonspecific, with similar symptoms emanating from different underlying endocrinological problems. Therefore, we include additional questions to be addressed that may assist in making referrals to the appropriate endocrine specialist in cases in which underlying endocrine pathology is suspected.

The endocrine system is one of the main structures responsible for our ability to regulate emotions, to control behavior within socially and environmentally acceptable frames, and to generate productive cognitive functions. Through the complexity of neurobiological hierarchies, the endocrine system regulates arousal, emotions in general, specific responses to stress, the quality and speed of motor activity, the life cycle, biological and circadian rhythms, and temperature regulation. Thus, stability in the balance between hormones is one of the leading factors contributing to cognitive and emotional well-being.

When the endocrine system is not functioning properly, patients can present with symptoms of distorted mood, cognitive impairment, behavioral change, or even frank psychosis. These symptoms may be directly linked to alterations in hormonal systems that affect mood, cognition, or behavior, or may represent true mood disorders or anxiety reactions that manifest secondary to the experience of living with a chronic medical illness. Moreover, endocrine pathology may develop secondary to perturbations in other medical conditions, such as hormonal changes that occur secondary to the presence of tumors, antibody stimulation, or the intentional stimulation of certain hormones to improve physical performance, such as anabolic androgenic steroids (Hartgens & Kuipers, 2004; Trenton & Currier, 2005).

There are five major endocrine systems with disorders that overlap in symptom presentation with psychiatric, psychological, and behavioral conditions: the adrenocorticoid system, thyroid system, parathyroid system, glucose regulation by the pancreas, and reproductive systems. As we describe these systems we present the most typical endocrine diseases associated with the dysfunction of each system and frames for differential diagnoses of psychopathology that might be associated with endocrine dysfunction. The diagnostic classification information we present in this chapter is based on the description of available epidemiological data, general psychological–psychiatric symptoms of the presented endocrine pathology, typical behavioral changes that might occur in the process of pathological development, and findings based on observations of patients with endocrine dysfunction. We also present a list of *DSM–IV* diagnoses to show the range of psychopathology and diagnostic clarification of psychological and behavioral symptoms in medically induced conditions.

THE ADRENOCORTICOID SYSTEM

Actions of the adrenocorticoid system are most clearly seen during times of extreme stress. The *fight or flight response* characteristic of an acute stress reaction involves increased production in the hypothalamus of corticotropin-releasing factor (CRF), which signals the pituitary to release adrenocorticotropic hormone (ACTH), which signals the adrenal glands to secrete cortisol. Activation of this system may also stimulate increased catecholamine output (i.e., neurotransmitters including dopamine, epinephrine, and norepinephrine), which activates the sympathetic nervous system to effect behavioral changes helpful in quick reactions such as heightened arousal, hypervigilance to threatening stimuli, increased heart rate, increased respiration, increased motor activity, decreased sleep, and decreased gastrointestinal motility (Nussey & Whitehead, 2001; Rasgon, Hendrick, & Garrick, 2004). The adrenocorticoid system is also central to the mobilization of anti-inflammatory responses in reaction to physical injury. Release of ACTH by the pituitary initiates the cascade of signals to the adrenal glands to secrete anti-inflammatory corticoids, which decrease dilation of blood vessels in the inflamed area and hence decrease reddening and swelling. Corticoid treatments are commonly used to reduce inflammation and control pain.

Hypercortisolism

Excess amounts of circulating cortisol, known as hypercortisolism, are most often found in people who use steroids (i.e., glucocorticoids) for treatment of autoimmune problems. Less commonly, hypercortisolism is associated with Cushing's disease and is caused by increases in ACTH secondary to a tumor in the pituitary gland. Finally, tumors in the adrenals or ectopic tumors that secrete ACTH may lead to high levels of circulating cortisol. Symptoms of hypercortisolism that is caused by Cushing's disease or medical conditions resulting in excess ACTH or CRF might resemble depression. Following exposure to large amounts of steroid treatments, there may be hypomanic-like symptoms; in some patients, bursts of uncontrolled aggressive behavior might be observed. There is also a vulnerable group of patients who might develop psychotic symptoms (Sonino, Bonnini, Fallo, Boscaro, & Fava, 2006).

Information for Diagnostic Classification of Psychological Symptoms in Hypercortisolism

The following psychiatric, cognitive and, behavioral changes reflect the broad range of symptoms that were monitored in patients with this endocrine pathology. Epidemiological information helps to identify the group of vulnerable population.

Epidemiology. Epidemiological data presented by the National Institutes of Health (NIH) and Centers for Disease Control and Prevention suggest that hypercortisolism affects mostly adults between the ages of 20 and 50 (NIH, 2002). Women can be more vulnerable to develop hypercortisolism than men, and environmental factors might be considered in some cases, but there are no clear data on this in research and epidemiologic literature. In the United States, from 10 to 15 cases per 1 million are diagnosed annually.

Psychiatric Symptoms. General psychiatric symptoms include emotional lability, irritability, anxiety, social withdrawal, decreased libido, disturbed sleep, circadian rhythm changes, and low tolerance to stress. In acute or medically uncontrolled conditions, paranoia, hallucinations, and depersonalization have been described (Nussey & Whitehead, 2001; Rasgon et al., 2004).

Cognitive Manifestations. Changes in performance are typically represented by hypersensitivity to stimuli, impaired concentration, impaired memory, heightened arousal, and hypervigilance.

Behavioral Observations and Common Complaints. Negative changes in appearance and facial expressions are considerable major complaints. Many patients develop a rounded face and increased fat around the neck, but arms and legs might appear comparatively thin. In women, excess hair growth on the face, chest, and thighs can be observed. The patient's skin is usually fragile, thin, easily bruised, and slow healing, and purple stretch marks are common. Behavioral reactivity expressed in uncontrolled facial muscle reactions to unpleasant stimuli (e.g., noise, light, crowded places) in some cases might be accompanied by pressured speech. Hypermotoractivity is typical and can be observed as sharp motor reaction with low productivity in daily functioning. Among typical complaints presented by patients with hypercortisolism are irregular cycles in women, decreased fertility in men, and diminished sexual drive. Patients might experience chronic pain and low backaches associated with bone weakening.

Diagnostic Considerations for Psychopathology in Hypercortisolism

The following diagnosis can be considered by the examiner during psychodiagnostic evaluation of patients with endocrine dysfunction indicated by excess amounts of circulating cortisol (American Psychiatric Association, 1994):

- 239.83: Mood Disorder Due to the General Medical Condition
- 293.9: Mental Disorder Not Otherwise Specified (NOS) Due to the General Medical Condition
- 310.1: Personality Changes Due to General Medical Condition

The most typical clusters of psychological and behavioral symptoms of hypercortisolism might mimic the following differential psychiatric diagnoses:

- 296.xx: Major Depressive Disorder
- 300.01: Panic Disorder
- 294.9: Cognitive Disorder NOS

Hypocortisolism

Damage to the cortex of the adrenals from an autoimmune disorder such as Addison's disease, infection, amyloidosis, hemochromatosis, or tumor growth may lead to low levels of circulating cortisol or hypocortisolism. Other causes of low cortisol may be poor functioning in the pituitary gland and withdrawal from treatment with glucocorticoids.

Information for Diagnostic Classification of Psychological Symptoms in Hypocortisolism

The following psychiatric, cognitive and, behavioral changes reflect the broad range of symptoms that were monitored in patients with this endocrine pathology. Epidemiological information helps to identify the group of vulnerable population.

Epidemiology. Epidemiological data presented by the Agency for Healthcare Research and Quality and the Centers for Disease Control and Prevention suggest the following: Hypocortisolism is a disorder that can equally affect males and females in all age groups (NIH, 2004). In certain circumstances, environmental factors might play significant role in the development of this endocrine pathology. Approximately 110 cases per 1 million are reported.

Psychiatric Symptoms. General psychiatric symptoms are usually expressed by emotional lability, irritability, social withdrawal, apathy, disturbed sleep, and lethargy. In some cases anorexia might develop. Chronic fatigue and significantly decreased tolerance for stress are typical for patients with hypocortisolism. In acute conditions, psychotic syndrome and delirium might occur (Nussey & Whitehead, 2001; Rasgon et al., 2004).

Cognitive Manifestations. Cognitive changes include long response latency, thought distortions, memory difficulties, limited attention span, and impaired concentration.

Behavioral Observations and Common Complaints. Behavioral observations, which are described in the literature as most typical, start with hyperpigmentation, skin darkening (i.e., a tanning effect); complaints of salt craving; significant weight loss; loss of body hair; masked or apathetic facial expression; changes in sexual activities (usually this complaint is presented by partners, not by a patient); irregularity in menstrual cycle or diminished or stopped cycle.

Diagnostic Considerations for Psychopathology in Hypocortisolism

The following diagnoses can be considered during psychodiagnostic evaluation of patients with endocrine dysfunction indicated by low level of cortisol circulation (American Psychiatric Assocation, 1994):

- 239.83: Mood Disorder Due to the General Medical Condition

- 293.9: Mental Disorder NOS Due to General Medical Condition
- 310.1: Personality Change Due to General Medical Condition

The most typical clusters of psychological and behavioral symptoms of hypocortisolism might mimic the fallowing differential psychiatric diagnoses:

- 296.xx: Major Depressive Disorder
- 294.9: Cognitive Disorder NOS
- 293.xx: Psychotic Disorder Due to General Medical Condition
- 298.9: Psychotic Disorder NOS

THE THYROID SYSTEM

The primary function of the hypothalamic–pituitary–thyroid system is to regulate metabolism. In reaction to environmental or physical stressors, thyroid-releasing hormone is released by the hypothalamus and signals the pituitary gland to release thyroid-stimulating hormone (TSH). TSH stimulates the release of thyroxine and triiodothyronine (T3) from the thyroid gland, which then bind to specific thyroid hormone receptors in the body to increase metabolic activity or indirectly stimulate centers in the central nervous system that regulate metabolic activity. Increased levels of T3 and TSH might be associated with psychopathic behavior and low level of adaptation to stress. In some studies, overactive T3 and TSH are linked to criminal behavior resulting from extremely poor social control.

Hyperthyroidism

Patients with elevations of thyroid hormone, or hyperthyroidism, present with weight loss, heart palpitations, shortness of breath, heat intolerance, and emotional control problems. Characteristic signs of Graves' disease are enlargement of the thyroid gland and increased fluid in the retro-orbital space that gives a characteristic bulging appearance to the eyes. If not treated early, significant ophthalmologic problems might develop. In the elderly most typical symptoms of the disease might be masked. Among the first symptoms of hyperthyroidism in the elderly are changes in psychomotor activity (i.e., multiple movements with an increased number of mistakes) and expressed cognitive impairment such as short-term memory decline, decreased level of attention, and an inability to perform multiple tasks without mistakes. Cognitive symptoms of untreated hyperthyroidism might be misdiagnosed as cognitive decline because of the development of dementia (Cappola et. al., 2006).

Information for Diagnostic Classification of Psychological Symptoms in Hyperthyroidism

Epidemiology. Reports by the Centers for Disease Control and Prevention and the NIH show that 0.5% of the general population have hyperthyroidism, and in 80% of cases symptom manifestations are provoked by Graves' disease (NIH, 2008). Hyperthyroidism is a frequent developmental pathology in teenage girls, but it can also occur during the ages of 30 to 40 and in older people. Gender plays a significant role in this type of endocrine pathology: Women and teenage girls develop the disease 4 times more than men, and some women (5%–9%) develop postpartum thyroiditis. Thyroid dysfunctions in some geographic regions might be identified as a regional pathology. Environmental factors should always be considered in the evaluation and assessment of thyroid disease.

Psychiatric Symptoms. General psychiatric symptoms are usually expressed by increased nervousness, fatigue, mood lability, dysphoria, restlessness, hyperactivity, irritability, and sleep disturbances. In untreated, acute cases visual hallucinations, paranoid ideation, and delirium might occur (Nussey & Whitehead, 2001; Rasgon et al., 2004).

Cognitive Manifestations. Changes in cognitive functioning usually include short attention span, impaired recent memory, exaggerated startle response, and changes in self-perception. In rare cases, disorganized thoughts and psychomotor retardation might be observed. Usually these symptoms manifest in patients with poor management of medications or predisposition to psychopathology. Psychomotor retardation is more typical for older patients, but in certain cases might be seen in young adults.

Behavioral Observations and Common Complaints. Behavioral presentation and main complaints reflect cognitive and physiological changes in patients with elevations of thyroid hormone. Typical observations are changes in eye expressions, facial expressions, behavioral reactivity to unpleasant stimuli (e.g., noise, light, crowded places) and sharp, poorly controlled motor reactions. Decreased productivity in daily functioning is typical for the patient in the first stages of treatment (e.g., inability to finish tasks, slowness in remembering words, inability to complete sentences, poor motivation and efforts to maintain verbal communication). Difficulty in tolerating crowded places, increased reactivity to noise and bright light, avoidance in personality characteristics, and decreased ability to tolerate stress are typical features for patients with hyperthyroidism.

Diagnostic Considerations for Psychopathology in Hyperthyroidism

The following diagnosis can be considered during psychodiagnostic evaluation of patients with endocrine dysfunction indicated by hyperactive thyroid (American Psychiatric Assocation, 1994):

- 293.89: Anxiety Disorder Due to the General Medical Condition
- 293.9: Mental Disorder NOS Due to General Medical Condition
- 310.1: Personality Change Due to General Medical Condition

The most typical clusters of psychological and behavioral symptoms of hyperthyroidism might mimic the following differential psychiatric diagnoses:

- 300.02: Generalized Anxiety Disorder
- 300.01: Panic Disorder
- 300.23: Social and Other Simple Phobias
- 239.83: Mood Disorder Due to General Medical Condition With Manic/Hypomanic Features

Hypothyroidism

Patients with deficiencies in circulating thyroid, or hypothyroidism, show a slowing of metabolic processes. Clinical features include modest weight gain; intolerance to cold; dry hair; brittle nails; loss of hair in the lateral third of the eyebrow; puffiness in legs, hands, and face; a hoarse voice; constipation; slowed heart rate; and excessive menstrual bleeding. Symptoms of hypothyroidism most closely resemble clinical depression.

Information for Diagnostic Classification of Psychological Symptoms in Hypothyroidism

The following psychiatric, cognitive and, behavioral changes reflect the broad range of symptoms that were monitored in patients with this endocrine pathology. Epidemiological information helps to identify the group of vulnerable population.

Epidemiology. Epidemiologic reports suggest that 0.1 % to 2.0% of the general population are affected by hypothyroidism and 3% to 7.5% have subclinical hypothyroidism (i.e., asymptomatic). Manifestations of clinically significant symptoms might occur in the years between ages 40 and 50 and in the older population. This pathology is more typical for women and rises with age. Environmental factors should be considered during assessment and evaluation. Dysfunction might be in the range of regional pathology (Nussey & Whitehead, 2001; Rasgon et al., 2004).

Psychiatric Symptoms. General psychiatric symptoms usually mimic the symptoms of depression and are expressed by depressed mood, apathy, decreased libido, rare suicidality, auditory hallucinations, paranoia, and even coma.

Cognitive Manifestations. Typical changes in cognition can be represented by impaired concentration and long response latencies.

Behavioral Observations and Common Complaints. Patients with low level thyroid functioning usually experience weight gain, body or figure changes, poor appetite, reduced hearing, unwillingness to communicate, significant decrease in social activities, low productivity, significant physical weakness, and loss of interest in sexual activities.

Diagnostic Considerations for Psychopathology in hypothyroidism.

The following diagnoses can be considered during psychodiagnostic evaluation of patients with endocrine dysfunction indicated by decreased thyroid hormone secretion (American Psychiatric Association, 1994):

- 239.83: Mood Disorder Due to General Medical Condition
- 293.9: Mental Disorder NOS Due to General Medical Condition
- 310.1: Personality Change Due to General Medical Condition

The most typical clusters of psychological and behavioral symptoms of hypothyroidism might mimic the following differential psychiatric diagnoses:

- 296.xx: Major Depressive Disorder
- 296.xx, 296.89, 296.80: Bipolar Disorder (i.e., after initial treatment)
- 294.9: Cognitive Disorder NOS

THE PARATHYROID SYSTEM

The parathyroid glands secrete parathyroid hormone (PTH), which is critical for the regulation of calcium levels in the blood. In combination with vitamin D and calcitonin, PTH increases gastrointestinal absorption of dietary calcium and stimulates bone resorption.

Hyperparathyroidism

Because neuronal cell membranes use calcium to function, abnormalities in the serum levels of this mineral can result in a wide variety of neurologic and psychiatric problems. Patients with excess parathyroid production, or hyperparathyroidism, have few signs of the disorder but exhibit a wide range of neuropsychiatric symptoms. Patients may complain of sad mood, anxiety, lethargy, change in sleep patterns, poor memory, and poor concentration and in the presence of hypomagnesia, auditory or visual hallucinations. Symptoms may or may not improve with surgical correction of the disorder.

Information for Diagnostic Classification of Psychological Symptoms in Hyperparathyroid Pathology

The following psychiatric, cognitive and, behavioral changes reflect the broad range of symptoms that were monitored in patients with this endocrine pathology. Epidemiological information helps to identify the group of vulnerable population.

Epidemiology. According to the reports of the NIH (2006a), 0.1 % to 2.0% of the general population of the United States are affected by hyperparathyroidism. Manifestations of the disease might occur in one's 40s or later in life. Typical age of onset in women (for hyperparathyroidism) is after age 60, and it is mostly due to other medical conditions. Gender is an important factor, as pathological development is more typical for women than men (2:1).

Psychiatric Symptoms. General psychiatric symptoms include nervousness, fatigue, mood lability, and irritability. In some cases delusions and suicidal thoughts might be observed (Nussey & Whitehead, 2001; Rasgon et al., 2004).

Cognitive Manifestations. Cognitive difficulties include short attention span and impaired recent memory. In some cases, changes in thought processing and changes in the typical structure of psychomotor activities might also occur.

Behavioral Observations and Common Complaints. Among general complaints, patients present almost constant feelings of weakness and/or thirst, increased urination (kidney stones might develop), and weight change. Some patients might develop more careful and slower movements because of the high risk of bone thinning and fractures. In some patients, facial expressions with signs of suffering (because of the development of chronic pain) might be observed. Avoidant behavior might be developed in the process of this disease because of the complex of medical symptoms.

Diagnostic Considerations for Psychopathology in Hyperparathyroidism

The following diagnoses can be considered during the psychodiagnostic evaluation of patients with endocrine dysfunction indicated by increased secretion of hormones in the parathyroid system (American Psychiatric Association, 1994):

- 293.89: Anxiety Disorder Due to General Medical Condition
- 293.9: Mental Disorder NOS Due to General Medical Condition
- 310.1: Personality Change Due to General Medical Condition

The most typical clusters of psychological and behavioral symptoms of hyperparathyroidism might mimic the following differential psychiatric diagnoses:

- 300.02: Generalized Anxiety Disorder
- 296.xx: Major Depressive Disorder
- 293.xx: Psychotic Disorder Due to General Medical Condition
- 298.9: Psychotic Disorder NOS
- 294.9: Cognitive Disorder NOS

Hypoparathyroidism

Insufficient levels of circulating parathyroid hormone, or hypoparathyroidism, may present with tingling sensations in the fingers, toes, and lips, muscle cramps, seizure activity, hyperventilation, and extrapyramidal symptoms. Neuroendocrine pathology is often accompanied by psychological and behavioral symptoms.

Information for Diagnostic Classification of Psychological Symptoms in Hypoparathyroid Pathology

The following psychiatric, cognitive and, behavioral changes reflect the broad range of symptoms that were monitored in patients with this endocrine pathology. Epidemiological information helps to identify the group of vulnerable population.

Epidemiology. Epidemiological reports suggest that hypoparathyroid dysfunction is a comparatively rare hormonal disease that can be congenital or acquired later in life. According to epidemiological information provided by the NIH (2006b), from 25% to 50% of members in families with a genetic predisposition might be affected with hypoparathyroidism; in many cases, parents might not present any symptoms of pathological parathyroid function. Some studies indicate the sex-linked inheritance in families with X chromosome defect (only boys would then be affected). Patients with genetic predisposition might present the signs of parathyroid pathology as early as age 2. The most typical age for acquired disease is during the 4th decade of life. A significant increase in cases is observed in the elderly population, secondary to multiple medical conditions. The effect of gender is minimal: Both women and men can be affected later in life. If the disease is congenital, the gender effect might be the factor in X chromosome defect. In epidemiologic reports no clear information is available regarding the impact of environmental factors on the development of hyporapathyroid conditions.

Psychiatric Symptoms. General psychiatric symptoms include increased irritability, poor emotional control, and decreased tolerance to stress. Psychotic symptoms might appear in medically uncontrolled conditions.

Cognitive Manifestations. Performance might be limited as a result of significant changes in attention and working memory, difficulties in executive function, slowness in processing information, and sensory perceptual agitation.

Behavioral Observations and Common Complaints. Mild nonspecific behavioral changes usually reflect more neurological signs such as lip movements described as a "feeling of tingling," and an inability to sit still for a long period of time. Hyperventilation might be observed as a response to minimal stress (i.e., positive and negative), and nonproductive activities (more like agitation) might be observed during multiple task performance.

Diagnostic Considerations for Psychopathology in Hypoparathyroidism

The following diagnoses can be considered during the psychodiagnostic evaluation of patients with endocrine dysfunction indicated by decreased secretion of hormones in the parathyroid system (American Psychiatric Association, 1994):

- 294.1: Dementia/Cognitive Disorder Due to General Medical Condition
- 293.9: Mental Disorder NOS Due to General Medical Condition
- 310.1: Personality Change Due to General Medical Condition

The most typical clusters of psychological and behavioral symptoms of hypoparathyroidism might mimic the following differential psychiatric diagnoses:

- 294.9: Cognitive Disorder NOS
- 296.xx: Mood Disorder
- 293.xx: Psychotic Disorder Due to General Medical Condition
- 298.9: Psychotic Disorder NOS

THE PANCREAS

Proper functioning of neuronal cells is dependent on a steady supply of glucose in the blood. Two hormones produced by the pancreas accomplish this task: insulin and glucagon. Insulin facilitates the entry of glucose into the cells of target tissues and helps convert glucose into glycogen, triglycerides, and protein for storage. Glucagon preserves glycogen and fatty acids from further conversion and increases the liver output of glucose. Together with other hormones, insulin and glucagons maintain a balance of glucose and fatty acids in the blood.

Imbalances in blood glucose levels are generally associated with either deficiencies or excesses of insulin and glucagons. Inability to produce adequate amounts of insulin to metabolize glucose is known as diabetes mellitus. In individuals with diabetes, glucose regulation is not automatic but must be monitored and controlled by external means. If daily injections of insulin are required, the disorder is known as insulin-dependent diabetes or Type 1 diabetes. Type 1 diabetes generally begins early in life, before age 40.

A second type of illness, known as Type 2 diabetes, typically begins later in life and is associated with the desensitization of insulin receptors after years of exposure to chronically high levels of blood glucose. Type 2 diabetes is typically controlled through careful monitoring of diet, exercise, and at times, through the use of oral hypoglycemic agents. Diet requirements for managing diabetes include restriction of foods and beverages high in fat or sugar content and restriction of alcohol intake. Eating small amounts of food more frequently increases the body's ability to handle the glucose that is ingested and maintain steady levels in the blood. Frequent monitoring of blood sugar levels is required to guide insulin, food, and exercise regimens. If not properly balanced, the deteriorating course of the illness will be hastened, and the patient is at risk for the development of severe and irreversible complications affecting the heart, kidney, nervous system, and retina (Kinmonth, Woodcock, Griffin, Spiegal, & Campbell, 1998). Psychological and behavioral symptoms in patients with diabetes might develop as a result of hormonal and metabolic destabilization and might also be associated with peripheral neuropathy, one of the most common complications in diabetes. Functional limitations, chronic pain, reduction in quality of life, and significantly limited stress tolerance can also develop (Vileikyte et al., 2005).

Hyperglycemia and Hypoglycemia

When blood sugars are too high, a condition known as hyperglycemia exists. Signs may include increased fluid intake, nausea or vomiting, dry mouth, dehydration, blurred vision, and fatigue. Severe hyperglycemia can lead to coma and acidosis. Psychiatric symptoms are common and might develop from mild to severe mood changes, lethargy, and slowed thought processes.

When blood sugars are too low, a condition known as hypoglycemia exists. Hypoglycemic states are associated with elevations in cortisol and epinephrine and the activation of the sympathetic nervous system, as seen in response to environmental stressors. Early signs include heart palpitations, increased sweating, dizziness, blurred vision, and hunger. Later symptoms include headache and mental confusion. If left untreated, hypoglycemia can lead to coma and death. Psychiatric symptoms in the range of anxiety disorders can be observed.

Information for Diagnostic Classification of Psychological Symptoms in Diabetes Mellitus

Epidemiology. The National Diabetes Education Program of the NIH reported that the number of cases diagnosed with Type 1 diabetes in the United States is around 700,000 (NIH, 2006b). One in every 500 children have Type 1 diabetes. Although the majority of cases start at age 10, all age groups are vulnerable. Diabetes affects both men and women. According to reports, the evidence of seasonal and regional impact in this pathology is significant but not leading. Autoimmune and genetic predispositions to the disease are very important.

Epidemiological data report that almost 13 million people in the United States have Type 2 diabetes. Clinical manifestation of symptoms is typical for adults age 40 and older and in younger populations with obesity problems. This pathology affects men and women, but the higher obesity rate in women makes them more vulnerable to developing Type 2 diabetes. According to epidemiological studies, the geographic–regional impact is significant. Manifestation of Type 2 diabetes is much higher among African Americans, Native Americans, Asian/Pacific Islanders, and Latin Americans and tends to be inversely related to socioeconomic status.

Psychiatric Symptoms. Mixed pathological development usually accompanies Type 1 and Type 2 diabetes; psychopathology, endocrine disease, and hypertension are the typical cluster of problems for adults with diabetes. Psychiatric symptoms include irritability, poor emotional control, anxiety, sleep disturbances, poor motivation, and decreased tolerance to stress. In acute conditions and when there is poor medical control over the symptoms, psychotic manifestations might occur (Nussey & Whitehead, 2001; Rasgon et al., 2004).

Cognitive Manifestations. The most typical problems of cognitive decline are based on sensory–perceptual activation with multiple functional limitations. Patients with diabetes usually show a decrease and slowness in movements because of developing neuropathies. Poor attention span resulting from sensory limitations, memory and learning difficulties, and extremely limited stress tolerance can also develop.

Behavioral Observations and Common Complaints. Adjustments to a new life structure include self-care and preventive measures, timely medication management, skin care, dental care, prevention and treatment of viral infections (e.g., ear infections), control over diet, and oversight of possible dehydration. In severe cases and with poor care, significant changes in patients' appearance can be noticed, including weight change, hearing loss, poor nail condition, poor skin condition, and red eyes. Social communication might be limited, and patients might feel isolated but unwilling to change the situation.

Psychological Factors Affecting Medical Condition. The most typical clusters of psychological and behavioral symptoms of diabetes mellitus might mimic the following differential psychiatric diagnoses:

- 296.xx and 296.89: Bipolar Disorder
- 295.xx: Schizophrenia
- 300.02: Generalized Anxiety Disorder
- 296.xx: Major Depressive Disorder
- 293.xx: Psychotic Disorder Due to General Medical Condition
- 298.9: Psychotic Disorder NOS

Among patients with these chronic psychiatric conditions, Type 2 diabetes is 3 times more prevalent, compared with the general population. Diabetes and bipolar disorder might be based on the same type of deregulations in immunologic, autonomic nervous system, and hormonal structure. That means that genetic predisposition or developed high risk factors for both diabetes and bipolar disorders might be the same (Taylor & MacQueen, 2006). Another path for the development of diabetes in patients with bipolar disorder is the impact of psychopharmacological treatment with psychotropic medication. In particular, many of the common mood stabilizing and antipsychotic medications prescribed to control symptoms of bipolar disorder result in significant weight gain and increased blood sugar levels and may eventually precipitate diabetes.

In addition to the main diagnoses, a number of differential diagnoses for patients with hypoglycemia and hyperglycemia should also be considered:

Hypoglycemia
- 307.50: Eating Disorder NOS
- 300.02: Generalized Anxiety Disorder
- 294.9: Cognitive Disorder NOS
- 298.8: Brief Psychotic Disorder

Hyperglycemia
- 296.90: Mood Disorder NOS
- 297.1: Delusional Disorder
- 294.9: Cognitive Disorder NOS

Diagnostic Considerations for Psychopathology in Diabetes Mellitus

The following diagnoses can be considered during psychodiagnostic evaluation of patients with diabetes mellitus (American Psychiatric Association, 1994):

- 293.83: Mood Disorder Due to General Medical Condition
- 293.9: Mental Disorder NOS Due to General Medical Condition
- 310.1: Personality Change Due to General Medical Condition

THE REPRODUCTIVE SYSTEM

The principal hormones produced by the ovaries and associated with the female reproductive system are estrogen and progesterone. During the reproductive years, a monthly cycle of hormonal changes regulates the maturation and release of follicles into eggs for fertilization. During the early or follicular phase of the cycle, estrogen is released by the ovaries in increasing quantities, which helps to build the endometrium in preparation for implantation. At midcycle, the brain stimulates the release of leutinizing hormone, which prompts the release of the mature egg from the ovary. If the egg is fertilized and implants in the uterus, estrogen levels continue to rise. If the egg does not implant, estrogen levels decline to a low over the final 2 weeks of the cycle. As the egg matures, it produces the hormone progesterone, which prepares the body for pregnancy. If pregnancy does not occur, the egg breaks down and progesterone levels decline sharply. Thus, the latter phases of the cycle are characterized by decreasing estrogen levels and rising, then falling, levels of progesterone produced by the egg. Commonly, the earlier high estrogen and low progesterone phases are associated with good energy and positive mood, whereas the latter stages of low estrogen and low progesterone are associated in some women with low mood and decreased energy. For some women, the latter parts of the cycle are associated with premenstrual syndrome, or PMS, characterized by low or irritable mood, fatigue, and changes in sleep and appetite. During the years just preceding the end of monthly cycling, the so-called perimenopause period, there may be wide oscillations in hormone functioning as the body prepares for menopause.

It is during this phase that women may report a wide variety of symptoms associated with mood, appetite, sleep, energy, and cognitive disturbances (Putman, Van Honk, Kessels, Mulder, & Koppeschaar, 2004). Changes in other interconnected hormonal systems, such as thyroid and adrenocorticoid, may also occur in reaction to changes in ovarian hormones and should be monitored. When the change is completed and cycling stops, menopause has occurred and the body functions with a low level of a different form of estrogen produced by fat tissue and the adrenal glands (Terrien et al., 2007). Because estrogen has been reported to function as a dopamine receptor blocker and an enhancer of serotonin functioning, decreases in naturally occurring estrogen may be associated with increases in anxiety, depression, irritability, and sleep disturbances in some women. Generally, depletions in serotonin levels are associated with depressed mood, irritability, anxiety, and sleep disturbances, whereas increases in dopamine levels are associated with poor reality testing and psychotic symptoms.

In males, testosterone is the principal hormone responsible for maturation of the reproductive system as well as secondary sexual characteristics. Although found in males and females, males produce testosterone at a rate that is 20 times that found in females. Healthy levels of testosterone are commonly associated with increased libido, energy, immune functioning, and promotion of muscle mass and bone growth. There is some thought that deficiencies in testosterone may be associated with decreased libido, decreased energy, poor muscle tone, and lack of initiative. Excess levels have been associated in some studies with increased aggression, particularly sexual aggression (Popma et. al., 2007). However, it is unclear how low or high levels must be to bring about these problems.

Stress-Provoked Endocrine Pathology

In addition to endocrine disorders that occur as primary medical conditions, exposure to certain psychosocial stressors can induce a cascade of physiologic responses that result in disturbances in the endocrine system. Exposure to stress provokes excessive activation of glands, production of biologically inactive hormones, activation of endocrine receptors without the presence of the relevant hormone, and even some activation of the receptors by antibodies. Predisposition toward these disturbances is likely to be under genetic control and may be primed by previous exposures to life stressors (Kaufer, Friedman, Seidman, & Soreq, 1998; Zhang, Zhou, Li, Ursano, & Li, 2006).

Diagnosis of stress-related hormonal conditions is difficult because laboratory testing may not be sufficiently sensitive to accurately measure hormones and the presenting symptoms may be mild or even postponed, making the etiological link with exposure to the stressor difficult to identify. Therefore, diagnostic evaluation of stress-related medical conditions is an investigation by exclusion in which the possibility of the hormonal impact should be ruled out. Initially, stress-related dysfunction in the neuroendocrine system may present with symptoms of acute anxiety, a wide range of fears with distortions in sensory perception, disturbed social behavior, or distress. It has been hypothesized that these symptoms can be associated with a specific overstimulation of the amygdala and an increase in adrenaline release (Adolphs & Tranel, 2004; LeDoux, 1998; Scott et al., 1997).

Elevation of glucocorticoids, inhibition of brain-derived neurotrophic factor, changes in serotonergic function associated with the reduction of hippocampal volume (ranging from 8% to 26% in different studies), and reduction of white matter may provoke distortion of emotional control, significant memory impairment, and slowing of the processing time of the complex cognitive functions (Bremner et al., 1995; Gurvits et al., 1996). Changes in thalamus and hypothalamus, known as the *gates* for sensory information, are associated with increased sensitivity and distortion in perception. The range of symptoms might be extremely broad, ranging from increased uncontrolled irritability to dissociations, typical for acute posttraumatic conditions and untreated hormonal hyperactivity.

CONSIDERATIONS FOR DIAGNOSIS

As previously outlined, a number of symptoms associated with endocrine pathology are also characteristic of certain types of psychiatric disorders (Brambilla, 1992; Samson, Levin, & Richardson, 1998). For example, the symptoms of altered mood, oversensitivity to stimuli, clouding of consciousness, and psychotic episodes or delirium might be triggered by endocrine or psychopathological conditions or might reflect the presence of comorbid endocrine and psychopathological disorders.

In this section, we present issues associated with making the distinction between primary psychiatric conditions and psychiatric conditions that are secondary to the presence of a medical condition, specifically endocrine pathology. We emphasize that in studies that routinely screen for endocrine disorder in psychiatric populations, the prevalence of endocrine disorder is reported between 5% and 10% of the population. However, although these numbers are not large they must be considered, especially in the case of illnesses that appear resistant to standard treatments.

In addition to thinking about the specific signs and symptoms presented, it is important to consider the context in which they are observed. Age or developmental phase plays a significant role in the manifestation of both endocrine and psychological symptoms and must be taken into account when interpreting signs and symptoms. For instance, during the adolescent period in girls, mood disorders, anxiety, cognitive changes, and some behavioral changes are expected because of changes associated with psychosocial development, but they may also be associated with unstable physiological development of the endocrine system or induced conditions. Among induced conditions are the use of dietary supplements and weight control products, unregulated day and night cycles, sleep deprivation, use of street drugs and stimulants, or incorrect use of contraceptives.

Psychological symptoms triggered by endocrine dysfunction in teenage boys is sometimes underdiagnosed because of the leading behavioral and cognitive manifestation of symptoms, which can also be explained by psychosocial factors. Endocrine triggers of behavioral and cognitive dysfunction in teenage boys include abnormalities in physiological development of the endocrine system, use of steroids by some athletes or bodybuilders, uncontrolled use of stimulants to improve cognitive performance, use of street drugs and alcohol, unregulated day and night cycles, and sleep deprivation (Hartgens & Kuipers, 2004; Trenton & Currier, 2005).

Pre- and postmenopausal women and men with prostate dysfunction show age-related changes in hormone secretion and a restructuring of the endocrine system. The intensity of endocrine disturbance in this group usually correlates with the time of the first manifestation of symptoms associated with psychiatric pathology. In patients with a history of psychiatric problems there may be an increase in severity of symptoms with the emergence of endocrine dysfunction, but the experience of the symptoms and the presentation might not be the same. A patient with a chronic psychiatric condition usually can feel this difference. These "new" symptoms of mood and anxiety disappear when the hormonal dysfunction is treated (e.g., through hormone replacement therapy). In rare cases, mood disturbance, anxiety, and psychotic disorders might occur for the first time during the pre- or postmenopausal period. Psychiatric conditions provoked by endocrine conditions are generally characterized by a shorter duration, and they resolve with treatment of the endocrine pathology, sometimes even without any psychopharmacological impact.

Older patients with multiple medical conditions and a history of treatment with hormonal therapy present the most complicated diagnostic challenge. Because of the overlapping symptoms, lifelong history of stress impact, development of vascular pathology, decline in immune and metabolic systems, multiple causes of pain, and sleep disturbance and cognitive changes, it is almost impossible to identify the leading cause of nonspecific psychological and behavioral symptoms. For this type of client, educational therapy and medication and treatment management might be the most productive first step in diagnosis. The importance of hormonal screening is extreme in this group.

Psychological and behavioral dysfunction secondary to various acute medical conditions may be manifested by hallucinations (primarily visual or olfactory), dissociation, aggressive and antisocial behavior, disturbing suicidal thoughts, acute manifestation of depression, and anxiety with expressed fears. These conditions are rare and might occur in the acute stages of endocrine pathology or when a patient is experiencing both endocrine pathology and psychopathology.

Psychotic symptoms that occur as a manifestation of endocrine disorder are extremely difficult to diagnose. According to epidemiological reports, from 5% to 20% of patients may express psychotic features primarily in extremely advanced conditions (Ferrier, 1987).

Psychotic-like symptoms usually appear when the severity of endocrine dysfunction is not controlled by treatment. Therefore, the clinician should examine for the following possibilities:

- There is no endocrine condition. Primary manifestation of psychotic features is the reason for medical emergency.
- An endocrine condition is identified, but the patient shows poor compliance with the treatment (typical for the older population).
- There is an acute endocrine dysfunction that is secondary to another medical pathology that exists.
- There is an untoward reaction caused by the use of stimulating herbal remedies, uncontrolled use of opiate pain medications, use of dietary supplements, and so on.

Assessment Guidelines for Differential Diagnosis

With the growing possibilities of advanced multilevel diagnostics, the structural investigative interview remains the most important and most frequently used technique. As we already mentioned, behavioral and psychological symptoms in endocrine disorders are rare and if manifested, are likely to be under control if the patient is in treatment with an endocrinologist and has no problems with compliance. However, when the medical condition is not disclosed, the "simple" cluster of behavioral and psychological symptoms is in the mild or moderate stage, or when endocrine disorders are treated but resistance to this treatment is obvious, specific reevaluation is advised.

Thus, the following guidelines for differential diagnosis are provided to rule out endocrine pathology as a cause of any cluster of psychopathological symptoms. Each of the following should be covered in the process of diagnostic investigation.

1. Comparative review of medical history and laboratory findings, including imaging.

(a) Before asking questions about medical conditions, ask the patient about physiological cycles: regularity; intensity; limitations, if any; impact on mood; and impact on daily activities or general functioning.

(b) Ask about medical problems in the past. Pay attention to the symptoms presented. In many cases, your patient will tell you, "It was not serious enough, and I never told my doctor about it" when describing symptoms such as heavy sweating, mild heart palpitation, occasional tremors, and so on.

(c) Never hesitate to consult the treating practitioner about the current condition and the history. You might be surprised to learn that your knowledge of the patient's history is more detailed than that of the physician because of the significance of the symptoms that patients do not report.

(d) You will help tremendously by reporting medical and or physiological symptoms to a primary care physician or treating psychiatrist. On the basis of our experience in outpatient practice, patients discuss much more in therapy than in their doctor's office.

(e) Examine for the presence of any significant medical conditions.

(f) Ask for any laboratory or test results received for the past year.

(g) Carefully monitor all current medications and previous prescriptions and always ask about any supplements, vitamins, or minerals.

2. Genetic predisposition to endocrine pathology.

(a) Evaluate and investigate family history of endocrine and other medical pathologies. Ask specifically about the presence of disorders in each of the endocrine areas for first degree relatives and, if known, for the extended family.

3. Exposure to environmental pathogens.

(a) Ask about geographical family history and whether there are any particular medical illnesses associated with any of the environments they have been exposed to (including occupational environments). Check into the region (if you do not know much about it) for regional pathologies.

4. Specific reactions to significant lifetime stress.

(a) Review the history of the onset to determine whether there are precipitating stressors. Evaluate for an exposure to a toxic psychosocial environment, such as exposure to domestic violence, wars, discrimination, and so on; evaluate how presented stress changed the patient's behavior, how intense the negative experience was, at what age the stress occurred, and so on; evaluate the content of recurrent thoughts, look for themes of guilt or trauma at the time of evaluation.

(b) Create a stress map.

Questions to ask: Stress Impact Mapping Interview.

1. What was the most stressful event or situation in your life?
2. How old were you when it happened?
3. How intense was this experience for you on the scale from 0 = *no impact*, to 5 = *the extreme, most intense negative emotions?*
4. Did you get a professional help at that time?
5. Did this stress change your behavior? If *yes*, what types of behavioral changes occurred?
6. How long did it last?
7. Did you experience problems in functioning (e.g., concentration, memory, planning, making decisions)?
8. How long did it last? Did it improve with time or treatment?
9. Did you experience any physical (i.e., health) problems within 6 months after the event?
10. Did you get medical treatment for these problems?
11. How often do you think about this event or situation?
12. Do you have any dreams about it?

(c) Was there any other stress-related experience in your life? If *yes*, repeat Questions 2 through 8 and fill out the chart for comparative review.

(d) Finally, ask your patient how he or she is reacting to stress now; monitor current physiological condition and any outstanding behavioral presentations.

5. Gender-related developmental endocrine status.

(a) Gender and age are the most significant aspects in hormonal development. Before assessing any pathology, get as much information as you can on developmental physiology: Teenage girls are vulnerable for manifestation of endocrine shifts, and pre- and postmenopausal women develop endocrine imbalance if not treated or controlled by medical professionals (pay special attention to patients with a history of gynecological surgeries).

(b) Another age group to consider is the older population: Decreases in hormones in this age group might provoke behavioral manifestations.

(c) Evaluate developmental milestones to identify any significant delays or perturbations; look for any gradual decline in function and compare against normative data for the patient's age, gender, and ethnicity.

6. History of psychological symptoms.

This part of your investigational work should determine when psychological and behavioral symptoms manifested for the first time.

(a) Is there a history of psychiatric diagnosis and treatment? If *yes*, rule out treatment with antipsychotic or mood stabilizing medications. If these medications were used, ask for monitoring methods (i.e., bloodwork). Rule out any endocrine pathology developed as a result of long-term treatment with antipsychotics or mood stabilizers (typical side effects include thyroid dysfunction, metabolic problems, predisposition to develop early diabetes, obesity, and high blood pressure). Always review these cases with the treating physician. Is the present psychiatric presentation similar to or different from episodes in the past? What treatments worked before, and are these treatments working now? Evaluate the onset and intensity of the symptoms. If the symptoms are similar to the past, but the onset, intensity, or quality of the symptoms is different, suspect a possible endocrine component. Patients with an extensive psychiatric condition will often report new symptoms that feel "different" from the past; this may be a mood disturbance that doesn't make sense in the context of current life circumstances and feels foreign or comes and goes quickly with a sudden onset and rapid escalation. Look for symptoms that appear to be ego dystonic.

If there is no history of psychiatric diagnosis and treatment, manifestation of psychological and behavioral symptoms has not previously occurred, assess the age and gender component as well as the other items in this set of guidelines for evidence of endocrine problems.

7. History of shifts in circadian rhythms.
This is an important factor in a number of metabolic conditions that might be accompanied by behavioral and cognitive manifestations. Identify the time when the shifts first occurred. Include detailed questions about specific times for sleeping and awakening as well as work shifts. If the patient has gotten into the habit of sleeping all day and staying up at night, ask the patient to try to establish a more normal sleep–wake cycle to determine whether presenting psychological symptoms remit with normalization of circadian rhythms. Evaluate the impact of the daily schedule and activities and examine for changes in patterns of eating, socializing, and rest. If abnormalities are reported, ask about the use of herbal supplements, exogenous steroids, and dietary supplements that might be affecting cycles.

(a) Ask whether your patient used or is currently using melatonin or other supplements to stabilize daily activities. In endocrine pathology, a shift in circadian rhythm is just one symptom and is usually presented only in response to questioning. For endocrine patients, this shift is not as significant as in psychopathology, when normalizing the rhythm can ameliorate the symptoms.

CONCLUSION

We hope that the guidelines outlined in this chapter will assist your differential diagnosis and add to your clinical armamentarium for a complete and accurate case formulation. In any case, if there is any question of endo-crine pathology, consult with the primary care physician about a simple screen-ing to rule out medical pathology. This simple act may save weeks and months of work if undiagnosed endocrine conditions exist.

REFERENCES

Adolphs, R., & Tranel, D. (2004). Impaired judgment of sadness but not happiness following bilateral amygdala damage. *Journal of Cognitive Neuroscience, 16,* 453–462.

American Psychiatric Association. (1994). *Diagnostic and statistical manual of mental disorders* (4th ed.). Washington, DC: Author.

Brambilla, F. (1992). Psychopathological aspects of neuroendocrine diseases: Pos-sible parallels with the psychoendocrine aspects of normal aging. *Psychoneuro-endocrinology, 17,* 289–291.

Bremner, J. D., Randall, P., Scott, T. M., Bronen, R. A., Seibyl, J. P., Southwick, S. M., et al. (1995). MRI-based measurement of hippocampal volume in pa-tients with combat-related posttraumatic stress disorder. *American Journal of Psychiatry, 152,* 973–981.

Cappola, A. R., Fried, L. P., Amold, A. M., Danese, M. D., Kuller, L. H., Burke, G. L., et al. (2006). Thyroid status, cardiovascular risk, and mortality in older adults: The cardiovascular health study. *The Journal of the American Medical Association, 295,* 1033–1041.

Ferrier, I. N. (1987). Endocrinology and psychosis. *British Medical Bulletin, 43,* 672–678.

Gurvits, T. V., Shenton, M. E., Hokama, H., Ohta, H., Lasko, N. B., Gilbertson, M. W., et al. (1996). Magnetic resonance imaging study of hippocampal volume in chronic, combat-related posttraumatic stress disorders. *Biological Psychiatry, 40,* 1091–1099.

Hartgens, F., & Kuipers, H. (2004). Effects of androgenic–anabolic steroids in ath-letes. *Sports Medicine, 34,* 513–554.

Kaufer, D., Friedman, A., Seidman, S., & Soreq, H. (1998). Acute stress facilitates long-lasting changes in cholonergic gene expression. *Nature, 393,* 373–377.

Kinmonth, A., Woodcock, A., Griffin, S., Spiegal, N., & Campbell, M. (1998, Oc-tober 31). Randomised controlled trial of patient-centered care of diabetes in general practice: Impact on current well-being and future disease risk. *BMJ, 317,* 1202–1208.

LeDoux, J. (1998). *The emotional brain.* New York: Touchstone.

National Institutes of Health. (2002). *Cushing's syndrome* (NIH Publication No. 02-3007). Retrieved March 18, 2007, from http://www.endocrine.niddk.nih.gov/pubs/cushings/cushings.htm

National Institutes of Health. (2004). *Addison's disease* (NIH Publication No. 04-3054). Retrieved March 18, 2007, from http://www.endocrine.niddk.nih.gov/pubs/addison/addison.htm

National Institutes of Health. (2006a). *Hyperparathyroidism* (NIH Publication No. 06-3425). Retrieved March 18, 2007, from http://www.endocrine.niddk.nih.gov/pubs/hyper/hyper.htm

National Institutes of Health. (2006b). *Your guide to diabetes type 1 and type 2.* Retrieved March 18, 2007, from http://diabetes.niddk.nih.gov/dm/pubs/type1and2

National Institutes of Health. (2008). *Hyperthyroidism* (NIH Publication No. 08-5415). Retrieved August 18, 2008, from http://www.endocrine.niddk.nih.gov/pubs/Hyperthyroidism/index.htm

Nussey, S. S., & Whitehead, S. A. (2001). *Endocrinology: An integrated approach.* London: Taylor & Francis.

Petrak, F., Hardt, J., Wittchen, H. U., Kulzer, B., Hirsch, A., Hentzelt, F., et al. (2003). Prevalence of psychiatric disorders in an onset cohort of adults with type I diabetes. *Diabetes Metabolism Research and Review, 19,* 216–222.

Popma, A., Vermeiren, R., Geluk, C. A., Rinne, T., van den Brink, W., Knol, D. L., et al. (2007). Cortisol moderates the relationship between testosterone and aggression in delinquent male adolescents [Abstract]. *Biological Psychiatry, 61,* 405–411.

Putman, P., Van Honk, J., Kessels, R. P., Mulder, M., & Koppeschaar, H. P. (2004). Salivary cortisol and short- and long-term memory for emotional faces in healthy young women. *Psychoneuroendocrinology, 29,* 953–960.

Rasgon, N., Hendrick, V., & Garrick, T. (2004). Endocrine and metabolic eisorders. In B. J. Sadock & V. A. Sadock (Eds.), *Kaplan and Sadock's comprehensive textbook of psychiatry* (8th ed., pp. 1806–1818). Philadelphia: Lippincott Williams & Wilkins.

Samson, J. A., Levin, R. M., & Richardson, G. S. (1998). Psychological symptoms in endocrine disorders. In P. M. Kleespies (Ed.), *Emergencies in mental health practice* (pp. 332–354). New York: Guilford Press.

Scott, S. K., Young, A. W., Calder, A. J., Hellawell, D. J., Aggleton, J. P., & Johnson, M. (1997). Impaired auditory recognition of fear and anger following bilateral amygdale lesions. *Nature, 385,* 254–257.

Sonino, N., Bonnini, S., Fallo, F., Boscaro, M., & Fava, G. A. (2006). Personality characteristics and quality of life in patients treated for Cushing's syndrome. *Clinical Endocrinology 64,* 314–318.

Taylor, V., & MacQueen, G. (2006). Associations between bipolar disorders and metabolic syndrome: A review. *Journal of Clinical Psychiatry, 67,* 1034–1041.

Terrien, F., Drapeau, V., Lupien, S. J., Beaulieu, S., Tremblay, A., & Richard, D. (2007). Awakening cortisol response in lean, obese, and reduced obese individuals: Effect of gender and fat distribution. *Obesity, 15,* 377–385.

Trenton, A. J., & Currier, G. W. (2005). Behavioral manifestations of anabolic steroid use. *CNS Drugs, 19,* 571–595.

Vileikyte, L., Leventhal, H., Gonzalez, J. S., Peyrot, M., Rubin, R. R., & Ulbrecht, J. S. (2005). Diabetic peripheral neuropathy and depressive symptoms: The association revisited. *Diabetes Care, 28*, 2378–2383.

Yehuda, R. (2004). Risk and resilience in posttraumatic stress disorder. *Journal of Clinical Psychiatry, 65*, 29–36.

Yehuda, R., Kahana, B., Binderbrynes, K., Southwick, S. M., Mason, J. W., & Giller, E. L. (1995). Low urinary cortisol excretion in holocaust survivors with posttraumatic stress disorder. *American Journal of Psychiatry, 152*, 982–986.

Zhang, L., Zhou, R., Li, X., Ursano, R. J., & Li, H. (2006). Stress-induced change of mitochondria membrane potential regulated by genomic and non-genomic GR signaling: A possible mechanism for hippocampus atrophy in PTSD. *Medical Hypotheses, 66*, 1205–1208.

VII

FOLLOW-UP TREATMENT OF PATIENTS AT RISK OF RECURRENT EMERGENCIES

15

THE PSYCHOSOCIAL TREATMENT OF SUICIDAL BEHAVIOR: A CRITIQUE OF WHAT WE KNOW (AND DON'T KNOW)

M. DAVID RUDD, THOMAS E. JOINER JR., DAVID TROTTER,
BEN WILLIAMS, AND LILIANA CORDERO

Suicide is consistently among the leading causes of death internationally, with almost 1 million lives lost each year (DeLao, Bertolote, & Lester, 2002). Over 30,000 lives are lost to suicide annually in the United States, and according to the Institute of Medicine (2002), suicides surpassed homicides by a rate of approximately 3:2 over the past 100 years. For a number of reasons, it is much more difficult to gather accurate data on suicide attempt rates. Conservative estimates, however, suggest that up to 5% of the U.S. population have made a suicide attempt (Kessler, Borges, & Walters, 1999). Rates of self-inflicted injuries have been estimated to be as high as 300 per 100,000 in the general population (Favazza, 1987; Walsh & Rosen, 1988). Rates of suicidal ideation vary greatly in the literature depending on the specific population being studied, but Linehan (1982) estimated that 31% of the clinical population and 24% of the general population have considered suicide at some point in their lives. It is clear that suicidality (i.e., death, attempts, and ideation) is a serious and persistent public health problem. Despite enduring high rates of suicide and open acknowledgment of the problem by those in the field and government alike, federal funding continues to be marginal at best, particularly when compared with funding for other major public health concerns (U.S. Department of Health and Human Services, 2001).

In this chapter we provide a critical review of the literature on the treatment of suicidality. We start by addressing some important conceptual and methodological issues, followed by a critical review and summary of available clinical trials. Finally, we provide a discussion of meaningful implications for day-to-day clinical practice.

QUESTIONS ABOUT TREATMENT IMPACT

What do we know about psychological and behavioral treatments of suicidal behavior? It is certainly a complicated question, and the available literature highlights this. As a reminder, we are not talking about efficacy studies targeting medications or broad-based (school or general population) prevention efforts. The focus here is simply psychotherapeutic interventions for suicidal behavior. The literature is replete with case examples and uncontrolled studies, all with considerable theoretical and methodological limitations. Accordingly, the ability to draw meaningful conclusions about clinical care is greatly hampered, if not impossible. There are far fewer randomized and controlled clinical trials, which are the focus of this brief chapter.

The central question to consider in examining the literature is, What treatments have been demonstrated to be effective specifically for suicidality? That is, which treatments have targeted suicidal behavior and associated symptoms, making use of appropriate inclusion and exclusion criteria? A persistent problem across studies is the exclusion of high-risk cases, that is, those making suicide attempts and multiple attempts. The studies we discuss in the following paragraphs have included the highest-risk patients, meaning those making suicide attempts and requiring immediate psychiatric care. This is a critical point: The focus is on treatments targeting those already manifesting suicidality, not those with symptoms commonly associated with suicidality (e.g., depression, hopelessness, anxiety, substance abuse). The intent is to be precise and specific about the high-risk nature of the sample and the intent of the treatment itself. Linehan (1997) previously estimated that 45% of treatment efficacy trials excluded high-risk patients. This is a simple but important point to consider when reviewing and evaluating the treatment outcome literature in suicidality.

With suicide and suicidal behavior as essential outcome markers, the treatment effect must endure for many years beyond treatment completion. Without longitudinal tracking after treatment, it will never be known whether effective treatments reduce suicide and attempt rates or just delay them for brief periods of time (e.g., 12–18 months). Certainly, none of the studies we review provide data with ideal long-term follow-up, but they have laid a solid foundation for ongoing tracking. Follow-up of 12 to 18 months is not convincing in this respect but is a step in the right direction. It is also important to mention that relatively brief follow-up periods are compounded by high attrition rates. Despite efforts to track patients for longer periods of time after treatment, high attrition rates create problems with statistical power and limit the ability to make meaningful inferences. It will simply take years, if not decades, to accumulate the data and numbers necessary to gain evidence about effective treatments.

Another important question in exploring the literature is, Are there emerging and identifiable core interventions or treatment techniques across treatment trials that are associated with positive outcomes? Are there similarities across treatments that have proven to be efficacious? Given the limited number of available clinical trials, it is important to look for similarities across trials. As illustrated in the following sections, there indeed appear to be identifiable common elements. The current literature provides limited data to address these two central questions (and hence are the focus of this chapter).

There are, of course, more detailed questions that must be asked. These include the following:

1. Does treatment setting (e.g., inpatient, outpatient, residential, day treatment) influence outcome? At present, there are no compelling data to support inpatient treatment as effective for suicidality (cf. Rudd, Joiner, & Rajab, 2004). Nonetheless, it continues to be readily accepted as the standard of care in high-risk cases. Hospitalization clearly plays an important role in treatment, and we would never seek to diminish its role, but there is no compelling evidence that it actually works (i.e., lowers the rates of subsequent suicides or suicide attempts) over the short or long term. Relatively few suicides occur in inpatient settings, but they do occur. Undeniably, the inpatient setting is safe. The question that has been left unanswered is, Does it reduce subsequent risk of a suicide attempt or death?

2. Are certain diagnostic entities (e.g., Axis I, Axis II, diagnostic comorbidity) more amenable and responsive to particular treatment interventions? The question of treatment matching is well beyond the scope of the extant literature.

3. Is there a minimum treatment duration for successful outcome? This question really gets to the issue of guidelines for psychotherapeutic care. That is, how long and how intense (e.g., How many times weekly or monthly?) should psychotherapy be for suicidal patients? As with other areas, there is simply inadequate data to address this question.

4. Are periodic booster sessions needed to maintain the treatment effect? Given the brief duration of follow-up (i.e., up to 18 months), there is also insufficient data to address this question.
5. Are retention rates and compliance better in some treatment approaches relative to others? Again, this question addresses issues of treatment matching.
6. Are some elements of treatment more effective than others? As you might imagine, the limited number of studies available has not allowed for treatment dismantling to explore active components of various treatments.

There certainly are many more questions relevant to treatment outcome for suicidality, but the literature is simply not expansive enough to address them at this point. The studies that are available provide limited (but important) insight into which treatments work for suicidal patients. In short, more controlled studies are needed, treating a greater number of patients across more diagnostic groupings (and comorbidity) with dramatically longer follow-up periods.

Despite a recent meta-analysis that concluded psychosocial interventions have essentially proven ineffective at reducing suicide rates (Crawford, Thomas, Khan, & Kulinskaya, 2007), there are hopeful signs in the literature over the past 2 decades. Frankly, we disagree with the conclusions offered by Crawford et al. (2007). They concluded, "results do not provide evidence that additional psychosocial interventions following self-harm have a marked effect on the likelihood of subsequent suicide" (p. 17). As has been mentioned elsewhere (Rudd, 2007), the conclusions are far too sweeping and definitive in light of considerable conceptual and methodological problems with their meta-analysis. Although they acknowledged a lack of statistical power (primarily because of brief follow-up periods and small sample sizes), the interventions included in the meta-analysis were neither developed nor intended to reduce suicide rates; rather, they targeted suicide attempts and associated symptoms such as suicidal ideation, hopelessness, and depression. It is also arguable that the studies included are not actually amenable to meta-analytic approaches given variable inclusion/exclusion criteria and outcome targets. The conclusions offered by Crawford et al. (2007) are simply inaccurate and not indicative of gains made over the past 2 decades, during which noticeable scientific progress has been made and cognitive–behavioral therapy (CBT) approaches offering the greatest promise in the treatment of suicidality have emerged.

A number of reviews are available in the literature, including Gunnell and Frankel (1994), Hepp, Wittmann, Schnyder, and Michel (2004), Linehan (1997), Rudd (2005), and several meta-analyses (Hawton, Arensman, et al., 1998; Hawton, Townsend, et al., 2005; van der Sande et al., 1997). These reviews are all extensive and detailed, particularly in pointing out considerable methodological limitations of available studies. Rather than repeat what is available elsewhere, this review critiques the extant literature and focuses on two essential elements of the suicidality treatment outcome literature: (a) evidence on what works and is suitable for clinical practice, and (b) which core interventions or identifiable similarities across treatments hold the most promise for future study and clinical application. The focus here is on randomized and controlled clinical trials targeting suicidal behaviors (i.e., attempts) and associated critical symptoms, such as hopelessness. Rather than address negative outcomes, the emphasis of this review is on promising approaches, hence the focus on CBT-based approaches. Our hope is that the reader will develop an appreciation for the difficulty of conducting clinical trials in this area, an emerging consensus on the efficacy of CBT-based approaches, identifiable similarities across different treatments, and the need for larger trials with dramatically longer follow-up periods.

Which Treatments Are Effective at Reducing Subsequent Suicide Attempts?

Although 13 randomized CBT trials have been conducted, only 4 (31%) have proven effective at reducing posttreatment suicide attempt rates (Brown et al., 2005; Linehan, Armstrong, Suarez, Allmon, & Heard, 1991; Linehan, Comotois, & Korslund, 2004; Salkovkis, Atha, & Storer, 1990). It appears that CBT approaches are emerging as a front-runner when it comes to effective treatments for suicidality. It is instructive to consider the success rates of various approaches. More specifically, across the major orientations (e.g., CBT, psychodynamic, interpersonal), what percentage of randomized–controlled treatment trials have demonstrated success in reducing subsequent attempt rates? Although a 31% success rate (i.e., 4 out of 13 studies) may seem low, only 2 other treatments (Guthrie et al., 2001; Wood, Trainor, Rothwell, Moore, & Harrington, 2001) have proven effective at lowering subsequent suicide attempt rates. Remember that quite a few treatments have been demonstrated to reduce associated symptoms such as depression, anxiety, hopelessness, and features of suicidal thinking (e.g., specificity, intensity). When talking about efficacy in treatment for suicidality, it is essential to focus on the two primary measures of treatment outcome: suicide attempts and deaths by suicide. By comparison, the success rate of non-CBT approaches is approximately 12% (i.e., 2 out of 16 clinical trials). Clearly, at this point in the treatment outcome literature, CBT approaches have the edge.

Salkovkis et al. (1990) examined the effectiveness of a brief CBT problem-solving intervention (5 sessions); Linehan, Armstrong, et al. (1991) and Linehan, Comotois, et al. (2004) compared dialectical behavior therapy (DBT) with treatment as usual; and Brown et al. (2005) compared brief cognitive therapy with enhanced treatment as usual. In all four studies reattempt rates were significantly lower, as were associated symptoms such as depression and hopelessness. Frequency of reported suicidal ideation was not lower in all trials, but this is not a surprising finding considering the issue of chronic suicidality (cf. Rudd et al., 2004) and the likelihood of enduring suicidal thoughts even with effective treatment. What is important is that the suicidal thinking is less severe or intense, with an associated drop in intent, something that becomes clear when there are significantly lower attempt rates. In Linehan, Armstrong, et al. (1991) and Linehan, Comotois, et al. (2004), reattempt rates were reduced by half, as were reattempt rates in the study by Brown et al. (2005). To date, DBT is the only effective treatment that has been replicated (Linehan, Comotois, et al., 2004; Turner, 2000; van den Bosch, Koeter, Stijnen, Verheul, & van den Brink, 2005). Follow-up in these studies ranged from 12 to 18 months. As mentioned earlier, longer follow-up periods are needed to resolve questions about simply delaying, rather than reducing, suicidal behaviors. Although previous CBT meta-analyses have had conflicting results (Hawton, Arensman, et al., 1998; van der Sande et al., 1997), the treatments in these four studies clearly worked.

Are There Identifiable Core Interventions or Treatment Techniques?

Although it is important that these four studies evidenced significant and enduring drops in suicide attempt rates following treatment, it is more meaningful for clinical practice to ask, what the treatments have in common. Are there identifiable elements that can be translated into any clinical practice? In other words, what can we carry away from the studies and apply in day-to-day clinical practice?

All four treatments have been identified by the authors as having cognitive–behavioral roots. What exactly does that mean? A review of these studies supports several conclusions about common elements, techniques, and interventions:

1. All four treatments are theoretically driven, targeting empirically supported risk factors, with proven associations with suicidality. The theoretical models identify cognitions, emotional processing, and associated behavioral responses as critical to understanding intent to die and altering the suicidal process. The models can be translated for patients in easy to understand language, with clear connections between thoughts, feelings, and behaviors. In other words, it is easy to explain to patients why they are thinking about or trying to kill themselves and what needs to be targeted in treatment to change those thoughts or behaviors. With the paucity of clinical trials in this area, whether or not the clarity of the model and ease of understanding for patients is critical to outcome is yet to be studied. It is clearly an important issue, however.

A number of other issues along these lines need to be considered. Does the clarity and ease of understanding of the theoretical model facilitate improved motivation for treatment? Does it enhance compliance? Does it facilitate skill development, acquisition, generalization, and retention? What about treatment fidelity among providers? Does the clarity of the treatment model provide for easier dissemination of effective treatments? At this point, there are simply inadequate data to answer these questions. As this list indicates, we know little about what works with suicidal patients or why it works.

2. All four studies included high-risk patients. They sought those at highest risk, including single and multiple suicide attempters in need of immediate treatment. As noted by others (cf. Linehan, 1997), issues regarding statistical power in clinical trials are of paramount importance. Accordingly, inclusion criteria need to be broad and inclusive, targeting those at highest risk. Undoubtedly, there will be times when hospitalization is essential (e.g., in cases of psychosis or intoxication or when there are medical complications secondary to an attempt), but the large majority of patients can be randomly assigned to treatment conditions. As these four studies indicate, even high-risk multiple attempters can be effectively and safely treated in outpatient settings if there is ready access to hospital and emergency care when indicated and needed. It is important for practicing clinicians to understand this fact. It is also important for this to be reflected in the standard of care, particularly because there are no available data indicating the hospital as efficacious in the treatment of suicidality.

3. In all treatments, clinicians were trained to a target standard of competence and supervised throughout (with variable formats), with treatment fidelity and adherence to the identified model a central concern. In short, the treatments were manual-driven, with appropriate supervision provided. The treatment approach could be articulated in a manual, with clear targets, specific interventions for each, and demonstrated clinical techniques. Clearly, the most complex treatment is DBT, with substantial training and supervision essential.

What is common across all four treatments is that suicidality is the central focus of treatment, not targeted disorders such as major depression, posttraumatic stress, or the like. Clinicians are trained and supervised to ensure the focus on suicidality as the specific target and outcome of treatment. The four studies conceptualized the treatment of suicidality as requiring unique competencies, consistent with the recent movement to identifiable core competencies in the assessment, management, and treatment of suicidality (Suicide Prevention Resource Center, 2006). Clearly, this is an important point for practicing clinicians. Assessing and treating suicidal behavior requires a unique clinical skill set that may well necessitate additional training and supervision.

4. The four treatments attended closely to issues of treatment compliance. All had specific interventions and techniques that targeted poor compliance and motivation for treatment. All recognized and emphasized the need for adequate treatment intensity and duration. Although no data are available to address the minimum duration or intensity required to ensure effective treatment, it is clear that continuity and consistency in treatment are essential for positive outcomes. In short, one of the treatment targets for suicidal patients is simply keeping them in treatment, something that practicing clinicians need to attend to with care. As has been demonstrated elsewhere, a considerable number of suicidal patients will withdraw prematurely from treatment despite continued distress and heightened risk (Rudd, Joiner, & Rajab, 1995). A strong therapeutic alliance is a common characteristic of good care, better treatment compliance, and positive outcomes.

5. The treatment interventions targeted clearly identifiable skill sets. Again, this is consistent with the clear theoretical models used. Patients were offered models for identifying and understanding skill deficits and how they would be targeted and modified. Interventions included emotion regulation skills training, problem solving, identifying and correcting cognitive distortions and related errors, interpersonal relationship skills (e.g., interpersonal assertiveness), and crisis management or response skills among others. In short, patients understood not only specific steps to take but also demonstrated competence in implementing the plans.

6. All treatments emphasized self-reliance, self-awareness, self-control, and issues of personal responsibility. As evident from the preceding points, self-reliance, awareness, and control were implicit and explicit in the treatment paradigms. Given the high rates of abuse and developmental trauma in suicidal populations (cf. Rudd et al., 2004), hopelessness often emerges secondary to chronically feeling incapable of resolving persistent dysphoria (including guilt and shame). In each treatment it was clear that if patients developed appropriate skills, the distress and upset tied to early events would diminish and associated suicidal urges would as well. It was also evident that

patients assumed a considerable degree of personal responsibility for their care. They recognized that the probability of treatment success was tied to their compliance and investment in care, including self-management of crisis and emergency situations. It is important for practicing clinicians to address these issues up front with suicidal patients as a part of the informed consent process. There are a range of models available for facilitating compliance and crisis management, but we encourage clinicians to consider use of the *commitment to treatment statement* (cf. Rudd, Mandrusiak, & Joiner, 2006). This approach is discussed in more detail later.

7. All treatments recognized the importance of crisis management and access to available emergency services during and after treatment. Each had clearly identified and practiced strategies for accessing crisis and emergency services when needed. Of particular importance, patients learned to clearly identify what characterizes a crisis or emergency and to use these services in judicious and appropriate fashion. For practicing clinicians, the importance of a clearly articulated crisis response plan cannot be overemphasized. It is also important to emphasize that the plan must be reviewed, practiced, and updated on a regular and predictable basis.

Considering what works in the treatment of suicidality can help alter the day-to-day nature of clinical practice. Each point summarized in this list can be integrated into practice regardless of one's theoretical approach and can be done in relatively seamless fashion. As the science of clinical suicidology moves forward, there are clearly intersections like this in which science can directly inform practice.

In addition to the CBT-oriented trials, two other studies have evidenced success at reducing suicidal behavior. Guthrie et al. (2001) demonstrated that brief in-home interpersonal psychotherapy was more effective than treatment as usual at reducing subsequent suicide attempts. The follow-up period for this study was only 6 months. Similarly, Wood et al. (2001) found that developmental group therapy was more effective at reducing suicide attempts in comparison to treatment as usual for adolescents. A review of both studies revealed elements very similar to those summarized in this list, despite that the studies were not described by the authors as CBT-oriented.

Informed Consent, Treatment Compliance, and Commitment to Treatment

As mentioned previously, a core intervention identified in the four CBT trials was facilitating compliance and general investment in care. An emerging area of interest in the treatment outcome literature for suicidality is the potential link between treatment compliance, investment in care, and eventual outcomes. It makes sense that improved compliance would facilitate a better outcome. One approach recommended by Rudd et al. (2004) is the commitment to treatment statement (CTS), integrated into the informed consent process. The CTS is a written agreement between the patient and clinician that articulates what it means to be committed or invested in treatment. It includes information such as the frequency of sessions, level of involvement, agreement to complete homework, experiment with new behaviors, and a crisis response plan (i.e., instructions about what to do in a suicidal crisis, including emergency calls or going to the emergency department). The CTS does not ask a patient to make an agreement not to kill him- or herself; rather, it asks the patient to make a commitment to living by being actively involved in all aspects of treatment and using a crisis response plan when necessary.

The critical difference between the CTS and the traditional no-suicide contract is that it minimizes potential adversarial tensions in the therapeutic relationship. It does not put the clinician in the potentially awkward and counterproductive position of having to restrict a patient's rights. It simply asks a patient to commit to the treatment process and then defines that process, including the use of a crisis response plan should a suicidal crisis emerge.

CONCLUSION

As evident in other extensive reviews available in the literature (cf. Gunnell & Frankel, 1994; Hepp, Wittmann, Schnyder, & Michel, 2004; Linehan, 1997; Rudd, 2005), we have a good understanding of what does not work in the treatment of suicidality. Among the most common criticisms of the clinical trials that have proven ineffective are poorly or vaguely defined treatment models; the lack of manuals to guide care; and limited supervision, oversight, and fidelity measures. Clinical practice needs a clearly articulated model of suicidality, one that the patient can understand and actively engage in. More important, though, there is a constellation of studies that suggest common elements or features of treatment that are effective at reducing suicidal behavior. Despite their CBT roots, these elements are flexible and amenable to integration across theoretical orientations.

Although only a limited number of treatments have proven efficacy to reduce suicidal behaviors, there are marked similarities among them that hold considerable promise for future work. It appears that there is indeed an emerging consensus about the efficacy of CBT-based approaches with suicidal patients.

REFERENCES

Brown, G. K., Have, T. T., Henriques, G. R., Xie, S. X., Hollander, J., & Beck, A. T. (2005). Cognitive therapy for the prevention of suicide attempts: A randomized controlled trial. *The Journal of the American Medical Association, 294,* 563–570.

Crawford, M. J., Thomas, O., Khan, N., & Kulinskaya, E. (2007). Psychosocial interventions following self-harm: A systematic review of their efficacy in preventing suicide. *The British Journal of Psychiatry, 190,* 11–17.

DeLao, D., Bertolote, J., & Lester, D. (2002). Self-directed violence. In E. G. Krugg, L. L. Dahlberg, J. A. Mercy, A. B. Zwi, & R. Lozano (Eds.), *World report on violence and health* (pp. 183–240). Geneva, Switzerland: World Health Organization.

Favazza, A. R. (1987). *Bodies under siege: Self-mutilation in culture and psychiatry.* Baltimore: Johns Hopkins University Press.

Gunnell, D., & Frankel, S. (1994, May 7). Prevention of suicide: Aspirations and evidence. *BMJ, 308,* 1227–1233.

Guthrie, E., Navneet, K., Mackway-Jones, K., Chew-Graham, C., Moorey, J., Mendel, E., et al. (2001, July 21). Randomised controlled trial of brief psychological intervention after deliberate self poisoning. *BMJ, 323,* 135–138.

Hawton, K., Arensman, E., Townsend, E., Bremner, S., Feldman, E., Goldney, R., et al. (1998, August 15). Deliberate self harm: Systematic review of efficacy of psychosocial and pharmacological treatment in preventing repetition. *BMJ, 317,* 441–447.

Hawton, K., Townsend, E., Arensman, E., Gunnell, D., Hazell, P., & Housed, A. (2005). Psychosocial and pharmacological treatments for deliberate self-harm. *Cochrane Database of Systematic Reviews, 3.* Available from http://www.cochrane.org

Hepp, U., Wittmann, L., Schnyder, U., & Michel, K. (2004). Psychological and psychosocial interventions after attempted suicide. *Crisis, 25,* 108–117.

Institute of Medicine. (2002). *Reducing suicide: A national imperative.* Washington, DC: National Academies Press.

Kessler, R. C., Borges, G., & Walters, E. E. (1999). Prevalence and risk factors for lifetime suicide attempts in the National Comorbidity Study. *Archives of General Psychiatry, 56,* 617–626.

Linehan, M. M. (1982). Suicidal behaviors among clients in an outpatient clinic versus the general population. *Suicide and Life-Threatening Behavior, 12,* 234–239.

Linehan, M. M. (1997). Behavioral treatments of suicidal behaviors: Definitional obfuscation and treatment outcomes. *Annals of the New York Academy of Sciences, 836,* 302–328.

Linehan, M. M., Armstrong, H. E., Suarez, A., Allmon, D., & Heard, H. L. (1991). Cognitive–behavioral treatment of chronically parasuicidal borderline patients. *Archives of General Psychiatry, 48,* 1060–1064.

Linehan, M. M., Comotois, K. A., & Korslund, K. E. (2004, August). Dialectical behavior therapy versus nonbehavioral treatment by experts in the community: Clinical outcomes. In J. R. Koum & N. Lindenboim (Chairs), *Advances in the treatment of suicidal behavior*. Symposium conducted at the 112th Convention of the American Psychological Association, Honolulu, HI.

Rudd, M. D. (2005). An update on the psychotherapeutic treatment of suicidal behavior. In J. Trafton & W. Gordon (Eds.), *Best practices in the behavioral management of chronic disease* (pp. 171–190). Palo Alto, CA: Institute for Brain Potential.

Rudd, M. D. (2007). Inaccurate conclusions based on limited data [Letter to the editor]. *The British Journal of Psychiatry, 190*. Available from http://bjp.rcpsych.org/cgi/eletters?lookup=by_date&days=30

Rudd, M. D., Joiner, T. E., Jr., Rajab, M. H. (1995). Help negation after acute suicidal crisis. *Journal of Consulting and Clinical Psychology, 63*, 499–503.

Rudd, M. D., Joiner, T. E., Jr., & Rajab, M. H. (2004). *Treating suicidal behavior* (2nd ed.). New York: Guilford Press.

Rudd, M. D., Mandrusiak, M., & Joiner, T. E., Jr. (2006). The case against no-suicide contracts: The Commitment to Treatment Statement as an alternative for clinical practice. *Journal of Clinical Psychology: In Session, 62*, 243–251.

Salkovkis, P. M., Atha, C., & Storer, D. (1990). Cognitive–behavioral problem solving in the treatment of patients who repeatedly attempt suicide: A controlled trial. *The British Journal of Psychiatry, 157*, 871–876.

Suicide Prevention Resource Center. (2006). *Assessing and managing suicide risk: Core competencies for mental health professionals*. Newton, MA: Author.

Turner, R. M. (2000). Naturalistic evaluation of dialectical behavior therapy–oriented treatment for borderline personality disorder. *Cognitive and Behavioral Practice, 7*, 413–419.

U.S. Department of Health and Human Services. (2001). *National strategy for suicide prevention: Goals and objectives for action* (Publication No. SMA01-3517). Washington, DC: Author.

van den Bosch, L. M., Koeter, M. W., Stijnen, T., Verheul, R., & van den Brink, W. (2005). Sustained efficacy of dialectical behavior therapy for borderline personality disorder. *Behaviour Research and Therapy, 43*, 1231–1241.

van der Sande, R., van Rooijen, L., Buskens, E., Allart, E., Hawton, K., & van der Graaf, Y. (1997). Intensive inpatient and community intervention versus routine care after attempted suicide: A randomised controlled intervention study. *The British Journal of Psychiatry, 171*, 35–41.

Walsh, B. W., & Rosen, P. M. (1988). *Self-mutilation: Theory, research and treatment*. New York: Guilford Press.

Wood, A., Trainor, G., Rothwell, J., Moore, J., & Harrington, R. (2001). Randomized trial of group therapy for repeated deliberate self-harm in adolescents. *Journal of the American Academy of Child & Adolescent Psychiatry, 40*, 1246–1253.

16

REDUCING THE RISK OF VIOLENCE AMONG PEOPLE WITH SERIOUS MENTAL ILLNESS: A CRITICAL ANALYSIS OF TREATMENT APPROACHES

KEVIN S. DOUGLAS, TONIA L. NICHOLLS, AND JOHANN BRINK

The relationship between serious mental illness (SMI) and violence to others has a long-standing and controversial history dating back millennia (Monahan, 1992). Current scientific opinion is divided on the point: Some scholars assert that a meaningful relationship does not exist (Bonta, Law, & Hanson, 1998; Quinsey, Harris, Rice, & Cormier, 2006), whereas others claim that it does (Silver, 2006). This divide is understandable because there is good quality research that has failed to find a robust association (Monahan et al., 2001) and there is other research that has found a relationship (Brennan, Mednick, & Hodgins, 2000). As Appelbaum (2006) recently reminded us, "violence and mental disorders—rightly or wrongly—appear to be irreversibly linked in the popular mind" (p. 1319).

Whether there is a systematic and independent association between SMI and violence is somewhat peripheral to the task of reducing risk of violence when it does exist. That is, some persons with mental illness act

351

violently, and mental health professionals are charged with managing this risk when confronted with it. This typically occurs in psychiatric and forensic settings, because one reason people end up in such settings is that they have acted violently. When studied at a nomothetic level, even if people with SMI pose no greater risk than others, society generally—and mental health professionals specifically—has a duty to reduce this risk when it occurs.

Clearly, a need exists for guidelines on evaluating and managing violence—or the threat of violence—among people with SMI. As we note, the empirical literature on violence reduction among people with SMI is underdeveloped. Therefore, in this chapter we focus on reviewing the research on general offending by discussing available studies that have used violence as an outcome. We analyze the problems resulting from generalizing many findings to violence and SMI and weigh which findings seem most likely to be generalizable. We conclude by identifying both a list of approaches that seem to have the greatest likelihood of success on the basis of the limited research available and a list of research needs that can provide an empirical basis for future guidelines.

SCOPE OF LITERATURE REVIEW: RISK FACTORS, VIOLENT BEHAVIOR, AND SERIOUS MENTAL ILLNESS

In this chapter our goal is to provide readers with a summary of empirical evidence for and against treatment procedures that have been applied to the reduction of violent behavior among persons with SMI. One broad approach to achieving this goal is to consider studies that have also targeted constructs that act as violence risk factors, such as psychotic symptomatology or substance use. Such an approach has an intuitive appeal in that reducing such factors should logically lead to a reduction of risk and hence violence. It is important to note that many of the same factors that elevate the risk of violence in nonill persons (i.e., substance use problems, antisocial peers, employment problems, antisocial or psychopathic personality traits) also elevate the risk of violence in people with SMI (Bonta et al., 1998; Feder, 1991). In addition, considerable evidence suggests that if there is an association between violence and factors unique to SMI, it is the acute positive symptoms that account for this risk (Swanson et al., 2006). Moreover, there are some associated features of SMI that elevate the risk of violence, including medication noncompliance (Swartz et al., 1998). This knowledge— that violence among persons with SMI may be due to general, associated, and SMI-specific violence risk factors—suggests that attempts to reduce violence risk must address all such domains of risk factors. Studies that have failed to do this have been relatively unsuccessful in reducing violence among persons with SMI.

Focusing on treatment studies that have targeted risk factors for violence, as opposed to targeting violence directly as the outcome variable, however, is too far removed from actual violence reduction to offer solid, empirically based evidence for treatment approaches that are likely to reduce violent behavior. One reason for this is that even if certain risk factors (e.g., substance use) are reduced, this does not guarantee that others (e.g., anger) will not remain active. There are many pathways to violence, and the only way to have confidence in the violence-reducing potential of an intervention is to measure violent behavior as an outcome. Therefore, rather than reviewing studies that target violence risk factors (e.g., substance use problems), we focus almost exclusively on studies that used violent behavior as the outcome variable.

We further limit our scope by focusing on studies of persons with SMI. Many treatment studies have been published on the topic of reducing violence, or crime more generally. However, many use samples of nonill criminal offenders; hence, their findings cannot be assumed to apply to people with SMI. As such, although we do not focus on these studies, we consider their relevance. We focus on the settings in which the risk of violence among persons with SMI is greatest—in civil and forensic psychiatric settings, both within institutions and in the community. We also draw on research conducted within prison settings with study participants who were mentally ill.

Before we present a review of empirical evidence for and against certain treatments, we point out the importance that theory plays in guiding such treatments. Theory is a necessary component of psychological science. Innumerable theories of violence have been espoused, and a number of treatments are based on these perspectives (e.g., social learning theory informs some variants of CBT-based treatment approaches). Theories are also essential to determine why interventions succeed or fail and to guide the development of improved interventions. Theoretical conceptualization of causes and correlates of violence is a powerful force in shaping the emphasis of treatment, guiding who or what is targeted by treatment and guiding policy changes in the criminal justice system (Hollin, 1999). Although in this chapter we cannot conduct a full discussion of theory, we encourage readers to consider its importance (see Akers & Sellers, 2004; Douglas & Skeem, 2005; Silver, 2006).

TREATMENT APPROACHES

We begin this section on treatment approaches with a caveat. Research on reducing violence in persons with SMI is in a seriously undeveloped stage. Most studies are not controlled and contain small samples. Furthermore it is difficult to make clean statements about the effectiveness of certain types of interventions because most include a host of approaches (e.g., social skills, problem solving, anger management, modeling), generally under the rubric of cognitive–behavioral therapy (CBT). Fortunately, the field is more mature when it comes to the treatment of offending in general (i.e., not limiting the target population to persons with SMI or the outcome to violence). We briefly describe this literature, although our focus is on what can be distilled from research conducted within psychiatric samples.

Cognitive and Behavioral Approaches

By far the most common systematically studied contemporary approach to crime and violence reduction is cognitive–behavioral in nature. As with CBT generally, these approaches include foci on both behavioral techniques (e.g., reinforcement contingencies, token economies, shaping, modeling, successive approximation, extinction) and cognitive techniques (e.g., correcting irrational cognitions, problem solving skills, social skills acquisition). In the crime and violence reduction arena, CBT is best construed as a broad umbrella framework under which a variety of related, though distinct, approaches have been developed and studied. As mentioned earlier, the majority of such studies have been conducted within general offender (and juvenile justice) samples and have used general criminal recidivism, as opposed to violence per se, as the outcome. We briefly describe the state of the discipline in this regard and then evaluate the extent to which these principles apply to (a) violence specifically, as distinguished from crime generally, and (b) persons with mental illness. We do so by introducing the concept of *risk–need–responsivity* (RNR; Andrews & Bonta, 2003; Andrews, Bonta, & Hoge, 1990).

Risk–Need–Responsivity

In the general correctional field, RNR has firm roots and solid support as a guiding treatment framework. The principles of risk, need, and responsivity link offender risk assessment with interventions designed to reduce recidivism. The risk principle holds that more intense services should be allotted to higher risk individuals. The need principle directs that services should be focused on *criminogenic needs,* or dynamic risk factors that "when changed, are associated with changes in the probability of recidivism" (Andrews & Bonta, 2003, p. 261). According to the responsivity principle, treatment should be tailored to the abilities and learning styles of the offender. Typically, this calls for structured approaches such as CBT and psychosocial techniques. More specifically, RNR-informed treatments adopt a variety of CBT-based principles, such as cognitive skills training (i.e., identifying and challenging cognitions that support or condone crime), problem solving (i.e., learning and practicing prosocial ways to deal with conflict and other challenges), anger management (i.e., identifying anger cues and strategies to cope with anger), behavior modification (i.e., applying reinforcement contingencies that reward prosocial behavior), and other behavioral techniques (e.g., modeling, shaping, role rehearsal). Typically, these programs are run within institutions and adopt group-based, psychoeducational formats. They may be supplemented with more specific programs that target common criminogenic needs (e.g., substance use treatment, anger management).

There have been numerous meta-analytic evaluations of RNR-based programs, sometimes with a comparison to non-RNR approaches. On the basis of a comprehensive review, Dowden and Andrews (2000) found that correctional treatment programs that focused on criminogenic needs (e.g., procriminal attitudes, anger and hostility, poor family supervision) were more effective in reducing recidivism than those focused on noncriminogenic needs (e.g., anxiety, depression, low self-esteem). Programs based on RNR have come to be described as using principles of effective correctional treatment (Gendreau & Goggin, 1996; Gendreau, Little, & Goggin, 1996).One meta-analysis (Pearson, Lipton, Cleland, & Yee, 2002) compared more behaviorally oriented approaches (e.g., behavioral contingency programs, token economies) with more cognitive–behavioral approaches (e.g., social skills training, cognitive skills, problem solving, social learning, relapse prevention, thinking errors). In total, there were 25 behavioral and 44 CBT studies. Generally, after the quality of the study was controlled, stronger support for CBT was reported, with a mean weighted effect size (r_w) of .14 (compared with r_w = .07). It is important to note that studies with higher quality (mostly experimental designs) tended to produce larger effect sizes. Some studies have shown that there may be a dose–response effect in RNR-based treatment (Bourgon & Armstrong, 2005). Although there is strong evidence for the effectiveness of CBT–RNR approaches to crime reduction, such evidence cannot be presumed to apply to the reduction of violence.

Do the Principles of Effective Correctional Treatment Apply to Violent as Well as General Recidivism? Most research on the RNR approach has used "general reoffending" as the outcome measure, without specifying whether the reoffending was violent or nonviolent. Dowden and Andrews (2000) conducted a meta-analysis of 35 unique samples that included violence as a dependent variable. The authors reported a small effect size of $r = .07$ across all studies; however, the range in correlations was considerable, from –.22 to .63. The authors also coded the extent to which studies subscribed to each of the three RNR principles, as well as a principle of *human service* (i.e., a provision of service, rather than solely punishment). Three of these four principles were associated with decreased violent recidivism; the risk principle was not. It is important to note that an aggregate score of the number of RNR–human service principles (0–4) reflected by the treatment study indicated that the studies that provided only punishment were essentially unrelated to violent recidivism ($r = -.01$), whereas those that provided human services that reflected each of the RNR principles were substantially more strongly related to reduction of violent recidivism ($r = .20$). The correlation between the number of RNR principles reflected in a study, on the one hand, and study effect size, on the other hand, was large ($r = .69$).

One RNR-based program and its evaluation is impressive for its size. In an unusually large sample of 44,000 offenders from Florida, those who went through an RNR-based program showed lower revocation rates (40%–50%) compared with those who did not (60%–63%; Leininger, 1998). This system has been shown to reduce violence as well. However, the sample was general population offenders, not people with SMI. The question remains, then—does this treatment approach work for people with SMI?

Do the Principles of Effective Correctional Treatment Apply to Persons With Mental Illness? There have been far fewer studies of RNR-based treatments conducted with persons with SMI, but we consider them in some detail. It is difficult, if not impossible, to categorize studies further because most include a variety of CBT/RNB-based approaches (e.g., social learning programs, social skills programs, cognitive skills programs). Some programs are based in institutions, whereas others are based in the community. Generally, one could conclude that such studies are consistent with the hypothesis that they will reduce violence. However, methodological problems are common, as reviewed in the following paragraphs.

In one study, Yates et al. (2005) applied a specialized CBT/cognitive skills–intensive inpatient training program for patients in state psychiatric facilities with persistent SMI and a history of crime or aggression. The program was informed by RNR treatment principles and enhanced with a behavioral reward system (i.e., increased liberties and rewards contingent on good behavior). It also included psychiatric management and 12-step substance use treatment. After patients reached a certain level or step in the program, they were assigned to a case manager who acted as a bridge between institution and community. After discharge, patients were followed in the community with case management and standard psychiatric aftercare. The core of the program was a cognitive skills training course, the purpose of which was to train patients on the "skills, values, and attitudes necessary for successful living in the community" (Yates et al., 2005, p. 215). It was administered in small group format. Skill modules included problem solving, creative thinking, social skills, critical reasoning, and management of emotions. Participants were 181 male and female patients with SMI (79% with psychosis) and histories of crime or violence. Most patients also had a substance-related diagnosis (69%) and a comorbid personality disorder (45% antisocial personality disorder; 12% borderline personality disorder). Approximately half the patients were able to complete the program ($n = 90$; 49.7%) and were discharged into the community. Although this is a low completion rate, the authors pointed out that the group of patients had been unable to complete previous treatment programs.

Kunz et al. (2004) followed 85 of the patients from the Yates et al. (2005) study into the community. Of these, 33 (39%) remained in the community without further hospitalizations or arrests (follow-up ranged from 6 months to 4 years). Thirty-five (42%) patients were rehospitalized, and 17 (20%) were arrested. In terms of violence, only 5 of the 17 patients who were rearrested had committed violent offenses. Although a fairly high proportion of the sample was rehospitalized or arrested, the authors argued that it was lower than for comparable patients who did not go through this treatment. Although on the surface this does appear to be the case, the authors conceded that the lack of a control group precludes firm conclusions about the actual difference in recidivism rates or the causal effect that treatment might have had on recidivism rates.

Lovell, Allen, Johnson, and Jemelka (2001) evaluated a residential treatment program for 448 offenders with SMI (i.e., schizophrenia, bipolar disorder, or depressive disorders). This program combined numerous approaches couched within a psychoeducational CBT model (consisting of case management, anger management, cognitive skills, life skills, stress management, symptom recognition, and relapse prevention). Using a pre–post design with a subgroup of 140 offenders, the authors evaluated the rates of staff and inmate assaults, as well as other institutional infractions, for inmates with at least 18 months of institutionalization prior to the program, 90 days in the program, and 18 months after the program. Staff assaults were significantly lower in the postperiod (from 15 to 5 in the 2 years pre- and posttreatment). Major infractions were generally reduced. Again, however, the study lacked a control group.

Other studies have been based more explicitly within a *social learning approach* that is based on social learning theory and assumes that principles of reinforcement and modeling will lead to a reduced risk of violence. For instance, Donnelly and Scott (1999) evaluated a social learning program originally used with offenders that applied the principles of a reasoning and rehabilitation cognitive skills model (Ross & Ross, 1995) to psychiatric patients with a history of crime or violence. This program taught cognitive and problem-solving skills and used behavioral methods and problem solving. It addressed self-control training, thinking style, emotion management, critical reasoning, and cognitive skills in the context of social learning theory. The program consisted of 54 group sessions that spanned 5 months. A small-scale evaluation of 24 patients (i.e., 12 in the intervention group and 12 in a comparison group), all of whom had records of previous violence and most of whom had diagnoses of schizophrenia, was limited to assessing changes in self-control, locus of control, problem-solving, social adjustment, and self-esteem (reoffending or aggression was not measured). Although the program led to relatively greater improvements in problem-solving abilities and the social adjustment in the treatment group, there were no similar improvements on other indexes. Thus, findings are equivocal.

Perhaps the most rigorous evaluation of a social learning program was reported by Paul and Lentz (1977). This study of chronic psychiatric inpatients included random assignment to the social learning program (compared with milieu therapy or traditional care) and also included a token economy, skills training, and other behavioral methods (e.g., shaping, modeling). Measures were collected every 6 months (approximately 4.5 years in the hospital, and 1.5 years in the community). There were 24 patients per group, who were replaced as necessary as a result of attrition. In addition to token reinforcement, patients were "punished" (i.e., secluded up to 48 hours) for assaultive behavior. Generally, both the social learning and the milieu groups showed greater reductions in assaultive behavior as well as increases in prosocial behavior, relative to the traditional care group. In addition, the social learning program was more effective than the milieu condition. In the social learning group, rates of assault dropped from approximately 30 per week at baseline to just over 10 per week at 2 years. In the milieu group, rates increased from approximately 25 per week to roughly 60 per week. An interesting quasi-experimental intervention arose from a state-mandated reduction in maximum seclusion time to 2 hours. Within 2 years after this state-mandated reduction, assaults had increased dramatically (from roughly 10 per week to approximately 75 per week in the social learning group, and much higher [i.e., 300+] in the milieu group). Because of this, the hospital sought and was granted permission to extend seclusion to 5:30 a.m. the day following an incident. Remarkably, assaultiveness decreased soon thereafter (in the final 6 months of the study), though not quite to its lowest levels.

Findings from Paul and Lentz's (1977) work have yet to be truly replicated owing to its complex design and inclusion of random assignment to conditions. However, a smaller scale study of 19 forensic psychiatric inpatients used an AB design in an attempt to conceptually replicate the program implemented and evaluated by Paul and Lentz (N. C. Beck, Menditto, Baldwin, Angelone, & Maddox, 1991). Participants were long-term (10+ years), chronically violent forensic inpatients with psychotic disorders. As with Paul and Lentz's design, the program included learning-based approaches to decreasing aggression and bizarre behavior and increasing self-care. It also included social and problem-solving skills programs as well as life skills training and the use of a closed token economy (all consumables and privileges were purchased with tokens). Actual or threatened violence or property destruction was punished by a 24-hour seclusion and a fine of 25 tokens. The program was implemented over 3 months.

N. C. Beck et al. (1991) reported a substantial and statistically significant decrease in aggressive behavior (defined as physical assault, threatened assault, and destruction of property). There were 49 acts of so-called intolerable behavior in the 3 months before the program was implemented and 43 during the 3-month implementation phase. During the next 18 months (during which the program was fully operational), there was a sharp decline in aggression (i.e., approximately 30 incidents in the next 3-month block, followed by approximately 15, 20, 20, 10, and 4 in subsequent 3-month time blocks). This represents a 92% decrease in aggression between baseline and the final 3-month block. As the authors duly acknowledged, it is not possible to draw causal inferences from this study because of the lack of experimental manipulation.

In tandem with the more comprehensive controlled trial reported by Paul and Lentz (1977), however, there appears to be strong evidence for the effectiveness of an intense social learning approach to institutional violence among chronically ill and aggressive inpatients. Furthermore, it is not possible to attribute the apparent success of the program to any of its constituent elements. On the basis of the findings from Paul and Lentz, it appears that the length of seclusion might be an important factor. However, such a conclusion is in need of systematic investigation through dismantling studies, which would be burdensome and ethically challenging to conduct.

A number of other studies have evaluated primarily cognitive-, social-, or life-skills-based programs with patients with SMI, although they suffer collectively from weak designs (i.e., no comparison group or even control for covariates; small N) or outcome measures of peripheral relevance to this chapter (i.e., self- or nurse-ratings of hostility, as opposed to violence per se; improved family relations; reduction of social anxiety; enhanced conversation skills; Benton & Schroeder, 1990; Derks, 1996; Fleck, Thompson, & Narroway, 2001; Hodel & West, 2003; Hogarty et al., 1991; Hornsveld, 2005; Liberman, Mueser, & Wallace, 1986; McMurran, Egan, Richardson, & Ahmadi, 1999; Timmerman & Emmelkamp, 2005; Wallace & Liberman, 1985). As a group, some (though not all) of these studies have reported positive findings (e.g., reduction in hostility ratings). However, not much credence can be given them for our purposes, given their methodological problems or peripheral relevance in terms of outcome measures, or both. We do not mean to dismiss such studies—empirical study in this area is difficult in terms of recruiting participants and implementing controlled designs. Although results typically are consistent with expectations, the studies are inherently limited for the reasons mentioned.

Anger Management

Anger is prevalent among individuals with a wide variety of psychiatric disorders (Novaco, 2000) and can be considered a criminogenic need among many violent individuals (Howells, Watt, Hall, & Baldwin, 1997). Anger management is premised on the belief that cognitive restructuring will reduce the skewed perceptions and negative thinking that predisposes some people to commit violence. Novaco's adaptation of Meichenbaum's Stress Inoculation Training (initially developed for the treatment of anxiety; Meichenbaum, 1985; Novaco, 1975) has been the focus of much of the accumulated research evidence. Reflecting a coping skills approach, stress inoculation consists of three principle components: cognitive preparation, skill acquisition, and application training (R. Beck & Fernandez, 1998). More generally, anger management often is a form of CBT intended to challenge attitudes, perceptions, and self-statements that can precede violence.

A meta-analysis of anger treatment studies demonstrated medium to large positive effects in terms of anger reduction (Edmondson & Conger, 1996). Examination of effect sizes by treatment type indicated that relaxation, social skills, and cognitive relaxation treatments yielded greater benefits than cognitive treatment (mean effect sizes were .82, .80, .76, and .64, respectively). R. Beck and Fernandez (1998), on the basis of their meta-analysis of 50 studies, reported that anger management clients were better off than 76% of control participants. The relevance of the findings to our discussion is limited, however, by highly heterogeneous samples and dependent variables that focused (understandably) on anger as opposed to violence. Despite these limitations, R. Beck and Fernandez's evaluation reflects more than 2 decades of research on anger treatment and suggests that anger management programs are an important component of interventions likely to yield moderate treatment gains.

Few studies have investigated the effectiveness of anger management directly for the reduction of violence among persons with SMI. Stermac (1986) compared a control group ($N = 20$) of forensic psychiatric patients with a group undergoing anger control treatment, including cognitive restructuring ($N = 20$). The treatment group reported lower levels of anger (but not impulsivity) and more adaptive coping strategies posttreatment compared with the control group. Because violence per se was not measured, findings are inconclusive, although they do suggest that this approach might reduce anger among persons with SMI.

A small study assigned 9 forensic inpatients with intellectual disabilities to a CBT-based anger management treatment group and 10 patients (who later received the treatment) to a wait-list control (Taylor, Novaco, Gillmer, & Thorne, 2002). Although patients who received the experimental treatment had lower self-reported anger reaction scores posttreatment than the wait-list control group did pretreatment, staff ratings of anger largely did not vary across groups. Verbal and physical aggression were rare in the post-treatment period for both groups; therefore, meaningful comparisons could not be made. Finally, Becker, Carney Love, and Hunter (1997) conducted four $N = 1$ studies of individualized anger management–behavior therapy approaches with formerly intractable forensic patients. The four patients had all been seriously and persistently violent in the past. Treatment applied various techniques, including classical and operant conditioning, affect modulation, shaping, and desensitization after a thorough assessment of the events, responses, emotions, and (sometimes delusional) perceptions that preceded violence, and a functional analysis of violence. In all cases, described in helpful detail, violence was substantially decreased.

As is clear, clinical interventions for anger have scarcely begun to evaluate anger management in the prevention of violence (as opposed to some index of anger), and this is particularly true for individuals with SMI. A blanket recommendation of anger management treatment for all individuals for whom violence is a concern is neither appropriate nor cost effective. In particular, anger management is likely to have limited relevance to individuals for whom anger arousal is unrelated to their use of violence (Watt & Howells, 1999).

Dialectical Behavior Therapy

Dialectical behavior therapy (DBT) was developed originally to treat chronically parasuicidal women with borderline personality disorder, a complex and difficult-to-treat population (Berzins & Trestman 2004). DBT is a comprehensive behavioral treatment predicated on Marsha Linehan's work addressing the etiology of borderline personality disorder and its associated behavioral patterns (Linehan, 1987). It combines basic strategies of behavior therapy and cognitive therapy techniques (Robins & Chapman, 2004) with Eastern mindfulness practices (Berzins & Trestman 2004). The core strategies are a balance and synthesis of validation (i.e., acceptance) and problem solving (i.e., change; Robins & Chapman, 2004). DBT is worthy of study in the attempt to reduce violence among persons with SMI because of its structured, problem-reduction approach to emotional dysregulation (McCann, Ball, & Ivanoff, 2000) and its empirical support with other challenging populations and problems (Lynch, Chapman, Rosenthal, Kuo, & Linehan, 2006). In one of the only known studies of DBT in a forensic sample, Evershed et al. (2003) examined the effectiveness of DBT in a high security hospital. The authors reported that DBT patients (*n* = 8) showed greater reductions on measures of cognitive, covert, and dispositional aspects of hostility and anger and were significantly better than the treatment as usual (TAU) group (*n* = 9) at managing outward expression of anger and hostility. Although the frequency of violent behaviors showed no significant change in this study, the seriousness of violent behaviors was reduced more in the DBT group than in the TAU group (i.e., a 53% vs. a 22% reduction). We encourage more research on DBT for the reduction of violence.

Approaches Not Based on Cognitive–Behavioral Therapy or Risk–Need–Responsivity

Generally, we would discourage the use of psychological interventions that are not grounded solidly within CBT or RNR approaches. For instance, therapeutic communities that are not based in either approach in which participants engage in a self-governing system of rule enforcement, as well as ostensible caring for and respect for other residents, have little support for the reduction of crime or violence (Quinsey et al., 2006). Furthermore, some studies have investigated interventions based on other theoretical approaches (e.g., personal construct theory and fuzzy logic systems, Goold & Kirchhoff,

1998; arts therapy, Smeijsters & Cleven, 2006). Although it is possible that such approaches could reduce violence, they have not convincingly demonstrated their ability to do so.

Some treatments or service approaches designed to operate primarily within the community may require the cooperation and involvement of legal players (e.g., mental health courts [MHCs]) or unfold within the context of legal supervision (e.g., outpatient commitment [OPC]). *Intensive case management* posits that if typical psychiatric aftercare, or psychiatric rehabilitation, is provided to persons with SMI but at an increased dose, outcomes will be more favorable. Findings are equivocal. For instance, Ventura, Cassell, Jacoby, and Huang (1998) examined the effect of the intensity of case management (administered within both the institution and the community) and 3-year recidivism rates among 261 persons (71% male participants) with SMI. Although most participants (78%) received case management in jail, the minority (29%) did so in the community. Receipt of case management was voluntary and subject to availability, another methodological weakness (though merely a reflection of reality). The median amount of case management services received in jail per client was a total of 40 minutes. Recidivism rates were generally high (72%), though expectedly lower for violent misdemeanors (23%) or violent felonies (11%). Recidivism rates for all these outcomes did not differ between those who did and did not receive case management in jail. However, those who received case management in the community were less likely to recidivate, both in general and in terms of violent recidivism. Controlling for numerous covariates using survival analysis, the receipt of community case management reduced the violent rearrest rate by 64%. However, the fact that assignment to groups was done on the basis of a voluntary sign-up procedure suggests that self-selection biases may have been operating.

In a large-scale randomized clinical trial study ($N = 708$) of intensive case management in which the only intervention was size of caseload (i.e., 10–15 patients in the intensive group vs. 30 in the standard group), Walsh et al. (2001) reported no differences in physical assaultiveness between groups (i.e., 22% in each group, over 2 years). Other studies have similarly failed to observe an effect of intensive case management for the reduction of violence (Solomon, Draine, & Meyerson, 1994) despite reasonably solid support for the reduction of more generic outcomes (e.g., rehospitalization; Johnson et al., 2005). This could stem from a lack of attention to criminogenic needs in such services, which tend to focus primarily on psychiatric services.

A related approach is *assertive community treatment* (ACT), in which service providers actively assist patients in meeting their needs in terms of treatment, housing, employment, and sustenance. Reviews of ACT generally indicate support for its effectiveness in terms of traditional clinical outcomes, though less so for criminal justice outcomes (Bond, Drake, Mueser,

& Latimer, 2001; Mueser, Bond, Drake, & Resnick, 1998). Few studies evaluate violence or crime per se as outcomes, and even methodologically solid studies that have done so have failed to yield promising results (Caslyn, Yonker, Lemming, Morse, & Klinkenberg, 2005; Killapsy et al., 2006). Some programs are designed specifically to reduce criminal justice outcomes and have somewhat more promising findings, though conclusions based on these studies tend to be limited by design characteristics such as lack of control groups or statistical control or failing to differentiate between violent and nonviolent outcome measures (Ford et al., 2001; McCoy, Roberts, Hanrahan, Clay, & Luchins, 2004; Wilson, Tien, & Eaves, 1995).

OPC is another community-based system approach to providing psychiatric services. This approach has reasonable support in terms of improving quality of life and reducing symptoms and hospitalizations, though less support has been demonstrated for the reduction of violence or other antisocial behaviors (O'Reilly, 2001). However, some research has yielded relatively favorable outcomes. Swanson et al. (2000) conducted a randomized clinical trial of OPC among 262 psychiatric patients with either serious psychotic or mood disorders. OPC was compared with being released from OPC. OPC continued for a minimum of 90 days and was renewed at the discretion of clinicians and the court. The study was limited by the mandated exclusion of patients with a history of serious violence in the year prior to hospitalization from the control group. With these patients excluded from analysis (to permit analysis of a truly randomized design), there was no effect of OPC on subsequent violence. When such patients were included in analyses and the OPC intervention was defined as having lasted for at least 6 months, OPC significantly reduced violence (26.7% vs. 41.6%). Factors enhancing the effectiveness of OPC, in addition to longer enrollment periods, included receipt of regular outpatient psychiatric services, medication compliance, and the absence of substance misuse (especially the combination of the latter two). Hough & O'Brien (2005) reported a decrease in violence from 18% to 7% associated with OPC in an ABA-designed study of 553 Australian patients.

Finally, MHCs have proliferated across the United States despite a relative paucity of evaluation research. Modeled after drug courts, MHCs typically enroll persons with SMI who have been charged with minor offenses (though there are exceptions). Christy, Poythress, Boothroyd, Petrila, and Shabnam, (2005) reported violence- and arrest-related outcome data associated with their evaluation of the Broward County MHC, the purpose of which is to increase mental health services for misdemeanants with mental illness and to reduce their contact with the criminal justice system, without risking public safety. Compared with matched participants from a different county, Christy et al. reported few differences in terms of criminal justice outcomes. However, there was a lower mean number of arrests in the MHC group and a smaller frequency of serious violent incidents detected through self-report (3% vs. 11%) than in the matched sample.

In contrast to the MHC evaluated by Christy et al. (2005), the MHC evaluated by Cosden, Ellens, Schnell, Yamini-Diouf, and Wolfe (2003) permitted random assignment to conditions (i.e., MHC vs. TAU—less intense case management and regular criminal justice system processing, respectively). This MHC also included a funded service delivery element (i.e., ACT), unlike the MHC evaluated by Christy et al. Furthermore, the Santa Barbara MHC received felony offenders as well as offenders postadjudication. Cosden et al. (2003) compared the 137 MHC clients with the 98 TAU offenders in terms of recidivism indexes at 12-months postintervention. They reported, inter alia, that those assigned to the MHC condition showed a significantly greater reduction in important risk factors such as drug use, as well as with criminal recidivism. Unfortunately, Cosden et al. did not report outcomes for different types of criminal activity (i.e., violent vs. nonviolent offenses). They did report that MHC and TAU clients were not significantly different in terms of having been booked or spent time in jail. However, the reasons underlying future criminal justice system contact differed—those in the MHC condition were more likely to have been arrested for probation violations as opposed to new charges, in comparison to the TAU group. Overall, a high proportion of both the MHC (76%) and the TAU (72%) conditions were booked at least once. Close to half of all MHC participants were convicted of a new crime (47%), although this was significantly lower than for the TAU group (60%). The differences between the two MHCs make comparisons difficult, if not impossible.

In summary, the evidence for community systemic approaches is best seen as encouraging yet mixed, with some studies reporting findings generally consistent with the expectation that such approaches should reduce violence. However, other studies have failed to report this, and some have not differentiated between violent and nonviolent outcomes. Furthermore, it is doubtful that these approaches systematically use RNR- or CBT-based interventions designed specifically to reduce violence. It also appears that for some approaches at least (i.e., OPC), there may be a dose–response relationship between treatment length and violence reduction that operates through enhancing medication adherence (Swanson et al., 2000), though other studies have failed to find a dose–response effect (Walsh et al., 2001). Because other studies of people with SMI have observed a dose–response effect on the reduction of violence (Skeem, Monahan, & Mulvey, 2002), it is worth pursuing whether treatment dose is systematically related to the reduction of violence among people with SMI. Unfortunately, Skeem et al. (2002) were not able to specify the type of treatments in their study, just the number of sessions that participants received in the community following discharge from hospital. It is important to note that a higher number of treatment sessions reduced violence not only in general but also for psychopathic individuals, who were at higher risk for violence in the study. As such, studying treatment dose may be particularly promising for higher risk individuals and would be consistent with the RNR principle that more intensive services should be allotted to higher risk people.

Nonpsychological Approaches

Psychological treatment of violence among persons with SMI is almost certain to take place in interdisciplinary settings (i.e., civil or forensic hospitals or community centers). For this reason, we briefly review research on three types of interventions or management strategies that tend not to be psychological in nature: (a) institutional policy or quality management, (b) staff training in crisis response or de-escalation, and (c) the role of psychotropic medication. Psychologists using such interventions must be able to coordinate their services with those of colleagues working within other professional disciplines.

Institutional Policies and Quality Management

Some approaches to violence risk reduction have focused not on the treatment of patients per se but on evaluating staff or agency intervention efforts. The premise underlying such approaches is that violence is not caused solely by factors internal to the patient but that situational or contextual variables can influence the probability of violence (Cooke, Wozniak, & Johnstone, in press). This reasoning would hold, for instance, that staff members who are trained to deal with agitated mentally disordered persons would be better able to prevent violent incidents than staff who are not so trained. Hunter and Carney Love (1996), for instance, used the principles of *total quality management* to reduce violence and other aggressive incidents in the dining room of a state forensic hospital. All interventions were pragmatic in nature (e.g., allowing patients with good behavior to leave after eating, rather than waiting for a designated time; allowing patients to choose the music that played; using plastic cutlery). Violence was reduced by 40%.

Drummond, Sparr, and Gordon (1989; see also Sparr, Drummond, & Hamilton, 1988) implemented and evaluated a *behavioral emergency committee*, which identified the most aggressive patients in a general Veterans Adminstration (VA) hospital (most of whom had psychiatric diagnoses), then implemented a computer flagging system along with risk management strategies for those patients who were flagged (e.g., having security near when interacting with these patients). There was a substantial decrease in violence and related events (e.g., weapon carrying) among these patients. Note that this policy was tested only for patients who were already flagged as being high risk. As Eichelman (1989) noted in response, the active ingredient in the effectiveness of this program is not clear. He also noted that without the support and resources of the hospital administration, this intervention likely would not have worked.

Staff Training

Needham et al. (2004) tested whether the adoption of a systematic risk assessment procedure and staff training in risk management (e.g., descriptive information about aggression, verbal de-escalation procedures) would reduce assaultive behavior in two psychiatric wards in Switzerland. The authors compared a baseline period with two postintervention periods, the first defined by the implementation of systematic risk assessment only and the second defined by the risk management training (hence, the second postintervention period involved the presence of both interventions). Findings showed that aggression was reduced on one ward but not on the other. Coercive staff measures decreased on the ward that showed no decline in aggression, but not on the other ward. Collapsing across wards, aggression did not decline, making the findings inconclusive. It should be pointed out, however, that simply assessing risk should not logically lead to a reduction of violence without an attendant risk management procedure that is tied to the assessment. In the present study, there was not a logical link between assessment and management (in fact, the management aspect of the study was not introduced for several months after assessment phase of the study).

Rice, Harris, Varney, and Quinsey (1989), however, showed that training in verbal de-escalation (e.g., calming and defusing skills, conflict resolution, interviewing skills, self-defense, and restraint training) can help to reduce tense or acute situations in which violence is highly likely to occur imminently and may result in less serious injuries (Rice, et al., 1989). Similar findings have been reported by others (Corrigan, Holmes, Luchins, & Basit, 1995; Infantino & Musingo, 1985), suggesting that people working in such settings should avail themselves of such techniques.

The Role of Psychotropic Medication

As we discussed earlier, violent behavior among persons with severe mental illness is an uncommon yet problematic and multiply determined phenomenon that challenges clinicians to use multifaceted treatment modalities. These modalities include the use of psychopharmacological advances, especially medications with proven efficacy and low or improved side-effect profiles. We make only a few observations on this point. First, medication alone will not effectively, or at least maximally, reduce violence. As noted earlier, most individuals with mental illness are not violent, and there are a host of other risk factors for violence among persons with SMI that must be managed. Second, evidence suggests that the majority of persons who are prescribed psychotropic medication will not adhere to it as prescribed. Although the effective treatment of psychosis includes the use of antipsychotic agents, reported rates of nonadherence range from 20% to 89%, with a mean rate of about 50% (Dolder, Lacro, Dunn, & Jeste, 2002; Fenton, Blyler, & Heinssen, 1997). In the National Institute of Mental Health Clinical Antipsychotic Trials of Intervention Effectiveness (CATIE), 74% of 1,432 participants discontinued medication before conclusion of the 18-month study period (Swanson et al., 2006).

Logistical and ethical challenges complicate the design and implementation of research protocols to establish a scientific basis for best-practice risk management models in the emergency setting. In response to this challenge, clinical consensus guidelines for the assessment, management, and treatment of agitated, psychotic, and potentially violent persons have been developed and are available (Allen, Currier, Carpenter, Ross, & Docherty, 2005; MacPherson, Dix, & Morgan, 2005; National Institute for Health and Clinical Excellence, 2002). Such measures, however, often necessitate urgent decision making on the basis of inadequate clinical information about diagnosis or medication history. This unfortunate yet unavoidable scenario may result in the administration of older antipsychotic agents such as haloperidol by intramuscular injection and on an involuntary basis, as well as the use of physical restraints. It is essential, therefore, that clinical stability and diagnostic clarity be attained as soon as possible after the emergency has dissipated to facilitate clinician–patient agreement about the implementation of appropriate, longer term medication strategies (which remain the cornerstone of treatment of SMI). Such an agreement typically depends on the interaction of various individual and psychosocial contextual variables, including symptom severity, illness awareness, prior medication experiences, and motivation for treatment adherence (Buckley et al., 2007; Fenton et al., 1997; Tait, Birchwood, & Trower, 2003).

For persons with schizophrenia, the atypical, so-called second generation antipsychotic agents such as olanzapine, risperidone, quetiapine, aripiprazole, and clozapine hold promise. Medication adherence rates have been reported to be moderately higher for atypical compared with typical antipsychotics (Dolder et al., 2002). In the CATIE trial, time to discontinuation of medication because of intolerable side effects was significantly longer for olanzapine compared with some but not all atypicals and did not differ from the first generation antipsychotic agent perphenazine (Lieberman et al., 2005). Debate continues over the perceived clinical superiority of atypical over typical medications and whether sufficient clinical and research evidence exists to support the 95% market share that these medications presently hold in developed countries. The high discontinuation rates and lack of evidence from the CATIE trial to support clear superiority in clinical efficacy between these medication groups (with the exception of the atypical agent clozapine) underscore the need for adjunctive evidence-based psychosocial interventions to support psychopharmacological strategies and optimize response rates in individual patients (Gilmer et al., 2004; Lieberman, 2006).

The literature on psychopharmacological interventions in aggression suggests that atypical agents, especially clozapine, are superior to typical antipsychotics in their antiaggressive effects, likely mediated through lower dopamine D_2 receptor affinity and greater affinity for specific serotonergic and norepinephrine neuroreceptors (Krakowski, Czobor, Citrome, Bark, & Cooper, 2006). In support of this hypothesis, a prospective, randomized parallel-group study of assaultive patients with schizophrenia or schizoaffective disorder demonstrated that clozapine was superior to both olanzapine and haloperidol in reducing violence in persons with schizophrenia (Krakowski et al., 2006; Volavka et al., 2004). Recent research has also found olanzapine to be more effective than risperidone in reducing aggression for those who remained on medication for at least a year (controlling for clinical and demographic variables; Swanson, Swartz, Elbogen, & Van Dorn, 2004). This was partly due to the improvement in medication compliance associated with olanzapine, which mediated the association between olanzapine and violence. This proposed model of neuroreceptor dysfunction and its psychopharmacological remedy may also be the mechanism by which other medication groups such as the selective serotonin reuptake inhibitors, and certain mood stabilizers (e.g., lithium, divalproex sodium) modulate aggression and reactive volatility across nosological dimensions (Coccaro, Astill, Herbert, & Schut, 1990; Glancy & Knott, 2002; Lee & Coccaro 2001; Lendenmayer, 2000; McElroy, 1999).

CONCLUSION

Although we covered a broad array of treatment studies in this chapter, we remain guarded in suggesting treatment approaches because of the lack of large-scale, well-controlled studies specifically dealing with SMI and violence. On the basis of the literature covered, however, and the broader literature on the principles of effective correctional treatment, we make the following conclusions about the treatment approaches with the greatest likelihood of success:

1. Psychosocial treatment should be informed by the principles of effective correctional treatment (i.e., RNR), and follow a CBT (e.g., social learning, cognitive skills) approach.
2. Treatment should focus on general (e.g., employment problems, substance use), associated (e.g., medication nonadherence), and specific (e.g., acute positive psychotic symptoms) criminogenic needs.
3. Multiple and coordinated treatment approaches should be used, including administrative (e.g., staff training in deescalation, institutional policies), psychosocial, and psychotropic approaches.

4. A sufficient dose of treatment should be administered.
5. Treatment integrity should be considered of utmost importance (e.g., well-trained treatment staff, supportive administration, well-coordinated evaluation mechanisms).
6. Treatment should be tailored individually (e.g., people who are not angry do not need anger management).

We conclude this chapter by indicating the areas we believe are in greatest need of research. First, more large-scale, controlled trials of RNR-based treatment are necessary. This has been accomplished in the general correctional and youth justice fields, but (save for Paul & Lentz, 1977) not yet with regard to violence and SMI. Second, studies need to disaggregate outcomes according to whether they are nonviolent or violent to make it possible to understand the reduction of violence, as opposed to crime, antisocial behavior, or self-reported hostility or anger. Third, community treatments (i.e., intensive case management) need to incorporate RNR-based principles if they hope to reduce violence in addition to improving general mental health outcomes. Fourth, dismantling studies should be used to identify the most effective elements of all-encompassing treatment programs. Fifth, factors that may reduce the effectiveness of treatment should continue to be studied. For instance, comorbid personality disorder, especially psychopathy, has been depicted as treatment-resistant (Quinsey et al., 2006), although with sufficient dosage, individuals may respond to treatment (Skeem et al., 2002). Other factors likely to reduce treatment effectiveness include poor treatment alliance (Beauford, McNiel, & Binder, 1997), substance abuse problems, and medication nonadherence (Swanson et al., 2000).

Finally, we emphasize the importance of bridging violence risk assessment and treatment. Efforts to reduce violence will fail, or at least underperform, if not informed first by comprehensive risk assessment procedures that identify for each individual the most salient violence risk factors present. Certain risk assessment–management approaches have been developed specifically to facilitate this bridging effort between assessment and treatment (Douglas & Kropp, 2002; Douglas, Webster, Hart, Eaves, & Ogloff, 2001; Webster, Douglas, Eaves, & Hart, 1997). We encourage treatment studies to evaluate such assessment approaches. We agree with Blackburn (2004), who lamented that "the literature does not yet permit empirically-based generalizations about treatment and rehabilitation efficacy" (p. 297). Yet we are optimistic that based on the corpus of literature viewed broadly and with continued research efforts, the principles of effective violence reduction treatment for people with SMI will be distilled.

REFERENCES

Akers, R. L., & Sellers, C. S. (2004). *Criminological theories: Introduction, evaluation, and application* (4th ed.). Los Angeles, CA: Roxbury Publishing.

Allen, M. H., Currier, G. W., Carpenter, D., Ross, R., & Docherty, J. (2005). The expert consensus guideline series: Treatment of behavioral emergencies. *Journal of Psychiatric Practice, 11,* 5–25.

Andrews, D. A., & Bonta, J. (2003). *The psychology of criminal conduct* (3rd ed.). Cincinnati, OH: Anderson.

Andrews, D. A., Bonta, J., & Hoge, R. D. (1990). Classification for effective rehabilitation: Rediscovering psychology. *Criminal Justice and Behavior, 17,* 19–52.

Appelbaum, P. (2006). Violence and mental disorders: Data and public policy. *American Journal of Psychiatry, 163,* 1319–1321.

Beauford, J. E., McNiel, D. E., & Binder, R. L. (1997). Utility of the initial therapeutic alliance in evaluating psychiatric patients' risk of violence. *American Journal of Psychiatry, 154,* 1272–1276.

Beck, N. C., Menditto, A. A., Baldwin, L., Angelone, E., & Maddox, M. (1991). Reduced frequency of aggressive behavior in forensic patients in a social learning program. *Hospital and Community Psychiatry, 42,* 750–752.

Beck, R., & Fernandez, E. (1998). Cognitive–behavioral therapy in the treatment of anger: A meta-analysis. *Cognitive Therapy and Research, 22,* 63–74.

Becker, M., Carney Love, C., & Hunter, M. E. (1997). Intractability is relative: Behavior therapy in the elimination of violence in psychotic forensic patients. *Legal and Criminological Psychology, 2,* 89–101.

Benton, M. K., & Schroeder, H. E. (1990). Social skills training with schizophrenics: A meta-analytic evaluation. *Journal of Consulting and Clinical Psychology, 58,* 741–747.

Berzins, L. G., & Trestman, R. L. (2004). The development and implementation of dialectical behavior therapy in forensic settings. *International Journal of Forensic Mental Health, 3,* 93–103.

Blackburn, R. (2004). "What works" with mentally disordered offenders. *Psychology, Crime & Law, 10,* 297–308.

Bond, G. R., Drake, R. E., Mueser, K. T., & Latimer, E. (2001). Assertive community treatment for people with severe mental illness. *Disease Management and Health Outcomes, 9,* 141–159.

Bonta, J., Law, M., & Hanson, R. K. (1998). The prediction of criminal and violent recidivism among mentally disordered offenders: A meta-analysis. *Psychological Bulletin, 123,* 123–142.

Bourgon, G., & Armstrong, B. (2005). Transferring the principles of effective treatment into a "real world" prison setting. *Criminal Justice and Behavior, 32,* 3–25.

Brennan, P. A., Mednick, S. A., & Hodgins, S. (2000). Major mental disorders and criminal violence in a Danish birth cohort. *Archives of General Psychiatry, 57,* 494–500.

Buckley, P. F., Wirshing, D. A., Bhushan, P., Pierre, J. M., Resnick, S. A., & Wirshing, W. C. (2007). Lack of insight in schizophrenia: Impact on treatment adherence. *CNS Drugs, 21,* 129–141.

Caslyn, R. J., Yonker, R. D., Lemming, M. R., Morse, G. A., & Klinkenberg, W. D. (2005). Impact of assertive community treatment and client characteristics on criminal justice outcomes in dual disorder homeless individuals. *Criminal Behaviour and Mental Health, 15,* 236–248.

Christy, A., Poythress, N. G., Boothroyd, R. A., Petrila, J., & Shabnam, M. (2005). Evaluating the efficiency and community safety goals of the Broward County Mental Health Court. *Behavioral Sciences & the Law, 23,* 227–243.

Coccaro, E. F., Astill, J. L., Herbert, J. L., & Schut, A. G. (1990). Fluoxetine treatment of impulsive aggression in *DSM–IV–R* personality disorder patients. *Journal of Clinical Psychopharmacology, 10,* 373–375.

Cooke, D. J., Wozniak, E., & Johnstone, L. (in press). Casting light on prison violence in Scotland: Evaluating the impact of situational risk factors. *Criminal Justice and Behavior.*

Corrigan, P., Holmes, E. P., Luchins, D., & Basit, A. (1995). The effects of interactive staff training on staff programming and patient aggression in a psychiatric inpatient ward. *Behavioral Interventions, 10,* 17–32.

Cosden, M., Ellens, J. K., Schnell, J. L., Yamini-Diouf, Y., & Wolfe, M. M. (2003). Evaluation of a mental health treatment court with assertive community treatment. *Behavioral Sciences & the Law, 21,* 415–427.

Derks, F. C. H. (1996). A forensic day treatment program for personality-disordered criminal offenders. *International Journal of Offender Therapy and Comparative Criminology, 40,* 123–134.

Dolder, C. R., Lacro, J. P., Dunn, L. P., & Jeste, D. V. (2002). Antipsychotic medication adherence: Is there a difference between typical and atypical agents? *American Journal of Psychiatry, 159,* 103–108.

Donnelly, J. P., & Scott, M. F. (1999). Evaluation of an offending behavior programme with a mentally disordered offender population. *British Journal of Forensic Practice, 1,* 25–32.

Douglas, K. S., & Kropp, P. R. (2002). A prevention-based paradigm for violence risk assessment: Clinical and research applications. *Criminal Justice and Behavior, 29,* 617–658.

Douglas, K. S., & Skeem, J. L. (2005). Violence risk assessment: Getting specific about being dynamic. *Psychology, Public Policy, and Law, 11,* 347–383.

Douglas, K. S., Webster, C. D., Hart, S. D., Eaves, D., & Ogloff, J. R. P. (Eds.). (2001). *HCR–20: Violence risk management companion guide.* Burnaby, British Columbia, Canada: Mental Health, Law, and Policy Institute, Simon Fraser University, and Department of Mental Health Law & Policy, University of South Florida.

Dowden, C., & Andrews, D. A. (2000). Effective correctional treatment and violent reoffending: A meta-analysis. *Canadian Journal of Criminology, 42,* 449–467.

Drummond, D. J., Sparr, L. F., & Gordon, G. H. (1989). Hospital violence reduction among high-risk patients. *The Journal of the American Medical Association, 261,* 2531–2534.

Edmondson, C. B., & Conger, J. C. (1996). A review of treatment efficacy for individuals with anger problems: Conceptual, assessment, and methodological issues. *Clinical Psychology Review, 16,* 257–275.

Eichelman, B. (1989). Proactive violence reduction: Successful quality assurance. *The Journal of the American Medical Association, 261,* 2546.

Evershed, S., Tennant, A., Boomer, D., Rees, A., Barkham, M., & Watsons, A. (2003). Practice-based outcomes of dialectical behavior therapy (DBT) targeting anger and violence, with male forensic patients: A pragmatic and noncontemporaneous comparison. *Criminal Behaviour and Mental Health, 13,* 198–213.

Feder, L. (1991). A comparison of the community adjustment of mentally ill offenders with those from the general prison population: An 18-month follow-up. *Law and Human Behavior, 15,* 477–493.

Fenton, W. S., Blyler, C. R., & Heinssen, R. K. (1997). Determinants of medication adherence in schizophrenia: Clinical and empirical findings. *Schizophrenia Bulletin, 23,* 637–651.

Fleck, D., Thompson, C. L., & Narroway, L. (2001). Implementation of the Problem Solving Skills Training Programme in a medium secure unit. *Criminal Behaviour and Mental Health, 11,* 262–272.

Ford, R., Barnes, A., Davies, R., Chalmers, C., Hardy, P., & Muijen, M. (2001). Maintaining contact with people with severe mental illness: 5-year follow-up of assertive outreach. *Social Psychiatry & Psychiatric Epidemiology, 36,* 444–447.

Gendreau, P., & Goggin, C. (1996). Principles of effective programming with offenders. *Forum on Corrections Research, 8,* 38–40.

Gendreau, P., Little, T., & Goggin, C. (1996). A meta-analysis of the predictors of adult recidivism: What works! *Criminology, 34,* 401–433.

Gilmer, T. P., Dolder, C. R., Lacro, J. P., Folsom, D. P., Lindamer, L., Garcia, P., & Jeste, D. (2004). Adherence to treatment with antipsychotic medication and health care costs among Medicaid beneficiaries with schizophrenia. *American Journal of Psychiatry, 161,* 692–699.

Glancy, G. D., & Knott, T. F. (2002). Part 1—The psychopharmacology of long-term aggression: Towards an evidence-based algorithm. *Canadian Psychiatric Bulletin, 34,* 13–18.

Goold, P., & Kirchhoff, E. (1998). Personal construing, fuzzy logic and group psychotherapy amongst men with schizophrenia in Broadmoor Hospital: An illustrative case study. *Criminal Behaviour and Mental Health, 8,* 51–65.

Hodel, B., & West, A. (2003). A cognitive training for mentally ill offenders with treatment-resistant schizophrenia. *Journal of Forensic Psychiatry & Psychology, 14,* 554–568.

Hogarty, G. E., Anderson, C. M., Reiss, D. J., Kornblith, S. J., Greenwald, D. P., Ulrich, R. F., & Carter, M. (1991). Family psychoeducation, social skills training, and maintenance chemotherapy in the aftercare treatment of schizophrenia: II. Two-year effects of a controlled study on relapse and adjustment: Environmental–Personal Indicators in the Course of Schizophrenia (EPICS) Research Group. *Archives of General Psychiatry, 48,* 340–347.

Hollin, C. R. (1999). Treatment programs for offenders: Meta-analysis, "what works," and beyond. *International Journal of Law and Psychiatry, 22,* 361–372.

Hornsveld, R. H. J. (2005). Evaluation of aggression control therapy for violent forensic psychiatric patients. *Psychology, Crime & Law, 11*, 403–410.

Hough, W. G., & O'Brien, K. P. (2005). The effect of community treatment orders on offending rates. *Psychiatry, Psychology and Law, 12*, 411–423.

Howells, K., Watt, B., Hall, G., & Baldwin, S. (1997). Developing programmes for violent offenders. *Legal and Criminological Psychology, 2*, 117–128.

Hunter, M. E., & Carney Love, C. (1996). Total quality management and the reduction of inpatient violence and costs in a forensic psychiatric hospital. *Psychiatric Services, 47*, 751–754.

Infantino, J. A., & Musingo, S. (1985). Assaults and injuries among staff with and without training in aggression control techniques. *Hospital and Community Psychiatry, 36*, 1312–1314.

Johnson, S., Nolan, F., Pilling, S., Sandor, A., Hoult, J., McKenzie, N., et al. (2005, September 17). Randomised controlled trial of acute mental health care by a crisis resolution team: The North Islington crisis study. *BMJ, 331*, 599–603.

Killaspy, H., Bebbington, P., Blizard, R., Johnson, S., Nolan, F., Pilling, S., & King, M. (2006, April 8). The REACT study: Randomised evaluation of assertive community treatment in north London. *BMJ, 332*, 815–820.

Krakowski, M. I., Czobor, P., Citrome, L., Bark, N., & Cooper, T. (2006). Atypical antipsychotic agents in the treatment of violent patients with schizophrenia and schizoaffective disorder. *Archives of General Psychiatry, 63*, 622–629.

Kunz, M., Yates, K. F., Czobor, P., Rabinowitz, S., Lindenmayer, J.-P., & Volavka, J. (2004). Course of patients with histories of aggression and crime after discharge from a cognitive–behavioral program. *Psychiatric Services, 55*, 654–659.

Lee, R., & Coccaro, E. (2001). The neuropsychopharmacology of criminality and aggression. *Canadian Journal of Psychiatry, 46*, 35–44.

Leininger, K. (1998). *Effectiveness of CMC.* Tallahassee: Florida Department of Corrections Research and Data Analysis.

Lendenmayer, J. P. (2000). Use of sodium valproate in violent and aggressive behaviors: A critical review. *Journal of Clinical Psychiatry, 61*, 123–128.

Liberman, R. P., Mueser, K. T., & Wallace, C. J. (1986). Social skills training for schizophrenic individuals at risk for relapse. *American Journal of Psychiatry, 143*, 523–526.

Lieberman, J. A. (2006). What the CATIE study means for clinical practice. *Psychiatric Services, 57*, 1075.

Lieberman, J. A., Stroup, T. S., McEvoy, J. P., Swartz, M. S., Rosenbeck, R. A., Perkins, D. O., et al. (2005). Effectiveness of antipsychotic drugs in patients with chronic schizophrenia. *The New England Journal of Medicine, 353*, 1209–1223.

Linehan, M. M. (1987). Dialectical behavioral therapy: A cognitive–behavioral approach to parasuicide. *Journal of Personality Disorders, 1*, 328–333.

Lovell, D., Allen, D., Johnson, C., & Jemelka, R. (2001). Evaluating the effectiveness of residential treatment for prisoners with mental illness. *Criminal Justice and Behavior, 28*, 83–104.

Lynch, T. R., Chapman, A. L., Rosenthal, M. Z., Kuo, J. R., & Linehan, M. M. (2006). Mechanisms of change in dialectical behavior therapy: Theoretical and empirical observations. *Journal of Clinical Psychology, 62*, 459–480.

MacPherson, R., Dix, R., & Morgan, S. (2005). A growing evidence base for management guidelines. *Advances in Psychiatric Treatment, 11*, 404–415.

McCann, R. A., Ball, E. M., & Ivanoff, A. (2000). DBT with an inpatient forensic population: The CMHIP forensic model. *Cognitive and Behavioral Practice 7*, 447–456.

McCoy, M. L., Roberts, D. L., Hanrahan, P., Clay, R., & Luchins, D. J. (2004). Jail linkage assertive community treatment services for individuals with mental illnesses. *Psychiatric Rehabilitation Journal, 27*, 243–250.

McElroy, S. L. (1999). Recognition and treatment of DSM–IV intermittent explosive disorder. *Journal of Clinical Psychiatry, 60*, 12–16.

McMurran, M., Egan, V., Richardson, C., & Ahmadi, S. (1999). Social problem solving in mentally disordered offenders: A brief report. *Criminal Behaviour and Mental Health, 9*, 315–322.

Meichenbaum, D. (1977). *Cognitive behavior modification.* New York: Plenum Press.

Monahan, J. (1992). "A terror to their neighbors": Beliefs about mental disorder and violence in historical and cultural perspective. *Bulletin of the American Academy of Psychiatry and the Law, 20*, 191–195.

Monahan, J., Steadman, H. J., Silver, E., Appelbaum, P. S., Robbins, P. C., Mulvey, E. P., et al. (2001). *Rethinking risk assessment: The MacArthur Study of Mental Disorder and Violence.* New York: Oxford University Press.

Mueser, K. T., Bond, G. R., Drake, R. E., & Resnick, S. G. (1998). Models of community care for severe mental illness: A review of research on case management. *Schizophrenia Bulletin, 24*, 37–74.

National Institute for Health and Clinical Excellence. (2002). *Clinical guideline 1: Schizophrenia: Core interventions in the treatment and management of schizophrenia in primary and secondary care.* London: Author.

Needham, I., Abderhalden, C., Meer, R., Dassen, T., Haug, H. J., Halfens, R. J. G., & Fischer, J. E. (2004). The effectiveness of two interventions in the management of patient violence in acute mental inpatient settings: Report on a pilot study. *Journal of Psychiatric and Mental Health Nursing, 11*, 595–601.

Novaco, R. W. (1975). Treatment of chronic anger through cognitive and relaxation controls. *Journal of Consulting and Clinical Psychology, 44*, 681.

Novaco, R. W. (2000). Anger. In A. Kazdin (Ed.), *Encyclopedia of psychology* (pp. 170–174). New York: Oxford University Press.

O'Reilly, R. L. (2001). Does involuntary outpatient treatment work? *Psychiatric Bulletin, 25*, 371–374.

Paul, G. L., & Lentz, R. J. (1977). *Psychosocial treatment of chronic mental patients: Milieu versus social-learning programs.* Cambridge, MA: Harvard University Press.

Pearson, F. S., Lipton, D. S., Cleland, C. M., & Yee, D. S. (2002). The effects of behavioral/cognitive–behavioral programs on recidivism. *Crime & Delinquency, 48*, 476–496.

Quinsey, V. L., Harris, G. T., Rice, M. E., & Cormier, C. A. (2006). *Violent offenders: Appraising and managing risk* (2nd ed.). Washington DC: American Psychological Association.

Rice, M. E., Harris, G. T., Varney, G. W., & Quinsey, V. L. (1989). *Violence in institutions: Understanding, prevention, and control.* Toronto, Ontario, Canada: Hans Huber.

Robins, C. J., & Chapman, A. L. (2004). Dialectical behavior therapy: Current status, recent developments, and future directions. *Journal of Personality Disorders 18*, 73–89.

Ross, R. R., & Ross, R. D. (Eds.). (1995). *Thinking straight: The reasoning and rehabilitation program for delinquency prevention and offender rehabilitation.* Ottawa, Canada: Air Training & Publications.

Silver, E. (2006). Understanding the relationship between mental disorder and violence: The need for a criminological perspective. *Law and Human Behavior, 30,* 685–706.

Skeem, J. L., Monahan, J., & Mulvey, E. P. (2002). Psychopathy, treatment involvement, and subsequent violence among civil psychiatric patients. *Law and Human Behavior, 26,* 577–603.

Smeijsters, H., & Cleven, G. (2006). The treatment of aggression using arts therapies in forensic psychiatry: Results of a qualitative inquiry. *The Arts in Psychotherapy, 33,* 37–58.

Solomon, P., Draine, J., & Meyerson, A. (1994). Jail recidivism and receipt of community mental health services. *Hospital and Community Psychiatry, 45,* 793–797.

Sparr, L. F., Drummond, D. J., & Hamilton, N. G. (1988). Managing violent patient incidents: The role of a behavioral emergency committee. *Quality Review Bulletin, 14,* 147–153.

Stermac, L. E. (1986). Anger control treatments for forensic patients. *Journal of Interpersonal Violence, 1,* 446–457.

Swanson, J. W., Swartz, M. S., Borum, R., Hiday, V. A., Wagner, H. R., & Burns, B. J. (2000). Involuntary outpatient commitment and reduction of violent behavior in persons with severe mental illness. *The British Journal of Psychiatry, 176,* 324–331.

Swanson, J. W., Swartz, M. S., Elbogen, E. B., & Van Dorn, R. A. (2004). Reducing violence risk in persons with schizophrenia: Olanzapine versus risperidone. *Journal of Clinical Psychiatry, 65,* 1666–1673.

Swanson, J. W., Swartz, M. S., Van Dorn, R. A., Elbogen, E. B., Wagner, H. R., Rosenheck, R. A., et al. (2006). A national study of violent behavior in persons with schizophrenia. *Archives of General Psychiatry, 63,* 490–499.

Swartz, M. S., Swanson, J. W., Hiday, V. A., Borum, R., Wagner, H. R., & Burns, B. J. (1998). Violence and severe mental illness: The effects of substance abuse and nonadherence to medication. *American Journal of Psychiatry, 155,* 226–231.

Tait, L., Birchwood, M., & Trower, P. (2003). Predicting engagement with services for psychosis: Insight, symptoms, and recovery style. *The British Journal of Psychiatry, 182,* 123–128.

Taylor, J. L., Novaco, R. W., Gillmer, B., & Thorne, I. (2002). Cognitive–behavioral treatment of anger intensity among offenders with intellectual disabilities. *Journal of Applied Research in Intellectual Disabilities, 15,* 151–165.

Timmerman, I. G. H., & Emmelkamp, P. M. G. (2005). The effects of cognitive–behavioral treatment for forensic inpatients. *International Journal of Offender Therapy and Comparative Criminology, 49,* 590–606.

Ventura, L. A., Cassel, C. A., Jacoby, J. E., & Huang, B. (1998). Case management and recidivism of mentally ill persons released from jail. *Psychiatric Services, 49,* 1330–1337.

Volavka , J., Czobor, P., Nolan, K., Sheitman, B., Lindenmayer, J. P., Citrome, L., et al. (2004). Overt aggression and psychotic symptoms in patients with schizophrenia treated with clozapine, olanzapine, risperidone, or haloperidol. *Journal of Clinical Psychopharmacology, 24,* 225–228.

Wallace, C. J., & Liberman, R. P. (1985). Social skills training for patients with schizophrenia: A controlled clinical trial. *Psychiatry Research, 15,* 239–247.

Walsh, E., Gilvarry, C., Samele, C., Harvey, K., Manley, C., Tyrer, P., et al. (2001, November 10). Reducing violence in severe mental illness: Randomised controlled trial of intensive case management compared with standard care. *BMJ, 323,* 1–5.

Watt, B. D., & Howells, K. (1999). Skills training for aggression control: Evaluation of an anger management programme for violent offenders. *Legal and Criminological Psychology, 4,* 285–300.

Webster, C. D., Douglas, K. S., Eaves, D., & Hart, S. D. (1997). *HCR–20: Assessing risk for violence* (Version 2). Burnaby, British Columbia, Canada: Mental Health, Law, and Policy Institute, Simon Fraser University.

Wilson, D., Tien, G., & Eaves, D. (1995). Increasing the community tenure of mentally disordered offenders: An assertive case management program. *International Journal of Law and Psychiatry, 18,* 61–69.

Yates, K., Kunz, M., Czobor, P., Rabinowitz, S., Lindenmayer, J.-P., & Volavka, J. (2005). A cognitive, behaviorally based program for patients with persistent mental illness and a history of aggression, crime, or both: Structure and correlates of completers of the program. *Journal of the American Academy of Psychiatry and the Law, 33,* 214–222.

17

PSYCHOLOGICAL–BEHAVIORAL TREATMENT WITH VICTIMS OF INTERPERSONAL VIOLENCE

MONICA M. FITZGERALD, MICHAEL R. McCART,
AND DEAN G. KILPATRICK

Violence is an inevitable part of human experience. Virtually no one escapes at least vicarious exposure to severe interpersonal conflict, and surveys of the general population suggest that 50% to 70% of individuals in the United States have experienced at least one form of interpersonal violence or criminal victimization during their lifetime (Kessler, Sonnega, Bromet, Hughes, & Nelson, 1995; Kilpatrick et al., 2003; Resnick, Kilpatrick, Dansky, Saunders, & Best, 1993). Interpersonal violence can take many forms—physical assault, robbery, intimate partner violence, sexual harassment, rape, and other sexual assault. Typically, interpersonal violence is defined to include violence between family members and intimate partners and violence between acquaintances and strangers that is not intended to further the aims of any formally defined group or cause. Thus, self-directed violence, war, state-sponsored violence, and other collective types of violence are excluded from this definition (Waters et al., 2004). Victims of interpersonal violence are at increased risk of developing a range of problems that impact emotional, psychological, behavioral, and physical health functioning (Felitti et al., 1998;

Riggs, Rothbaum, & Foa, 1995). Interpersonal violence also has a tremendous economic cost for societies in which it occurs (Bureau of Justice Statistics, 2002; Centers for Disease Control and Prevention, 2003; National Institute of Justice, 1996; Waters et al., 2004).

The most common adverse consequences for victims of interpersonal violence include extreme levels of anxiety and depression and impaired interpersonal and vocational functioning (Coker et al., 2002; Nelson et al., 2002; Resnick et al., 1993). Research indicates that most individuals will experience a decrease in psychological symptoms within a few days or weeks of a traumatic event (Bonanno, 2004). However, up to 33% of adult victims of interpersonal violence may go on to develop more chronic psychiatric problems, particularly posttraumatic stress disorder (PTSD; Kessler et al., 1995; Kilpatrick et al., 2003). For these individuals, formal treatment is often needed to facilitate recovery to healthy levels of functioning.

According to the *Diagnostic and Statistical Manual of Mental Disorders* (*DSM–IV–TR*; 4th ed., text rev.; American Psychiatric Association, 2000), PTSD is characterized by (a) reliving the traumatic event or frightening elements of it; (b) avoidance of thoughts, memories, people, and places associated with the event; (c) emotional numbing; and (d) symptoms of elevated arousal that persist for more than 1 month following a traumatic stressor. Individuals who experience interpersonal victimization are at greater risk of developing PTSD compared with victims of other types of trauma, such as motor vehicle accidents and natural disasters (Resnick et al., 1993). Individuals exposed to multiple types of interpersonal victimization are also at greater risk of developing PTSD than those exposed to a single event (Hedtke et al., 2008; Saunders, 2003). Furthermore, individuals with lower levels of social support are typically at greater risk of the development of PTSD compared with those with higher levels of support (Acierno et al., 2007; Norris & Kaniasty, 1996). Other common psychiatric correlates of interpersonal victimization that are often comorbid with PTSD include major depression and substance abuse or dependence (Cascardi, O'Leary, & Schlee, 1999; Kilpatrick et al., 1997, 2000, 2003). In fact, national epidemiological research has shown that 80% of individuals with lifetime PTSD also experience lifetime depression, another anxiety disorder, or chemical abuse or dependence (Foa, Keane, & Friedman, 2000).

A number of promising cognitive–behavioral interventions implemented soon after a traumatic event (i.e., within 4 weeks) appear to accelerate the recovery process among victims of trauma and reduce their risk of developing longer term mental health problems such as PTSD (e.g., see Bryant et al., 2006; Foa, Hearst-Ikeda, & Perry, 1995). These early interventions are described in detail in chapter 8 of this volume; however, in this chapter we limit our discussion to evidence-based treatments (EBTs) that are typically recommended when at least 1 month has passed since the index event. Victims of interpersonal violence often do not seek treatment until many months or years after the traumatic event has occurred and many experience PTSD symptoms for an extended period of time. Fortunately, a number of interventions are currently available that reduce chronic PTSD symptoms among these victims. In this chapter we begin by describing important aspects of creating a safe, therapeutic environment for victims to engage in assessment and treatment. Next, we describe core treatment components and strategies effective for adult victims of interpersonal violence with PTSD, as well as three empirically supported treatment programs that incorporate some or all these techniques into a single intervention package. We also briefly discuss commonly used interventions that have limited theoretical and empirical support. Finally, we discuss several integrated EBTs for individuals with comorbid psychiatric disorders.

INITIATING ASSESSMENT AND TREATMENT WITH VICTIMS

The Therapeutic Environment

An important aspect of effective assessment and treatment for victims of interpersonal violence is providing and ensuring safety. Victims of violence often feel vulnerable to danger, and they navigate their environment with a compromised sense of safety (Briere & Scott, 2006; Herman, 1997). In addition, victims seeking treatment may live in a chaotic, unsafe setting. Therefore, before initiating formal treatment it is important for a clinician to assess the victim's perceived sense of safety and the actual likelihood of physical danger within his or her environment (Little, 2000). At this time, the clinician should also assess any current medical problems or concerns, such as physical injuries or medical conditions that require immediate attention.

Another immediate safety concern for clinicians to assess is whether the victim is suicidal or a potential danger to others. Before initiating formal treatment, a clinician should routinely assess the presence of suicidal and homicidal ideation, self-destructive and impulsive behaviors, as well as any severe psychosis such as thought disturbances, delusions, and hallucinations. These behaviors require immediate interventions focused on stabilization and often require referrals or triage to emergency medical or psychiatric services, law enforcement, or social service resources. Chapter 8 of this volume contains a more detailed discussion of strategies for managing acute safety concerns among victims of violence.

Initial and Ongoing Assessment

The purpose of the initial screening and assessment process is to make decisions regarding the most appropriate first intervention or referral for victims of violence. Initial assessment involves gathering information about an individual's current safety level, victimization history, mental health status, functional impairment, and current substance use. Ongoing assessment is also important and should be a standard part of any type of treatment. A victim's symptoms and concerns may, and we hope will, change over the course of therapy. It is often helpful for a victim to observe the progress he or she is making in treatment, and ongoing assessment will make that possible.

When assessing for PTSD and other psychiatric problems experienced by victims, use of validated assessment measures is important. As assessment needs change, measurement selection may also change. For example, some measures are specifically designed to facilitate clinical diagnoses, whereas others may correspond less directly to *DSM–IV–TR* criteria. If a measure is being selected for diagnostic purposes, clearly an interview that corresponds to *DSM–IV–TR* criteria is warranted. If sensitivity to treatment change is a key goal, a measure with a reasonably short time frame for symptom endorsement (e.g., the past week) and the ability to allow symptom scaling (e.g., intensity rating of 0–7 for a given symptom) is preferable to a measure that uses a longer time frame (e.g., past 6 months). In sum, three domains should be considered when choosing an assessment measure: (a) reliability and validity, (b) diagnostic sensitivity and specificity, and (c) sensitivity to treatment change. The last point is critical for treatment providers using assessment measures as markers of treatment progress. Both the rating scale and variability and the time frame of the measure should be considered (see Acierno, Byrne, Resnick, & Kilpatrick, 1998, for a more detailed discusison). Examples of brief, well-validated self-report measures for assessing trauma related symptomatology in adults include the PTSD Symptom Scale—Self-Report (Foa, Riggs, Dancu, & Rothbaum, 1993), the Trauma Assessment for Adults—Self-Report (Resnick, Falsetti, Kilpatrick, & Freedy, 1996), the Impact of Event Scale—Revised (Weiss & Marmar, 1997), the Beck Anxiety Inventory (Beck & Steer, 1991), and the Beck Depression Inventory (Beck, Ward, Mendelson, Mock, & Erbaugh, 1961). Examples of useful self-report measures that correspond directly to *DSM–IV–TR* symptom criteria for PTSD include the Posttraumatic Diagnostic Scale (Foa, Cashman, Jaycox, & Perry, 1997), the PTSD Checklist (Gorski, 2001), and the Davidson Trauma Questionnaire (Davidson et al., 1997). A variety of semistructured interviews are also currently available to assess symptoms of PTSD in adults, such as the Clinician-Administered PTSD Scale (Blake et al., 1995; Weathers, Keane, & Davidson, 2001) and the PTSD Symptom Scale—Interview Version (Foa et al., 1993). The topic of PTSD assessment is well described in the literature (see Briere, 2004; Orsillo, 2001; Wilson & Keane, 2004).

Other features associated with PTSD that should be considered during the assessment process include difficulties in interpersonal relationships; problems with modulation of affect; "survivor guilt"; self-destructive and impulsive behaviors; dissociative symptoms; somatic complaints; feelings of shame, anger, despair, and hopelessness; and social withdrawal (Andrews, Brewin, Rose, & Kirk, 2000; van der Kolk, Roth, Pelcovitz, Sunday, & Spinazzola, 2005). Furthermore, PTSD is associated with higher rates of major depressive disorders, substance abuse, panic disorder, agoraphobia, obsessive–compulsive disorder, social phobia, specific phobia, and somatization disorder (Foa, Keane, & Friedman, 2000). The temporal relationship of onset among these disorders is unclear, however. That is, traumatic events may increase the risk of multiple types of mental health problems, developing PTSD may create a vulnerability to other forms of psychological difficulties, or the presence of other psychopathology may create a vulnerability to PTSD. Overall, good clinical practice dictates that the best treatment for victims experiencing PTSD and comorbid symptoms is one that might be expected to ameliorate both (Foa et al., 2000). Thus, when conducting psychological assessment with victims of interpersonal violence, clinicians should assess a wide range of trauma-related disturbances and routinely administer more general, standardized measures of anxiety, depression, and panic (see Briere & Scott, 2006, for a review of available measures). Finally, clinicians should be aware of the impact of culture on the experience of trauma and expression of posttraumatic stress symptoms and familiarize themselves with culture-bound syndromes (Marsella, Friedman, Gerrity, & Scurfield, 1996).

Initiating Treatment: Clinical Considerations

As discussed previously, PTSD-specific treatment is begun only after the victim has been safely removed from a crisis situation. Similarly, if a victim is severely depressed or suicidal, is experiencing extreme panic or disorganized thinking, or is in need of drug or alcohol detoxification, it is important to address these crisis problems as a part of the first phase of treatment. Most PTSD-specific intervention protocols recommend that treatment be initiated only when victims have achieved a few months of sobriety, but data do not exist to support the notion that concurrent treatment for substance abuse and PTSD is contraindicated. One set of cognitive–behavioral approaches used with trauma victims involves dealing directly with strong emotions and painful memories and exposure of individuals (either in vivo or in imagination) to feared stimuli that are associated with the traumatic event during therapy. This process facilitates reduced responding to the traumatic event and related stimuli and promotes recovery (Foa & Rothbaum, 1998; Resick & Schnicke, 1996). Thus, individuals who live in extreme poverty (e.g., having no shelter or food) or actively use substances to relieve stress or avoid unpleasant emotions may not be able to tolerate the additional distress sometimes activated by the exposure component (Briere & Scott, 2006). Victims may become overwhelmed and use substances to cope with unpleasant feelings, cognitions, or painful memories that arise in therapy (Resick & Schnicke, 1996). Therefore, if severe chemical abuse or dependency is present, it should be addressed before PTSD treatment is initiated (Foa et al., 2000). Most existing treatment programs do not attempt to treat the two disorders simultaneously. However, trauma-focused intervention protocols that integrate PTSD and substance abuse treatments are evolving (e.g., see Back, Dansky, Carroll, Foa, & Brady, 2001; Brady, Dansky, Back, Foa, & Carroll, 2001; Najavits, 2002).

Establishing a Collaborative Relationship

Establishing a working relationship that is genuinely collaborative is essential for supporting effective psychological assessment and treatment with victims of violence (Foa & Rothbaum, 1998). The willingness of a client to open up and express his or her concerns, fears, anger, sadness, and other reactions related to the traumatic events he or she has experienced is likely to be increased by a positive, collaborative relationship and to be decreased by an evaluative, hierarchical, or coercive relationship. Moreover, effective interventions are based on imaginal and in vivo exposure to feared stimuli, and a good therapeutic relationship characterized by high levels of trust will likely result in elevated motivation and adherence to uncomfortable or anxiety-provoking treatment procedures. However, victims may have difficulties entering into and sustaining a working relationship with a clinician because of a difficulty trusting others, especially authority figures (Briere & Scott, 2006). Thus, a clinician should consistently attempt to promote and communicate respect, empathy, safety, and support, as well as refrain from judgment. Focusing on rapport building to initiate a therapeutic alliance and maintaining a positive and consistent therapeutic relationship will serve the clinician well in engaging the victim across the course of treatment. In fact, a strong therapeutic alliance is associated with positive therapeutic outcomes (Lambert & Bergin, 1994) such as decreased treatment dropout rates, more reliable session attendance, greater treatment adherence and medication compliance, less avoidance and more capacity to tolerate painful thoughts and feelings (e.g., see American Psychiatric Association, 2001; Farber & Hall, 2002; Rau & Goldfried, 1994). Finally, taking into consideration a victim's sociocultural background, ethnicity, and religious beliefs is also an important part of forming a therapeutic alliance and collaborative therapeutic relationship. The effectiveness of treatment may depend on the extent to which victims or their families see therapy as sensitive to, and consistent with, their values (Kinzie, 2004; Marsella et al., 1996).

Psychotherapy Treatment Components

There are several core treatment components shared among different evidence-based, trauma-focused interventions that are effective in improving outcomes among victims of interpersonal violence with PTSD and other psychological sequelae (Amstadter, McCart, & Ruggiero, 2007; Foa, Davidson, & Frances, 1999; Foa et al., 2000; Rothbaum, Meadows, Resick, & Foy, 2000). These techniques include (a) *psychoeducation*, (b) *anxiety management training* (AMT), (c) *exposure therapy*, and (d) *cognitive therapy*. These four techniques are rarely used in isolation and are more commonly used in combination in the context of various interventions. These components may be conceptualized as the "active ingredients" of empirically supported treatments or EBTs, or "treatments that work." EBTs are those with written protocols that have been tested in well-controlled clinical trials and generate better outcomes than passage of time, usual care, or alternative interventions (see Borkovec & Castonguay, 1998, for a discussion about EBTs). EBTs are structured, behavioral, and goal-oriented. They involve working with individuals to identify target problems, set goals, measure progress toward goals, build specific coping skills through practice, and give specific behavioral assignments. EBTs involve manualized treatment protocols that are sometimes criticized as too rigid and less useful for real-world clinical practice for clinicians treating individuals with complex presentations. However, these treatment protocols can be powerful tools when they are tailored to meet specific characteristics and concerns of the individual (Castonguay, Schut, Constantino, & Halperin, 1999; Cloitre, Koenen, Cohen, & Han, 2002). Tailoring mental health treatment to each victim's needs while maintaining adequate fidelity to evidence-based components within the treatment protocol likely contributes to the optimal mental health outcomes.

CORE INTERVENTION TECHNIQUES

Psychoeducation

Psychoeducation involves providing victims with accurate information about the nature and prevalence of interpersonal victimization and common reactions after a traumatic event (McFarlane, 2001). The cognitive and emotional reactions experienced by victims of interpersonal violence often include anxiety, shock, anger, confusion, and self-blame. Victims of violence may have misinformation that is feeding into their cognitive and emotional responding. Psychoeducation can help validate clients' experiences, normalize their reactions, and dispel faulty beliefs, all of which are associated with positive posttrauma functioning. The major topics covered in the psychoeducation process include describing the prevalence of the trauma, common myths associated with trauma and its effects, the most common reasons perpetrators engage in interpersonal violence, and common immediate and long-term reactions to trauma (Briere & Scott, 2006). Psychoeducation is often presented to victims early in treatment. However, psychoeducation should also be provided on an ongoing, as needed basis whenever victims may benefit from additional information or evince cognitive distortions about the trauma. Typically, clinicians provide psychoeducation verbally. However, printed materials and handouts outlining common reactions to victimization and its effects are helpful tools for educating victims and are widely available to consumers and clinicians on the Internet (e.g., see http://www.istss.org). However, handouts should not be considered stand-alone sources of information; instead, clinicians should tailor the information to make it relevant to the victim. Overall, it is most helpful if the exchange of information is didactic and interactive. For examples of how to present psychoeducation to victims, see Briere and Scott (2006), Foa and Rothbaum (1998), and Resick and Schnicke (1996).

Anxiety Management Training

AMT involves teaching strategies to victims to reduce overall levels of anxiety and cope with trauma-related distress (Briere & Scott, 2006; Foa & Meadows, 1997). These techniques may help victims' ability to cope with acute, destabilizing emotions and symptoms that emerge throughout treatment. AMT techniques may also build victims' general emotion regulation skills or their skills for handling negative feelings and managing distress. These approaches are sometimes termed *distress reduction skills training* or *affect regulation skills training* (Cloitre, Heffernan, Cohen, & Alexander, 2001; Linehan, 1993). One widely used AMT-based intervention is stress inoculation training (Meichenbaum, 1974). Regardless of the label, anxiety management approaches all focus on "the client's increased capacity to tolerate and downregulate painful emotional states, both during treatment and in his or her ongoing life" (Briere & Scott, 2006, p. 96). Anxiety management interventions are typically introduced early in treatment and are used throughout the treatment process. AMT most often involves teaching victims relaxation skills such as *breathing retraining* (or diaphragmatic breathing) and *progressive muscle relaxation* (PMR). As part of AMT, clinicians also work with victims on increasing their capacity to regulate emotions in their daily lives and how to counter negative cognitions, given that they often exacerbate or trigger trauma-related emotions (Cloitre et al., 2002).

Breathing Retraining

Teaching breathing techniques to victims is important because individuals with anxiety-related problems often show signs of hyperventilation (or overbreathing; Craske, Barlow, & O'Leary, 1992). When distressed, these individuals breathe with rapid, shallow breaths in the upper chest region. Some temporarily stop breathing altogether. This type of breathing can disrupt the balance of oxygen and carbon dioxide in the body, leading to strong somatic sensations (e.g., dizziness, blurred vision) and heightened anxiety. Breathing exercises aim to reduce hyperventilation or inappropriate ventilation by teaching clients to engage in slow, regular, rhythmic abdominal breathing whenever they experience elevated levels of tension or stress. When individuals learn to breathe more efficiently, they often experience a calming effect. Clinicians typically begin breathing retraining by guiding individuals through basic breathing exercises so they become more attuned to their breathing patterns and increase their capacity to modulate and calm their respiration. Often clinicians teach individuals repetitive associations and relaxation cues (e.g., choosing a calming word) to facilitate breathing control and relaxation. Victims initially practice using these skills in nonstressful situations so they can apply them successfully in stressful situations, such as times they encounter a trauma cue (e.g., see someone who looks like the perpetrator of violence). There are a number of other useful strategies recommended to facilitate the mastery of breathing control and relaxation (e.g., see Best & Ribbe, 1995), and many resources are available for clinicians using trauma treatment, including manuals with written scripts, music, and guided relaxation tapes (e.g., see Davis, Eshelman, & McKay, 2000; Foa & Rothbaum, 1998; Payne, 2005).

Progressive Muscle Relaxation

PMR is another commonly used anxiety management technique that involves teaching clients to distinguish between feelings of tension and relaxation by engaging in different tension-reduction exercises for each major muscle group. During PMR, individuals are guided to contract and then release muscles sequentially from head to toe until the entire body reaches a relaxed state (Rimm & Masters, 1979). Individuals are also taught to pair cue words (e.g., *relax, calm*) or a pleasant image (e.g., the beach) with feelings of relaxation, and they are encouraged to focus on these cues whenever they experience anxiety or distress (e.g., see Davis et al., 2000; Payne, 2005).

Additional Anxiety Management Training Components

In addition to breathing retraining and PMR, clinicians often work with individuals on increasing their general emotion regulation skills (e.g., see Cloitre et al., 2002). Helping individuals correctly label and discriminate their feeling states is a key component of successful affect regulation (Linehan, 1993). Victims of chronic interpersonal violence may have difficulty identifying what they are feeling in emotionally arousing situations and may have an overly simplistic understanding of their feeling states (e.g., "I feel bad") and inaccurate differentiation of their primary or secondary emotions (e.g., differentiating anger from fear, sadness, or disappointment). Thus, a beneficial component of treatment may be to help victims develop emotional awareness and build their skills for handling unpleasant feeling states and managing distress (Cloitre et al., 2002). AMT may also integrate cognitive interventions given that thoughts often exacerbate or trigger trauma-related emotions. For example, the technique of cognitive restructuring involves helping victims identify and counter unhelpful cognitions and gain a more realistic, positive perspective. These skills help victims gain an ability to forestall extreme emotional reactivity and regulate emotional experience (Briere & Scott, 2006). Cognitive interventions are described in more detail in the cognitive therapy section later in this chapter.

Clinical Considerations

In the treatment of victims of interpersonal violence with PTSD, anxiety management techniques (e.g., breathing retraining, PMR) alone are not likely to significantly reduce trauma-related symptoms. Other key therapeutic activities such as exposure are required (Rothbaum et al., 2000). Furthermore, some victims may have negative reactions, increased anxiety, or dissociative reactions to induced relaxation or may not be able to achieve a relaxed state (Allen, 2001). For example, relaxation training may be less helpful for victims who are chronically overwhelmed by flashbacks and other reexperiencing symptoms (Taylor, 2003). Overall, relaxation training may be helpful for many victims, but clinicians should monitor victims' responses and any increased arousal during these exercises (Briere & Scott, 2006).

Exposure Therapy

Exposure therapy is a cognitive–behavioral intervention technique that involves direct exposure of individuals, either in vivo or in imagination, to feared stimuli that are associated with the traumatic event. These feared stimuli (i.e., trauma cues) can include objects, people, places, situations, or information that reminds victims of the traumatic event or upsetting memories or thoughts of the traumatic event. Exposure therapy should occur in the context of a safe and supportive therapeutic environment. During exposure exercises, individuals are exposed only to stimuli that are objectively harmless (e.g., do not conduct in vivo exposure exercises in dangerous locations).

As mentioned, imaginal and in vivo forms of exposure therapy are often used for victims with PTSD. Imaginal exposure is often described as "reliving the trauma." This procedure involves the use of careful, repeated, detailed imagining of the traumatic event(s) in a safe, controlled context to help victims face and gain control of the fear and distress that was overwhelming during the traumatic event(s). To use conditioning terminology, participants in exposure-based treatments are taught to expose themselves to the conditioned trauma cues until the conditioned anxiety response is extinguished. More specifically, during imaginal exposure the client is instructed to describe the traumatic event in as much detail as possible and focus on the cognitions and emotions he or she experienced during the trauma. Repeated imaginal exposure is thought to facilitate extinction, which refers to the gradual reduction in anxiety over time. This process of deliberately confronting a feared memory in a supportive therapeutic setting may also foster feelings of mastery and courage, and it helps clients realize that the trauma memory is not dangerous. Exposure exercises can also involve victims writing about the traumatic events and reading what they wrote to the clinician (Cloitre et al., 2002; Foa & Rothbaum, 1998; Resick & Schnicke, 1996).

During in vivo exposure, individuals are taught to expose themselves to trauma-related stimuli that cause distress and perpetuate avoidance. Victims typically create a hierarchy of real-life cues such as people, places, or situations that have been paired with the trauma, and they practice exposing themselves to those cues in a graduated fashion. It is critical for victims to expose themselves only to situations that are actually safe. Therefore, the clinician should evaluate the safety of each situation and only safe situations should be included on the hierarchy list (Foa & Rothbaum, 1998). For example, if a rape victim avoids walking in the area in which she was assaulted and the danger level of this neighborhood is relatively high during the day and night, she should not be encouraged to expose herself to this situation.

When engaging victims in any type of exposure therapy, clinicians should routinely measure the victim's distress level before, during, and after each exercise. Rating scales, or "anxiety thermometers," such as Wolpe's (1958) Subjective Units of Discomfort Scale (SUDS; 0–100), are extremely helpful in monitoring individual's discomfort level and progress during exposures inside and outside of session. Exposure exercises should be graduated or titrated on the basis of the intensity of fear the different situations or recalled material provoke.

It is not surprising that many treatment-seeking victims may be wary of activities that involve intentionally "reliving" the trauma and confronting feared situations. This may seem counterintuitive and unsafe to the victim. Before engaging in imaginal or in vivo exposure exercises, it is critical that clinicians provide a strong rationale for the use of exposure and a clear explanation of the process of extinction. The rationale should touch on the importance of repeated exposure for extinction, discrimination between remembering and being retraumatized, and increased mastery (see Foa & Rothbaum, 1998, p. 161). It is helpful to provide victims with several neutral examples and analogies of how exposure and extinction works so they understand that exposure to anxiety-producing situations will result in an eventual decrease in anxiety (see Foa & Rothbaum, 1998, for helpful suggestions and scripts for teaching exposure). It is also important to discuss victims' concerns or any misinformation they may have about engaging in this process. Explaining the gradual and systematic nature of exposures and the collaborative creation of hierarchies may reduce victims' anxiety level related to initiating the process. In addition, clinicians should allow the victim to set the pace and level of detail with which he or she recalls the traumatic event in the initial exposure sessions, and clinicians may want to be available to talk with the victim by telephone between sessions if the exposure exercises cause extreme distress (Foa & Rothbaum, 1998).

Cognitive Therapy

Traditional cognitive therapy aims to alter maladaptive thought patterns that are correlated with individuals' appraisals of their world, other people, and themselves (Beck, 1976). Cognitive theorists assert that when individuals change the way they think about certain events, they may also alter emotional experiences and behavior associated with those events. In trauma-focused treatment, cognitive interventions try to reduce trauma-related anxiety and distress by teaching clients to become aware of negative and maladaptive beliefs associated with their trauma experience (e.g., responsibility, self-blame) and to analyze and modify them through cognitive restructuring techniques. Cognitive restructuring entails teaching clients how to identify, challenge, and alter unhelpful or dysfunctional cognitions. Distorted beliefs that are prevalent among individuals with PTSD include thinking that the world is unsafe, that others are untrustworthy, and that oneself is incompetent (Foa & Riggs, 1993; Janoff-Bulman, 1992). Cognitive processing interventions also help victims integrate the traumatic event with previously constructed schemata or their beliefs about themselves and the world (Resick & Schnicke, 1996). Furthermore, trauma-focused cognitive interventions encourage victims to explore how prior experiences and beliefs were affected by the traumatic experience and influenced their reactions (Resick & Schnicke, 1996).

EMPIRICALLY SUPPORTED TREATMENTS FOR POSTTRAUMATIC STRESS DISORDER

The four core intervention components—psychoeducation, AMT, exposure therapy, and cognitive therapy—are key elements of EBTs for PTSD. To some extent, they are grounded in distinct but overlapping theoretical frameworks and have varying levels of empirical support. Often these components have not been isolated in efficacy research. Rather, various combinations of these strategies have been used in comprehensive treatment approaches designed for victims of violence. We now briefly describe three empirically supported treatment programs for PTSD that incorporate some or all of the four core treatment techniques into a single intervention package: *prolonged exposure* (PE), *cognitive processing therapy* (CPT), and *stress inoculation training* (SIT). We also briefly discuss three other interventions that are often used with traumatized populations but have limited theoretical and empirical support for the treatment of trauma-related symptoms in adults: *eye movement desensitization and reprocessing* (EMDR), *hypnotherapy*, and *psychodynamic therapy* (Amstadter et al., 2007).

Prolonged Exposure

PE (Foa & Rothbaum, 1998) has received considerable empirical support in the treatment of crime-related PTSD (see reviews by Foa, Davidson,

& Frances 1999; Foa et al., 2000). In addition to reducing PTSD symptoms, PE also reduces symptoms of depression, anxiety (Foa, Davidson, & Frances, 1999; Foa et al., 2005; Foa, Rothbaum, Riggs, & Murdock, 1991), and guilt (Resick, Nishith, Weaver, Astin, & Feuer, 2002). Furthermore, the effectiveness of PE has been established in both academic and community clinic settings (Foa et al., 2005), supporting the applicability of this intervention approach.

Generally, PE involves 8 to 12 sessions, each lasting 60 to 120 minutes. Clients are initially presented with a conceptualization that PTSD symptoms are a learned set of fear-related behavioral responses, and exposure therapy is based on unlearning these responses. Psychoeducation is provided through various stages of the intervention and is featured toward the beginning of treatment. Diaphragmatic breathing and other anxiety management techniques may also be taught in the early phases of treatment. The remaining sessions are devoted to imaginal and in vivo exposure exercises. During imaginal exposure, the client is instructed to close his or her eyes and imagine the traumatic event in great detail, attending to cues in all five senses. He or she is instructed to describe the event in vivid detail using first person present tense while providing periodic ratings of distress using a SUDS ranging from 0 (*no anxiety/distress*) to 100 (*highest anxiety/distress imaginable*). The therapist encourages the client to focus on "hot spots" in the traumatic event narrative, or areas that elicit the most emotion. In a typical therapy session, exposure exercises last 45 to 60 minutes. After a significant decrease in distress has been achieved, a cool-down phase begins that prepares the client for leaving the clinic. Often the trauma narrative is audio-recorded and the client is instructed to listen to the tape at home between sessions. Therapists also have clients construct a hierarchy of fearful activities to be used as in vivo homework assignments throughout treatment. For many clients, this combination of AMT, imaginal exposure, and in vivo exposure is sufficient to yield a reduction in PTSD symptoms. Others, however, may continue to experience dysfunctional thoughts about their traumatic event that produce feelings of guilt and shame (Andrews et al., 2000). For these individuals, cognitive restructuring techniques may be needed to help modify automatic negative thoughts and cognitive distortions (Foa & Rothbaum, 1998).

Many misconceptions regarding exposure-based interventions exist (e.g., exposure elevates symptoms, exposure results in a high dropout rate compared with other interventions, exposure is not tolerated well). These positions have limited empirical backing. First, rigorous scientific investigations have not yielded evidence that exposure intensifies client distress or PTSD symptoms over time (e.g., see Foa, Davidson, & Frances, 1999; Foa et al., 1991, 2005; Foa, Zoellner, Feeny, Hembree, & Alvarez-Conrad, 2002). Moreover, the initial increase in distress in the early sessions is actually associated with superior posttreatment outcomes (Foa et al., 2002). Second, studies comparing exposure therapy to other interventions show that dropout is comparable (e.g., Resick et al., 2002). A recent meta-analysis of PTSD treatments reported equal attrition rates across the different intervention types (Van Etten & Taylor, 1998). Third, exposure therapy had higher perceived treatment desirability compared with medication or no treatment options (Zoellner, Feeny, Cochran, & Pruitt, 2003).

A few client characteristics have been associated with the overall efficacy of exposure therapy for PTSD. These characteristics include anger, substance abuse, and dissociative symptoms. Symptoms of anger and irritability are common among adults with PTSD, and clients often experience a reduction in these symptoms following PE (Cahill, Rauch, Hembree, & Foa, 2003). However, if anger is too extreme, it can interfere with one's ability to experience other trauma-related emotions such as anxiety and fear (Foa, Riggs, Massie, & Yarczower, 1995). One strategy for addressing this problem is to encourage clients to suspend any discussion of their anger until exposure-based exercises are complete (Coffey, Schumacher, Brimo, & Brady, 2005). Adults who find this difficult may benefit from anger management techniques prior to initiating exposure therapy. Clients with severe dissociative symptoms may also experience limited benefit during exposure-based treatment. Grounding techniques aimed at reducing cognitive avoidance can be used to enhance the effectiveness of exposure for these clients (Coffey et al., 2005). Examples of grounding techniques include squeezing an object, counting items in a room, or any other activity that heightens clients' awareness of the immediate environment. Research is limited with regard to the efficacy of PE for individuals with comorbid substance abuse. If substances are used as an avoidance strategy, the initial distress that often occurs during the early stages of exposure may increase risk of drug or alcohol use. Foa and Rothbaum (1998) recommended at least 90 days of sobriety and ongoing support from substance abuse treatment providers before initiating PE. However, this remains a controversial issue, one that research has not yet adequately resolved (Back et al., 2001; Brady et al., 2001).

Cognitive Processing Therapy

CPT (Resick & Schnicke, 1992) is a cognitive–behavioral treatment that has received empirical support for use with rape victims. CPT significantly reduces PTSD and depressive symptoms when compared with a wait-list control group (Resick & Schnicke, 1992). In a more recent randomized controlled trial, Resick et al. (2002) compared CPT and PE for rape victims with PTSD. Both treatments were equally effective and superior to a minimal attention comparison condition. Resick (2001) has also adapted CPT for more general use with individuals who experienced other types of traumatic events and traumatic bereavement.

CPT typically consists of 12 sessions conducted in an individual or group-based format. Treatment begins with psychoeducation regarding PTSD responses, information processing theory, and basic emotions. After the first session, clients are instructed to write a brief summary of their thoughts and feelings regarding the traumatic event. In this summary, they are asked to consider any effects the traumatic event may have had on their attitudes about the world, others, and themselves. Clients are also encouraged to comment on changes they have experienced regarding their beliefs about safety, trust, power, competence, esteem, and intimacy. Over the next few sessions, clients practice using A-B-C (i.e., activating events, beliefs, and consequences) worksheets to become more aware of the connections between their thoughts, feelings, and behavior. Additional sessions focus on the creation of a trauma narrative. Clients are instructed to write about their traumatic experience(s) and to include information on sensations, thoughts, and feelings that were present at the time of the event. This is a form of exposure to traumatic fear cues. Clients read their narrative aloud in session, and the clinician encourages them to confront "stuck points" using cognitive restructuring techniques. Stuck points reflect conflicting beliefs or frightening thoughts that interfere with acceptance of the event. The trauma-writing assignment is repeated to facilitate exposure. During the remaining sessions, clients learn how to confront common faulty thinking patterns (e.g., overgeneralization, mind reading, emotional reasoning). Cognitive restructuring techniques are also used to address any remaining thinking patterns related to the themes of safety, trust, power, esteem, and intimacy.

Many client characteristics that are related to the overall efficacy of PE (e.g., severe anger, dissociation, substance abuse problems) may also interfere with the emotional and cognitive processing that takes place during CPT. Resick and Schnicke (1996) highlighted two additional client populations requiring special consideration during treatment: marital rape victims and clients with a comorbid diagnosis of borderline personality disorder (BPD). In addition, people with limited cognitive abilities may have difficulties engaging in cognitive restructuring techniques.

Marital rape victims are likely to have a history of multiple sexual assaults, and they often present to therapy in the middle of complicated divorce or custody battles. These individuals may require more than the standard 12 sessions of CPT because multiple trauma narratives are often needed to cover the range of assaults that were experienced. More extensive work is also recommended for clients who blame themselves for their repeat victimization and criticize themselves for not leaving their husbands sooner (Resick & Schnicke, 1996).

Trauma victims presenting with a diagnosis of BPD also require special consideration during treatment. Because these clients are generally considered poor candidates for group-based interventions, CPT is more likely to be effective if it is delivered in an individualized format. If the client with BPD has difficulty remaining focused on his or her trauma or presents with frequent parasuicidal behavior, he or she may need to be referred to a longer term treatment program that focuses more directly on the borderline tendencies (e.g., dialectical behavior therapy; Linehan, 1993).

Stress Inoculation Training

SIT (Meichenbaum, 1974) is a multifaceted cognitive–behavioral intervention for anxiety that has been effectively adapted for use with crime victims (e.g., see Veronen & Kilpatrick, 1983). Existing data provide a moderate level of support for the efficacy of SIT in reducing symptoms of PTSD in female sexual assault survivors (Foa et al., 1991; see also Foa et al., 2000, for a review). A study examining the differential effectiveness of SIT, PE, and the combination of SIT and PE with a sample of women who had experienced either sexual or nonsexual assault found that the three interventions produced similar reductions on measures of PTSD and depression, and all were superior to a wait-list control group. Nevertheless, PE was more effective than SIT and PE–SIT on several other key measures of treatment outcome (Foam, Dancu, et al., 1999).

Generally, SIT entails 8 to 15 sessions, with booster sessions occurring for up to a year posttreatment. According to the developers of SIT, individuals may experience excessive anxiety when they perceive themselves as unable to cope with environmental stressors. Thus, SIT aims to reduce anxiety by fostering clients' stress management skills.

SIT has three phases: (a) conceptualization, (b) skill acquisition, and (c) application (Meichenbaum, 1994). The conceptualization phase is aimed at providing psychoeducation regarding relations between behavior, emotions, cognitions, and environmental stressors. During the skill acquisition phase, clients learn a variety of emotion-relevant and cognitive coping techniques (e.g., emotion regulation, relaxation, cognitive restructuring). During the application phase, clients are provided with opportunities to apply their skills in anxiety provoking situations. When applied to victims of crime, clients use their SIT skills to manage symptoms of PTSD. These skills are thought to reduce distress and, collaterally, make avoidance of trauma-relevant cues less likely.

Although a handful of studies (two well-controlled studies) provide support for the effectiveness of SIT, all these studies included female sexual assault survivors. Therefore, the efficacy of SIT with other trauma populations is unknown at this time (Rothbaum et al., 2000).

Other Treatments for Posttraumatic Stress Disorder

PE, CPT, and SIT have all received support for efficacy in the context of methodologically rigorous research (i.e., well-designed randomized controlled trials). However, there are other interventions that are often used with traumatized populations in real world settings that have achieved varying levels of empirical support for the treatment of trauma-related symptoms in adults: EMDR (Shapiro, 1989, 1995), hypnotherapy (Brom, Kleber, & Defres, 1989), and psychodynamic therapy (Marmar, Foy, Kagan, & Pynoos, 1994). For a review of expert consensus on these treatments and guidelines on best practices in the treatment of PTSD, see Foa, Davidson, and Frances (1999) and Foa et al. (2000).

Comorbidity

Given the high prevalence of comorbidity between PTSD and other psychiatric disorders (Kessler et al., 1995; McFarlane, 2001), such as major depression (Kessler et al., 1995), panic disorder (Falsetti, Resnick, Dansky, Lydiard, & Kilpatrick, 1995), and substance use disorder (Dansky, Saladin, Brady, Kilpatrick, & Resnick, 1995), there is a growing body of research on interventions for treating dual diagnoses. Emerging data suggest that trauma-focused interventions such as PE and CPT may be sufficient to reduce symptoms of depression and prevalence of depression comorbidity among adult victims of crime (Foa, Davidson, and Frances, 1999; Resick, Nishith, et al., 2002). However, panic disorder symptoms and substance abuse problems tend to be less responsive to trauma-focused interventions, and the literature points to the value of combined intervention techniques for these comorbid psychological problems (Falsetti, Resnick, & Davis, 2005; Kofoed, Friedmen, & Peck, 1993). *Multiple-channel exposure therapy* (M-CET) represents an example of an integrated intervention technique that was specifically designed to target emotional, behavioral, and physiological symptoms experienced by individuals with PTSD and panic attacks (Falsetti & Resnick, 1997a, 1997b). This 12-session intervention combines elements of panic control treatment, a widely used treatment for panic developed by Barlow and Craske (1988), and CPT (Resick & Schnicke, 1996) for PTSD. M-CET was developed because interventions aimed solely at PTSD are unlikely to address the physiological cues that can trigger anxiety and panic attack symptoms in individuals with panic disorder. In a randomized controlled trial, M-CET was superior to a wait-list control condition in reducing symptoms of PTSD and panic among women exposed to different traumatic events (e.g., natural disasters, sexual assault, physical assault; Falsetti, Resnick, Davis, & Gallagher, 2001). Other integrated EBTs for PTSD and comorbid disorders, such as substance abuse problems, also have received preliminary support (Brady et al., 2001; Najavits, 2002).

CONCLUSION

In summation, a substantial proportion of adults who have experienced interpersonal violence develop mental health problems and are in need of effective treatments. Mental health intervention with victims can ameliorate current problems and reduce the likelihood that others will develop. Fortunately, a number of effective, EBTs are available for adults who have experienced traumatic events, and clinicians may draw on many resources to provide the highest quality of mental health services to their clients in a variety of settings.

REFERENCES

Acierno, R., Byrne, K., Resnick, H., & Kilpatrick, D. G. (1998). Adult victims of physical assault. In A. S. Bellack & M. Hersen (Eds.), *Comprehensive clinical psychology* (Vol. 9, pp. 307–324). New York: Pergamon Press.

Acierno, R., Ruggiero, K. J., Galea, S., Resnick, H. S., Koenen, K., Roitzsch, J., et al. (2007). Psychological sequelae resulting from the 2004 Florida hurricanes: Implications for postdisaster intervention. *American Journal of Public Health, 97*(Suppl. 1), 103–108.

Allen, J. G. (2001). *Traumatic relationships and serious mental disorders.* Chichester, England: Wiley.

American Psychiatric Association. (2000). *Diagnostic and statistical manual of mental disorders* (4th ed., text rev.). Washington, DC: Author.

American Psychiatric Association. (2001). *Practice guideline for the treatment of patients with borderline personality disorder.* Washington, DC: Author.

Amstadter, A. B., McCart, M. R., & Ruggiero, K. J. (2007). Psychosocial interventions for adults with crime-related PTSD. *Professional Psychology: Research and Practice, 38,* 640–651.

Andrews, B., Brewin, C. R., Rose, S., & Kirk, M. (2000). Predicting PTSD symptoms in victims of violent crime: The role of shame, anger, and childhood abuse. *Journal of Abnormal Psychology, 109,* 69–73.

Back, S., Dansky, B. S., Carroll, K., Foa, E. B., & Brady, K. T. (2001). Concurrent treatment of PTSD and cocaine dependence. *Journal of Substance Abuse Treatment, 21,* 35–45.

Barlow, D. H., & Craske, M. G. (1988). *Mastery of your anxiety and panic treatment manual.* Albany, NY: Graywind.

Beck, A. T. (1976). *Cognitive therapy and the emotional disorder.* New York: International University Press.

Beck, A. T., & Steer, R. A. (1991). Relationship between the Beck Anxiety Inventory and the Hamilton Anxiety Rating Scale with anxious outpatients. *Journal of Anxiety Disorders, 5,* 213–223.

Beck, A. T., Ward, C. H., Mendelsohn, M., Mock, J., & Erbaugh, J. (1961). An inventory for measuring depression. *Archives of General Psychiatry, 4,* 561–571.

Best, C. L., & Ribbe, D. P. (1995). Accidental injury: Approaches to assessment and treatment. In J. R. Freedy & S. E. Hobfoll (Eds.), *Traumatic stress: From theory to practice* (pp. 315–337). New York: Guilford Press.

Blake, D. D., Weathers, F. W., Nagy, L. M., Kaloupek, D. G., Gusman, F. D., Charney, D. S., & Keane, T. M. (1995). The development of a Clinician-Administered PTSD Scale. *Journal of Traumatic Stress, 8*, 75–90.

Bonanno, G. A. (2004). Loss, trauma, and human resilience: Have we underestimated the human capacity to thrive after extremely aversive events? *American Psychologist, 59*, 20–28.

Borkovec, T. D., & Castonguay, L. G. (1998). What is the scientific meaning of empirically supported therapy? *Journal of Consulting and Clinical Psychology, 66*, 136–142.

Brady, K. T., Dansky, B. S., Back, S., Foa, E. B., & Carroll, K. (2001). Exposure therapy in the treatment of PTSD among cocaine-dependent individuals: Preliminary findings. *Journal of Substance Abuse Treatment, 21*, 47–54.

Briere, J. (2004). *Psychological assessment of adult posttraumatic stress: Phenomenology, diagnosis, and measurement* (2nd ed.). Washington, DC: American Psychological Association.

Briere, J., & Scott, C. (2006). *Principles of trauma therapy. A guide to symptoms, evaluation, and treatment.* Thousand Oaks, CA: Sage.

Brom, D., Kleber, R. J., & Defres, P. B. (1989). Brief psychotherapy for posttraumatic stress disorder. *Journal of Consulting and Clinical Psychology, 57*, 607–612.

Bryant, R. A., Moulds, M. L., Nixon, R. D. V., Mastrodomenico, J., Felmingham, K., & Hopwood, S. (2006). Hypnotherapy and cognitive–behaviour therapy of acute stress disorder: A 3-year follow-up. *Behaviour Research and Therapy, 44*, 1331–1335.

Bureau of Justice Statistics. (2002). *National crime victimization survey: Personal and property crimes, 2000.* Washington, DC: U.S. Department of Justice.

Cahill, S. P., Rauch, S. A., Hembree, E. A., & Foa, E. B. (2003). Effect of cognitive–behavioral treatments for PTSD on anger. *Journal of Cognitive Psychotherapy, 17*, 113–131.

Campbell, R., Sullivan, C. M., & Davidson, W. S. (1995). Women who use domestic violence shelters: Changes in depression over time. *Psychology of Women Quarterly, 19*, 237–255.

Cascardi, M. A., O'Leary, K. D., & Schlee, K. A. (1999). Co-occurrence and correlates of posttraumatic stress disorder and major depression in physically abused women. *Journal of Family Violence, 14*, 227–249.

Castonguay, L. G., Schut, A. J., Constantino, M. J., & Halperin, G. S. (1999). Assessing the role of treatment manuals: Have they become necessary but nonsufficient ingredients of change? *Clinical Psychology: Science and Practice 6*, 449–455.

Centers for Disease Control and Prevention. (2003). *Costs of intimate partner violence against women in the United States.* Atlanta, GA: Author.

Cloitre, M., Heffernan, K., Cohen, L., & Alexander, L. (2001). *A phase-based treatment for the multiply traumatized.* Unpublished manual, Weill Medical College, Cornell University, Ithaca, New York.

Cloitre, M., Koenen, K. C., Cohen, L. R., & Han, H. (2002). Skills training in affective and interpersonal regulation followed by exposure: A phase-based treatment for PTSD related to childhood abuse. *Journal of Consulting and Clinical Psychology, 70,* 1067–1074.

Coffey, S. F., Saladin, M. E., Drobes, D. J., Brady, K. T., Dansky, B. S., & Kilpatrick, D. G. (2002). Trauma and substance cue reactivity in individuals with comorbid posttraumatic stress disorder and cocaine or alcohol dependence. *Drug and Alcohol Dependence, 65,* 115–127.

Coffey, S. F., Schumacher, J. A., Brimo, M. L., & Brady, K. T. (2005). Exposure therapy for substance abusers with PTSD: Translating research into practice. *Behavior Modification, 29,* 10–38.

Coker, A. L., Davis, K. E., Arias, I., Desai, S., Sanderson, M., Brandt, H. M., & Smith, P. (2002). Physical and mental health effects of intimate partner violence for men and women. *American Journal of Preventive Medicine, 23,* 260–268.

Craske, M. G., Barlow, D. H., & O'Leary, T. A. (1992). *Mastery of your anxiety and panic.* New York: Graywind.

Dansky, B. S., Saladin, M. E., Brady, K. T., Kilpatrick, D. G., & Resnick, H. S. (1995). Prevalence of victimization and posttraumatic stress disorder among women with substance use disorders: Comparison of telephone and in-person assessment samples. *International Journal of Addictions, 30,* 1079–1099.

Davidson, J. R. T., Book, S. W., Colket, J. T., Tupler, L. A., Roth, S. H., David, D., et al. (1997). Assessment of a new self-rating scale for posttraumatic stress disorder. *Psychological Medicine, 27,* 153–160.

Davis, M., Eshelman, E. R., & McKay, M. (2000). *The relaxation and stress reduction workbook* (5th ed.). Oakland, CA: New Harbinger.

Falsetti, S. A., & Resnick, H. S. (1997a). *Multiple channel exposure therapy: Patient manual.* Charleston: Medical University of South Carolina.

Falsetti, S. A., & Resnick, H. S. (1997b). Trauma, posttraumatic stress disorder, and panic attacks: Frequency, severity, and implications for treatment. *Journal of Traumatic Stress, 10,* 683–689.

Falsetti, S. A., Resnick, H. S., Dansky, B. S., Lydiard, R. B., & Kilpatrick, D. G. (1995). The relationship of stress to panic disorder: Cause or effect? In C. M. Mazure (Ed.), *Does stress cause psychiatric illness?* (pp. 111–147). Washington DC: American Psychiatric Press.

Falsetti, S. A., Resnick, H. S., & Davis, J. (2005). Multiple channel exposure therapy: Combining cognitive–behavioral therapies for the treatment of posttraumatic stress disorder with panic attacks. *Behavior Modification, 29,* 70–94.

Falsetti, S. A., Resnick, H. S., Davis, J., & Gallagher, N. G. (2001). Treatment of posttraumatic stress disorder with comorbid panic attacks: Combining cognitive processing therapy with panic control treatment techniques. *Group Dynamics: Theory, Research, and Practice, 5,* 252–260.

Farber, B. A., & Hall, D. (2002). Disclosure to therapists: What is and is not discussed in psychotherapy. *Journal of Clinical Psychology, 58,* 359–370.

Felitti, V. J., Anda, R. F., Nordenberg, D., Williamson, D. F., Spitz, A. M., Edwards, V., et al. (1998). Relationship of childhood abuse and household dysfunction to many of the leading causes of death in adults: The Adverse Childhood Experiences (ACE) Study. *American Journal of Preventive Medicine, 14,* 245–258.

Foa, E. B., Cashman, L., Jaycox, L., & Perry, K. (1997). The validation of a self-report measure of posttraumatic stress disorder: The Posttraumatic Diagnostic Scale. *Psychological Assessment, 9,* 445–451.

Foa, E. B., Dancu, C. V., Hembree, E. A., Jaycox, L. H., Meadows, E. A., & Street, G. P. (1999). A comparison of exposure therapy, stress inoculation training, and their combination for reducing posttraumatic stress disorder in female assault victims. *Journal of Consulting and Clinical Psychology, 67,* 194–200.

Foa, E. B., Davidson, J. R. T., & Frances, A. (Eds.). (1999). The expert consensus guidelines series: Treatment of posttraumatic stress disorder [Special issue]. *Journal of Clinical Psychiatry, 60*(Suppl. 16).

Foa, E. B., Hearst-Ikeda, D., & Perry, K. J. (1995). Evaluation of a brief cognitive–behavioral program for the prevention of chronic PTSD in recurrent assault victims. *Journal of Consulting and Clinical Psychology, 63,* 948–955.

Foa, E. B., Hembree, E. A., Cahill, S. P., Rauch, A. M., Riggs, D. S., Feeny, N. C., & Yadin, E. (2005). Randomized trial of prolonged exposure for posttraumatic stress disorder with and without cognitive restructuring: Outcome at academic and community clinics. *Journal of Consulting and Clinical Psychology, 73,* 953–964.

Foa, E. B., Keane, T. M., & Friedman, N. J. (2000). *Effective treatments for PTSD: Practice guidelines from the International Society for Traumatic Stress Studies.* New York: Guilford Press.

Foa, E. B., & Meadows, E. A. (1997). Psychosocial treatment for posttraumatic stress disorder: A critical review. In J. Spence, J. M. Darley, & D. J. Foss (Eds.), *Annual review of psychology* (Vol. 48, pp. 449–480). Palo Alto, CA: Annual Reviews.

Foa, E. B., & Riggs, D. S. (1993). Post-traumatic stress disorder in rape victims. In J. Oldham, M. B. Riba, & A. Tasman (Eds.), *American Psychiatric Press review of psychiatry* (Vol. 12, pp. 273–303). Washington, DC: American Psychiatric Press.

Foa, E. B., Riggs, D. S., Dancu, C. V., & Rothbaum, B. O. (1993). Reliability and validity of a brief instrument for assessing post-traumatic stress disorder. *Journal of Traumatic Stress, 6,* 459–473.

Foa, E. B., Riggs, D. S., Massie, E. D., & Yarczower, M. (1995). The impact of fear activation and anger on efficacy of exposure treatment for PTSD. *Behavior Therapy, 26,* 487–499.

Foa, E. B., & Rothbaum, B. O. (1998). *Treating the trauma of rape: Cognitive–behavior therapy for PTSD.* New York: Guilford Press.

Foa, E. B., Rothbaum, B. O., Riggs, D., & Murdock, T. (1991). Treatment of post-traumatic stress disorder in rape victims: A comparison between cognitive-behavioral procedure and counseling. *Journal of Consulting and Clinical Psychology, 59,* 715–723.

Foa, E. B., Zoellner, L. A., Feeny, N. C., Hembree, E. A., & Alvarez-Conrad, J. (2002). Does imaginal exposure exacerbate PTSD symptoms? *Journal of Consulting and Clinical Psychology, 70,* 1022–1028.

Gorski, T. (2001). *PTSD Checklist Civilian version (PCL).* Retrieved July 29, 2008, from http://www.tgorski.com/Terrorism/ptsd_checklist_civilian_version.htm

Hedtke, K. A., Ruggiero, K. J., Fitzgerald, M. M., Zinzow, H. M., Saunders, B. E., Resnick, H. S., & Kilpatrick, D. G. (2008). A longitudinal investigation of interpersonal violence in relation to mental health and substance use. *Journal of Consulting and Clinical Psychology, 76,* 633–647.

Herman, J. L. (1997). *Trauma and recovery: The aftermath of violence—From domestic abuse to political terror.* New York: Basic Books.

Janoff-Bulman, R. (1992). *Shattered assumptions: Toward a new psychology of trauma.* New York: Free Press.

Keane, T. M., Fairbank, J. A., Caddell, J. M., & Zimmering, R. T. (1989). Implosive (flooding) therapy reduces symptoms of PTSD in Vietnam combat veterans. *Behavior Therapy, 20,* 245–260.

Kessler, R. C., Sonnega, A., Bromet, E., Hughes, M., & Nelson, C. B. (1995). Post-traumatic stress disorder in the National Comorbidity Survey. *Archives of General Psychiatry, 52,* 1048–1060.

Kilpatrick, D. G., Acierno, R., Resnick, H. S., Saunders, B. E., & Best, C. L. (1997). A 2-year longitudinal analysis of the relationship between violent assault and alcohol and drug use in women. *Journal of Consulting and Clinical Psychology, 65,* 834–847.

Kilpatrick, D. G., Acierno, R., Saunders, B., Resnick, H. S., Best, C. L., & Schnurr, P. P. (2000). Risk factors for adolescent substance abuse and dependence: Data from a national sample. *Journal of Consulting and Clinical Psychology, 68,* 19–30.

Kilpatrick, D. G., & Resnick, H. S. (1993). PTSD associated with exposure to criminal victimization in clinical and community populations. In J. R. Davidson & E. B. Foa (Eds.), *Post-traumatic stress disorder in review: Recent research and future directions* (pp. 113–143). Washington, DC: American Psychiatric Press.

Kilpatrick, D. G., Ruggiero, K. J., Acierno, R., Saunders, B. E., Resnick, H. S., & Best, C. L. (2003). Violence and risk of PTSD, major depression, substance abuse/dependence, and comorbidity: Results from the National Survey of Adolescents. *Journal of Consulting and Clinical Psychology, 71,* 692–700.

Kinzie, D. J. (2004). Cross-cultural treatment of PTSD. In J. Wilson, M. J. Friedman, & J. D. Lindy (Eds.), *Treating Psychological Trauma & PTSD* (pp. 255–277). New York: Guilford Press.

Kofoed, L., Friedman, M. J., & Peck, R. (1993). Alcoholism and drug abuse in patients with PTSD. *Psychiatric Quarterly, 64,* 151–171.

Lambert, M. J., & Bergin, A. E. (1994). The effectiveness of psychotherapy. In A. E. Bergin & S. C. Garfield (Eds.), *Handbook of psychotherapy and behavior change* (4th ed., pp. 143–189). New York: Wiley.

Linehan, M. M. (1993). *Cognitive–behavioral treatment of borderline personality disorder.* New York: Guilford Press.

Little, K. J. (2000). Screening for domestic violence. Identifying, assisting, and empowering adult victims of abuse. *Postgraduate Medicine, 108*, 135–141.

Marmar, C. R., Foy, D., Kagan, B., & Pynoos, R. S. (1994). An integrated approach for treating posttraumatic stress. In R. S. Pynoos (Ed.), *Posttraumatic stress disorder: A clinical review* (pp. 99–132). Lutherville, MD: Sidran Press.

Marsella, A. J., Friedman, M. J., Gerrity, E. T., & Scurfield, R. M. (Eds.). (1996). *Ethnocultural aspects of posttraumatic stress disorder: Issues, research, and clinical applications*. Washington, DC: American Psychological Association.

McFarlane, A. C. (2001). Dual diagnosis and treatment of PTSD. In J. P. Wilson, M. J. Friedman, & J. D. Lindy (Eds.), *Treating psychological trauma and PTSD* (pp. 237–254). New York: Guilford Press.

Meichenbaum, D. (1974). *Cognitive behavior modification*. Morristown, NJ: General Learning Press.

Meichenbaum, D. (1994). Stress inoculation training for coping with stressors. *The Clinical Psychologist, 49*, 4–7.

Najavits, L. M. (2002). *Seeking safety: A treatment manual for PTSD and substance abuse*. New York: Guilford Press.

National Center for Victims of Crime & Crime Victims Research and Treatment Center. (1992). *Rape in America: A report to the nation*. Arlington, VA: National Center for Victims of Crime.

National Institute of Justice. (1996). *Victim costs and consequences: A new look*. Washington, DC: U.S. Department of Justice.

Nelson, E. C., Heath, A. C., Madden, P. A., Cooper, M. L., Dinwiddie, S. H., Bucholz, K. K., et al. (2002). Association between self-reported child sexual abuse and adverse psychosocial outcomes: Results from a twin study. *Archives of General Psychiatry, 59*, 139–145.

Norris, F. H., & Kaniasty, K. (1996). Received and perceived social support in times of stress: A test of the social support deterioration deterrence model. *Journal of Personality and Social Psycholog, 71*, 498–511.

Orsillo, S. (2001). Measures of acute stress disorder and posttraumatic stress disorder. In M. M. Antony, S. Orsillo, & L. Roemer (Eds.), *Practitioner's guide to empirically based measures of anxiety* (pp. 255–307). New York: Kluwer Academic/Plenum Publishers.

Payne, R. A. (2005). *Relaxation techniques: A practical handbook for the health care professional* (3rd ed.). New York: Elsevier.

Rau, P. J., & Goldfried, M. R. (1994). The therapeutic alliance in cognitive–behavior therapy. In A. O. Horvath & L. S. Greenberg (Eds.), *The working alliance: Theory, research, and practice* (pp. 131–152). New York: Wiley.

Resick, P. A. (2001). *Cognitive processing therapy generic version*. Unpublished manual, Center for Trauma Recovery, University of Missouri—St. Louis.

Resick, P. A., Nishith, P., Weaver, T. L., Astin, M. C., & Feuer, C. A. (2002). A comparison of cognitive processing therapy with prolonged exposure and a waiting list condition for the treatment of chronic posttraumatic stress disorder in female rape victims. *Journal of Consulting and Clinical Psychology, 70*, 867–879.

Resick, P. A., & Schnicke, M. K. (1992). Cognitive processing therapy for sexual assault victims. *Journal of Consulting and Clinical Psychology, 60*, 748–756.

Resick, P. A., & Schnicke, M. K. (1996). *Cognitive processing therapy for rape victims: A treatment manual.* Newbury Park, CA: Sage.

Resnick, H. S., Falsetti, S. A., Kilpatrick, D. G., & Freedy, J. R. (1996). Assessment of rape and other civilian trauma-related posttraumatic stress disorder: Emphasis on assessment of potentially traumatic events. In T. W. Miller (Ed.), *Stressful life events* (pp. 231–266). Madison, WI: International Universities Press.

Resnick, H. S., Kilpatrick, D. G., Dansky, B. S., Saunders, B. E., & Best, C. L. (1993). Prevalence of civilian trauma and PTSD in a representative national sample of women. *Journal of Consulting and Clinical Psychology, 61*, 984–991.

Riggs, D., Rothbaum, B. O., & Foa, E. B. (1995). A prospective examination of symptoms of post-traumatic stress disorder in victims of non-sexual assault. *Journal of Interpersonal Violence, 2*, 201–214.

Rimm, D. C., & Masters, J. (1979). *Behavior theory* (2nd ed.). New York. Academic Research.

Rothbaum, B. O., & Foa, E. B. (1993). Subtypes of posttraumatic stress disorder and duration of symptoms. In J. R. T. Davidson & E. B. Foa (Eds.), *Posttraumatic stress disorder: DSM–IV and beyond* (pp. 23–35). Washington, DC: American Psychiatric Press.

Rothbaum, B. O., Meadows, E. A., Resick, P., & Foy, D. W. (2000). Cognitive–behavioral therapy. In E. B. Foa, T. M. Keane, & M. J. Friedman (Eds.), *Effective treatments for PTSD: Practice guidelines from the International Society for Traumatic Stress Studies* (pp. 60–83). New York: Guilford Press.

Saunders, B. E. (2003). Understanding children exposed to violence: Toward an integration of overlapping fields. *Journal of Interpersonal Violence, 18*, 356–376.

Shapiro, F. (1989). Efficacy of the eye movement desensitization procedure in the treatment of traumatic memories. *Journal of Traumatic Stress, 2*, 199–223.

Shapiro, F. (1995). *Eye movement and desensitization and reprocessing: Basic principles, protocols, and procedures.* New York: Guilford Press.

Taylor, S. (2003). Outcome predictors for three PTSD treatments: Exposure therapy, EMDR, and relaxation training. *Journal of Cognitive Psychotherapy, 17*, 149–162.

van der Kolk, B. A., Roth, S., Pelcovitz, D., Sunday, S., & Spinazzola, J. (2005). Disorders of extreme stress: The empirical foundation of a complex adaptation to trauma. *Journal of Traumatic Stress, 18*, 389–399.

Van Etten, M. L., & Taylor, S. (1998). Comparative efficacy of treatments for post-traumatic stress disorder: A meta-analysis. *Clinical Psychology and Psychotherapy, 5*, 125–144.

Veronen, L. J., & Kilpatrick, D. G. (1983). Stress management for rape victims. In D. Meichenbaum & M. E. Jaremko (Eds.), *Stress reduction and prevention* (pp. 341–374). New York: Plenum Press.

Waters, H., Hyder, A., Rajkotia, Y., Basu, S., Rehwinkel, J. A., & Butchart, A. (2004). *The economic dimensions of interpersonal violence*. Geneva, Switzerland: World Health Organization.

Weathers, F. W., Keane, T. M., & Davidson, J. R. T. (2001). Clinician-Administered PTSD Scale: A review of the first ten years of research. *Depression and Anxiety, 13,* 132–156.

Weiss, D., & Marmar, C. R. (1997). The Impact of Event Scale—Revised. In J. Wilson & T. Keane (Eds.), *Assessing psychological trauma and PTSD* (pp. 399–411). New York: Guilford Press.

Wilson, J., & Keane, T. (Eds.). (2004). *Assessing psychological trauma and PTSD: A practitioner's handbook* (2nd ed.). New York: Guilford Press.

Wolpe, J. (1958). *Psychotherapy by reciprocal inhibition*. Palo Alto, CA: Stanford University Press.

Zoellner, L. A., Feeny, N. C., Cochran, B., & Pruitt, L. (2003). Treatment choice for PTSD. *Behaviour Research and Therapy, 41,* 879–886.

VIII

LEGAL AND
PSYCHOLOGICAL RISKS
IN TREATING PEOPLE WITH
BEHAVIORAL EMERGENCIES

18

LEGAL AND ETHICAL RISK MANAGEMENT WITH BEHAVIORAL EMERGENCIES

WENDY PACKMAN, HOURI ANDALIBIAN, KERRY EUDY,
BROOKE HOWARD, AND BRUCE BONGAR

Many mental health practitioners are apprehensive about treating patients who are at a high risk of self-harm or violence. The fear stems from not only the thought of losing a patient or having a patient harm another but also the consequences that may directly affect mental health practitioners themselves.[1] When a mental health practitioner's conduct falls below the standard of care, there can be legal ramifications. Complaints can also be filed with state licensing boards or the American Psychological Association (APA) Ethics Committee (if the psychologist is a member of APA), in which the complaining party alleges that the psychologist was not competent ("Ethical Principles of Psychologists and Code of Conduct" [hereinafter APA Ethics Code]; APA, 2002, Ethical Standards 2.01, 2.03; www.apa.org/ethics/code2002.html) and his or her work was not based on established scientific and professional knowledge (Ethical Standard 2.04). Complaints filed with

---

[1]Throughout this chapter, the terms *mental health practitioner* and *clinician* refer to both psychologists and psychiatrists. Note that psychologists and psychiatrists may be held to different standards of care. However, the theories of liability, case law, and risk management guidelines are sufficiently similar to warrant addressing them together.

the APA Ethics Committee could result in the most serious sanction of expulsion from the association. Legally, mental health practitioners may be sued for malpractice. Mental health practitioners often question whether they can be sued in a particular instance. Unfortunately, the answer is always *yes*. However, whether a mental health practitioner can be sued successfully depends on the facts of the case. In this chapter, we first discuss the elements of medical malpractice. We then discuss the legal areas of liability in working with suicidal patients and violent patients.

OUTLINE OF LEGAL STANDARD: ELEMENTS OF NEGLIGENCE AND MALPRACTICE

Legal cases involving risk management with behavioral emergencies are usually medical malpractice cases filed against a mental health practitioner (i.e., the defendant; Andalibian et al., 2006). The main legal theory in malpractice complaints is *negligence*. Therefore, in almost all cases in which risk management for a suicidal or violent patient is of concern, negligence will be the main legal issue. The following is an overview of negligence law provided to shed light on how each of the four elements of the law is applied in these cases (Andalibian et al., 2006).

Negligence is "the failure to exercise the standard of care that a reasonably prudent person would have exercised in a similar situation" (Black, 1996, p. 1405). The area of negligence law falls under the broader scope of tort law. A *tort* is a civil wrong committed by one individual (i.e., the defendant), which has caused some injury to another individual (i.e., the plaintiff; Packman & Harris, 1998). Unlike intentional torts, negligence does not require any intent on the part of the defendant. This means that, for example, in a tort case of *battery* (i.e., the use of force against another resulting in harmful or offensive contact; Black, 1996), the defendant must intend to harm the victim for liability to occur. In a negligence case, the defendant may bear no intentions of harm and still be held liable. This area of law essentially provides compensation for people when harm is done to them because someone (i.e., the defendant) did something they should not have done (i.e., *act of commission*) or failed to do something they should have done (i.e., *act of omission*; Simon, 1988), even when there was no harm intended. The lack of a requirement of intent is of crucial importance because it leaves health care practitioners vulnerable to liability even when they have the best intentions (Andalibian et al., 2006).

Specifically, to recover on a claim of negligence, the plaintiff must prove four elements: damages, causation, duty, and breach of duty (Prosser, 1971).[2]

---

[2]In legal references, the customary order of the elements of negligence is (a) duty, (b) breach of duty, (c) causation, and (d) damages. Whether there was a duty is determined first by the court; if there is no duty on the part of the defendant, there can be no negligence. For the purpose of this chapter, the

It should be noted that the plaintiff must show all four elements. By refuting just one element, the defendant can safeguard him- or herself from liability (Andalibian et al., 2006). Indeed, attempting to refute one or more elements of the claim is the primary method practitioners and their legal counsel will use in preventing liability.[3] Regarding the primary elements of negligence, we begin with the most basic element—damages—and end with duty and breach of duty.

Understanding Damages

Generally, when a plaintiff files a negligence lawsuit, the element of damages is usually satisfied. It essentially reflects the law's requirement that the plaintiff suffer some harm in order to be compensated (Packman, Pennuto, Bongar, & Orthwein, 2004). Simply put, a defendant may be negligent, but he or she is not liable unless this negligence results in injury. For example, if a practitioner's negligence leads to a patient's unsuccessful suicide attempt and the attempt results in minimal psychological or physical harm, then the practitioner is not liable. In most cases, a completed suicide or physical and psychological injuries from a suicide attempt easily satisfy the damages requirement. In addition, violent patients whose behavior results in harm to self or others should also satisfy the element of damages. Thus, in these cases the more salient issue in court is usually the amount of damages that resulted from the negligence (Andalibian et al., 2006). The amounts are determined by the courts and are fact-specific to each case.

Understanding Causation: Cause in Fact and Proximate Cause (Foreseeability)

Causation refers to the elements of both *cause in fact* and *proximate cause*. Cause in fact refers to the basic requirement that the defendant's negligence must cause the damages to evoke liability (Packman, Pennuto, et al., 2004).

---

elements are addressed in a different order. This is because damages and causation are generally easily met in malpractice suits and are therefore explained first. The crux of the issue hinges on whether there was a duty on the part of the clinician and whether it was breached. We, the chapter authors, discuss these issues secondarily, and at length.

[3]The other form of defense that is used is referred to in a legal sense as an *affirmative defense*. Affirmative defenses are legal defenses that can excuse the defendant from liability even after all elements of the tort have been met (Black, 1996). Essentially, this means that the court can find that the tort (i.e., negligence) has been committed, but the wrongdoer (i.e., the defendant) will not be held liable because he or she has a legally viable excuse. Affirmative defenses against negligence do exist; however, they rarely prevent full liability and serve mainly to mitigate it (Andalibian et al., 2006). Affirmative defenses include assumption of the risk and comparative liability. The former relates to the theory that the defendant assumed some or all of the risk going into the treatment and, as such, the clinician should not be held liable (Black, 1996). *Comparative liability* is more commonly used as a defense and refers to the idea that the plaintiff's own actions were also at fault and thus the liability of the defendant should be lessened (Black, 1996). Legal theories of assumption of risk and comparative liability are outside the scope of this chapter; practitioners who want a more thorough understanding should consult other legal sources.

Essentially, a negligent act is said to be the cause in fact of the harm when "the resulting harm would not have occurred without the party's conduct" (Black, 1996, p. 81).

The element that limits liability for the defendant who causes harm is the second half of causation: proximate cause. Proximate cause deals mainly with the requirement that the harm be reasonably *foreseeable*. In the area of suicide, the foreseeability of the suicide often becomes the heated issue in court. If the court decides that the suicide was foreseeable, liability is often likely. However, if the court determines that the suicide was not reasonably foreseeable given the circumstances, then the practitioner may not be liable even when providing substandard care (Andalibian et al., 2006).

It is important to distinguish foreseeability of suicide from predictability. Mental health practitioners cannot predict suicidal behavior reliably and validly without a high degree of false positives (Berman & Jobes, 1991). Thus, foreseeability involves a comprehensive and reasonable assessment of the risk. Nevertheless, once in court the difference between foreseeability and predictability may be blurred: "When a suicide is viewed through the lens of hindsight, it can take on a quality of apparent predictability" (Schultz, 2000, p. 15). This can give the plaintiff an advantage and is one reason we recommend that practitioners practice within and even above the applicable standard of care (Packman, Pennuto, et al., 2004).

Because the law tends to assume that a foreseeable suicide is preventable in many cases, a clinician who fails to either reasonably assess risk level or implement appropriate preventative measures is potentially vulnerable if the patient is harmed (Simon, 1998). The same reasoning may apply to violent patients. As such, it is of crucial importance to carefully review the patient's history and determine the specific risk factors.

In *Stallman v. Robinson* (1953), the decedent's husband sued for the death of his wife, who committed suicide while an inpatient at a private hospital. During her 4-day stay, the patient tore off strips of fabric from her nightgowns and successfully committed suicide by hanging herself. In finding the hospital liable, the court reasoned, "the most important single factor in determining whether a hospital was negligent in failing to prevent suicide of a patient is whether hospital authorities under the circumstances could have reasonably anticipated that the patient might harm himself." The court added, "whether these determinative factors are present depends on the detailed facts and circumstances of the particular case" (p. 747) The patient in *Stallman* was preliminarily diagnosed prior to her death as either manic–depressive or schizophrenic with paranoid ideas. In addition, the patient had a history of four previous suicide attempts. In the court's view, suicide was foreseeable given the patient's history and specific risk factors. It is this foreseeability that opens the door to liability when a suicide attempt is made and substandard care is found on the part of the practitioner.

Understanding Duty and Breach of Duty

The elements of *duty* and *breach of duty* are the fundamental basis of negligence law because they establish the standard of care that, when not met, renders a defendant negligent (Packman, Pennuto, et al., 2004). When considering the first element of duty, the courts primarily consider whether the defendant owed the plaintiff a duty. A particular relationship established between the two parties can create the duty to exercise reasonable care. As this pertains to our discussion, any health practitioner will owe a duty to his or her patient simply by taking on the role of health practitioner. In the case of *Stallman v. Robinson* (1953) referred to previously, the court noted, "the doctors in the case were specialists in care and treatment of the mentally ill and accepted the patient in the hospital operated by such doctors, and therefore owed the patient a specific duty" (p. 743). Simply put, a mental health practitioner will almost always owe a duty to his or her patient. What the specific duty actually requires becomes the crux of the matter (Andalibian et al., 2006).

Negligence is defined by a failure to operate within a particular standard of care. Following this standard of care is the duty that the health practitioner owes his or her patient. When the practitioner fails to do so, it is the breach of duty that essentially defines negligence. It is also the single element of negligence that the health practitioner actually has control over after accepting the patient. The other elements can be debated and refuted by the parties' legal counsel after a case has been filed, but the practitioner does not determine what the duty requires, whether a behavioral emergency is actually foreseeable, or results in damages. In contrast, the practitioner is entirely in control of whether he or she breaches his or her duty (Andalibian et al., 2006). Therefore, to provide patients with proper care and minimize liability, practitioners must understand and examine what clearly constitutes their duty (i.e., practicing within the standard of care). It is against this legal background that we discuss what usually constitutes breach of duty by a mental health practitioner in behavioral emergencies.

LEGAL AREA OF LIABILITY: SUICIDE

Common Failure Examples

Bongar, Maris, Berman, and Litman (1998) outlined common failure scenarios in the case of inpatient and outpatient suicide. These scenarios represent some of the different factual patterns under which a mental health practitioner would be vulnerable to a malpractice action (Baerger, 2001). What is crucial in these scenarios is the practitioner's thoroughness in assessing the relative degree of risk of suicide and implementing a treatment plan to reduce or eliminate the risk (Baerger, 2001; Packman & Harris, 1998).

Failure to Properly Diagnose the Risk of Suicide

Mental health practitioners are expected to reach the proper diagnosis and not misdiagnose patients. That is, if the clinician had exercised ordinary and accepted care in reaching a diagnosis, the clinician would have ascertained that the patient was suicidal (*Dillmann v. Hellman*, 1973). Liability under this theory may also be referred to as "failure to predict," indicating that the clinician should have been able to predict the patient's suicidal tendencies if adequate steps and procedures had been employed (Packman, Pennuto, et al., 2004).

Several cases address the clinician's responsibility to accurately diagnose a patient. *Misdiagnosis* refers to a negligent failure to recognize the nature of the patient's condition and then implement proper measures before harm occurs (Packman, Cabot, & Bongar,1994). In a well-known treatise, Gutheil and Appelbaum (1982) commented that misdiagnosis of psychiatric conditions "is a ripe area for future litigation and for consciousness raising" (p. 151) in the mental health profession. In *O'Sullivan v. Presbyterian Hospital in City of New York at Columbia Presbyterian Medical Center* (1995), the court found that the psychiatrist failed to properly diagnose the extent of depression suffered by a man who committed suicide. Specifically, the survivor's expert illustrated that the psychiatrist failed to diagnose a major depression, formulate a treatment plan, detect the severity and acuteness of the patient's problem, order a physical examination, consult the patient's treating physician about the patient's weight loss, assign the patient a therapist, or refer him for psychotropic medication. Given this evidence of deficient diagnosis and treatment, the court held there was no basis to conclude that the psychiatrist conducted a competent evaluation (Packman, Pennuto, et al., 2004). In short, practitioners must conduct a competent evaluation as part of their duty to the patient.

Failure to Take Adequate Protective Measures

Adequate protective measures may refer to a variety of techniques, procedures, or methods. Liability under this legal theory may include the failure to observe or supervise and assess, the failure to medicate, the failure to control, and the failure to restrain (Packman, Pennuto, et al., 2004). A general rule is that the clinician must take adequate precautions against patient suicide, consistent with accepted psychotherapeutic practices and on the basis of his or her knowledge and thorough assessment of the patient (see *Dimitrijevic v. Chicago Wesley Memorial Hospital*, 1968; *Topel v. Long Island Jewish Medical Center*, 1981). VandeCreek and Knapp (1989) cited the case of *Dinnerstein v. United States* (1973), which held that clinicians are liable when a treatment plan overlooks or neglects the patient's suicidal tendencies. VandeCreek and Knapp also noted that courts will generally not find a psychotherapist liable when the patient's suicide attempt was not foreseeable. This is in line with our earlier analysis of negligence, requiring proximate cause to be met to find liability on the part of the defendant.

A primary protective measure that is required is supervision and assessment. In fact, VandeCreek, Knapp, and Herzog (1987) found that hospitals and clinicians are not typically found liable if reasonable steps were taken to supervise and assess the patient. In situations in which the hospital did know or should have known about a patient's suicidal tendencies but was negligent by allowing the patient to be in a high-risk situation, adequate supervision or assessment has not been met. Liability has been frequently imposed in these situations (Packman, Pennuto, et al., 2004b). The legal lesson is that a reasonably prudent practitioner would not allow a known suicidal patient (or any patient whom the practitioner should have known was suicidal) to be in a high-risk situation. Therefore, doing so would be a breach of their duty. Following are examples of such breaches.

In *Meier v. Ross General Hospital* (1968), a physician in charge of the psychiatric wing of a hospital was held liable for the death of a patient because he had assigned him to a psychiatric wing on the second floor after the patient had attempted to commit suicide by slashing his wrists. Following the assignment, the patient jumped head first through an open window of his room. The court reasoned that the facts of the case supported a duty on the part of the practitioner to protect the decedent from his own actions, voluntary or involuntary. The practitioner was held liable on the basis of his failure to do so.

Failure to properly supervise was also the legal theory that led to liability in *Fatuck v. Hillside Hospital* (1974). Here, an action was brought claiming that the hospital was negligent in failing to prevent a patient from escaping the grounds approximately 2 to 3 hours before the patient committed suicide by jumping from the roof of a building. Evidence included a 14-year history of mental health problems and recently expressed suicidal threats. During the patient's 9-day hospital stay, notations were made in his record stating that he was not to be permitted to wander off. The patient was also placed on 15-minute checks for 2 days after admission; however, there was no notation that the checks were ever conducted. The court held that the evidence established negligence on the part of the hospital. In other words, they failed to meet their duty of adequate supervision (Packman, Pennuto, et al., 2004).

Failure to Disclose or Warn

The duty to warn the patient or patient's family of a risk of suicide differs from the duty to warn of a risk of danger to another (see discussion on *Tarasoff v. The Regents of the University of California*, 1974, 1976, regarding a violent patient, later in this chapter). In some cases, the courts have found liability for the failure of a physician or psychiatrist to warn family members of a patient's condition or to disclose pertinent information regarding the patient's condition to the patient (Packman, Pennuto, et al., 2004). In *Wozniak v. Lipoff* (1988), the court found fault on the part of an internist for a patient's suicide. The internist had diagnosed and treated the patient for Graves' disease, a thyroid condition. He did not tell her or her family that people with Graves' disease become anxious and irritable, engage in inappropriate behavior, and might develop serious psychiatric problems or deep depression. This omission on the part of the internist constituted a breach of the duty to disclose or warn.

In contrast, in *Bellah v. Greenson* (1978) liability was not established for failing to warn particular persons of the patient's condition. The parents of Tammy Bellah (who died by an overdose of pills) brought an action against their daughter's outpatient therapist. The court found that the plaintiff's complaint was legally legitimate by alleging the existence of a psychiatrist–patient relationship, knowledge by the psychiatrist of the patient's suicidal propensity, and the psychiatrist's failure to take adequate steps to prevent the suicide. However, the court rejected the parents' contention that the psychiatrist's duty included breaching the confidence of the doctor–patient relationship by revealing to the parents disclosures made by their daughter about conditions that might cause her to commit suicide. The court reasoned that imposing a duty on a psychiatrist to disclose to others vague or even specific manifestations of suicidal tendencies on the part of the patient who is being treated in an outpatient setting could inhibit psychiatric treatment. The court added that the dynamics of the interaction between the psychotherapist and the patient seen in office visits are highly complex and subtle, with intimate privacy being a virtual necessity for successful treatment. Although the *Bellah* court did not impose a *Tarasoff*-type duty to warn relatives of potential suicide risk, it remains an option that clinicians should consider seriously when a patient presents as at risk of suicide (Bongar, 2002; Fremouw, de Perczel, & Ellis, 1990).

Failure to Commit or Confine and Negligent Release of Patient

Along the same lines as the duty to take protective measures, discussed previously, clinicians can be found liable for failing to commit or confine a patient at high risk of suicide. This includes negligently allowing a patient to leave a confined environment to go on a pass and releasing a patient prematurely. The issue, as with the other duty scenarios, is whether the mental health practitioner operated below the standard of care or made a valid professional judgment (Andalibian et al., 2006). In *Tabor v. Doctors Memorial Hospital* (1990), an emergency department physician failed to admit a suicidal patient because his parents could not pay the hospital's $400 deposit. The patient was depressed and had taken a dangerous amount of sleeping pills. The court held that the doctor's decision not to admit the patient in an emergency, due to the parents' inability to pay the $400 deposit, constituted a failure to follow the appropriate standard of care.

Allowing a patient to leave a confined environment without properly assessing and documenting one's reasoning may also give rise to legal liability. In *Foster v. Charter Medical Group* (1992), the court held the psychiatrist liable after considering whether he or she was negligent in allowing the patient to leave the facility. In coming to its decision, the court considered the patient's expressions of suicidal intent on earlier passes, his anxiety immediately before leaving the facility, and the psychiatrist's failure to notify the man's family that he would be temporarily leaving the facility.

In a related vein, hospitals have also been found negligent in releasing a suicidal patient. In *Bell v. New York City Health and Hospital Corporation* (1982), a physician recommended the release of a psychiatric patient despite the presence of the patient's potentially harmful delusions. The physician failed to investigate the previous psychiatric history of the patient, the patient's delusions, or an incident that occurred the evening before the patient's release during which the patient had to be restrained. The court held that the hospital was negligent in releasing the patient and that it was the cause of his suicide following his release.

As noted, on the one hand, a clinician may be found liable for the early release of a patient if the release is negligent and not a valid exercise of professional judgment (Robertson, 1988). On the other hand, Fremouw et al. (1990) pointed out that when a clinician makes a reasonable assessment of danger and believes a risk no longer exists, he or she is not held liable for the death of a patient after discharge. For example, in *Johnson v. United States* (1981) and *Paradies v. Benedictine Hospital* (1980), the courts did not find psychiatrists responsible for the postdischarge suicides of their patients because the psychiatrists had assessed the patients and had reasonably concluded that the benefits of release outweighed the potential risks of danger. In *Johnson*, the court observed that "accurate prediction of dangerous behavior, and particularly of suicide and homicide, are almost never possible" (Fremouw et al., 1990, p. 8). This holding again highlights the importance of reasonableness in all negligence cases. Practitioners who use caution and document their reasoning when making decisions regarding the confinement, supervision, and release of their patients have the best protection against liability.

Failure to Obtain and Maintain Adequate History and Records

Clinicians must obtain an adequate history of each patient and maintain up-to-date documentation regarding changes for each patient. History gathering is properly completed upon intake of the patient and needs to include information involving past suicide attempts, prior incidents of self-harm, past suicidal ideation or impulses, as well as information about attempted and completed suicides in the patient's family (Baerger, 2001).

Obtaining a complete history should also entail gathering past records and risk assessment data (Packman & Harris, 1998). Maintaining appropriate records is simply an exercise in accurate documentation. In *Abille v. United States* (1980), the status of a psychiatric inpatient was changed, which allowed the patient to leave the unit unattended. The treating clinician did not record a written order changing the patient's status and did not prepare documentation stating reasons for the lowered precautions. The patient committed suicide while away from the unit. The court found the clinician negligent, stating that the "failure to maintain contemporaneous notes, orders or other records adequately recording and explaining his action in reclassifying [the patient] fell below the applicable standard of care" (p. 709). This case illustrates how the success or failure of a lawsuit can hinge on the documentation and reasoning behind the practitioner's behavior. The requirement of maintaining adequate records cannot be overstated.

LEGAL AREA OF LIABILITY: VIOLENT PATIENTS

The *Tarasoff* Rulings

Background on an Affirmative Duty to Act

As stated earlier, cases involving patients with behavioral emergencies are analyzed under the theory of negligence, which is part of the broader area of law called torts. According to tort law (Restatement (Second) of Torts § 315, 1965), there is no duty to control the conduct of a third party to prevent him or her from causing physical harm to another. That is, there is no liability if the individual fails to exercise his ability to control the actions of a third person to protect another person from even the most serious harm. This is true even if the individual has the ability to exercise control and could do so with ease. Although this is the general rule, many jurisdictions provide an exception. A duty may be imposed on the individual to control a third party if a special relationship exists between the individual and the third party. This may then give rise to a duty to control the third party's conduct (Restatement (Second) of Torts § 315, 1965).

Tarasoff: Case Background and the Duty to Warn

In *Tarasoff v. The Regents of the University of California* (1974, 1976) the court applied this exception extending an affirmative duty to therapists. Tatianna Tarasoff's parents brought a malpractice suit against the Regents of the University of California, who employed the outpatient therapist treating Prosenjit Poddar. The legal suit was based on the theory of negligence, outlined earlier. In this case, Poddar killed Tatiana Tarasoff, a fellow student at the University of California at Berkeley. Two months prior to the murder,

Poddar had expressed his intention to kill Tatiana to his treating psychologist at Cowell Memorial Hospital, Dr. Moore. During his therapy session, Poddar had communicated to Dr. Moore his intentions to kill a girl, readily identifiable as Tatiana Tarasoff, when she returned from Brazil. Acting on this information, Dr. Moore notified campus police of his belief of Poddar's risk of harm to himself or others. The campus police arrested Poddar but released him when he appeared rational and promised to stay away from Tatiana Tarasoff. No further attempts were made to hospitalize Poddar, and he discontinued treatment with Dr. Moore. On October 27, 1960, Poddar drove to Tarasoff's home, shot her with a pellet gun, and stabbed her to death.

Tarasoff's parents brought suit against the University of California under two theories: failure of defendants to (a) warn plaintiffs of the impending danger and (b) bring about Poddar's confinement under California's civil commitment statute (Lanterman-Petris-Short Act, Welf. & Inst. Code, § 5000ff). Initially, in 1974 the California Supreme Court held that

> when a doctor or a psychotherapist, in the exercise of his professional skill and knowledge, determines, or should determine, that a warning is essential to avert danger arising from the medical or psychological condition of his patient, he incurs a legal obligation to give that warning. (*Tarasoff v. Regents of the University of California*, 13 Cal. 3d 177, 1974)

This rule not only impacted mental health practice but also created a dilemma. Given mental health practitioners' inability to accurately predict future acts of violence, practitioners were concerned with the extension of their duty. In addition, this affirmative duty to act created a conflict with mental health professionals' ethical duty of confidentiality. It was feared that the impact resulting from informing patients of the limits of confidentiality when the duty to warn arose would inhibit patients from discussing feelings and thoughts that could rise to the level of danger to self or others. Mental health practitioners argued that the results could have a paradoxical effect of increasing the very danger courts sought to prevent (Givelber, Bowers, & Blitch, 1984).

Expansion on the Duty to Warn

Duty to Use Reasonable Care to Protect

Despite the mental health practitioners' concerns, the court subsequently reheard the *Tarasoff v. Regents of University of California* (1976) case and further expanded the duty to warn. The court held that

> when a therapist determines, or pursuant to the standards of his profession should determine, that his patient presents a serious danger of violence to another, he incurs an obligation to use reasonable care to protect the intended victim against such danger. (*Tarasoff v. Regents of University of California*, 17 Cal. 3d 431, 1976)

This rule extended the duty imposed on therapists from merely warning a potential victim to the active protection of the identifiable victim (*Tarasoff v. Regents of University of California*, 1976). In the court's decision, it also recognized that a mental hospital may be liable for the negligent release of dangerous patients.

Expansion of Duty to Treating Psychiatrists

In *McIntosh v. Milano* (1979), the duty to warn rule was extended to include psychiatrists. The issue before the court was whether a psychiatrist had a duty to warn a potential victim of the danger posed by one of the psychiatrist's patients. In *McIntosh*, the plaintiff filed a wrongful death action against Dr. Milano, the psychiatrist who treated Lee Morgenstein for approximately 2 years. Morgenstein was 15 years old when he was referred to the psychiatrist for his involvement with drugs. During the course of treatment, he expressed many fantasies to the psychiatrist regarding his neighbor, Kimberley McIntosh. Throughout treatment, Morgenstein informed Dr. Milano that he had experiences with Ms. McIntosh. He also related that he had fired a weapon at Ms. McIntosh's car, exhibited a knife, forged a prescription, and verbalized threats toward Ms. McIntosh and her boyfriend. Morgenstein eventually shot and killed Ms. McIntosh. Her parents instituted a wrongful death action against the psychiatrist, alleging that he had a duty to warn Kimberly McIntosh, her parents, or appropriate authorities that Morgenstein posed a physical threat or danger to decedent. The court held that a psychiatrist or therapist has a duty to take

> whatever steps are reasonably necessary to protect an intended or potential victim of his patient when he determines, or should determine, in the appropriate factual setting and in accordance with the standards of his profession established at trial, that the patient is or may present a probability of danger to that person. (*McIntosh v. Milano*, 168 N.J. Super. 466, 1979)

Liability for Unintended Victims

After the imposition of the duty to warn a potential victim, courts continue to expand the *Tarasoff* obligation on mental health practitioners. In *Hedlund v. Superior Court* (1983), the California court extended the *Tarasoff* duty to include prevention of forseeable harm to unintended victims. In *Hedlund*, a mother was shot while her son sat next to her. The mother and son filed suit against the psychologists who had treated the gunman for failure to warn them of a threat made by his patient. The petitioners claimed that the psychologists had failed to warn the victims after the patient had disclosed that he had intentions to commit serous bodily injury to the mother. The son claimed the duty extended to him as well. The court agreed and extended *Tarasoff* to include a duty on the part of the practitioner to protect not only the person against whom the threat was made but also other persons who may be injured or emotionally damaged if the threat is carried out. In determining whether a duty is owed to the unintended party, the court considered the following factors: (a) whether the unintended injured party (i.e., the plaintiff) was located near the scene of the intended injury or was a distance away from the scene; (b) whether the plaintiff's damage was the result of a direct emotional impact on the plaintiff "from the sensory and contemporaneous observance" (p. 49) of the accident or whether the plaintiff learned about the accident from others after it happened; and (c) whether the plaintiff and victim were closely related or whether there was a distant relationship or absence of any relationship.

Patient or Family Member as Informant

The information of a threat that is given to a practitioner does not necessarily have to come from the patient to trigger the duty to protect. In *Ewing v. Goldstein* (2004), Geno Colello, a severely depressed patient, completed a murder–suicide when he shot and killed Keith Ewing and then himself. Colello's father informed the treating therapist that Colello had threatened to kill an ex-girlfriend's new boyfriend. Colello's parents contended that the information relayed to the therapist by Colello's father should have triggered the duty to warn of impending harm. The court held that

> when the communication of a serious threat of grave physical harm is conveyed to the psychotherapist by a member of the patient's immediate family, and is shared for the purpose of facilitating the patient's treatment, the fact that the family member is not a patient of the psychotherapist is not material. (*Ewing v. Goldstein*, 120 Cal. App. 4th 807, 2004)

Limitations on the Duty to Warn and Protect

Requirement of a Threat

In general, a mental health practitioner is not required to take action until he or she knows or has reason to know that a potential victim is endangered. In addition, he or she is not required to take any action beyond that which is reasonable under the circumstances. (Restatement (Second) of Torts, § 314A). For instance, according to Massachusetts law, the duty to warn a patient's potential victims is triggered when

> (a) the patient has communicated to the licensed mental health professional an explicit threat to kill or inflict serious bodily injury upon a reasonably identified victim or victims and the patient has the apparent intent and ability to carry out the threat . . . or (b) the patient has a history of physical violence which is known to the licensed mental health professional and the mental health professional has a reasonable basis to believe that there is a clear and present danger that the patient will at-

tempt to kill or inflict serious bodily injury against a reasonably identified victim or victims. (Massachusetts General Laws ch. 123: § 36B)

Most states require that there be a threat to inflict serious bodily harm or kill. In some jurisdictions these affirmative duties imposed on mental health practitioners are not triggered unless the threat is imminent or explicit. In some cases, it is when in the professional judgment of the practitioner, he or she determines that the patient has the intent and ability to carry out the threat (Grann, Belfrage, & Tengstrom, 2000).

All threats to kill or threats to inflict serious bodily injury are serious and should not be taken lightly. However, the kind of threat made and the degree to which the individual is likely able to carry out the threat must be weighed before taking the necessary reasonable steps prescribed by statute (Grann et al., 2000). For instance, if an individual is committed to a maximum security mental facility for 1 year and on his arrival threatens to kill his mother, claiming to use "magical, special powers" that he possesses, the duty to protect the patient's mother is likely not triggered. However, the duty to protect would likely arise if a patient with a history of violence enters the therapist's office brandishing a weapon and states that he is going to his ex-girlfriend's home to "give her what she finally deserves." Although most cases are not as clear as this last example, further inquiry into the patient's threat, likelihood of carrying out the threat, and history of violence are all factors to be considered when determining whether the duty to protect will apply.

Requirement of Foreseeability

In *Lipari v. Sears, Roebuck & Co.* (1980) the court held that a therapist's liability is limited to those persons foreseeably endangered by a hospital's negligent conduct. In *Lipari*, Mr. Cribbs Jr. had previously been committed to a mental institution and had been receiving psychiatric care from the Veterans Administration (VA). He discontinued treatment and later entered a nightclub and fired a shotgun into a crowded dining room, killing Lipari and seriously wounding his wife. Ms. Lipari brought suit against Sears, claiming damages by the negligence of Sears in selling the gun to one whom Sears knew or should have known was mentally ill or had been committed to a mental institution. Sears filed a third-party complaint against the United States alleging Sears should be indemnified for any damages. Sears alleged that the VA knew or should have known that Mr. Cribbs was a danger to himself or others, and the VA failed "to take those steps, and to initiate those measures and procedures customarily taken or initiated for the care and treatment of mentally ill and dangerous persons by mental health professionals practicing in the community" (p. 187).

Ms. Lipari then filed a second complaint outlining the same allegations against the VA and included in the allegation that the hospital failed to detain Mr. Cribbs or failed to initiate civil commitment proceedings against him. In *Lipari v. Sears, Roebuck & Company* (1980), the court determined that "Nebraska law imposes a duty on a psychotherapist to take reasonable precautions to protect potential victims of his patient when the psychotherapist knows or should know that his patient presents a danger to others" (p. 187). The requirement that the psychotherapist's duty is triggered when he knows or should know of a danger refers to the basic requirement of foreseeability in all negligence cases, as outlined earlier.

The Lipari case has been criticized as imposing a duty to protect the public at large. In *Leedy v. Hartnett* (1981) a voluntary outpatient who had been treated for paranoid schizophrenia and alcoholism at a VA hospital assaulted a couple who had befriended him while he was a patient at the hospital. Hospital personnel knew the patient had a history of violent outbursts and knew of his relationship with the victims. The court held that the hospital had no duty to warn the victims because even if it was foreseeable, the danger posed to the victims was no different from the danger posed to anyone with whom he might be in contact when he became violent. Therefore, there was no foreseeable readily identifiable group of victims to whom the hospital owed a duty.

Requirement of a Reasonably Identifiable Victim

In addition to foreseeability of the danger, identifiability of the victim is also necessary. In California, the legislature restricted the scope of *Tarasoff* liability under California Civil Code § 43.92(a). A duty to warn and protect from a patient's threatened violent behavior arises only "where the patient has communicated to the psychotherapist a serious threat of physical violence against a reasonably identifiable victim or victims."

Confidentiality

Confidentiality is one of the cornerstones of psychotherapy. Many mental health practitioners have argued that the duty to protect breaches this duty of confidentiality and will interfere with the treatment of the dangerous individual. In addition, there have been concerns that the affirmative duty to act would deter mental health practitioners from treating potentially violent patients for fear of possible malpractice claims. Although confidentiality is essential to the psychotherapist–patient relationship, it nevertheless continues to be encroached on by competing societal interests. In the process, the need for the public to know of potential victims threatened with violence took precedence over confidentiality. To account for such breach in confidentiality, the APA Ethics Code allows practitioners the discretion to breach confidentiality to protect the patient or others from harm (APA, 2002). Specifically, Section 4.05 of the APA Ethics Code provides that a psychologist may disclose confidential information without the patient's consent only as mandated or permitted by law for a valid purpose such as to protect the patient or others from harm. To ameliorate the dangers of breaching confidentiality under the appropriate circumstances, it is important to understand when the requirement of confidentiality begins. Most states require that the practitioner inform patients at the initiation of treatment about the limits of confidentiality. The APA Ethics Code (§ 4.02) requires that the practitioner inform the patient of the limits of confidentiality. This discussion occurs at the outset of the relationship unless it is not feasible or is contraindicated.

Examples of Duty to Warn and Protect Laws

In some states, the mental health practitioner's duty is satisfied when the therapist contacts the police and warns the victim. Examples from California, Utah, and Louisiana are as follows:

California Civil Code § 43.92 (2006)
§ 43.92. Psychotherapist's duty to warn of patient's violent behavior; Immunity from liability
(b) If there is a duty to warn and protect under the limited circumstances specified above, the duty shall be discharged by the psychotherapist making reasonable efforts to communicate the threat to the victim or victims and to a law enforcement agency.

Utah Code Ann. § 78-14a-102 (2006)
§ 78-14a-102. Limitation of therapist's duty to warn
(1) A therapist has no duty to warn or take precautions to provide protection from any violent behavior of his client or patient, except when that client or patient communicated to the therapist an actual threat of physical violence against a clearly identified or reasonably identifiable victim. That duty shall be discharged if the therapist makes reasonable efforts to communicate the threat to the victim, and notifies a law enforcement officer or agency of the threat.

La. R.S. 9:2800.2 (2006)
This duty shall be discharged by the psychologist, psychiatrist, or marriage and family therapist, or licensed professional counselor, or social worker if the treating professional makes a reasonable effort to communicate the threat to the potential victim or victims and to notify law enforcement authorities in the vicinity of the patient's or potential victim's residence.

However, in other states, such as Massachusetts, mental health practitioners are given some discretion in deciding which appropriate steps to take. A Massachusetts statute (Chapter 112: § 129A. Confidential communications [2]) allows the professional to take one or more of the following protective actions:

1. Communicate a threat of death or serious bodily injury to a reasonably identified person.

2. Notify an appropriate law enforcement agency in the vicinity in which the patient or any potential victim resides.
3. Arrange for the patient to be hospitalized voluntarily.
4. Take appropriate steps to initiate proceedings for involuntary hospitalization pursuant to law.

CLINICAL RISK MANAGEMENT

Assessment and Risk Variables for Suicidal Patients

One of the duties for practitioners is to properly assess the patient's risk level and predict a foreseeable suicide. McNiel and Binder (1987) reiterated what many clinicians have experienced in clinical practice: that predicting suicide is more challenging and even less accurate than predicting future violence. On the basis of the literature, it is unrealistic to expect clinicians to predict suicide; however, the obligation of clinicians to conduct appropriate suicide risk assessments still remains (Bongar et al., 1998; Packman & Harris, 1998). As noted earlier, clinicians are expected to gather information about the patient's clinical characteristics and make informed decisions about a patient's likelihood to be dangerous to self. Knowing the recognized methods of assessing the potential for suicide is the first step in taking prudent measures to assess and prevent it (Packman, Marlitt, Bongar, & Pennuto, 2004). Assessment methods and risk variables are detailed in chapters 3 and 4 of this volume.

Assessing Future Acts of Violence

For the past 2 decades a continuing debate has existed regarding whether "dangerousness" can be predicted with sufficient accuracy to justify the deprivation of one's liberty. Although clinical predictions of violence may be imperfect, the legal system continues to expect mental health clinicians to form opinions regarding an individual's risk of future dangerousness (*Barefoot v. Estelle*, 1983). More detailed descriptions of assessment procedures for dangerousness are outlined in the chapters regarding the evaluation and management of potentially violent adults and violent youth (chaps. 6 and 7, respectively, this volume).

Overall Risk Management Guidelines

In our view, coping with malpractice and legal complexities is manageable if risk management procedures are integrated into clinical practice. The risk management procedures outlined will also assist mental health practitioners testifying as expert witnesses in suicide and violence cases to evaluate whether the practitioner (i.e., the plaintiff or the defendant) operated within the standard of care (Packman, Pennuto, et al., 2004). The procedures are general enough to apply to all practicing clinicians, but are particularly relevant for those working with suicidal and violent patients.

Consultation

Clinicians should routinely consult colleagues who have expertise with suicidal and dangerous patients (Packman & Harris, 1998). It is advisable for clinicians to also seek consultation or supervision on cases that are outside their competence area (or refer the patient out; Bongar, 2002). This needs to be done to ensure that services provided are indeed competent. Both clinician and consultant should provide written notes for the record, as consultation can provide legal evidence for the reasonableness of selected diagnostic and treatment plans (VandeCreek, Knapp, & Herzog, 1987). Clinicians should make appropriate referrals for medication evaluations if they are not physicians themselves and should be knowledgeable about the effects of psychotropic medications (Bongar, 1991).

Documentation

Perhaps the most important risk management technique is good record keeping (Packman & Harris, 1998). In a legal context, "if it isn't written down, it didn't happen" (Gutheil, 1980, p. 482). Inadequate documentation can cripple a legal case, even if there was no actual negligence (VandeCreek & Knapp, 1989). Thus, if a clinician fails to record an action in the records, the jury may assume the clinician failed to carry out the treatment completely (Packman & Harris, 1998). In fact, clinicians "who make bad decisions but whose reasoning [is clearly articulated]" may come out more favorably than clinicians "who have made reasonable decisions but whose poor documentation leaves them vulnerable" (Gutheil, 1984, p. 3). A thorough record should document interactions, consultations, and professional judgments (Halleck, 1980). The signed informed consent for treatment and documentation of confidentiality considerations should also be included (Packman & Harris, 1998). It is also beneficial to document steps not taken, along with reasoning. Gutheil (1980, p. 482) referred to this as "thinking out loud" for the record.

Finally, tampering with records by inserting new material after-the-fact can destroy any chances of winning a case (Monahan, 1993).

Know the Legal and Ethical Responsibilities

Knowing one's legal and ethical responsibilities helps clinicians recognize risk before it becomes a liability. Confidentiality and informed consent are two salient issues (Packman & Harris, 1998). All APA members and student affiliates are required to follow the APA Ethics Code regardless of the jurisdiction in which they practice. In many jurisdictions, the code or similar ethics provisions are also codified in laws or regulations.

Know the Risk Factors

Clinicians must know what the literature and experts say about the management of suicidal and dangerous patients in order to exercise good clinical judgment in such a situation (Packman & Harris, 1998). Clinicians who treat such patients should be familiar with community resources, voluntary and involuntary hospital admissions, and crisis centers (Bongar, 2002).

Obtain Risk Assessment Data

A thorough clinical assessment of elevated risk must be performed and recorded in a careful, professional manner (Packman & Harris, 1998). Suicide potential and the potential for violence should be evaluated several times during the treatment process, including the time of admission, transfer to less restrictive areas, before home visits, and before discharge (Vandecreek & Knapp, 1983).

Determine Competence

Clinicians are limited as to their specific areas of professional competence (Welch, 1989). Competence varies greatly, depending on education, training, and experience. Thus, clinicians must be aware of their own proficiencies and emotional tolerance levels in treating suicidal and violent patients (Bongar, 2002). If a clinician decides not to treat suicidal or violent patients, a list should be developed of colleagues to whom the clinician can refer these high-risk patients (Packman & Harris, 1998).

Obtain Adequate History and Treatment Records

When working with suicidal patients, historical information should include details regarding past suicide attempts, prior incidents of self-harm, past suicidal ideation and impulses, as well as information about attempted and completed suicides in the patient's family (Baerger, 2001). Peruzzi and Bongar (1999) stated the importance of also obtaining information about the medical seriousness or lethality of all prior patient attempts. In a related vein, when working with violent patients it is important to be cognizant of historical, clinical, dispositional, and other risk management factors (see chaps. 6 and 7, this volume). A thorough risk assessment is also warranted (see chaps. 1–5, this volume).

When mental health practitioners work with suicidal or violent patients or confront potential *Tarasoff* situations, their records should be highly detailed. Records should include a risk–benefit analysis that details all the actions the practitioner considered, as well as the reasoning process that led him or her to take some actions and reject others (Packman & Harris, 1998).

In all instances, the clinician should make reasonable efforts to obtain patients' previous treatment records (Packman & Harris, 1998).

Determine Diagnostic Impression

Clinicians need to master the diagnostic system from the latest version
of the *Diagnostic and Statistical Manual of Mental Disorders* (4th ed., text rev.;
American Psychiatric Association, 2000), as well as use it appropriately
(Packman & Harris, 1998). Underdiagnosing a patient to protect the patient
from stigmatization is legally risky and is not an advisable risk management
procedure (Packman & Harris, 1998).

Involve the Family

In our view, it is advisable to inform the patient's support system of the
patient's suicide or violence potential and to increase their involvement in
management and treatment (VandeCreek & Knapp, 1989). From an ethical
perspective, when we talk about involving the family, it is assumed that pursuant to Ethical Standard 4.05, the psychologist has the consent of the patient. If the psychologist does not have the consent of the patient, he or she
could disclose this information to protect the patient or others from harm if
such disclosure was mandated or permitted by law (Ethical Standard 4.05).
The clinician must judge, however, whether such interactions with family
members would be beneficial or whether the patient needs protection from
them for the time being (Jacobson, 1999). Legally speaking, the family is less
likely to initiate litigation against the clinician when good relations have
been achieved (Bongar, 2002).

RESOURCES FOR CLINICIANS

Throughout this chapter, case law has been presented to demonstrate
the current legal trends in interpreting a clinician's legal duties to the patient or third parties. It is important to note that issues such as the duty to
warn a third party, established from cases such as *Tarasoff*, vary among different states. There is no federal statute or case that establishes (or invalidates)
a duty to warn. Therefore, clinicians must look to the applicable law in his or
her own state to determine what the legal duty includes and omits in the
state. When a court rules on an issue within the state in question, the previous ruling is considered legal precedent. This means that future courts should
follow the same ruling if the facts are similar. Rulings from a different state
can still be presented, but the holding of the case does not set a precedent
that the court must follow. Instead, cases out of state provide persuasive authority. This means that the court may hear the argument and should grant
some deference to it, but must not follow it the way it must if it had set a legal
precedent (from the same state).

Depending on the state and importance of the issue at hand, an out-of-state case can carry little to great persuasive authority. A landmark case such as *Tarasoff*, in which a California court ruled that a psychologist has a duty to protect an identifiable victim, would be considered very persuasive in all states. Indeed, many states have held similarly in future cases. Table 18.1 provides a list of cases by state that have ruled on the *Tarasoff* issue of a duty to warn or protect. The list is intended as a starting-off point for clinicians interested in researching the applicable state law for his or her state. It is not intended as a complete list and does not include relevant statutes that may have been enacted on a state level. To prevent malpractice, clinicians should be aware of the current court rulings in their own state to be sure they are not breaching their duty.

Equally important is that many states' legislatures follow landmark cases' rulings by enacting statutes that codify the rulings. After *Tarasoff*, the California legislature created an exception to the psychotherapist–patient privilege rule of evidence. Many other states have enacted similar statutes. State statutes are available to the public and may be found online or at government libraries. Clinicians should search the evidence codes of their own state to determine whether a similar exception exists. This legal research, although it may appear daunting, is imperative in determining the current applicable law. Without a clear understanding of what the state requires of the clinician, the clinician cannot be certain whether he or she is appropriately breaking rules of confidentiality. A current understanding of the applicable law to his or her state can, at most, protect the clinician from malpractice lawsuits, and at the very least, arm the clinician with information necessary to defend his or her actions when faced with a suit.

CONCLUSION

In conclusion, it is clear that many mental health practitioners are uneasy about the clinical assessment and treatment of patients at risk of harm to themselves or others. This anxiety stems from not only the disturbing possibility that the patient or another individual could be harmed but also the negative ramifications to the clinician. Consequences for clinicians could include complaints filed with state licensing boards, complaints to the APA Ethics Committee, or suits for malpractice. Depending on the outcome of these proceedings, a mental health practitioner is at risk of substantial monetary liability, expulsion from professional organizations, or the loss of the license to practice.

In this chapter we reviewed both the legal and the ethical standards by which a clinician's conduct is assessed when determining liability or breach of ethical duties and detailed risk management techniques that should be used to mitigate the risk to patients and their clinicians. First, the elements

TABLE 18.1
Tarasoff Cases by State

State	Case
Alabama	*King v. Smith*, 539 So. 2d 262 (Ala. 1989)
California	*Hedlund v. Superior Court*, 34 Cal. 3d 695, 194 Cal. Rptr. 805, 669 P.2d 41, 41 A.L.R.4th 1063 (1983)
	Mavroudis v. Superior Court, 102 Cal. App. 3d 594, 162 Cal. Rptr. 724 (1st Dist. 1980)
	Tarasoff v. Regents of University of California, 17 Cal. 3d 425, 131 Cal. Rptr. 14, 551 P.2d 334, 83 A.L.R.3d 1166 (1976)
Colorado	*Brady v. Hopper*, 751 F.2d 329 (10th Cir. 1984) (construing Colorado law)
	Brady v. Hopper, 570 F. Supp. 1333 (D. Colo. 1983) (applying Colorado law)
Connecticut	*Garamella for Estate of Almonte v. New York Medical College*, 23 F. Supp. 2d 167 (D. Conn. 1998) (applying Connecticut law)
Florida	*O'Keefe v. Orea*, 731 So. 2d 680 (Fla. Dist. Ct. App. 1st Dist. 1998)
Iowa	*Cole v. Taylor*, 301 N.W.2d 766 (Iowa 1981)
	Votteler's Estate, Matter of, 327 N.W.2d 759 (Iowa 1982)
Louisiana	*Doyle v. U.S.*, 530 F. Supp. 1278 (C.D. Cal. 1982) (applying Louisiana law)
	Dunnington v. Silva, 916 So. 2d 1166 (La. Ct. App. 1st Cir. 2005)
	Durapau v. Jenkins, 656 So. 2d 1067 (La. Ct. App. 5th Cir. 1995)
Michigan	*Bardoni v. Kim*, 151 Mich. App. 169, 390 N.W.2d 218 (1986)
	Soutear v. U.S., 646 F. Supp. 524 (E.D. Mich. 1986) (applying Michigan law)
	Swan v. Wedgwood Christian Youth and Family Services, Inc., 230 Mich. App. 190, 583 N.W.2d 719 (1998)
Mississippi	*Evans v. U.S.*, 883 F. Supp. 124 (S.D. Miss. 1995) (applying Mississippi law)
Missouri	*Bradley v. Ray*, 904 S.W.2d 302 (Mo. Ct. App. W.D. 1995)
Nebraska	*Lipari v. Sears, Roebuck & Co.*, 497 F. Supp. 185 (D. Neb. 1980) (construing Nebraska law)
	Munstermann ex rel. Rowe v. Alegent Health-Immanuel Medical Center, 271 Neb. 834, 716 N.W.2d 73 (2006)
New Hampshire	*Carlisle v. Frisbie Memorial Hosp.*, 152 N.H. 762, 888 A.2d 405 (2005).
	Powell v. Catholic Medical Center, 145 N.H. 7, 749 A.2d 301 (2000)
New Jersey	*McIntosh v. Milano*, 168 N.J. Super. 466, 403 A.2d 500 (Law Div. 1979)
	Runyon v. Smith, 163 N.J. 439, 749 A.2d 852 (2000)
New Mexico	*Weitz v. Lovelace Health System, Inc.*, 214 F.3d 1175, 46 Fed. R. Serv. 3d 1364 (10th Cir. 2000) (applying New Mexico law)

New York	*Wagshall v. Wagshall*, 148 A.D.2d 445, 538 N.Y.S.2d 597 (2d Dep't 1989)
North Carolina	*Currie v. U.S.*, 644 F. Supp. 1074 (M.D. N.C. 1986) (applying North Carolina law)
Ohio	*Jenks v. City of West Carrollton*, 58 Ohio App. 3d 33, 567 N.E.2d 1338 (2d Dist. Montgomery County 1989)
	Littleton v. *Good Samaritan Hosp. & Health Center*, 39 Ohio St. 3d 86, 529 N.E.2d 449 (1988)
	Morgan, Estates of v. *Fairfield Family Counseling Ctr.*, 77 Ohio St. 3d 284, 1997-Ohio-194, 673 N.E.2d 1311 (1997)
Pennsylvania	*Dunkle v. Food Service East Inc.*, 400 Pa. Super. 58, 582 A.2d 1342 (1990)
South Carolina	*Bishop v. South Carolina Dept. of Mental Health*, 331 S.C. 79, 502 S.E.2d 78 (1998)
Tennessee	*Turner v. Jordan*, 957 S.W.2d 815 (Tenn. 1997)
Texas	*Thapar v. Zezulka*, 994 S.W.2d 635 (Tex. 1999)
Vermont	*Peck v. Counseling Service of Addison County, Inc.*, 146 Vt. 61, 499 A.2d 422 (1985)

of a malpractice claim under the legal theory of negligence were reviewed. Components of this claim that must be understood by mental health practitioners include damages, elements of causation, the duty of the clinical professional, and the consequences of breach of this duty. Next, two specific areas of clinical concern were reviewed in light of negligence theory. Under liability for patient suicide, common failure scenarios were enumerated, including issues of diagnosis, protection, disclosure, commitment, and treatment history. Under liability for patient violence toward others, the landmark *Tarasoff* decision was reviewed and the legal precedents established in this case were examined. In addition, both subsequent expansions to the duty to warn and limitations to this legal theory of liability were discussed, with the impact on clinical care highlighted. Because the specific nature of these duties differs according to state law, examples of different state statutes were included. Finally, strategies for clinical risk management, in light of legal and ethical duties, were discussed. This included the overall assessment of risk of harm as well as seven specific steps all clinicians should include in their clinical practice with high-risk patients to minimize risk by the patient and subsequent negative ramifications for the clinician.

REFERENCES

Abille v. United States, 482 F. Supp. 703 (N.D. Cal. 1980).

American Psychiatric Association. (2000). *Diagnostic and statistical manual of mental disorders* (4th ed., text rev.). Washington, DC: Author.

American Psychological Association. (2002). Ethical principles of psychologists and code of conduct. *American Psychologist, 47*, 1597–1611.

Andalibian, H., Howe, L., Milner, M., Eudy, K., Bongar, B., & Packman, W. (2006). Medical–legal aspects of treating suicidal schizophrenic patients. In R. Tatarelli, M. Pompili, & P. Girardi (Eds.), *Suicide and schizophrenia* (pp. 1–16). Hauppauge, NY: Nova.

Baerger, D. R. (2001). Risk management with the suicidal patient: Lessons from case law. *Professional Psychology: Research and Practice, 32,* 359–366.

Barefoot v. Estelle, 463 U.S. 880, 103 S. Ct. 3383 (1983).

Bell v. New York City Health and Hospitals Corporation, 90 A.D.2d 270, 456 N.Y.S.2d 787 (1982).

Bellah v. Greenson, 81 Cal. App. 3d 614, 146 Cal. Rptr. 535 (1978).

Berman, A. L., & Jobes, D. A. (1991). *Adolescent suicide: Assessment and intervention.* Washington, DC: American Psychological Association.

Black, H. C. (1996). *Black's law dictionary.* St. Paul, MN: West.

Bongar, B. (1991). *The suicidal patient: Clinical and legal standards of care.* Washington, DC: American Psychological Association.

Bongar, B. (2002). *The suicidal patient: Clinical and legal standards of care* (2nd ed.). Washington, DC: American Psychological Association.

Bongar, B., Maris, R. W., Berman, A. L., & Litman, R. E. (1998). Outpatient standards of care and the suicidal patient. In B. Bongar, A. L. Berman, R. W. Maris, M. M. Silverman, E. A. Harris, & W. L. Packman (Eds.), *Risk management with suicidal patients* (pp. 4–33). New York: Guilford Press.

California Civil Code § 43.92 (2006).

Dillmann v. Hellman, 283 So.2d 388 (Fla. Dist. Ct. App. 1973).

Dimitrijevic v. Chicago Wesley Memorial Hospital, 92 Ill.App.2d 251, 236 N.E.2d 309, (Ill.App. 1 Dist. 1968).

Dinnerstein v. United States, 486 F. 2d 34 (1973).

Ewing v. Goldstein, 15 Cal. Rptr. 3d 864 (Cal.App. 2 dist., 2004).

Fatuck v. Hillside Hospital, 45 A.D. 2nd 708, 356 N.Y.S.2d 105 (New York, 1974).

Foster v. Charter Medical Group, 601 So.2d 435 (Ala. 1992).

Fremouw, W. J., de Perczel, M., & Ellis, T. E. (1990). *Suicide risk: Assessment and response guidelines.* New York: Pergamon Press.

Givelber, D. J., Bowers, W. J., &. Blitch, C. L. (1984) *Tarasoff,* myth and reality: An empirical study of private law in action. *Wisconsin Law Review,* 443–497.

Grann, M., Belfrage, H., & Tengstrom, A. (2000). Actuarial assessment of risk for violence: Predictive validity of the VRAG and the historical part of the HCR–20. *Criminal Justice and Behavior, 27,* 97–114.

Gutheil, T. G. (1980). Paranoia and progress notes: A guide to forensically informed psychiatric recordkeeping. *Hospital and Community Psychiatry, 31,* 479–482.

Gutheil, T.G. (1984). Malpractice liability in suicide. *Legal Aspects of Psychiatric Practice, 1,* 1–4.

Gutheil, T. G., & Appelbaum, P. S. (1982). *Clinical handbook of psychiatry and the law.* New York: McGraw-Hill.

Halleck, S. (1980). *Law in the practice of psychiatry*. New York: Plenum Press.

Hedlund v. Superior Ct., 669 P.2d 41 (1983).

Jacobson, G. (1999). The inpatient management of suicidality. In D. G. Jacobs (Ed.), *The Harvard Medical School guide to suicide assessment and intervention* (pp. 383–405). San Francisco: Jossey-Bass.

Johnson v. United States, 409 F. Supp. 1283 (M.D. Fl. 1981).

La. R.S. 9:2800.2 (2006).

Lanterman-Petris-Short Act, Welf. & Inst. Code, Sect 5000ff.

Leedy v. Hartnett, 510 F.Supp. 1125, (D.C.Pa. 1981).

Lipari v. Sears, Roebuck & Co., 497 F. Supp. 185 (D. Neb. 1980).

Massachusetts General Laws Chapter 123: § 36B.

Massachusetts Statute Chapter 112: § 129A. Confidential Communications (2).

McIntosh v. Milano, 403 A.2d 500 (N.J. 1979).

McNiel, D. E., & Binder, R. L. (1987). Predictive validity of judgments of dangerousness in emergency civil commitment. *American Journal of Psychiatry, 144,* 197–200.

Meier v. Ross General Hospital, 69 Cal.2d 420, 445 P.2d 519, 71 Cal.Rptr. 903 (Cal. 1968).

Monahan, J. (1993). Limiting therapist exposure to *Tarasoff* liability: Guidelines for risk containment. *American Psychologist, 48,* 242–250.

O'Sullivan v. Presbyterian Hosp. in City of New York at Columbia Presbyterian, 217 A.D.2d 98, 634 N.Y.S.2d 101 (1995).

Packman, W. L., Cabot, M. G., & Bongar, B. (1994). Malpractice arising from negligent psychotherapy: Ethical, legal, and clinical implications of *Osheroff v. Chestnut Lodge. Ethics and Behavior, 4,* 175–197.

Packman, W. L., & Harris, E. A. (1998). Legal issues and risk management in suicidal patients. In B. Bongar, A. L. Berman, R. W. Maris, M. M. Silverman, E. A. Harris, & W. L. Packman (Eds.), *Risk management with suicidal patients* (pp. 150–186). New York: Guilford Press.

Packman, W. L., Marlitt, R. E., Bongar, B., & Pennuto, T. O. (2004). A comprehensive and concise assessment of suicide risk. *Behavioral Sciences & the Law, 22,* 667–680.

Packman, W. L., Pennuto, T. O., Bongar, B., & Orthwein, J. (2004). Legal issues of professional negligence in suicide cases. *Behavioral Sciences & the Law, 22,* 697–713.

Paradies v. Benedictine Hospital, 77 A.D.2d 757, 431 N.Y.S.2d 175 (1980).

Peruzzi, N., & Bongar, B. (1999). Assessing risk for completed suicide in patients with major depression: Psychologists' views of critical factors. *Professional Psychology: Research and Practice, 30,* 576–580.

Prosser, W. L. (1971). *Handbook of the law of torts* (4th ed.). St. Paul, MN: West.

Restatement (Second) of Torts §314(A) & §315 (1965).

Robertson, J. D. (1988). *Psychiatric malpractice: Liability of mental health professionals*. New York: Wiley.

Schultz, D. (2000). Defending the psychiatric malpractice suicide. *Health Care Law*, 13–26.

Simon, R. I. (1988). *Concise guide to clinical psychiatry and the law*. Washington, DC: American Psychiatric Press.

Simon, R. I. (1998). *Concise guide to psychiatry and law for clinicians*. Washington, DC: American Psychiatric Press.

Stallman v. Robinson, 364 Mo. 275, 260 S.W.2d743. (1953).

Tabor v. Doctors Memorial Hospital, 563 So.2d 233 (La. 1990).

Tarasoff v. Regents of the University of California, 13 Cal. 3d 177 (1974).

Tarasoff v. Regents of the University of California, 17 Cal.3d 425 (1976).

Topel v. Long Island Jewish Medical Center, 431 N.E.2d. 293 (1981).

Utah Code Ann. § 78-14a-102 (2006).

VandeCreek, L., & Knapp, S. (1983). Malpractice risks with suicidal patients. *Psychotherapy: Theory, Research, Practice, Training, 20,* 274–280.

VandeCreek, L., & Knapp, S. (1989). Tarasoff *and beyond: Legal and clinical considerations in the treatment of life-endangering patients*. Sarasota, FL: Professional Resource Exchange.

VandeCreek, L., Knapp, S., & Herzog, C. (1987, October). Malpractice risks in the treatment of dangerous patients. *Psychotherapy: Theory, Research, Practice, Training, 24,* 145–153.

Welch, B. (1989). A collaborative model proposed. *Monitor on Psychology, 20*(10), 28.

Wozniak v. Lipoff, 242 Kan. 583, 750 P.2d 971 (Kan. 1988).

19

THE STRESS AND EMOTIONAL IMPACT OF CLINICAL WORK WITH THE PATIENT AT RISK

PHILLIP M. KLEESPIES AND ALLISON N. PONCE

One patient in your private practice is a young man in his late 20s. He dropped out of school in the 11th grade but was subsequently able to get a general education diploma. You have been seeing him for chronic depression marked by low self-esteem and for anger control problems manifest by occasions of road rage. He works as a custodian at a local high school, and his supervisor has been critical of his work. One day between therapy sessions, he calls you and he sounds upset. He states that his supervisor has given him a very poor performance appraisal. He feels that his job is threatened and he has been struggling with impulses to assault his supervisor. You help him to talk, delay his impulses, and consider other options such as requesting transfer to another work site or to another supervisor. He seems calmer and says that he is in better control and no longer plans to hurt his supervisor.

This chapter builds on and updates a previous article on the stress of behavioral emergencies on clinicians. From "The Stress of Patient Emergencies for the Clinician: Incidence, Impact, and Means of Coping," by P. M. Kleespies and E. Dettmer, 2000, *Journal of Clinical Psychology*, 56, pp. 1353–1369. Copyright 2000 by Wiley. Adapted with permission.

431

Several days later, you receive a call from a local emergency department. The emergency department clinician states that she has your patient's permission to speak with you. She reports that your patient got into a violent confrontation with his supervisor, pulled a knife, and stabbed the supervisor in the shoulder. He then ran to the men's room and cut his own wrists. The supervisor was able to call 911 and he and your patient were taken to separate ERs. You are thankful that neither your patient nor his supervisor sustained fatal injuries, but you begin to have many thoughts and reactions: "How could this happen? He seemed to be working on his issues and on managing his anger"; "Did I miss how deeply threatened and volatile he really was?"; "I'm so sorry for him; this will change things"; "Am I to blame for not foreseeing how much of a risk he was to himself and his supervisor?"; and "This will be in the news. What will my colleagues think?"

Dealing with patient emergencies and crises such as this can be very stressful. As noted in the Introduction to this book, however, such stress is not only in the province of the emergency department or crisis clinic practitioner. In fact, in a scenario such as the one described, we suggest that the patient's therapist is likely to have greater distress than the emergency department clinician who has no prior experience with the patient.

In this chapter we discuss the frequency or incidence in clinical practice of patient suicidal behavior, patient violent behavior, and patients as victims of interpersonal violence. We further discuss the impact that such events can have on the clinician and how he or she might cope with the emotional aftermath.

BEHAVIORAL EMERGENCIES IN CLINICAL PRACTICE: INCIDENCE

When taken cumulatively, the incidence of behavioral emergencies in clinical practice is perhaps greater than commonly recognized. For clarity of presentation, we discuss each type of emergency separately in the sections that follow.

Patient Suicidal Behavior

The well-known reference to patient suicide as an "occupational hazard" for therapists (Chemtob, Bauer, Hamada, Pelowski, & Muraoka, 1989, p. 294) continues to be an apt description of the personally and professionally taxing experience of losing a client to self-inflicted death. Over 30,000 people die by suicide each year in the United States (Hoyert, Kung, & Smith, 2005), and about one third of suicide completers had contact with mental health services within a year of their death, and one in five had contact within their last month of life (Luoma, Martin, & Pearson, 2002). This leaves a significant number of mental health practitioners affected by the suicide of patients, especially in light of the fact that many patients have more than one mental health provider. In addition, there are many instances of patient suicide attempts or nonfatal self-injurious behaviors, some of which can be very stressful for the clinician (Jacobson, Ting, Sanders, & Harrington, 2004; Kleespies, Penk, & Forsyth, 1993).

Traditionally, the bulk of the literature on suicidal behavior in clinical practice focused on psychologists and psychiatrists, although this trend is changing. The incidence of suicide in the practice of professional counselors (McAdams & Foster, 2000) and social workers (Jacobson et al., 2004) has been increasingly explored.

Ruskin, Sakinofsky, Bagby, Dickens, and Sousa (2004) established that 50% of the 239 psychiatrists and psychiatry residents in their sample experienced at least one suicide of a patient. This finding is consistent with the 51% rate noted by Chemtob, Hamada, Bauer, Kinney, and Torigoe (1988). Psychologists report lower rates of patient suicide: Pope and Tabachnick (1993) found that 28.8% of psychologists experienced a patient suicide, and Chemtob, Hamada, Bauer, Torigoe, and Kinney (1988) found a rate of 22%. Investigations of patient suicide incidents among social workers and counselors demonstrate numbers similar to those of psychologists. In a large national random sample of social workers engaged in mental health services, approximately one third of the respondents reported having a client complete suicide (Jacobson et al., 2004), and 23% of professional counselors in a study by McAdams and Foster (2000) reported the same experience.

Those in training status have not necessarily been immune or protected from having a patient suicide. Approximately one third of the psychiatrist respondents in Ruskin et al.'s (2004) investigation experienced a patient suicide while in training, and Kleespies et al. (1993) reported that 11.3% of psychology predoctoral trainees had experienced a patient suicide and another 29% had a patient who made a suicide attempt. McAdams and Foster (2000) found that 24% of their sample of counselors who experienced suicide did so during their training.

To better understand the occurrence of suicide among the patients of mental health providers, there has been an emphasis in the literature on identifying clinician or practice variables associated with this outcome. Clinicians who work in inpatient, emergency, or outpatient mental health agency settings appear to be at higher risk (Chemtob et al., 1989; Ruskin et al., 2004), as do those who work with patients who abuse substances and have organic, affective, or psychotic disorders. Additionally, psychiatrists who are oriented toward pharmacotherapy or ECT have substantially higher risk of patient suicide (Ruskin et al., 2004). It is hypothesized that these practitioners are more likely to see patients who have severe mental disorders and have a higher incidence of suicidal ideation with intent. Additionally, they have a higher volume of patients and may be more likely to prescribe medication that can be used in a suicide by overdose.

Patient Violent Behavior

Patient violence can be considered another occupational hazard for psychologists. In a national survey, Pope and Tabachnick (1993) found that 89% of their sample of psychologists reported episodes in which they were afraid that a patient might attack a third party, and 60.7% reported having had a patient who had actually attacked a third party physically. In addition, Whitman, Armao, and Dent (1976) reported that during a 1-year period of practice, 81% of their sample of psychologists perceived a patient of theirs as a threat to others.

The threat of a patient harming a third party is distressing, but Guy and Brady (1998) asserted that few challenges facing psychotherapists are more upsetting than the possibility of patient violence toward the clinician. In terms of the incidence of violence directed at therapists, Tryon (1986) reported on a national survey that revealed that 12% of therapists in private practice and 24% in hospitals and clinics had been victims of patient violence at some point in their careers. Moreover, 81% of those surveyed had experienced some form of verbal abuse or threat. In another national survey, Guy, Brown, and Poelstra (1990) reported that nearly 50% of their sample of psychologists had been threatened with physical attack by a patient and 40% indicated that they had actually been attacked. The data from these studies suggest that 35% to 40% of psychologists in clinical practice may be at risk of being assaulted by a patient at some time during their graduate school and professional careers.

Of course, psychologists are not the only mental health professionals who experience patient violence or threatening behavior. In a mail survey of mental health providers in Georgia (including clinical social workers, licensed counselors, psychiatrists, and psychologists), Arthur, Brende, and Quiroz (2003) reported that 61% of the respondents had been victims of violent acts of a psychological (e.g., stalking, harassment) or physical nature. Moreover, 29% of the sample said that they had feared for their lives at some point while they worked with clients or patients. In a national survey of social workers, Jayaratne, Croxton, and Mattison (2004) found that social workers frequently experienced physical threats (22.8% of the sample) and verbal abuse (49.3% of the sample). Flannery, Stone, Rego, and Walker (2001), in a report on assault data gathered in a public mental health system as part of an ongoing, peer-help crisis intervention program (i.e., the Assaulted Staff Action Program [ASAP]), found that psychiatric nurses were second only to mental health workers as victims of patient assault.

Guy et al. (1990) found that a majority of reported attacks on psychologists occurred in inpatient psychiatric settings; that is, 41% in public psychiatric hospitals and 22% in private psychiatric facilities. Studies with other mental health professionals, however, have found that a lesser but still significant number of attacks occurred in residential, outpatient, and private practice settings (Bernstein, 1981; Flannery et al., 2001; Jayaratne et al., 2004). Such findings suggest that clinicians must be aware of the possibility of patient violence in virtually any setting.

Although any clinician can become a victim, some findings suggest that the risk is greater for newer and perhaps less experienced clinicians. Thus, Jayaratne et al. (2004) reported that being young and male placed social workers at greater risk, and Guy et al. (1990) found that 46% of all attacks on psychologists involved graduate students or trainees, and another 33% occurred in the first 5 years after completing the doctoral degree. These data suggest that nearly 80% of patient assaults on psychologists occur in their first 8 to 10 years in the field. Guy and Brady (1998) hypothesized that there may be a number of reasons for this phenomenon. Newer therapists may be less alert to cues of violence. They may set fewer limits and allow aggressive behavior to escalate. They may be more likely to work in inpatient settings in which more severely impaired patients tend to be assigned to clinicians in training.

Although there have been instances in which a patient assault resulted in serious injury or death to the clinician, most patient attacks seem to result in minor injury or no injury (Arthur et al., 2003). In their national survey, Guy et al. (1990) reported that only 30% of those assaulted suffered any physical injury, and only 10% reported moderate injury. Usually, the emotional distress was far more disturbing than any physical injury. Aside from years of clinical experience, little in the literature suggests a set of characteristics attributable to a typical therapist victim (Guy & Brady, 1998).

Patients as Victims of Interpersonal Violence

According to the National Crime Victimization Survey statistics updated in 2007, about 23 million crimes per year impact U.S. residents over age 12 (U.S. Department of Justice, 2007). Violent crimes account for about 5.2 million of these, and include murder, rape and sexual assault, robbery, and assault, all of which are violence of an interpersonal nature. The prevalence of childhood victimization has also been studied extensively. Briere and Elliott (2003) found that about 32% of women and 14% of men in their national sample reported surviving childhood sexual abuse, and 22% of women and 24% of men experienced childhood physical abuse. Among respondents who endorsed a history of abuse, about 21% experienced both types (i.e., sexual and physical). These figures are comparable to those of several other investigations (Briere & Elliott, 2003).

Interpersonal relationship violence among adults is also of concern; nonfatal intimate violence affects approximately 627,000 individuals per year (U.S. Department of Jusice, 2007). Although these crimes, perpetrated by current or former spouses, boyfriends, or girlfriends, have declined in recent years, they still pose serious physical and emotional risk.

Not all individuals who experience trauma have negative outcomes; however, it has been well established that many victims are at risk of psychological difficulties. Among other problems, both major depression and post-traumatic stress disorder (PTSD) are related to interpersonal violence (Nixon, Resick, & Nishith, 2004) as are alcohol and drug use (Kaslow et al., 2002). Stark and Flitcraft (1996) reported that 35% to 40% of female victims of interpersonal violence report a history of multiple suicide attempts.

The sequelae of interpersonal violence have the potential to lead victims to treatment in which therapists are confronted with the need to address the impact of the victimization. Moreover, the literature also indicates that the existence of a serious mental illness (SMI) makes some individuals vulnerable to victimization, creating the need for professionals to be aware of the potential of violence against those already in their care.

Teplin, McClelland, Abram, and Weiner (2005) compared rates of violence against adults with SMI with those reported in the National Crime Victimization Survey and found that violent crime against this vulnerable group was almost 12 times higher than in the general population. More than 25% of participants with SMI reported victimization in the year preceding the interviews. Assault and personal theft are among the more common forms of violence they experience. Lifetime history of victimization among persons with SMI reaches to nearly 88%, with 46% reporting lifetime incidence of PTSD (McFarlane, Schrader, Bookless, & Browne, 2006). It is important to note that comorbid PTSD is frequently underdiagnosed in this population, although the effects of victimization can have a significant impact on prognosis (McFarlane et al., 2006). Given the knowledge that psychotherapy can be useful for individuals who have experienced interpersonal trauma and that positive reactions from providers are associated with benefits after some traumatic experiences (Borja, Callahan, & Long, 2006), it is important for clinicians to be aware of the potential for patient victimization and to know how to address it.

BEHAVIORAL EMERGENCIES IN CLINICAL PRACTICE: IMPACT ON THE CLINICIAN

As Kleespies and Dettmer (2000) noted, the very sensitivity that enables individuals to become excellent clinicians may also leave them vulnerable to the emotional distress that can follow negative clinical events such as patient suicidal behavior or patient violence.

Impact of Patient Suicidal Behavior

There is now accumulating, albeit retrospective, evidence that when confronted with a patient suicide, clinicians from virtually all mental health disciplines (e.g., psychology, psychiatry, social work) often report feelings of shock, disbelief, failure, self-blame, guilt, shame, helplessness, anxiety, and depression (Brown, 1987; Chemtob, Hamada, Bauer, Kinney, & Torigoe, 1988; Chemtob, Hamada, Bauer, Torigoe, & Kinney, 1988; Grad, Zavasnik, & Groleger, 1997; Hendin, Haas, Maltsberger, Szanto, & Rabinowicz, 2004; Jacobsen et al., 2004; Kleespies et al., 1993; Kleespies, Smith, & Becker, 1990; Ruskin et al., 2004; Sanders, Jacobson, & Ting, 2005; Ting, Sanders, Jacobson, & Power, 2006). A number of studies have found elevations on the Intrusion and Avoidance scales of the Impact of Event Scale (Horowitz, Wilner, & Alvarez, 1979) suggesting that clinicians who have a patient suicide frequently struggle with intrusive thoughts about the event or make efforts to avoid reminders of it (Chemtob, Hamada, Bauer, Kinney, & Torigoe, 1988; Chemtob, Hamada, Bauer, Torigoe, & Kinney, 1988; Jacobsen et al., 2004; Kleespies et al., 1990, 1993; Ruskin et al., 2004). Among mental health social workers, Jacobsen et al. (2004) found that female therapists were more likely to have elevations on intrusive thoughts, whereas male therapists were more likely to have elevations on avoidance. Brown (1987) and Kleespies et al. (1993) found that these intense emotional reactions usually diminish substantially over a period of weeks or months, but some emotional effects (particularly anxiety when evaluating suicidal patients) can remain for years for some clinicians.

Hendin et al. (2004) conducted in-depth personal interviews with 34 therapists who had a patient suicide. They found that one third of them reported severe distress in the aftermath. The four factors that were most frequently mentioned as the sources of this distress are as follows: (a) failure to hospitalize a suicidal patient who then killed him- or herself, (b) making a treatment decision that may have contributed to a patient's suicide, (c) negative reactions from the therapist's institution after a patient suicide, and (d) fear of a lawsuit by relatives who blamed the therapist. Hendin et al. noted that therapists who were less distressed compared with those who were severely distressed appeared to have a greater capacity to view the situation as a learning opportunity, rather than an occasion for self-reproach.

Brown (1987) suggested that clinicians in training who have a patient suicide may be protected from negative emotional effects because they are under supervision and do not bear ultimate ethical or legal responsibility. Others, however, have suggested the opposite, that trainees are more likely to assume responsibility for "fixing the client" (Rodolfa, Kraft, & Reilley, 1988, p. 47) and thus have stronger feelings of inadequacy when treatment interventions are unsuccessful. There is some evidence that those in training tend to be more distressed by patient suicide than those at the professional level (Ruskin et al., 2004). In addition, Kleespies et al. (1993) reported a negative relationship between intrusive thoughts and images and the year in training in which a patient suicide was experienced (i.e., the earlier in training the suicide occurred, the greater the perceived impact). It is hypothesized that trainees who are less experienced may feel less prepared, less secure in their roles, or more surprised or shocked by patient suicidal behavior than more experienced trainees and professionals.

Impact of Patient Violent Behavior

The impact of patient violence on mental health staff was of sufficient magnitude in a public mental health care system in Massachusetts that Flannery, Fulton, Tausch, and DeLoffi (1991) initiated the ASAP. As mentioned earlier in this chapter, ASAP is a voluntary, system-wide, peer-help crisis intervention program to assist staff in coping with the psychological sequelae of patient violence. In terms of psychological sequelae, those involved with the ASAP program noted that a significant number of staff victims have reported a disruption in a sense of mastery of their work, a disruption of their caring attachments, and distress about the meaning of the event.

The findings of Flannery et al. (2001) seem consistent with earlier findings reported by Guy, Brown, and Poelstra (1991). In a national survey of the consequences of patient violence directed at psychotherapists, these investigators found that 40% of clinicians who reported one or more instances of patient violence experienced a dramatically increased sense of vulnerability in the aftermath. The greater the extent of any physical injury, the greater the sense of fear and vulnerability that followed. Some clinician victims reported a decrease in overall emotional well-being and in a sense of professional competency. As noted in the section on incidence of patient violence, because many victims of patient attacks are students or those early in their postdoctoral years, it is easy to see how a sense of self-doubt and incompetence can be heightened, even though our actual ability to predict patient violence is limited.

Most clinicians in the survey by Guy et al. (1991) did not reduce their workload after a patient attack, but many engaged in protective measures. The most common protective measure was to refuse to accept patients whom they perceived as having potential for violence. This more cautious approach was especially true of clinicians who believed they could have predicted or prevented the previous episode of violence. Their tendency was to refer such patients to other clinicians. Therapist victims also reported being more active about setting limits on patient behavior and about formulating contingency plans for obtaining assistance in the event another incident occurred. Some were reported to have relocated to a safer building or office or to have their home phone number unlisted. Others avoided working alone in the office, hired a secretary, or had a security alarm system installed.

Some episodes of patient violence required that the clinician be active in his or her self-defense or have the patient physically restrained. As Guy and Brady (1998) pointed out, these practitioners sometimes have lingering fears about possible litigation or malpractice claims. In reality, however, it is the rare patient who files a complaint against a clinician whom he or she has physically assaulted.

Impact of Working With Victims of Violence

Although therapy is vitally important to the recovery of individuals who have experienced trauma, research and common knowledge lead us to understand that therapists who provide this treatment are at risk of experiencing a range of personal difficulties. Working with individuals in crisis can lead trauma therapists to be concerned about their competency and ability to help those who are suffering (Astin, 1997), and they may develop anxiety, intrusive thoughts about the client's experiences, and emotional numbing. They may also use avoidance strategies to dodge traumatic material in sessions (McCann & Pearlman, 1990).

These negative experiences happen with sufficient frequency to have become identified by a number of names, including *vicarious trauma* (VT) and *secondary traumatic stress* (STS), also known as *compassion fatigue*. *Burnout* is another term that describes negative reactions on the part of the clinician in response to difficult work; however, it differs from the others in that it is not generally linked to specific client traumas (Trippany, Kress, & Wilcoxon, 2004).

The terms STS and VT are often used interchangeably; however, there are, in fact, some differences. VT emphasizes cognitive disruptions for the therapist, whereas STS, or compassion fatigue, focuses on emotional or social disturbances (Jenkins & Baird, 2002). The concept behind STS is that the clinician experiences trauma symptoms secondary to working with trauma survivors and these symptoms are identical to the symptoms of PTSD. Figley (1995) described three domains of this construct, including reexperiencing the client's trauma event, avoidance or numbing in response to reminders of the trauma, and arousal. VT describes disturbances in beliefs or cognitive schemas related to intimacy, trust, safety, control, and esteem (Saakvitne & Pearlman, 1996) and is based on constructivist self-development theory (CSDT). Schemas organize and direct how people experience the world and are reinforced and influenced by others (McCann & Pearlman, 1990). In essence, the experience of hearing about clients' traumatic events can result in the disruption of cognitive schemas, impacting how the clinician perceives the environment and regards her- or himself and others. Despite the distinctions between STS and VT, at their core they both are ways of understanding distress that trauma therapists experience (Bober & Regehr, 2006).

The Traumatic Stress Institute Belief Scale (McCann & Pearlman, 1990) has been used widely to measure VT in terms of disruptions consistent with CSDT. Counselors who work with sexual assault survivors appear to have more disrupted beliefs (Schauben & Frazier, 1995), a finding echoed by Bober and Regehr (2006) and VanDeusen and Way (2006), who respectively found an increase in cognitive disruptions for rape counselors and counselors who work with sexual abuse survivors.

Saakvitne and Pearlman (1996) outlined specific examples of how VT can affect the clinician. For example, those affected by VT may have trouble accessing emotions, often experience guilt, and may find it difficult to be intimate with their partners because of intrusive thoughts of clients' abuse. Grief is another common reaction for trauma therapists, and this can lead to feeling alienated from others (Herman, 1992). Psychotherapy itself can be compromised by the clinician's VT, even leading to lower quality of care (Raquepaw & Miller, 1989). The therapist may be irritable, less able to attend to stimuli, and more prone to misdiagnosis (Munroe, 1990).

COPING WITH THE AFTERMATH OF BEHAVIORAL EMERGENCIES

The research summarized earlier in this chapter has shown that patient suicidal behavior and patient violence and victimization can be quite disturbing to the mental health clinician. Certainly, patient suicidal behavior and patient violence are behaviors that can arouse feelings of self-doubt, self-blame, and failure in the clinician. They can destroy so-called rescue fantasies and leave the clinician with a sense of helplessness. Yet, as Jones (1987) pointed out, "The tragedy of patient suicide can also be an opportunity for us as therapists to grow in our skills at assessing and intervening in suicidal crisis" (p. 141). It is this perspective on crisis as an opportunity for growth that seemed to distinguish those therapists in the study by Hendin et al. (2004), who seemed to cope while engaging in less self-reproach. It would seem that framing difficult events as both a crisis and an opportunity should be encouraged.

Patient Suicidal Behavior

It should be noted that efforts to cope with the impact of patient suicide or suicidal behavior can be complicated by the nature of our relationship with the patient. As both Farberow (1993) and Jones (1987) suggested, patient suicidal behavior can bring about both a personal crisis and a professional crisis for the clinician. On a personal level, the clinician often comes to know the most intimate feelings of the patient and so may have intense reactions to the patient's self-destructiveness. On the professional level, however, the clinician may have concerns about responsibility, malpractice suits, censure from colleagues, damage to reputation, and so forth. The professional concerns can thus complicate and inhibit the clinician's personal reactions. They can cause the therapist to withdraw from colleagues and to become isolated from potential sources of support.

Symptomatic of these professional concerns is the cautionary note sounded by Bongar (1991, 2002) and Ruben (1990); that is, intern discussions with a supervisor or postmortem case reviews in the wake of such events as a patient suicide may be open to the legal discovery process in the event of a malpractice suit. As a protective measure, Bongar (2002) suggested that such discussions "be confined to the context of a psychotherapeutic or legal consultation" (p. 250). This position, although legally conservative, would seem to have the effect of deterring the student therapist from accessing sources of support and professional development. In fact, in their survey of patient suicidal behavior during psychology training, Kleespies et al. (1993) found that the greatest percentage of psychology graduate students and interns in their sample sought support from their case supervisors following a patient suicide or suicide attempt. These same graduate students and interns rated discussions with their case supervisors as the most beneficial form of case review as they attempted to understand the patient's behavior and their own functioning.

Ellis and Dickey (1998) sought legal consultation on this issue, and although caution was advised, they reported that there seemed to be no legal precedent for a supervisor being required by a court to divulge information from a postsuicide debriefing or review in a malpractice proceeding. They also noted that programs might be at equal or greater legal risk if they failed to try to examine and understand the events leading to a patient's suicide. From an ethical perspective, Behnke (2005) reminded us that when the therapist is a trainee, the legal responsibility for the patient's or client's treatment resides with the supervisor. He also informs us that the supervisor not only protects the client's welfare but also helps the trainee to attain competence as a treatment provider.

Yet, the position expressed by Bongar (1991, 2002) and others would seem to prevent the supervisor from working with the trainee to understand what happened with the treatment and from fulfilling his or her responsibility to determine whether remedial education or skill development is needed.

From our perspective, the issue seems similar to what has been referred to as *defensive practice*. In defensive practice, the clinician either over- or underresponds to a potentially suicidal patient, not out of concern for the patient's well-being but primarily to protect him- or herself from future potential legal action. It seems as though there can also be *defensive supervision* in which the processing and review of critical clinical events is discouraged or suppressed because of an uncertain legal risk. If such an approach is adopted, the clinician-in-training is likely to be deprived of the support and learning that can come from the opportunity to share his or her feelings and reactions with those who are in a position to help. Unless they have engaged in some egregious behavior in the therapy, trainees or interns need their supervisor's support to deal with and learn from such sad and unsettling events.

There have been a number of single case reports of what proved helpful to clinicians in coping with the aftermath of a patient suicide (e.g., see Alexander, 1991; Berman, 1995; Spiegelman & Werth, 2005). Other investigators have attempted to gather data from larger samples on this topic. Thus, Kleespies et al. (1990, 1993) found that former psychology interns reported coping with patient suicide primarily by the use of support systems and case reviews. As mentioned earlier, the greatest percentage turned to their case supervisors for emotional support, followed by seeking out peers, other staff members, and finally family or significant others. They also found discussions of the case with their supervisor very beneficial.

Talking with a colleague who knew the patient or who had a similar experience with a patient has been reported as beneficial in reducing isolation and providing support (Alexander, 1991; Berman, 1995; Spiegelman & Werth, 2005). At times, this sort of discussion has happened in a group format. Thus, Kolodny, Binder, Bronstein, and Friend (1979) reported how meaningful it was for four therapists to meet over the course of a year to discuss their reactions to patient suicides that each had recently experienced. In addition, Jones (1987) described a successful self-help support group for therapist–survivors. The group provides a nonjudgmental atmosphere in which therapists can share their feelings and issues related to patient suicide.

Patient Violent Behavior

Many suggestions for coping with the aftermath of patient suicidal behavior also apply to coping with the aftermath of patient violent behavior. Some clinicians seem to go through a natural recovery process and prefer to cope on their own. Others may wish to do as suggested by Guy and Brady (1998) and find a trusted colleague with whom to discuss the issues and sort through feelings of guilt or responsibility for the patient's behavior. As reported by Guy et al. (1991), it is not unusual for some clinicians who were attacked by a patient to enter or reenter personal psychotherapy following the incident. Psychological issues regarding personal vulnerability and safety can be activated by a physical assault. A therapist can assist the clinician–victim in dealing with the concerns that can arise and in reducing the possibility that these concerns can bleed through into the individual's professional work.

As noted earlier, Flannery et al. (1991) developed a voluntary program in a state mental health system (i.e., the ASAP). Initially, this program included *critical-incident stress debriefing* as one of its services to staff victims (Flannery et al., 1991). Given the controversy in recent years, however, over whether such intense debriefings shortly after a traumatizing event are helpful or harmful (Tuckey, 2007), the program now emphasizes a response that is more consistent with a supportive, or so-called psychological first aid, approach (Flannery, Juliano, Cronin, & Walker, 2006). When a patient assault occurs, an ASAP team member responds to the individual staff member to offer support and see whether any needed medical care is being provided. The team member discusses whether the victim feels able to manage his or her feelings and continue to work. The staff victim might be referred to a weekly support group for assaulted staff members. The team member offers to call back in 3 days and 10 days to see how the victim is doing.

Patient Victimization

Schauben and Frazier (1995) surveyed female psychologists and counselors who worked with victims of sexual violence regarding how they coped emotionally with hearing about such events. Some, usually those with greater levels of distress reported disengaging from the patient, but most reported using active strategies such as working hard to solve problems with the patient and seeking out their own support systems. In discussing work with self-injuring trauma survivors, Deiter, Nicholls, and Pearlman (2000) as well as Trippany et al. (2004) emphasized attending to professional needs such as continuing education, ongoing supervision, and consultation from trauma-sensitive colleagues. They recommended balancing this type of work with other types and with play and rest. In discussing the stress of hearing about the trauma experienced by combat veterans, Munroe (1990) also suggested that therapists may need to learn to use supervision and consultation to address potential secondary traumatization. He felt that the review of therapist responses to trauma material should be a regular function of supervision and consultation. He also recommended that trauma therapists do their work as part of a clinical team in which team members have an awareness of the stress of this work and are supportive of each other.

Although trauma therapists tend to believe that these coping strategies will be helpful, Bober and Regehr (2006) did not find an association between traumatic stress scores and time devoted to leisure, self-care, or supervision. They recommended a focus on structural changes to protect therapists, a suggestion also put forth by Bell, Kulkarni, and Dalton (2003). A significant change, for example, might include distributing workloads in a manner that limits exposure to trauma.

CONCLUSION

In this chapter we presented evidence that psychologists and other mental health practitioners frequently work with patients or clients who are at risk of suicidal behavior, of violence, or of becoming the victims of violence. This work can be stressful in itself, but when there is a negative outcome (e.g., the patient commits suicide or becomes violent), the impact on the clinician can be considerable. We noted ways that clinicians have found to cope with such events on an individual basis. Efforts to cope, however, can be supported or made difficult by the environment or system within which one works. As Kleespies and Dettmer (2000) noted, clinical sites and training programs need to be sensitive to clinicians who undertake the stress-inducing task of treating patients or clients who are at high risk. Thus, clinics and hospitals can try to foster a health-promotive environment (Stokols, 1992) in which clinicians and clinicians-in-training feel supported and protected in their efforts to work with and discuss difficult cases, or they can be primarily focused on defending institutional interests, narrowly defined. It is our contention that those that take the former approach will ultimately reap the benefit of having clinicians who are less stressed and better able to function to their fullest capacities.

REFERENCES

Alexander, V. (1991). *Words I never thought to speak: Stories of life in the wake of suicide.* New York: Lexington Books.

Arthur, G., Brende, J., & Quiroz, S. (2003). Violence: Incidence and frequency of physical and psychological assaults affecting mental health providers in Georgia. *The Journal of General Psychology, 130,* 22–45.

Astin, M. (1997). Trauma therapy: How helping rape victims affects me as a therapist. *Women & Therapy, 20,* 101–109.

Behnke, S. (2005, May). The supervisor as gatekeeper: Reflections on Ethical Standards 7.02, 7.04, 7.05, 7.06, and 10.01. *Monitor on Psychology, 36*(5), 90–91.

Bell, H., Kulkarni, S., & Dalton, L. (2003). Organizational prevention of vicarious trauma. *Families in Society: The Journal of Contemporary Human Services, 84,* 463–470.

Berman, A. (1995). "To engrave herself on all our memories; to force her body into our lives": The impact of suicide on psychotherapists. In B. Mishara (Ed.), *The impact of suicide* (pp. 85–99). New York: Springer Publishing Company.

Bernstein, H. (1981). Survey of threats and assaults directed toward psychotherapists. *American Journal of Psychotherapy, 35,* 542–549.

Bober, T., & Regehr, C. (2006). Strategies for reducing secondary or vicarious trauma: Do they work? *Brief Treatment and Crisis Intervention, 6,* 1–9.

Bongar, B. (1991). *The suicidal patient: Clinical and legal standards of care.* Washington, DC: American Psychological Association.

Bongar, B. (2002). *The suicidal patient: Clinical and legal standards of care* (2nd ed.). Washington, DC: American Psychological Association.

Borja, S. E., Callahan, J. L., & Long, P. J. (2006). Positive and negative adjustment and social support of sexual assault survivors. *Journal of Traumatic Stress, 19,* 905–914.

Briere, J., & Elliott, D. M. (2003). Prevalence and psychological sequelae of self-reported childhood physical and sexual abuse in a general population sample of men and women. *Child Abuse & Neglect, 27,* 1205–1222.

Brown, H. (1987). Patient suicide during residency training: Incidence, implications, and program response. *Journal of Psychiatric Education, 11,* 201–216.

Chemtob, C., Bauer, G., Hamada, R., Pelowski, S. R., & Muraoka, M. Y. (1989). Patient suicide: Occupational hazard for psychologists and psychiatrists. *Professional Psychology: Research and Practice, 20,* 294–300.

Chemtob, C., Hamada, R., Bauer, G., Kinney, B., & Torigoe, R. (1988). Patients' suicides: Frequency and impact on psychiatrists. *American Journal of Psychiatry, 145,* 224–228.

Chemtob, C., Hamada, R., Bauer, G., Torigoe, R., & Kinney, B. (1988). Patient suicide: Frequency and impact on psychologists. *Professional Psychology: Research and Practice, 19,* 416–420.

Deiter, P., Nicholls, S., & Pearlman, L. (2000). Self-injury and self-capacities: Assisting an individual in crisis. *Journal of Clinical Psychology, 56,* 1173–1191.

Ellis, T., & Dickey, T. (1998). Procedures surrounding the suicide of a trainee's patient: A national survey of psychology internships and psychiatry residency programs. *Professional Psychology: Research and Practice, 29,* 492–497.

Farberow, N. (1993). Bereavement after suicide. In A. Leenaars, A. Berman, P. Cantor, R. Litman, & R. Maris (Eds.), *Suicidology: Essays in honor of Edwin Shneidman* (pp. 337–345). Northvale, NJ: Jason Aronson.

Figley, C. R. (1995). Compassion fatigue as secondary traumatic stress disorder: An overview. In C. R. Figley (Ed.), *Compassion fatigue: Coping with secondary traumatic stress disorder in those who treat the traumatized* (pp. 1–20). New York: Brunner/Mazel.

Flannery, R., Fulton, P., Tausch, J., & DeLoffi, A. (1991). A program to help staff cope with psychological sequelae of assaults by patients. *Hospital and Community Psychiatry, 42,* 935–938.

Flannery, R., Juliano, J., Cronin, S., & Walker, A. (2006). Characteristics of assaultive psychiatric patients: Fifteen-year analysis of the Assaulted Staff Action Program (ASAP). *Psychiatric Quarterly, 77,* 239–249.

Flannery, R., Stone, P., Rego, S., & Walker, A. (2001). Characteristics of staff victims of patient assault: Ten year analysis of the Assaulted Staff Action Program (ASAP). *Psychiatric Quarterly, 72,* 237–248.

Grad, O., Zavasnik, A., & Groleger, U. (1997). Suicide of a patient: Gender differences in bereavement reactions of therapists. *Suicide and Life-Threatening Behavior, 27,* 379–386.

Guy, J., & Brady, J. L. (1998). The stress of violent behavior for the clinician. In P. M. Kleespies (Ed.), *Emergencies in mental health practice: Evaluation and management* (pp. 398–417). New York: Guilford Press.

Guy, J., Brown, C., & Poelstra, P. (1990). Who gets attacked? A national survey of patient violence directed at psychologists in clinical practice. *Professional Psychology: Research and Practice, 21,* 493–495.

Guy, J., Brown, C., & Poelstra, P. (1991). Living with the aftermath: A national survey of the consequences of patient violence directed at psychotherapists. *Psychotherapy in Private Practice, 9*, 35–44.

Hendin, H., Haas, A., Maltsberger, J., Szanto, K., & Rabinowicz, H. (2004). Factors contributing to therapists' distress after the suicide of a patient. *American Journal of Psychiatry, 161*, 1442–1446.

Herman, J. L. (1992). *Trauma and recovery*. New York: Basic Books.

Horowitz, M., Wilner, N., & Alvarez, W. (1979). Impact of Event Scale: A measure of subjective stress. *Psychosomatic Medicine, 41*, 209–218.

Hoyert, D. L., Kung, H., & Smith, B. L. (2005). Deaths: Preliminary data for 2003. *National Vital Statistics Report, 53*(15). Hyattsville, MD: National Center for Health Statistics.

Jacobsen, J., Ting, L., Sanders, S., & Harrington, D. (2004). Prevalence and reactions to fatal and nonfatal client suicidal behavior: A national study of mental health social workers. *Omega, 49*, 237–248.

Jayaratne, S., Croxton, T., & Mattison, D. (2004). A national survey of violence in the practice of social work. *Families in Society: The Journal of Contemporary Social Services, 85*, 445–453.

Jenkins, S. R., & Baird, S. (2002). Secondary traumatic stress and vicarious trauma: A validational study. *Journal of Traumatic Stress, 15*, 423–432.

Jones, F., Jr. (1987). Therapists as survivors of client suicide. In E. Dunne, J. McIntosch, & K. Dunne-Maxim (Eds.), *Suicide and its aftermath: Understanding and counseling the survivors* (pp. 126–141). New York: Norton.

Kaslow, N. J., Thompson, M. P., Okun, A., Price, A., Young, S., Bender, M., et al. (2002). Risk and protective factors for suicidal behavior in abused African American women. *Journal of Consulting and Clinical Psychology, 70*, 311–319.

Kleespies, P. M., & Dettmer, E. (2000). The stress of patient emergencies for the clinician: Incidence, impact, and means of coping. *Journal of Clinical Psychology, 56*, 1353–1369.

Kleespies, P. M., Penk, W., & Forsyth, J. (1993). The stress of patient suicidal behavior during clinical training: Incidence, impact, and recovery. *Professional Psychology: Research and Practice, 24*, 293–303.

Kleespies, P. M., Smith, M., & Becker, B. (1990). Psychology interns as patient suicide survivors: Incidence, impact, and recovery. *Professional Psychology: Research and Practice, 21*, 257–263.

Kolodny, S., Binder, R., Bronstein, A., & Friend, R. (1979). The working through of patients' suicides by four therapists. *Suicide and Life-Threatening Behavior, 9*, 33–46.

Luoma, J. B., Martin, C. E., & Pearson, J. L. (2002). Contact with mental health and primary care providers before suicide: A review of the evidence. *American Journal of Psychiatry, 159*, 909–916.

McAdams, C., & Foster, V. (2000). Client suicide: Its frequency and impact on counselors. *Journal of Mental Health Counseling, 22*, 107–121.

McCann, I. L., & Pearlman, L. A. (1990). Vicarious traumatization: A framework for understanding the psychological effects of working with victims. *Journal of Traumatic Stress, 3*, 131–149.

McFarlane, A., Schrader, G., Bookless, C., & Browne, D. (2006). Prevalence of victimization, posttraumatic stress disorder, and violent behavior in the seriously mentally ill. *Australian and New Zealand Journal of Psychiatry, 40*, 1010–1015.

Munroe, J. (1990). *Therapist traumatization from exposure to clients with combat-related post-traumatic stress disorder: Implications for administration and supervision.* Unpublished doctoral dissertation, Northeastern University, Boston, MA.

Nixon, R. D., Resick, P. A., & Nishith, P. (2004). An exploration of comorbid depression among female victims of intimate partner violence with posttraumatic stress disorder. *Journal of Affective Disorders, 82*, 315–320.

Pope, K., & Tabachnick, B. (1993). Therapists' anger, hate, fear, and sexual feelings: National survey of therapist responses, client characteristics, critical events, formal complaints, and training. *Professional Psychology: Research and Practice, 24*, 142–152.

Raquepaw, J., & Miller, R. (1989). Psychotherapist burnout: A componential analysis. *Professional Psychology: Research and Practice, 20*, 32–36.

Rodolfa, E., Kraft, W., & Reilley, R. (1988). Stressors of professionals and trainees at APA-approved counseling and VA medical center internship sites. *Professional Psychology: Research and Practice, 19*, 43–49.

Ruben, H. (1990). Surviving a suicide in your practice. In S. Blumenthal & D. Kupfer (Eds.), *Suicide over the life cycle: Risk factors, assessment, and treatment of suicidal patients* (pp. 619–636). Washington, DC: American Psychiatric Press.

Ruskin, R., Sakinofsky, I., Bagby, R., Dickens, S., & Sousa, G. (2004). Impact of patient suicide on psychiatrists and psychiatry trainees. *Academic Psychiatry, 28*, 104–110.

Saakvitne, K. W., & Pearlman, L. A. (1996). *Transforming the pain: A workbook on vicarious traumatization.* New York: Norton.

Sanders, S., Jacobson, J., & Ting, L. (2005). Reactions of mental health social workers following a client suicide completion: A qualitative investigation. *Omega, 51*, 197–216.

Schauben, L., & Frazier, P. (1995). Vicarious trauma: The effects on female counselors of working with sexual violence survivors. *Psychology of Women Quarterly, 19*, 49–64.

Spiegelman, J. S., & Werth, J. L., Jr. (2005). Don't forget about me: The experiences of therapists-in-training after a client has attempted or died by suicide. *Women and Therapy, 28*, 35–57.

Stark, E., & Flitcraft, A. (1996). *Women at risk: Domestic violence and women's health.* Thousand Oaks, CA: Sage.

Stokols, D. (1992). Establishing and maintaining healthy environments: Towards a social ecology of health promotion. *American Psychologist, 47*, 6–22.

Teplin, L. A., McClelland, G. M., Abram, K. M., & Weiner, D. A. (2005). Crime victimization in adults with severe mental illness: Comparison with the National Crime Victimization Survey. *Archives of General Psychiatry, 62,* 911–921.

Ting, L., Sanders, S., Jacobson, J., & Power, J. (2006). Dealing with the aftermath: A qualitative analysis of mental health social workers' reactions after a client suicide. *Social Work, 51,* 329–341.

Trippany, R. L., Kress, V. E. W., & Wilcoxin, S. A. (2004). Preventing vicarious trauma: What counselors should know when working with trauma survivors. *Journal of Counseling & Development, 82,* 31–37.

Tryon, G. (1986). Abuse of therapist by patient: A national survey. *Professional Psychology: Research and Practice, 17,* 357–363.

Tuckey, M. (2007). Issues in the debriefing debate for emergency services: Moving research outcomes forward. *Clinical Psychology: Science and Practice, 14,* 106–116.

U.S. Department of Justice. (2007). *Bureau of Justice Statistics: Crime and victim statistics.* Retrieved May 7, 2007, from http://www.ojp.usdoj.gov/bjs/cvict.htm

VanDeusen, K. M., & Way, I. (2006). Vicarious trauma: An exploratory study of the impact of providing sexual abuse treatment on clinicians' trust and intimacy. *Journal of Child Sexual Abuse, 15,* 69–85.

Whitman, R., Armao, B., & Dent, O. (1976). Assault on the therapist. *American Journal of Psychiatry, 133,* 426–429.

AUTHOR INDEX

Numbers in italics refer to listings in the references.

Bell v. New York City Health and Hospitals
     Corporation, 413, 428
Bender, D. S., 276, 279
Bender, M., 446
Benjamin, M., 119
Bennett, L., 200, 204
Benoit, J., 132, 142
Benson, S., 144
Benton, M. K., 359, 370
Berchick, R. J., 72, 75
Bergin, A. E., 382, 398
Berglund, J., 152, 161, 162
Berglund, M., 242, 253
Berglund, P., 16, 30
Beringer, L., 98
Berkman, B., 120, 308
Berman, A., 10, 442, 444
Berman, A. L., 62, 77, 83, 86, 97, 408, 409,
     428
Bernstein, H., 435, 444
Bernston, G. G., 258, 280
Bertolote, J., 339, 349
Berzins, L. G., 361, 370
Besson, J. A. O., 300, 307
Best, C. L., 168, 169, 171, 182, 185, 187,
     377, 385, 394, 398, 400
Best, S. R., 167, 187
Bhushan, P., 370
Bienvenu, O. J., III, 284
Biering-Sorensen, F., 113, 118, 119
Bille-Brahe, U., 100
Binder, R., 442, 446
Binder, R. L., 126–128, 130–136, 138–140,
     141–144, 370, 421, 429
Binderbrynes, K., 335
Binswanger, O., 294, 305
Bioulac, S., 259, 268, 270, 280
Birchwood, M., 367, 375
Bird, E. D., 300, 305
Birmaher, B., 88, 99
Bisson, J., 20, 31, 168, 187
Bisson, J. I., 28
Bisson, J. L., 174, 182
Björkenstam, C., 106, 107, 117
Bjornaas, M. A., 237, 253
Black, D. W., 268–270, 280
Black, H. C., 406, 407n.3, 408, 428
Black, K., 113, 117
Black, M. C., 168, 182
Blackburn, R., 369, 370
Blair-West, G. W., 280
Blake, D. D., 380, 395

Blake, S. M., 84, 97
Blane, H. T., 193, 195, 205
Blaustein, M., 217, 232
Bleich, A., 279
Blitch, C. L., 415, 428
Blizard, R., 373
Block, C., 203
Block, M., 301, 306
Blum, N., 280
Blumer, D., 109, 117, 303, 305
Blyler, C. R., 269, 271, 281, 367, 372
Boardman, A. P., 260, 280
Bober, T., 439, 443, 444
Bodner, E., 19, 30
Bogel, C., 299, 308
Bola, J., 36, 54
Boldsen, J., 110, 120
Bonanno, G. A., 18, 28, 167, 168, 170, 174,
     182, 378, 395
Bond, G. R., 362, 363, 370, 374
Bond, J., 237, 245, 253
Bongar, B., 5, 7, 10, 60, 63–65, 67, 70, 75,
     76, 78, 407, 409, 410, 412, 421–424,
     428, 429, 441, 444
Bonnin, J. M., 280
Bonnini, S., 313, 334
Bonta, J., 351, 352, 354, 370
Book, S. W., 396
Bookless, C., 436, 447
Boomer, D., 372
Boothroyd, R. A., 363, 371
Borges, G., 66, 76, 80, 99, 245, 253, 282,
     339, 349
Borja, S. E., 436, 444
Borkovec, T. D., 383, 395
Borum, R., 136, 141, 145, 147–152, 155,
     157, 158, 160, 160, 161–163, 375
Boscaro, M., 313, 334
Bostrom, A. G., 68, 78, 275, 283
Bostwick, J. M., 269, 273, 280
Boudreaux, E., 171, 182
Boudreaux, E. D., 245, 253
Bourgeois, M., 280
Bourgon, G., 355, 370
Bowen, J., 121
Bowen, J. D., 297, 308
Bowers, W. J., 415, 428
Boxer, P., 147, 162
Boyer, R., 30, 283
Boyle, E., 203
Brady, J. L., 36, 53, 434, 435, 438, 442,
     445

Brady, K. T., 171, *184*, 382, 390, 393, *394–396*

Brambilla, F., 327, *333*

Brandt, H. M., *183, 396*

Brandt, J., 300, *305*

Brasch, J., 5, *10*

Breiter, H. C., *307*

Bremner, J. D., 327, *333*

Bremner, S., *349*

Brende, J., 434, *444*

Brennan, P. A., 128, *141*, 351, *370*

Brent, D., 88, *99*

Brent, D. A., 81–83, 85–86, *97*, 264, *280*

Breslau, N., 169, 171, *182*

Brewer, D., *162*

Brewin, C. R., 19, *31*, 173, 174, 178, *182*, 187, 381, *394*

Bridge, J., 81, *97*, *280*

Bridge, J. A., 85, *97*

Briere, J., 213, 216, 230, 379–384, 386, *395*, 435, *445*

Brimo, M. L., 390, *396*

Brink, J., 135, *144, 145*

Brinkerhoff, M. B., 194, *203*

Brison, R., 113, *119*

Britt, G. C., 250, *253*

Brock, K., 220, *230*

Brom, D., 393, *395*

Bromet, E., 16, *30*, 168, *185*, 192, *205*, 377, *398*

Bronen, R. A., *333*

Bronisch, T., 18, *28*

Bronish, T., 87, *101*

Bronnum-Hansen, H., 110, 111, 113, *117*, *118*

Bronselaer, K., *255*

Bronstein, A., 442, *446*

Brook, J. S., *98*

Brown, C., 284, 434, 438, *445, 446*

Brown, G., 72, *75*

Brown, G. K., 343, 344, *349*

Brown, H., 437, *445*

Brown, J., *98*

Brown, L., 80, *101*

Brown, L. M., 64, 65, *75*

Brown, R., 269, 272, *284*

Brown, R. A., *207*

Browne, D., 436, *447*

Bryant, R. A., 18, 20, *28*, *30*, 168, 170, 172, 174, 175, 178–180, *182*, *183, 185*, *186*, 378, *395*

Bucholz, K. K., *399*

Buckley, P. F., 367, *370*

Bunch, J., 263, *279*

Bureau of Justice, *52*

Bureau of Justice Statistics, 133, *141*, 378, *395*

Burgess, P., 128, *145*

Burgess, P. M., 266, 267, *282*

Burke, G. L., *333*

Burns, A., 300, *305*

Burns, B. J., *145, 375*

Burns, T., *144*

Busch-Iversen, H., 130, 134, *142*

Buskens, E., *350*

Butchart, A., *401*

Butollo, W., *28*

Buylaert, W., *285*

Bylsma, F. W., 293, *306*

Byrd, D., 62, *78*

Byrne, C. A., 195, *203*, *207*

Byrne, C. M., *186*

Byrne, K., 380, *394*

Byrnes, H. F., 245, *255*

Cabot, M. G., 410, *429*

Cacioppo, J. T., 258, *280*

Caddell, J. M., *398*

Cadsky, O., 194, *204*

Cahill, S. P., 390, *395, 397*

Cahn, T. S., 194, *206*

Caine, E., *53*, 111, *117*

Caine, E. D., 258, 259, *281, 282*, 299–301, *305*

Calder, A. J., *334*

Calhoun, L. G., 18, *28*

California Civil Code § 43.92, 419, 420, *428*

Calkins, D. R., 241, *254*

Callahan, C., 153, *161*

Callahan, J., 15, 19, 25, *28*

Callahan, J. L., 436, *444*

Calof, D. L., 215, 216, 222, *231*

Camargo, C. A., Jr., 245, *253*

Campanella, G., *117*

Campayo, A., 295, *305*

Campbell, D., *203*

Campbell, J., *203*

Campbell, J. C., 170, *183*, 191, 199, 200, 202, *203*

Campbell, M., 323, *333*

Campbell, R., *395*

Campling, P., 268, 270, *281*

Cannon-Bowers, J. A., 33, 34, *52*

Cantor, C. H., *280*

Caplan, G., 15, 28
Cappola, A. R., 316, 333
Caralis, P., 36, 52
Cardena, E., 24, 30, 179, 183
Caringi, J., 229, 233
Carlson, J. G., 18, 29
Carney, D. P., 133, 141
Carney Love, C., 360, 365, 370, 373
Carpenter, D., 367, 370
Carpenter, R., 40, 52
Carroll, K., 382, 394, 395
Carson, A. J., 257, 280
Carter, M., 372
Cascardi, M. A., 197, 199, 203, 378, 395
Cashman, L., 380, 397
Caslyn, R. J., 363, 370
Caspi, A., 191, 197, 203, 206
Cassel, C. A., 362, 376
Cassem, E., 113, 114, 117
Cassens, G. P., 308
Castello, M. F., 280
Castonguay, L. G., 383, 395
Castro-Blanco, D., 14, 29
Catalano, R., 162
Catalano, S. M., 167, 169, 183
Caton, C. L. M., 236, 253
Cauffman, E., 148, 163
Causby, V., 192, 206
Cavanagh, J. T., 257, 261, 263, 264, 280
Celesia, G. G., 298, 305
Centers for Disease Control and Prevention, 87, 97, 169, 170, 183, 378, 395
Centers for Medicare and Medicaid Services, 138, 141
Chae, B.-J., 297, 305
Chalmers, C., 372
Chamberlain, J. R., 140, 143
Chan, C. L., 280
Chan, K. A., 259, 260, 280
Chan, K. -L., 295, 305
Chan, S. S., 280
Chan, S. S. M., 285
Chan, W. S., 280
Chandler, J. H., 301, 307
Chang, H., 119
Chapman, A. L., 361, 374, 375
Charlifue, S., 113, 117
Charney, D. S., 395
Chase, G. A., 300, 306
Chauncey, D. L., 272, 286
Chawky, N., 281, 282
Chelminski, I., 266, 286

Chemtob, C., 432, 433, 437, 445
Chemtob, C. M., 18, 29, 75, 174, 183
Chen, J., 168, 182
Chen, L., 119
Chen, T., 81, 97
Chen, Y. H., 264, 280
Cheng, A. T. A., 259, 260, 266, 267, 280
Cheng, Q., 111, 117
Cherpitel, C., 237, 245, 253
Chertow, G., 108, 119
Chew-Graham, C., 349
Chi, I., 285
Chiappetta, L., 81, 97
Chilcoat, H. D., 182
Chiles, J. A., 72, 77
Chiu, H. F. K., 285
Choi, C., 105, 120
Cholo, A. B., 26, 29
Choo, I. H., 306
Chou, S. P., 281
Christensen, M. L., 106, 121
Christy, A., 363, 364, 371
Chu, M., 119
Ciokajlo, M., 26, 29
Ciraulo, A., 41, 54
Ciraulo, D., 40, 41, 52, 54
Citrome, L., 138, 141, 368, 373, 376
Clark, D., 47, 53, 114, 117
Clark, D. C., 73, 75
Clark, E., 120, 308
Classen, C., 23, 24, 30, 172, 179, 183, 186
Classen, C. C., 169, 172, 183
Clay, R., 363, 374
Clayton, P. C., 268, 279
Cleary, K., 64, 65, 75
Cleary, P., 36, 52
Cleland, C. M., 355, 374
Clements, A., 282
Clery, C., 213, 231
Cleven, G., 362, 375
Cloitre, M., 383–385, 387, 395, 396
Clough, J. B., 153, 163
Clum, G. A., 173, 187
Cobb, T., 5, 10
Coccaro, E., 368, 373
Coccaro, E. F., 368, 371
Cochran, B., 390, 401
Cochrane, K. J., 253
Coffey, S. F., 390, 396
Cohan, S. L., 247, 255
Cohen, D., 279
Cohen, E., 98

Cohen, L., 384, 395
Cohen, L. R., 383, 396
Cohen, P., 98
Cohen, S., 23, 29
Coid, J., 266, 276, 280
Coker, A. L., 170, 171, 183, 378, 396
Cole, G., 292, 305
Colket, J. T., 396
Collins, B., 170, 187
Collins, B. S., 196, 206
Comotois, K. A., 343, 344, 350
Compton, W. M., 172, 183
Comstock, B., 51, 53
Conger, J. C., 360, 371
Conneally, P. M., 117, 299, 305
Conner, K. R., 261, 280
Connolly, J., 85, 97, 280
Connors, R., 213, 230, 233
Connors, R. E., 215, 231
Conrad, S. D., 216, 232
Constantino, M. J., 383, 395
Conterio, K., 213, 231
Conwell, Y., 37, 53, 66, 75, 258, 259, 261,
    263, 264, 266, 268, 269, 272–274,
    276, 280–282, 285, 286
Conybeare, R., 119
Cook, P. J., 153, 161
Cooke, D. J., 365, 371
Cooper, J., 260, 279
Cooper, M. L., 399
Cooper, T., 368, 373
Cormier, C. A., 128, 144, 201, 204, 205,
    351, 375
Corona-Vazquez, T., 297, 306
Corrigan, P., 366, 371
Cosden, M., 364, 371
Costa, P. T., Jr., 284
Costello, E., 234
Cottle, C., 149, 161
Cottler, L. B., 171–173, 183, 184
Cottrell, S. S., 297, 305
Cournos, F., 127, 144
Courtois, C., 231
Cowen, P. J., 262, 283
Cox, C., 53
Cramer, V., 266, 285
Crane, D. F., 240, 254
Craske, M. G., 384, 393, 394, 396
Craven, D., 204
Craven, M., 120
Crawford, E., 64, 65, 75
Crawford, M. J., 342, 349

Creed, F., 144
Creelman, W., 40, 52
Cremniter, D., 174, 183
Crime Victims Research and Treatment Cen-
    ter, 399
Cronin, S., 442, 445
Crow, T. J., 299, 305
Crowell, N. A., 148, 162
Croxton, T., 434, 446
Cummings, J. L., 112, 119, 292, 299, 305
Cupples, L. A., 120, 308
Currier, G., 40, 52
Currier, G. W., 237, 253, 312, 328, 334, 367,
    370
Curry, M. A., 203
Cutting, J. C., 262, 283
Czbor, P., 127, 142
Czobor, P., 368, 373, 376

Daffern, M., 130, 134, 135, 144
Dalton, L., 443, 444
Daly, M., 199, 208
Dancu, C. V., 380, 392, 397
Danese, M. D., 333
Dang, S. T., 179, 180, 182, 183
Daniel, S. S., 98
Danielson, K. K., 197, 203
Dansky, B. S., 167, 171, 184, 187, 377, 382,
    393, 394–396, 400
Dassen, T., 374
David, D., 396
Davidsen, M., 110, 117
Davidson, J., 275, 285
Davidson, J. R. T., 380, 383, 388, 389, 393,
    396, 397, 401
Davidson, L., 67, 76
Davidson, R. T., 307
Davidson, W. S., 395
Davies, J. M., 216, 222, 231
Davies, K., 117
Davies, R., 372
Davies, S., 268, 270, 281
Davis, B., 36, 52
Davis, G. C., 182
Davis, J., 126, 142, 393, 396
Davis, J. M., 31
Davis, K. E., 183, 396
Davis, M., 385, 396
Davis, R., 83, 100
Dawson, D. A., 281
Day, A., 281
Deahl, M., 174, 184

Eichelman, B., 365, 372
Eickelberg, S. J., 247, 253
Eisner, J., 131, 143
Eisner, J. P., 131, 143
Ekeberg, Ø., 106, 118, 253
Ekouevi, D. K., 280
Elbogen, E. B., 130, 141, 368, 375
Elitzur, A., 4, 5, 10
Ellens, J. K., 364, 371
Elliott, D., 148, 161
Elliott, D. M., 435, 445
Ellis, T., 10, 441, 445
Ellis, T. E., 412, 428
Elofsson, S., 268, 272, 284
Emmelkamp, P. M. G., 20, 32, 359, 376
Endicott, J., 283
Engberg, A., 110, 121
Engelhard, I. M., 173, 184
Engholm, G., 106, 121
Epstein, A., 36, 52
Erbaugh, J., 179, 182, 380, 394
Erickson, D. J., 186
Eror, E. A., 293, 305
Eshelman, E. R., 385, 396
Espinosa, G., 249, 254
Essock, S. M., 145
Estroff, S. E., 132, 142
Eudy, K., 428
Even, C., 117
Everly, G. S., 18, 19, 31, 174, 184, 186
Evershed, S., 361, 372
Ewing v. Goldstein, 417, 428
Exner, J. E., 71, 75
Eyeson-Annan, M. L., 280
Eyman, J. R., 70, 71, 75
Eyman, S. K., 70, 71, 75

Fahy, T., 144
Fairbank, J. A., 205, 398
Fallo, F., 313, 334
Falsetti, S. A., 170, 171, 176, 179, 184, 187, 380, 393, 396, 400
Fals-Stewart, W., 195, 199, 206, 245, 253, 255
Faragher, B., 260, 279
Farahmand, B., 119
Farber, B. A., 382, 396
Farberow, N., 440, 445
Farrell, L. E., 207
Farrell, R. B., 297, 306
Farrer, L. A., 112, 117
Farrington, D., 162

Fatuck v. Hillside Hospital, 411, 428
Fava, G., 119
Fava, G. A., 313, 334
Favazza, A. R., 212, 213, 231, 339, 349
Fawcett, J., 47, 53, 62, 67, 73, 75, 114, 117
Fazel, S., 128, 142
Feder, L., 352, 372
Feeny, N. C., 389, 390, 397, 398, 401
Fein, R., 149, 152, 155, 161
Feinstein, A., 111, 117
Feld, S. L., 194, 195, 204
Feldman, E., 349
Feldman, M. E., 203
Felitti, V. J., 377, 397
Felmingham, K., 183, 395
Fenger, K., 112, 120
Fenton, W. S., 269, 271, 281, 367, 372
Ferguson, B., 60, 77
Fergusson, D. M., 82, 84, 97, 98
Fernandez, E., 359, 360, 370
Ferrier, I. N., 329, 333
Feuer, C. A., 389, 399
Figley, C. R., 439, 445
First, M. B., 262, 284
Fischer, J. E., 374
Fischman, A. J., 307
Fisher, P., 85, 98
Fiszbein, A., 272, 282
Fitzgerald, M. M., 398
Flannery, R., 434, 435, 438, 442, 445
Fleck, D., 359, 372
Flitcraft, A., 436, 447
Flory, M., 85, 98, 101
Fluch, A., 279
Foa, E. B., 178, 180, 184, 187, 378, 380–385, 387–390, 392, 393, 394, 395, 397, 398, 400
Fogg, L., 73, 75
Foley, K., 115, 117
Folsom, D. P., 372
Folstein, M., 49, 53
Folstein, M. F., 293, 299–301, 305–307
Folstein, S., 49, 53
Folstein, S. E., 299–301, 305–307
Foltynie, T., 298, 309
Fonagy, P., 217, 218, 231, 276, 279
Fong, G. T., 152, 162
Forbes, N., 53
Ford, J. D., 217–219, 228, 231
Ford, R., 363, 372
Fordwood, S. R., 143
Forsyth, J., 433, 446

Forsyth, J. P., 59, 76
Forth, A., *161*
Foster, T., 260, 264, 265–267, *281*
Foster, V., *446*
Foster, V. A., 59, *77*
Foster v. Charter Medical Group, 413, *428*
Fowler, R., 114, *120*
Fowler, R. C., *284*
Foy, D., 393, *399*
Foy, D. W., 27, *31*, 197, 203, 383, *400*
Frances, A., 383, 389, 393, *397*
Franck, J., *253*
Franke, T., 153, *163*
Frankel, H., 113, *118*
Frankel, S., 342, 348, *349*
Frankenburg, F. R., 272, 285, *286*
Franus, N., *285*
Franz, M. L., 300, *306*
Frawley, M. G., 216, 222, *231*
Frazier, J., *98*
Frazier, P., 439, 443, *447*
Frazier, P. H., *98*
Fredrickson, B. L., 18, *29*
Fredrikson, S., 111, *117*
Freedy, J. R., 176, *187*, 380, *400*
Fremouw, W. J., 412, 413, *428*
Freud, S., 258, *281*
Freyer, C., *28*
Fried, H., 22, *29*
Fried, L. P., *333*
Friedman, A., 327, *333*
Friedman, D. H., 196, *206*
Friedman, M. J., *186*, 378, 393, 398, *399*
Friedman, N. J., 381, *397*
Friend, A., *97*, *280*
Friend, R., 442, *446*
Fritz, G., 80, *101*
Fritze, J., *284*
Frost, A. K., *98*
Frye, L. H., 240, *254*
Fullerton, C. S., 18, *32*
Fulton, F. M., 139, *143*
Fulton, P., 438, *445*

Galea, S., *394*
Gallacher, F., *54*, 104, *118*
Gallagher, N. G., 393, *396*
Galvin, D. M., 250, *256*
Gamble, S., 220, *233*
Ganju, V. K., 127, *145*
Garcia, P., *372*
Gardner, W., 126, *142*, *144*

Garfinkel, B. D., 83, *98*
Garofalo, R., 84, *98*
Garre, J., *117*
Garrick, T., 313, *334*
Garrison, B., 63, *75*
Gatsonis, C., 81, *99*
Geller, B., 82, *98*
Gelles, R. J., 194, *207*
Geluk, C. A., *334*
Gendreau, P., 355, *372*
Gergely, G., 217, *231*
Gerhart, K., 113, *117*
Gerhart, U. C., 25, *29*
Gerrity, E. T., 381, *399*
Gerson, S., 34, *53*
Ghaziuddin, N., *99*
Giaconia, R. M., 83, *98*
Gibbon, M., 262, *284*
Gibertson, M. W., *333*
Gil, E., 213, 216, *230*
Gill, M., 106, *119*
Giller, E. L., *335*
Gillespie, K., 260, 264, 265, *281*
Gillham, A. B., 19, *29*
Gilliland, B. E., 20, 25, *29*
Gillmer, B., 360, *376*
Gilmer, T. P., 367, *372*
Gilovich, T., 136, *142*
Gilvarry, C., *376*
Girardi, P., 109, *120*
Givelber, D. J., 415, *428*
Glancy, G. D., 368, *372*
Glassmire, D. M., 70, *76*
Glick, R. L., 5, *10*
Glinski, J., 86, *100*
Goeb, J., 111, *117*
Goetz, C. G., 299, *308*
Goggin, C., 355, *372*
Gohier, B., *117*
Golan, N., 15, 16, 20, 25, *29*
Goldfried, M. R., 382, *399*
Golding, J. M., 192, 197, *204*
Golding, S., 136, *141*
Goldman Consensus Group, 111, *118*
Goldney, R., *349*
Goldstein, C. E., *97*
Goldston, D., 81, *99*
Goldston, D. B., 82, *98*
Gonzales, B., *280*
Gonzalez, A., 247, 249, *253*
Gonzalez, J. S., *335*
Goodenow, C., *97*

Hokama, H., *333*
Holden, G., 152, *161*
Hollander, J., *349*
Hollin, C. R., 353, *372*
Holmberg, E. B., 89, *100*
Holmes, E. P., 366, *371*
Holt, P. E., 178, *185*
Holtzworth-Munroe, A., 196, *205*
Holzer, C. E., 127, *145*
Hooks, S., 250, *254*
Hope, T., 105, *118*, 261, 264, *281*
Hopfer, C., 250, *254*
Hopwood, S., *183, 395*
Hornsveld, R. H. J., 359, *373*
Horowitz, M., 437, *446*
Horton-Deutsch, S., 114, *117*
Horwood, L. J., 84, *98*
Hotaling, G. T., 196–198, *205, 207*
Hoth, K. F., *119*
Hough, R. L., *205*
Hough, W. G., 363, *373*
Houghton, A. B., 201, *208*
Hoult, J., *30, 373*
Housed, A., *349*
Houston, K., *282*
Hovda, K. E., *253*
Hoven, C., 104, *118*
Howard, M. O., 149, *162*
Howe, L., *428*
Howell, J., 149, *162*
Howells, K., 359, 361, *373, 376*
Howieson, D. B., 302, *306*
Hoy, J., *118*
Hoyert, D. L., 432, *446*
Huang, B., 362, *376*
Huang, M. T., *186*
Huber, S. J., 298, *306*
Hughes, D., *54*, 104, *118*
Hughes, E. M., *307*
Hughes, M., 16, *30*, 168, *185*, 192, *205*, 377, *398*
Huizinga, D., 148, *161*
Hulsbosch, A. M., 20, *32*
Hunt, R. D., 300, *305*
Hunter, M. E., 360, 365, 370, *373*
Huntington, G., 112, *118*
Huntington, G. W., 301, *306*
Hurlbert, D. F., 196, *205*
Hurt, S. W., 259, *284*
Huss, M. T., 130, *141*
Hutchinson, G., 196, *205*
Hyden, H., 199, *205*

Hyder, A., *401*

Iancu, I., 19, *30*
Ilgen, M. A., 245, *255*
Imai, K., 112, *118*
Infantino, J. A., 366, *373*
Inskip, H., 113, *118*
Institute of Medicine, 339, *349*
Iosifescu, D., 113, *118*
Isaac, A., 192, *206*
Isaac, M., *281*
Isometsä, E. T., 62, 66, 76, 99, *100*, 264, 267, *282*
Itoh, I., *307*
Iucci, S., *30*
Ivanoff, A., 361, *374*

Jackson, H. J., 266, 267, *282*
Jacobs, G. A., 18, *31*
Jacobsen, D., *253*
Jacobsen, J., 437, *446*
Jacobson, G., 424, *429*
Jacobson, J., 433, 437, *447, 448*
Jacoby, J. E., 362, *376*
Jacoby, R., 105, *118*, 261, 264, *281*
Jaeger, T. M., 242, *254*
James, R. K., 20, 25, *29*
Jamison, S., 114, *118*
Janca, A., 172, *183*
Jankowski, M. K., 127, *144*
Jannes, S., *285*
Janoff-Bulman, R., 22, *29*, 388, *398*
Janosik, E. H., 20, *30*
Jayaratne, S., 434, 435, *446*
Jaycox, L., 380, *397*
Jaycox, L. H., 172, 173, *184, 185, 397*
Jemelka, R., 357, *373*
Jemmott, J. B., III, 152, 154, *162*
Jemmott, L. S., 152, *162*
Jen, I., *119*
Jenike, M. A., *307*
Jenkins, P. L., 28, 174, *182*
Jenkins, R., 262, *283*
Jenkins, S. R., 439, *446*
Jensen, B. A., 300, *306*
Jensen, P. S., *283*
Jenson, J. M., 149, *162*
Jesse, S., 37, *53*
Jeste, D., 62, 78, 367, *372*
Jeste, D. V., *371*
Jhoo, J. H., *306*
Jia, H., 235, *255*

Myrick, H., 242, *254*

Nagy, L. M., *395*
Najavits, L. M., 382, 393, *399*
Nakashima, J., 18, *29*
Napolitano, G., *117*
Naranjo, C. A., 236, 240, *255*
Narroway, L., 359, *372*
Nathan, J. S., 91, *100*
National Center for PTSD, 175, *186*
National Center for Victims of Crime, *399*
National Child Traumatic Stress Network, 175, *186*
National Institute for Health and Clinical Excellence, 367, *374*
National Institute of Justice, 378, *399*
National Institute of Mental Health, 18–20, *31*, 173, 175, *186*
National Institutes of Health, 313, 315, 317, 320, 321, 323, *333, 334*
Navneet, K., *349*
Naylor, M., *99*
Neblett, C., *184*
Needham, I., 366, *374*
Neeleman, J., 259, 274, *283*
Nehl, C., 112, *119*
Neidig, P. H., 196, *206*
Nelson, B., 263, *279*
Nelson, C. B., 16, *30*, 168, *185*, 192, *205*, 377, *398*
Nelson, E. C., 378, *399*
Ness, R., *253*
Nestadt, G., *284*
Nicholls, S., 213, *231*, 443, *445*
Nicholls, T. L., 127, 134, 135, *141, 144, 145*
Nicholson, K., 290, *307*
Nicolas, G., *117*
Nielsen, S. L., 72, *77*
Nijenhuis, E. R., *231*
Niles, B., 4, *10*, 34, *53*
Niles, B. L., *232*
Nilsson, L., *119*
Nishith, P., 389, 393, *399*, 436, *447*
Nixon, R. D., 436, *447*
Nixon, R. D. V., 180, *183*, *395*
Nock, M. K., 89, *100*
Nogue, S., 249, *254*
Nolan, F., *30*, *373*
Nolan, K., *376*
Nordenberg, D., *397*
Nordentoft, M., 84, *96*
Norris, F. H., 173, *186*, 378, *399*

Nortstrom, T., 267, *283*
Norwood, A. E., 18, *32*
Novaco, R. W., 131, *144*, 359, 360, *374, 376*
Novins, D. K., 84, *100*
Nowlis, D., 269, 272, *284*
Nussey, S. S., 313–315, 317, 318, 320, 324, *334*
Nutt, D. J., 247, 249, *253*
Nyenhuis, D. S., 298, 301, *308*

O'Brien, C. P., 242, *255*
O'Brien, K. P., 363, *373*
O'Campo, P., *183*
O'Connor, M., *281*
O'Connor, P. G., 242, *254, 255*
O'Connor, W. A., 127, *142*
Odegard, O., 112, *120*
Odgers, C., *144*
O'Farrell, T., 245, *255*
O'Farrell, T. J., 195, 199, 202, *206*
Offord, D. R., *283*
Ogloff, J. P., 134, *141*
Ogloff, J. R. P., 127, 130, 134, 135, *144*, 369, *371*
Ohta, H., *333*
Ojehagen, A., *253*
Ojo, A., 108, *119*
Okun, A., *446*
O'Leary, K. D., 193–197, 199, *203, 204, 206, 207*, 378, 384, *395, 396*
Oliver, J. E., 300, *305, 307*
Olson, S., 191, *208*
Oltmanns, T. F., 213, *232*
Omer, H., 4, 5, *10*
Oney, K. M., 71, *78*
Ong, J., 236, *255*
Opler, L. A., 272, *282*
Orbach, I., 5, *10*, *96*
Oregon Death With Dignity Act, 104, 115n.1, *119*
Oregon Department of Human Services, Health Services, 115, *119*
O'Reilly, R. L., 363, *374*
Oreskovich, M. R., 240, 241, *255*
Orlando, M., 173, *185*
Orsillo, S., 179, *186*, 380, *399*
Orthwein, J., 407, *429*
Osher, F. C., *145*
Osman, A., 89, *100*
Osman, J. R., *100*
O'Sullivan v. Presbyterian Hosp. in City of New York at Columbia Presbyterian, 410, *429*

Sar, V., 213, *234*
Sarason, S. B., 275, 278, *284*
Sargk, D., *284*
Saugstad, L., 112, *120*
Saunders, B., *398*
Saunders, B. E., 168, 169, 171, *182, 185, 187,*
       377, 378, *398, 400*
Saunders, D. G., 194, 197, 200, *207, 208*
Saunders, K., 195, *204*
Savage, C. R., *307*
Savas, H. A., 213, *234*
Sawyer, R., *97*
Sax, D. S., *120*, 298, *308*
Scalora, M. J., 130, *141*
Schanzer, W. B., *253*
Schauben, L., 439, 443, *447*
Scheftner, W., *283*
Scheftner, W. A., 73, *75*
Schell, T. L., 172, *184*
Schettler, P., *283*
Schiffer, R. B., 297, *308*
Schlaerth, K. R., 236, *255*
Schlee, K. A., 378, *395*
Schlenger, W. E., *205*, 250, *256*
Schmidt, U., 275, *285*
Schmidtke, A., *100*
Schmitz, B., 109, *120*
Schnabel, A., *284*
Schneider, B., 259, 262, 264–266, *284*
Schneider, F., *284*
Schneiderman, J., 236, 240, *255*
Schnell, J. L., 364, *371*
Schnicke, M. K., 381, 384, 387, 388, 390,
       391, 393, *400*
Schnurr, P. P., *398*
Schnyder, U., 342, 348, *349*
Schoenfeld, M., 112, *120*, 301, *308*
Schollenberger, J., *183*
Schore, A. N., 217, *233*
Schrader, G., 436, *447*
Schroeder, H. E., 359, *370*
Schubert, C., *144*
Schultz, D., 408, *430*
Schultz, L. R., *182*
Schumacher, J. A., 193–198, *207*, 390, *396*
Schumann, A., 169, *185*
Schuster, M., 153, *163*
Schut, A. G., 368, *371*
Schut, A. J., 383, *395*
Schwab-Stone, M., *98*
Schwartz, R., 83, *97*
Schwid, S., 111, *117*

Scott, C., 79, 99, 379, 381–384, 386, *395*
Scott, J., 129, *144*
Scott, M. F., 357, *371*
Scott, S. K., 327, *334*
Scott, T. M., *333*
Scurfield, R. M., 381, *399*
Searle, M. M., 19, *29*
Sedlak, A. J., 198, *207*
Seeley, J. R., 80, *99*
Segal, H., *99*
Segal, S., 36, *54*
Seguin, M., *281, 282*
Seibyl, J. P., *333*
Seidenschnur, A., 113, *118*
Seidman, L. J., 303, 304, 306, *308*
Seidman, S., 327, *333*
Sellbom, M., 214, *233*
Sellers, C. S., 353, *369*
Sellers, E. M., 236, 240, *255*
Senchak, M., 195, *206*
Senol, S., 259, 268, 271, *284*
Sepaher, I., 70, *78*
Seymour, A. K., 171, *185*
Shabnam, M., 363, *371*
Shader, R., 40, 41, *52, 54*
Shaffer, D., 80–83, 85, 98, *101*, 214, *231*
Shapiro, F., 393, *400*
Shapiro, J. P., 153, *163*
Sharkansky, E. J., *186*
Sharpe, M., 257, *280*
Shaw, E. C., 126, *142*
Shaw, S., 157, *162*
Shea, C., 35–37, 47, *54*
Shea, M. T., *234, 279, 284*
Sheitman, B., *376*
Sheley, J., 153, *163*
Shenton, M. E., *333*
Shepperd, R., *282*
Shneidman, E. S., 63, 67, *78*
Shopshire, M. S., 138, 139, *144*
Shoptaw, S., 249–251, *255*
Shoulson, I., 299–301, 305, *308*
Shrout, P. E., *253*
Shuman, D. W., 60, *78*
Shuttleworth, E. C., 298, *306*
Siegert, R., 111, *120*
Siegler, I. C., 268, *285*
Siever, L., 219, *232*
Silk, K. R., 272, *285*
Silva, P. A., 197, *203*
Silver, E., *54*, 127, 131, *144, 145*, 254, 351,
       353, *374, 375*

Sugarman, A., 94, 99
Sugarman, D. B., 196–198, *205, 207*
Suicide Prevention Resource Center, 346, *350*
Sullivan, C. M., *395*
Sullivan, G. R., 59, 60, 64, 65, *75, 78*, 128, *143*
Sullivan, J. T., 236, 240, *255*
Sullivan, L., *162*
Sunday, S., 216, *233*, 381, *400*
Sunderland, M., 217–219, *233*
Sutker, P. B., 18, *31*
Swanson, J., 150, *161*
Swanson, J. W., 127–129, *145*, 352, 363, 364, 367–369, *375*
Swartz, M., 150, *161*
Swartz, M. S., 132, *145*, 352, 368, *375*
Sweet, R. A., 293, *305*
Sykora, K., 236, 240, *255*
Szalai, J. P., 66, 76
Szanto, K., 437, *446*

Tabachnick, B., 38, *54*, 433, 434, *447*
Tabor v. Doctors Memorial Hospital, 412, *430*
Tait, L., 367, *375*
Taliaferro, E., *205*
Tanaka, H., 107, *121*
Tanaka, Y., *307*
Tanner, C. M., 299, *308*
Tanney, B., 50, *54*
Tarasoff v. Regents of the University of California, 411, 414–416, *430*
Tarasoff v. Regents of University of California, 139, *145*
Tardiff, K., 40, 41, *54*, 128, 137, 140, *145*
Target, M., 217, *231*
Tatarelli, G., *120*
Tatarelli, R., 109, *120*
Tate, R., 109, *120*
Tatemichi, T. K., 295, *308*
Tausch, J., *445*
Taylor, A. E., 289, *307*
Taylor, J. L., 360, *376*
Taylor, R. L., 247, *255*
Taylor, S., 386, 390, *400*
Taylor, V., 325, *334*
Teasdale, B., 131, *145*
Teasdale, T., 110, *121*
Tedeschi, R. G., 18, *28*
Telch, C., 196, *208*
Tengstrom, A., 269, 271, *283*, 418, *428*

Tennant, A., *372*
Teplin, L. A., 436, *448*
Terr, L., 17, *31*
Terrien, F., 326, *334*
Testa, M., 199, *208*
Thelander, S., *253*
Thoennes, N., 169, 170, *187, 191, 208*
Thomas, J., *184*
Thomas, J. T., 19, *29*
Thomas, O., 342, *349*
Thompson, C. L., 359, *372*
Thompson, M. P., 169, *184, 446*
Thompson, P. J., 303, *308*
Thompson, S., 275, *285*
Thorne, I., 360, *376*
Thorvaldsen, P., 110, *117*
Tidemalm, D., 268, 269, 272, 273, *284*
Tien, G., 363, *376*
Tiett, Q. Q., 245, *255*
Timmerman, I. G. H., 359, *376*
Ting, L., 433, 437, *446–448*
Tjaden, P., 169, 170, *187, 191, 208*
Tocker, T., 174, *182*
To-Figueras, J., 249, *254*
Tolman, R. M., 200, *208*
Tolosa, E., 298, *308*
Tomas, S., 174, *183*
Tomkins, A. J., 130, *141*
Tomson, T., 109, *119*
Topel v. Long Island Jewish Medical Center, 410, *430*
Torbet, P., 148, *161*
Torgersen, S., 266, *285*
Torigoe, R., 433, 437, *445*
Tortolero, S. R., 84, *101*
Tousignant, M., *281*
Townsend, E., 342, *349*
Trainor, G., 343, *350*
Tranel, D., 327, *333*
Trautman, M. P., 80, *101*
Trautman, P. D., *101*
Trautmann, K., 213, 230, *233*
Tremblay, A., *334*
Trenton, A. J., 237, *253*, 312, 328, *334*
Trestman, R. L., 361, *370*
Trezza, G., 37, *54*
Trezza, G. R., 235, 240, 244, *256*
Trimble, M. R., 303, *308*
Tripp, J. E., 171, *184*
Trippany, R. L., 439, 443, *448*
Tritt, D., 193, *207*
Trofatter, J. A., *117*

Trower, P., 367, *375*
Trull, T. J., 130, *145*
Tryer, P., *144*
Tryon, G., 434, *448*
Trzepacz, P. T., 300, *308*
Tsoh, J. M. Y., 263, *285*
Tsukuma, H., *121*
Tu, X., *285*
Tubb, T., *205*
Tuckey, M., 442, *448*
Tudor, J., 36, *55*
Tudor, W., *55*
Tugade, M. M., 18, *29*
Tupler, L. A., *396*
Turecki, G., 263, *279, 281, 282*
Turkheimer, E., 213, *232*
Turkington, D., 243, *256*
Turner, A., 111, *121*
Turner, A. P., 297, *308*
Turner, R. M., 344, *350*
Turner, S., 36, *55*
Tutkun, H., 213, *234*
Tuzun, U., 213, *234*
Tyano, S., *96*
Tyree, A., 194, 196, *206, 207*
Tyrer, P., 262, 263, 266, 275, 276, 280, *285,*
    376

Uddo, M., 18, *31*
Ulbrecht, J. S., *335*
Ullrich, S., 266, *280*
Ulrich, R. F., *372*
United Nations Office on Drugs and Crime,
    251, *256*
Ursano, R. J., 18, *32,* 327, *335*
U.S. Department of Health and Human Ser-
    vices, 148, 149, *163,* 340, *350*
U.S. Department of Justice, 435, *448*
Useda, J. D., 263, *285*
Utah Code Ann. § 78-14a-102, 420, *430*

Vaiva, G., 275, *285*
Vale, A., 64, *77*
VandeCreek, L., 410, 411, 422–424, *430*
van den Bosch, L. M., 344, *350*
van den Brink, W., *334,* 344, *350*
van den Hout, M. A., 173, *184*
van der Graaf, Y., *350*
van der Hart, O., *231*
van der Kolk, B. A., 216–219, 222, 227, *233,*
    381, *400*
van der Sande, R., 342, 344, *350*

VanDeusen, K. M., 439, *448*
Van de Voorde, W., *255*
Van Dorn, R. A., 368, *375*
van Emmerik, A. A. P., 20, *32*
Van Etten, M. L., 390, *400*
van Heeringen, K., 275, *284*
van Herringen, C., *285*
Van Honk, J., 326, *334*
van Hutton, V., 195, *206*
Vanier, C., 282, *283*
Van Leeuwen, J. M., 250, *254*
van Remoortel, J., *285*
van Rooijen, L., *350*
Varney, G. W., 366, *375*
Varra, E., 220, *230*
Vasterling, J. J., 299–301, *308*
Velting, D. M., 81, 83, 85–88, 98, *101*
Ventura, L. A., 362, *376*
Verhaagen, D., 147–149, 157, *161*
Verheul, R., 344, *350*
Vermeiren, R., *335*
Veronen, L. J., *185,* 392, *400*
Vesselinov, R., 126, *142*
Victor, B. J., 269, 271, *281*
Victor, M., 297, 303, *308*
Vijayakumar, L., 259, 261, *285*
Vileikyte, L., 323, *335*
Vitaliano, P. P., 194, *206*
Vitanza, S., 197, *208*
Vivian, D., 193, 197, 199, *203, 207, 208*
Vogel, L. C. M., 197, *208*
Volavka, J., 128, 129, *145,* 368, *373, 376*
Volkmar, F. R., 83, *101*
Vossekuil, B., 149, 152, 155, *161*

Waelde, L. C., 179, *183*
Waern, M., 268, 272, *284*
Wagner, B. C., 194, *206*
Wagner, B. M., 85, *101*
Wagner, E. E., 91, *100*
Wagner, H. R., *145, 375*
Waldner-Haugrud, L. K., 192, *208*
Walker, A., 434, 442, *445*
Walker, J., 113, *119*
Walker, R. L., 73, *76*
Wallace, C., 128, 129, *145*
Wallace, C. J., 359, *373, 376*
Wallin, M., 111, *121*
Walsh, B. W., 213, 215, 218, 219, *234,* 339,
    350
Walsh, E., *144,* 362, 364, *376*
Walsh, J., *120*

Walsh, P. G., 237, *253*
Walters, E. E., 16, *30*, 66, *76*, 80, 99, 245, *253, 282, 339, 349*
Wan, N., 245, *253*
Wanamaker, W. M., 298, *305*
Wang, L. J., *285*
Ward, C. H., 179, *182, 380, 394*
Ward, D. B., 193, *207*
Wartella, M. E., *97*
Wasserman, D., 111, *117*
Waternaux, C., 83, 99, 215, *232*
Waters, H., 377, 378, *401*
Watson, M., 36, *54*
Watson, P. J., *186*
Watsons, A., *372*
Watt, A., 62, *78*
Watt, B., 359, *373*
Watt, B. D., 361, *376*
Waugh, C. E., 18, *29*
Way, I., 439, *448*
Weathers, F. W., 195, *207, 380, 395, 401*
Weaver, C. M., 133, *143*
Weaver, T. L., 173, *187*, 389, *399*
Webb, M., 300, *308*
Webster, C. D., 134, 135, *144, 145*, 201, *205*, 369, *371, 376*
Webster, D., *203*
Wedin, I., 201, *204*
Weiderhorn, N., *203*
Weil, G., 174, *182*
Weimbs, R., *28*
Weiner, D. A., 436, *448*
Weingartner, H., 300, *305*
Weisaeth, L., 216, *233*
Weiss, D., 380, *401*
Weiss, D. S., 167, *187, 205*
Weissman, J., 36, *52*
Weissman, M., 109, *120*
Weissman, M. M., 274, *284*
Weisz, A. N., 200, 201, *208*
Weitkamp, L. R., 297, *308*
Weizman, R., *96*
Welch, B., 423, *430*
Welker, C. J., 153, *163*
Wellford, C., 153, *163*
Werth, J. L., Jr., 442, *447*
Wessely, S., 20, *31*
Wessley, S., 168, *187*
Wesson, D. R., 236, 243, *256*
West, A., 359, *372*
Wetterling, T., *284*
White, B., *207*

White, B. W., 192, *206*
White, I. R., *30*
White, J. D., 247, *255*
White, R. F., 297–299, 301, *308*
Whitehead, S. A., 313–315, 317, 318, 320, 324, *334*
Whitlock, F., 104, *121*
Whitlock, J. L., 213, *234*
Whitman, R., 434, *448*
Whittaker, K. E., 196, *205*
Whittingham, D., 135, *142*
Wichstrom, L., 79, *101*
Widiger, T. A., 130, *145*
Widom, C. S., 148, *162*
Wiichen, H. U., 87, *101*
Wilcoxin, S. A., 439, *448*
Wilken, J., 111, *121*
Wilkins, J. N., 251, *256*
Wilkinson, D. L., 198, *208*
Williams, B., *98*
Williams, B. I., 84, 98, *162*
Williams, J. B. W., 262, *284*
Williams, K. R., 201, *208*
Williams, L., 110, *121*
Williams, M., *98*
Williams, R., 111, 112, *121*
Williams, R. A., 194, *207*
Williams, R. M., 297, *308*
Williams-Gray, C. H., 298, *309*
Williamson, D. F., *397*
Willmott, S., 260, *280*
Wilner, N., 437, *446*
Wilson, D., 363, *376*
Wilson, J., 380, *401*
Wilson, M., 199, *208*
Wilson, S. A. K., 297, *305*
Wilt, S., 191, *208*
Wineman, N. M., 297, *308*
Wing, J. K., 270, *285*
Winters, J., 199, *206*
Wirshing, D. A., *370*
Wirshing, W. C., *370*
Wissow, L. S., 84, *98*
Wittchen, H. U., *334*
Wittmann, L., 342, 348, *349*
Witztum, E., 174, *182*
Wold, C. I., 275, *283*
Wolf, R. C., 84, *98*
Wolfe, J., *186*
Wolfe, M. M., 364, *371*
Wolfe, N., 295, *309*
Wolfe, R., *119*

SUBJECT INDEX

Agitation, 295
Agitation–excitement, 130
AIDS. *See* HIV/AIDS
Alabama, 426
Alarm center, 218–219, 228
Alcohol dependence
    and partner violence, 245
    as suicide risk factor, 64
    and victimization, 171–172
Alcohol use. *See also* Intoxication
    and benzodiazepines, 41
    and GHB, 249
    and Huntington's disease, 300–301
    and intimate partner violence, 195, 199
    and ketamine, 251
    measures of, 237
    overdose from, 248
    as risk marker for IPV, 92, 199
    as suicide risk factor, 83, 244
    and victimization, 171–172
    and violence, 129
    withdrawal from, 238–242
Alcohol withdrawal syndrome (AWS), 240–242
Alexythymia, 222
Alzheimer's disease (AD), 292–294
American Association for Emergency Psychiatry, 5
American Indians. *See* Native Americans
American Psychological Association (APA), 5, 60
American Society of Addiction Medicine, 242
Amphetamines
    intoxication from, 239, 244
    overdose from, 248
    popularity of, 251
    withdrawal from, 239
AMT. *See* Anxiety management training
Amygdala, 218, 327
Amyl, 250
Amyotrophic lateral sclerosis, 115
Anabolic steroids, 312
Anger
    with ITLE, 304
    and prolonged exposure therapy, 390
    in victims of violence, 176, 177
    as violence risk factor, 131
    and working-alliance formation, 36–37
Anger management
    for violence reduction, 359–361

violence risk management with, 138–139
Animals, self-injury among, 213–214
Anosagnosia, 296
Anticholinergic drugs, 299
Anticipation, of recurrence, 93
Antidepressants, 46
Antihypertensive medications, 46
Anti-inflammatory responses, 313
Antipsychotics, 40, 137–138, 331, 367–368
Antiretroviral therapies, 105, 106
Antisocial disorders, 83
Antisocial personality disorder, 272n.
    as suicide risk factor, 259, 264, 266, 269, 270, 276
    violence during normal functioning of persons with, 27
    as violence risk factor, 129
Antisocial traits, 130
Anxiety
    clinician's, with suicide assessment, 60
    and self-injury, 214
    as suicide risk factor, 62
    in victims of violence, 180
Anxiety disorders, 82–83
Anxiety management training (AMT), 384–386
Anxiety thermometers, 387
APA. *See* American Psychological Association
APA Ethics Code, 405, 419–420, 422–423
APA Ethics Committee, 405–406
Apathy, 293, 295, 300
Aphasia, 294
Appraisal, 21
Aripiprazole, 367
ASAP. *See* Assaulted Staff Action Program
ASD. *See* Acute stress disorder
Asians
    with diabetes, 324
    suicide risk among, 84
Assaulted Staff Action Program (ASAP), 434, 438, 442–443
Assertive community treatment (ACT), 362–363
Assessment. *See specific* assessment; e.g. Suicide risk assessment
Assessment measures, selection of, 380
Assisted suicide, 114–116
Ativan, 40
Attachment, 217–218
Attention-deficit disorder, 291

Attitude(s)
    constructive, 8–9
    violence supported by/facilitating, 152–153
Attributional style, 131
Atypical antipsychotic agents, 368
Auditory hallucinations, 293, 296, 298
Auschwitz concentration camp, 22
Australia, 105
Authenticity, 35
Authoritarianism, 196
Authority, persuasive, 424–425
Autoimmune problems, 313
Autonomy, loss of, 115
Availability, of potential victims of violence, 132
Avoidant personality disorder, 258, 266, 274
AWS. *See* Alcohol withdrawal syndrome

Balkan conflict, 21–22
Barbiturates, 238, 240
Bardoni v. Kim, 426
Barefoot v. Estelle, 421
Baseline level of functioning, 25
Battery, 406
BDI–II. *See* Beck Depression Inventory
Beck Anxiety Inventory, 180, 380
Beck Depression Inventory (BDI–II), 71–72, 89, 180, 380
Beck Hopelessness Scale (BHS), 72
Behavioral Assessment Scales for Children, 89
Behavioral couples treatment, 245
Behavioral emergency(-ies)
    coping with aftermath of, 440–443
    defined, 4, 13
    description of, 3
    evaluation of. *See* Evaluation, of behavioral emergency(-ies)
    impact on clinicians of, 436–440
    incidence of, 432–436
    model curriculum for, 5–7
    training for, 7–9
    types of, 4, 13
    without crises, 27
Behavioral emergency committee, 365
Behavioral factors, high-risk, 91–92
Behavior-based queries, 176
"Being in a K-hole," 251
Belief, in personal invulnerability, 22
Belief system, 68
Bellah, Tammy, 412

Bellah v. Greenson, 412
Bell v. New York City Health and Hospital Corporation, 413
Benadryl, 252
Benjamin Rush Center for Problems of Living in Los Angeles, 20, 21
Benzodiazepines
    for agitated behavior, 40–41
    with antipsychotic medication, 138
    with other drugs, 252
    respiratory depression/coma induced by, 248
    withdrawal from, 238–242
    withdrawal management with, 249
Benztropine, 40
BHS (Beck Hopelessness Scale), 72
Bias, of clinician, 135–136
Biliary passage cancer, 107
Binswanger's disease, 294
Biological factors, of suicide risk, 68
Biopsychosocial approach, 42–43
Biopsychosocial risk factors, for suicide, 61–69, 80–87
    academic difficulties, 87
    accessible means of suicide, 85–86
    biological–genetic–dispositional, 68
    demographic factors, 67, 84
    family dysfunction/parental psychopathology, 85
    firearms access, 65
    functional impairment from disease/injury, 87
    lack of protective factors, 68, 69
    life events, 64, 86
    medical illness, 65–66
    mental disorders, 81–84
    prior suicide attempts, 66, 81
    psychache/hopelessness, 63
    psychiatric diagnosis, 61–62
    recent losses, 64
    sexual/physical abuse, 87
    social isolation, 67–68
    social milieu, 86–87
    stress, 64, 86
    substance use, 64, 65
    suicidal communication, 67
    suicidal ideation, 66, 85
Biopsychosocial risk factors, for youth violence, 149–150
Bipolar disorder
    and diabetes, 324–325
    as suicide risk factor, 82

and violence, 128
Bishop v. South Carolina Dept. of Mental Health, 427
"Blaming the victim," 169–170
Blood samples, 238, 247
Bodily functions, loss of control of, 115
Bone resorption, 319
"Booty bumping," 250
Borderline personality disorder (BPD), 272n.
    baseline level of functioning of persons with, 25
    and cognitive processing therapy, 391–392
    DBT for, 361
    and intimate partner violence, 194, 195
    stable instability of persons with, 27
    as suicide risk factor, 61, 83, 259, 264, 266–273, 276, 277
    as violence risk factor, 130
Bradley v. Ray, 426
Brady v. Hopper, 426
Brain cancer, 107
Brain development, 217–218
Brain lesions, 294–295
Brain tumors, 291
Breach of duty, negligence and, 409
Breathing retraining, 384–385
Bronchus cancer, 107, 115
Broset Violence Checklist, 134
Broward County MHC, 363–364
Buccal cavity cancer, 107
Bullying, 156
Buprenorphine, 243
Bureau of Justice Statistics, 169
Burnout, 439
1,4-Butanediol, 249
Butyl nitrate, 250

Caffeine, 238
Calcium, 319
California, 251, 416, 419, 420, 425, 426
California Supreme Court, 415
Canada, 106, 267
Cancer
    and assisted suicide, 115
    suicide risk assessment in people with, 106–108
    as suicide risk factor, 65
Cannabis, 251
Capacity for violence, 153
Captivity, 17
Carbon monoxide poisoning, 86

Cardiac irregularities, 40
Caregivers
    and brain development, 217–218
    as targets of violence, 131
Carlisle v. Frisbie Memorial Hosp., 426
Case formulation, developing, 49–50
Case management, 356, 362
Castro-Blanco, D., 14
Catecholamines, 313
CATIE (Clinical Antipsychotic Trials of Intervention Effectiveness), 367
Causation, negligence and, 407–408
Cause in fact, 407–408
Cause of Death Registry (Denmark), 111
CBT. *See* Cognitive–behavioral therapy
Centers for Disease Control and Prevention (CDC), 79, 169, 313, 316
Central nervous system (CNS), 248, 252
Cerebral contusion, 110
Cerebrovascular disease (CVD), 294–297
Chief complaint, patient's, 44
Child abuse
    by caregivers, 218
    effects of, 216
Child development
    and self-injury, 217–218
    and youth violence, 148
Childhood abuse, 169
    prevalence of, 435
    as suicide risk factor, 87
Children. *See also* Suicide risk assessment, in children and adolescents
    with diabetes, 323
    as protective factor against suicide, 68
    suicide risk assessment of. *See* Suicide risk assessment, in children and adolescents
China, 277
CHIs. *See* Closed head injuries
Chorea, 299
Chronic heart failure, 291
Chronic medical problems, 45
Circadian rhythms, 332
"Circuit parties," 249
CISD. *See* Critical Incident Stress Debriefing
CISM (critical incident stress management), 19
CIWA (Clinical Institute Withdrawal Assessment Scale for Alcohol), 236
CIWA-AD. *See* Clinical Institute Withdrawal Assessment Scale for Alcohol

Commitment, to plan of action, 92
Commitment to treatment statement (CTS), 347–348
Communication
    couple's style of, 194
    parent–child, 85
    of school violence intent, 155
    suicidal, 67
    of threat, 417
Community-based strategies, for violence reduction, 158, 361–365
    assertive community treatment, 362–363
    intensive case management, 362
    mental health courts, 363–364
    outpatient commitment, 363
Community resources, 423
Comorbidity
    with PTSD, 381, 393
    as suicide risk factor, 83–84
    in victims of IPV, 393
    with violence, 129
Comparative liability, 407n.3
Compassion fatigue, 439
Competence
    clinician's, 422
    determining patient's, 423
Complaints, to APA Ethics Committee, 405–406
Compliance
    with prescribed medications, 45–46
    with suicidal behavior treatment, 347–348
Concentration camps, 17, 22
Concussion, 110
Confidentiality
    with adolescent suicidal patients, 92
    documentation of considerations with, 422
    knowledge of state law on, 425
    and liability with suicidal patients, 412
    and liability with violent patients, 415, 419–420
    limits of, 420–421
Confine, failure to, 412–413
Confusion, 295, 298
Congenital disease, 321
Connecticut, 426
Connection
    and CSDT, 225
    as CSDT goal, 227
    inner, 221

Constructive attitude, 8–9
Constructive self-development theory (CSDT), 220–229, 439
    and clinician's self-care, 228–229
    inner-connection ability in, 221
    long-term goals of, 226–227
    sense-of-self-worth ability in, 222–223
    short-term goals of, 223–225
    strong-affect ability in, 221–222
    and trauma's effects on body, 227–228
Consultation, 443
    in risk management, 422
    and violence risk, 136
Contact, with adolescent suicidal patients, 94
Contagion, suicide, 68, 87
Containment, 34–42
    engagement principles for, 34–35
    and patient's loss of self-control, 38–39
    and reducing risk of harm, 39–42
    for violence, 138, 157, 158
    working-alliance issues in, 35–38
Control
    guilt and illusion of, 22
    with restraints/seclusion, 41–42
    working-alliance formation and loss of, 38
Coping
    assessment of, 25–26
    psychoeducation about, 178
    role of, 23
Coping mechanisms, 20, 21
Coping skills, 359
Correctional treatment programs, 355–356
Cortex, 219
Corticoids, 313
Corticotropin-releasing factor (CRF), 312–313
Cortisol, 172, 313
Court rulings, 424–427
COVR (Classification of Violence Risk), 133
Cowell Memorial Hospital, 415
COWS. See Clinician Administered Opiate Withdrawal Scale
CPT. See Cognitive processing therapy
Cranial fractures, 110
"Crash" state, 250
CRF. See Corticotropin-releasing factor
Crime
    and substance-related violence, 129
    violent, 167, 435
Crime victim's compensation, 177–178

with ITLE, 304
with medical illness, 113–114
and MS, 111
with MS, 297
with Parkinson's disease, 298
with PTSD, 393
and self-injury, 214
and stroke, 110–111
as suicide risk factor, 61, 62, 64, 68, 82, 83, 113–114
in victims of violence, 176, 180
Designer drugs
detection of, 247
intoxication state from, 246
overdose from, 248–252
withdrawal from, 239, 244
Developmental crises, 15
Developmental history, 290–291
Dextromorphan, 252
Diabetes, 291
Diabetes mellitus, 322–325
Diagnose risk of suicide, failure to, 410
Diagnosis. *See also* Psychiatric diagnosis mis-, 410
rapid differential, 137
Diagnostic and Statistical Manual of Mental Disorders (DSM), 258–259
Diagnostic and Statistical Manual of Mental Disorders (DSM–III–R), 240
Diagnostic and Statistical Manual of Mental Disorders (DSM–IV), 16, 172, 311
Diagnostic and Statistical Manual of Mental Disorders (DSM–IV–TR), 171, 378, 424
Diagnostic impression, 424
Dialectical behavior therapy (DBT)
for self-injury, 228
for suicidal behavior, 343–345
for violence reduction, 361
Dialysis, 108
Diaphragmatic breathing, 178, 384–385
Diazepam, 252
Dignity, loss of, 115
Dimitrijevic v. Chicago Wesley Memorial Hospital, 410
Dinnerstein v. United States, 410
Diphenhydramine, 252
Direct inquiries, in suicide risk assessment, 69–70
Disclose, failure to, 411–412
Disclosure
in group debriefings, 174

of previous violence, 126
in psychological first aid, 175–176
Disease, functional impairment from, 87
Disinhibition, 129
Disorganized attachment, 218
Disorganized patients, 37
Dispositional factors, of suicide risk, 68
Disrupted spirituality, 229
Disruptive disorders, 83
Dissociation, 222
Dissociative amnesia, 24
Dissociative symptoms, 16
Distal risk factors, of suicide, 81–85
affective/anxiety disorders, 82–83
alcohol/substance use disorders, 83
comorbid disorders, 83–84
demographic factors, 84
disruptive/antisocial disorders, 83
ethnicity, 84
family dysfunction/parental psychopathology, 85
gender, 84
mental disorders, 81–84
personality disorders, 83
prior suicide attempts, 81
sexual orientation, 84
socioeconomic status, 84
temporally and structurally, 258
Distress, tolerating, 92–93, 228
Distress reduction skills. *See* Anxiety management training
Divalproex sodium, 368
Documentation
of consultation, 136
failure to maintain, 413–414
of professional actions/judgment, 413
in risk management, 422
of suicide risk assessment, 74
in violence risk management, 159–160
Domestic violence, 244
Domestic violence hotlines and shelters, 178
Domestic Violence Supplementary Report (DVSR), 201
Dopamine, 313
Dopamine D_2 receptor affinity, 368
Dopamine receptor blocker, 326
Dosage, 244
Dose–response effect, 364
Doyle v. U.S., 426
Dress, 137
Drug Abuse Warning Network, 247

Drug dependence
    baseline level of functioning of persons
        with, 25
    stable instability of persons with, 27
Drug interaction, 46
Drug use. *See* Substance use and abuse
DSM. *See Diagnostic and Statistical Manual of
        Mental Disorders*
Dunkle v. Food Service East Inc., 427
Dunnington v. Silva, 426
Durapau v. Jenkins, 426
Duty, negligence and, 409
Duty of psychiatrists, 416
Duty to protect
    failure in, 410–411
    limitations on, 417–420
    reasonable care in, 415–416
    and suicide risk management, 410–411
    and violence risk management, 139–
        140, 415–420
Duty to warn, 414–415, 417–420
DVSR (Domestic Violence Supplementary
        Report), 201
Dynamic Appraisal of Situational Aggression
        (DYAS), 135
Dyskinesia, 299

EBTs. *See* Evidence-based treatments
Ecstasy, 239, 249–251
ED. *See* Emergency department
Education. *See* Psychoeducation
Educational history, 290–291
Education level, 115
Elderly persons
    completed suicide among, 80, 259
    suicide risk among, 66
    violence among, 127
Elitzur, A., 4–5
EMDR, 393
Emergencies in Mental Health Practices
        (Kleespies), xiii
Emergency cards, 94
Emergency department (ED), 170, 191, 235–
        237, 245
Emergency intervention
    defined, 13–14
    determining need for, 51–52
    goals of, 14
    integration of crisis intervention and,
        23–27
    without crisis intervention, 27
Emergency interview, 44–50

about acute/chronic medical problems,
    45
case formulation from, 49–50
about chief complaint, 44
current functional status during, 45
lethality assessment from, 46–47
and limits of risk prediction, 50
about medications, 45–46
about mental health/substance use his-
    tory, 45
mental status exam in, 47–49
about precipitating factors, 44–45
semistructured, 44
tasks in, 34
validity of information from, 47
Emergency response personnel, 19, 174
Emotional abuse, 194
Emotion regulation, 385
Empathetic preface statements, 176
Empathic understanding, 5
Empathy, 24, 25, 35–37, 176
Employee assistance programs, 277
Empowerment, 177
Endocrine disorders, 311–332
    of adrenocorticoid system, 312–316
    diagnostic considerations with, 327–332
    function of, 312
    hypercortisolism, 313–314
    hyperglycemia/hypoglycemia, 323–325
    hyperparathyroidism, 319–320
    hyperthyroidism, 316–318
    hypocortisolism, 315–316
    hypoparathyroidism, 321–322
    hypothyroidism, 318–319
    of pancreas, 322–325
    of parathyroid system, 319–322
    prevalence of, 328
    of reproductive system, 325–327
    stress-provoked endocrine pathology,
        326–327
    of thyroid system, 316–319
End-stage renal disease (ESRD), 108
Engagement, 34–35
England, 105
Environment
    for psychological first aid, 175–176
    for substance withdrawal, 242
Environmental pathogens, 330
Epilepsy, 109, 290–291, 303–304
Epinephrine, 313
Esophageal cancer, 107
ESRD (end-stage renal disease), 108

Estrogen, 325–326
Ethiopia, 191
Ethnicity
    as suicide risk factor, 84
    and working-alliance formation, 36
Evaluation, of behavioral emergency(-ies),
        33–52
    containment of emotional turmoil in,
        34–42
    problem definition in, 42–44
    risk assessment in, 44–50
    training in, 8
    treatment considerations in, 50–52
Evans v. U.S., 426
Evidence-based treatments (EBTs), 378, 383
Ewing, Keith, 417
Ewing v. Goldstein, 417
Exits, 39, 150–151
Exposure therapy, 386–387
Extrapyramidal side effects, 40
Eye contact, 36

Face-to-face emergency intervention, 23–24
Failure to commit or confine, 412–413
Failure to diagnose risk of suicide, 410
Failure to disclose or warn, 411–412
Failure to obtain and maintain history and
        records, 413–414
Failure to protect, 410–411
False positives, 73
Family conflict, 131
Family dysfunction, 85
Family history, 68
Family intervention, 139
Family member(s)
    failure to warn, 411–412
    as informant, 417
    risk-management involvement of, 424
    suicidal communication to, 67
    suicide of, 87
    as targets of violence, 127, 131
Family of origin violence, 196, 198
Family therapy, 139
Fantasies, violent, 126
Fatty acids, 322
Fatuck v. Hillside Hospital, 411
Fear, extreme, 173
Femicide, 202
Fight or flight response, 312
Fights, youth, 148
Finland, 267
Firearms access

securing, 92
    as suicide risk factor, 65, 85–86
    as violence risk factor, 133, 153
Firearms screening, 133
Flagging system, 365–366
Flexeril, 252
Florida, 356, 426
Flumazenil. *See* Flunitrazepam
Flunitrazepam, 248, 250–252
Follow-up, violence risk management with,
        159
Follow-up letters, 69
Ford, J. D., 219
Forensic evidence, from sexual assault, 178
Foreseeability requirement
    for liability with violent patients, 418–
        419
    predictability vs. foreseeability, 408
Foster v. Charter Medical Group, 413
France, 259, 267
Friends, suicide among, 87
Frontal cortex, 218, 219, 228
Frontal lobe dementias, 294
Frontal system dysfunction, 295
Frontotemporal dementia, 294
Full agonist opioids, 247
Functional impairment, 15, 87
Functional status, 45

GHB. *See* Gamma hydroxybutyrate
Gait disturbance, 292, 298
Gamma butyrolactone, 249
Gamma hydroxybutyrate (GHB), 239, 247,
        249, 250
*Garamella for Estate of Almonte v. New York
        Medical College*, 426
Gas chromatography, 247
Gates, for sensory information, 327
Gender differences
    with alcohol and violence issues, 245
    with cancer and suicide risk, 107
    with clinician responses to behavioral
        emergencies, 437
    with criminal victimization, 171
    with endocrine disorders, 328, 331
    with hypercortisolism, 313–314
    with hyperparathyroidism, 320
    with hyperthyroidism, 317
    with hypoparathyroidism, 321
    with intimate partner violence, 191
    with MS, 111
    with school violence, 155

with suicide risk, 67, 84
with traumatic brain injury, 110
with violence risk, 127
with violent victimization, 168–169
and working-alliance formation, 36
in youth violence, 148
Genetic factors
of endocrine disorders, 330
of suicide risk, 68
Geographic differences, in suicide rates, 264, 267, 277
Georgia, 434
Germany, 259
GHB. *See* Gamma hydroxybutyrate
Giving-up syndrome, 114
Glucagon, 322
Glucocorticoids, 313, 327
Glucose, 322–323
Glycogen, 322
Graves' disease, 316, 317, 412
Grief, 440
Grounding techniques, 390
Group debriefing, 174
Group therapy, 347
Guilt, 22, 294
Gulf War veterans, 18
Gun control, 274
Gustatory hallucinations, 296–297
Gynecological problems, 170

HAART. *See* Highly active antiretroviral therapy
Haldol, 40
Hallucinations
with Alzheimer's disease, 293
command, 62, 131
with CVD, 296
with Huntington's disease, 301
with Parkinson's disease, 298
Hallucinogens, 244
Haloperidol, 40, 367, 368
Hanging, suicide by, 86
Harassment, 156
Harkavy-Asnis Suicide Survey, 89
Harm reduction, strategies for, 39–42
pharmacological intervention, 40–41
physical restraint/seclusion, 41
verbal limits, 39
HCR–20 (Historical, Clinical, Risk Management—20), 134
HD. *See* Huntington's disease
Head injury, 66, 128–129

Health insurance, 115
Heat sensitivity, 292
Hedlund v. Superior Court, 416, 426
Helpless dependence, 60
Help seeking, 275
Hematopoietic cancer, 107
Heterosexual couples, 191
Highly active antiretroviral therapy (HAART), 105, 106
High-risk approaches, 275–276
High-risk behavioral factors, reducing, 91–92
High-risk situations, 411
Himmelsbach's Point System for Measuring Opioid Abstinence Syndrome Intensity by the Day or Hour, 242
Hippocampus, 218
Hispanics
and intimate partner violence, 193
and violent victimization, 169
Historical, Clinical, Risk Management–20 (HCR—20), 134
History of victimization, 127
History of violence
as violence risk factor, 126
in youth violence assessment, 151–152
Histrionic personality disorder, 267
HIV/AIDS
and assisted suicide, 115
and crystal meth use, 250
and GHB, 249
suicide risk assessment in people with, 105–106
as suicide risk factor, 65
withdrawal seizures in people with, 240
Homelessness, 133
Homicidality, 176–177
Homicide, 50
and intimate partner violence, 191
juvenile, 147, 148
racial differences in victims of, 169
Homosexual couples, 192
Homosexuality, 84
Hope
and CSDT, 225
offering, 25
restoring, 90–91
Hopelessness
as suicide risk factor, 63
in victims of violence, 177
Hormones, 312
Hospital-based internship, 9

and violence, 128–129
Lethality potential, 46–47
Leukoariosis, 294
Leutinizing hormone, 325
Life events, 64, 86, 267
Life-threatening events, 15–16
Limbic system, 217
Limitations on duty to warn/protect, 417–420
Limits, setting, 36–37, 39, 137, 438
Linehan, Marsha, 361
Linehan Reasons for Living (LRFL), 72–73
Lipari v. Sears, Roebuck & Co., 418–419, 426
"Liquid X." *See* Gamma hydroxybutyrate
Lithium, 368
Littleton v. Good Samaritan Hosp. & Health Center, 427
Liver cancer, 107
Liver disease, 41
Lorazepam, 40, 41, 138
Los Angeles, California, 236
Losses, recent, 62, 64
Louisiana, 420, 426
Lovers' quarrels, 199
LRFL. *See* Linehan Reasons for Living
Lung cancer, 107, 115
Lymphatic cancer, 107

MacArthur Violence Risk Assessment Study, 244–245
Magnetic resonance imaging (MRI), 294
Making a threat, 149, 150
Mallory-Weiss syndrome, 242
Malpractice, 406–409
Managing behavioral emergencies, 8
Manchester VA Medical Center, 241
Mania
    and Alzheimer's disease, 293
    with closed head injuries, 303
    with Huntington's disease, 300
    with MS, 297
    with Parkinson's disease, 299
    and violence, 128
Marital rape victims, 391
Marital status, 67–68, 131–132
Massachusetts, 417–418, 420–421, 438
Mass spectrometry, 247
Mastery, sense of, 9
Maturational crises, 15
Mavroudis v. Superior Court, 426
M-CET (multiple-channel exposure therapy), 393

McFarlane, A. C., 216
McIntosh, Kimberley, 416
McIntosh v. Milano, 416, 426
McNally, R. J., 21–22
MDMA. *See* Ecstasy
Meaning
    of event to client, 24
    search for, 22–23
    in self-injury, 215
Media coverage, 86
Medical examination, 178
Medical history
    and endocrine disorders, 330
    failure to obtain, 413–414
    as neurological-disorder indicator, 291
    in risk management, 423–424
Medical illness, suicide risk and, 63, 65–66. *See also* Suicide risk assessment, in people with medical illness
Medical problems
    gathering information about patient's, 45
    in victims of violence, 170
Medical records, 413–414
Medical University of South Carolina, 181
Medications. *See also* Pharmacological interventions
    gathering information about patient's, 45–46
    Parkinson's disease and side effects of, 298–299
Meier v. Ross General Hospital, 411
Melatonin, 332
Menopause, 326, 328, 331
Mental disorders
    and intimate partner violence, 191–192
    as suicide risk factor, 81–84
    with traumatic brain injury, 109–110
    as violence risk factor, 128–130
Mental health courts (MHCs), 363–364
Mental health crisis, 14–15
Mental health history, 45
Mental health problems, 171–172
Mental illness, serious. *See* Serious mental illness
Mental retardation, 128
Mental status exam (MSE), 47–49, 130
Mentor model, 8
Mentors, 34
Metabolism, 316, 318
"Meth." *See* Methamphetamine
Methadone, 243, 248

Methamphetamine, 129, 249–251
3,4-Methylenedioxymethamphetamine
(MDMA). *See* Ecstasy
MHCs. *See* Mental health courts
Michigan, 426
Mindfulness, 361
Mini-Mental State Exam, 49
Minnesota Multiphasic Personality Inventory—2 (MMPI-2), 70–71
Misdiagnosis, 410
Mississippi, 426
Missouri, 426
Mitchell, Jeffrey, 18–19
MMPI-2. *See* Minnesota Multiphasic Personality Inventory—2
Mobile crisis team, 9
Model curriculum, 5–7
Mood stabilizers, 331
Morgan, Estates of v. Fairfield Family Counseling Ctr., 427
Morgenstein, Lee, 416
Motor system
    disorders involving, 292
    and Huntington's disease, 299
    and MS, 297
    and Parkinson's disease, 298
Motor vehicle accidents, 18
MRI (magnetic resonance imaging), 294
MS. *See* Multiple sclerosis
MSE. *See* Mental status exam
Multiple-channel exposure therapy (M-CET), 393
Multiple sclerosis (MS)
    as neurological disorder, 297–298
    and suicide, 66, 111–112
    symptoms of, 292
Multiple suicide attempts, 436
Multiple traumas, 173, 176
Munstermann ex rel. Rowe v. Alegent Health-Immanuel Medical Center, 426
Myelin sheaths, 297

Naloxone, 247, 248
Narcissistic personality disorder, 267
National Alliance for the Mentally Ill, 139
National Bureau of Health (Denmark), 110
National Center for PTSD, 175
National Child Traumatic Stress Network, 175, 181
National Comorbidity Survey, 18
National Crime Victimization Survey (NCVS), 167, 169, 435, 436

National Crime Victims Research and Treatment Center (NCVC), 181
National Crime Victimization Survey, 190, 191
National Diabetes Education Program, 323
National Huntington's Disease Register, 112
National Institute of Mental Health (NIMH), 18, 20, 367
National Institutes of Health (NIH), 313, 316
National Vietnam Veterans Readjustment Survey, 195
National Violence Against Women Survey (NVAWS), 169–170, 190–191
National Women's Survey (NWS), 171
Native Americans
    with diabetes, 324
    suicide risk among, 84
    and violent victimization, 169
NCVC (National Crime Victims Research and Treatment Center), 181
NCVS. *See* National Crime Victimization Survey
Nebraska, 419, 426
Need principle, 354
Negative press, 63
Neglect, 216
Negligence
    causation element of, 407–408
    damages element of, 407
    defined, 406
    duty/breach-of-duty elements of, 409
    legal elements of, 406–409
Negligent release of patient, 412–413
Negotiating conflicts, 25
Neocortex, 217
Neuritic plaques, 292
Neurofibrillary tangles, 292
Neurological disorders, 289–304
    Alzheimer's disease, 292–294
    cerebrovascular disease, 294–297
    developmental/educational-history factors of, 290–291
    epilepsy, 109
    frontal lobe dementias, 294
    Huntington's disease, 112, 299–301
    idiopathic temporal lobe epilepsy, 303–304
    medical-history factors of, 291
    multiple sclerosis, 111–112, 297–298
    Parkinson's disease, 298–299
    physical symptoms of, 291–292

social/occupational-history factors of, 291

spinal cord injury/disorder, 112–113

stroke, 110–111

suicide risk assessment in people with, 109–113

traumatic brain injury, 109–110, 301–303

Neurotoxins, exposure to, 290, 291

New Hampshire, 426

New Jersey, 426

New Mexico, 426

New York, 427

New York City, 236

Nicotine, 238

NIH. *See* National Institutes of Health

NIMH. *See* National Institute of Mental Health

Nitrous oxide, 250

N-methyl-D-aspartate. *See* Ketamine

No-harm contracts, 74

Noncompliance, with risk reduction, 154–155

Nonpsychological violence reduction strategies, 365–368

institutional policies/quality management, 365–366

psychotropic medication, 366–368

staff training, 366

Norepinephrine, 313

Norepinephrine neuroreceptors, 368

Normative crises, 16

Normative stress, 15

North Carolina, 427

Norway, 106, 107

No-suicide contract, 348

Numbing, 219, 222

Numbness, 292

NVAWS. *See* National Violence Against Women Survey

NWS (National Women's Survey), 171

Obesity, 323–324

Occupational history, 291

ODARA (Ontario Domestic Assault Risk Assessment), 201

ODDA. *See* Oregon Death with Dignity Act

Ohio, 427

O'Keefe v. Orea, 426

Oklahoma City bombing, 17, 19

Oklahoma City Police Department, 19

Olanzapine, 40, 367, 368

Olfactory hallucinations, 293, 296–297

Omer, H., 4–5

Omission, act of, 406

Ontario Domestic Assault Risk Assessment (ODARA), 201

OPC (outpatient commitment), 363

Open-ended questioning, 24, 44

Open head injuries, 301

Ophthalmologic problems, 316

Opiate full agonists, 243

Opiate replacement therapy, 243

Opiates, 236, 242–243

Opiate system, 219

Opioids, 239, 248

Optimism, 25, 177, 297

Orbach, I., 5

Orbitomedial frontal lobe, 128–129

Oregon Death with Dignity Act (ODDA), 115–116

Oregon Department of Human Services, 115

Oslo, Norway, 237

O'Sullivan v. Presbyterian Hospital in City of New York at Columbia Presbyterian Medical Center, 410

Others' reactions and responses, 154

Out-of-state rulings, 424–425

Outpatient commitment (OPC), 363

Outpatient management, 50–51

Outpatients, 273

Ovaries, 325

Overdose, 246–252

from alcohol/opioids/amphetamines/cocaine, 248

defined, 246–247

from designer drugs, 248–252

general management of, 246–248

as suicide method, 86

Overmedication, 240

Oxazepam, 41

OxyContin, 250

Pacific Islanders

with diabetes, 324

suicide risk among, 84

Pagers, 94

Pain, 63, 66

Pain control, 115, 313

Pain insensitivity, 219

Pancreas disorders, 322–325

Pancreatic cancer, 107

Panic attacks

as suicide risk factor, 62, 82

in victims of violence, 171, 172, 180
Panic button or message, 137
Panic disorders, 171, 393
Paradies v. Benedictine Hospital, 413
Paranoia
    with closed head injuries, 303
    risk of violence with, 39
    and working-alliance formation, 37
Paranoid delusions
    with cerebrovascular disease, 295–296
    with Huntington's disease, 301
    with Parkinson's disease, 298
Paranoid personality disorder, 266, 267, 269,
    272, 272n., 276
Paranoid psychosis, 304
Paraplegia, 113
Parasuicidal behavior. *See* Self-injury
Parathyroid hormone (PTH), 319, 321
Parathyroid system disorders, 319–322
Parental psychopathology, 85
Parents, adolescent suicide risk and, 89
Paresthesias, 292
Parkinson's disease (PD)
    as neurological disorder, 298–299
    symptoms of, 292
Partial agonists, 243
Passive avoidant coping, 23
Passive problem-focused coping, 23
Past victimization, 169–170
Patient, as informant, 417
PCL–R (Psychopathy Checklist—Revised),
    130
PCP (phenylcyclidine), 129
PD. *See* Parkinson's disease
PE. *See* Prolonged exposure
Peck v. Counseling Service of Addison County,
    Inc., 427
Peer-help crisis intervention program, 434,
    438
Peers
    suicide among, 87
    and youth violence, 149
Pelcovitz, D., 216
Pennsylvania, 427
Peptic ulcer, 66
Perceived danger, 200
Perception
    of meaning of event, 26
    role of, 21–23
Perimenopause, 326
Peripheral nervous system, 292
Peripheral neuropathy, 323

Perphenazine, 367
Personal invulnerability, belief in, 22
Personality disorders, 272n. *See also* Suicide
    risk assessment, in people with per-
    sonality disorders
    as suicide risk factor, 83
    as violence risk factor, 129–130
Persuasive authority, 424–425
Perturbation, 63
Pharmacological interventions
    harm reduction via, 40–41
    for self-injuring behavior, 219
    for violence, 137–138
Pharyngeal cancer, 107
Phenylcyclidine (PCP), 129
Phenylcyclidine hydrochloride, 251
Physical abuse, 87
Physical aggression, 151
Physical assault, 168–171
Physical Reactions Scale, 180
Physical restraint, 41
Physician-assisted suicide, 115
Pick's disease, 294
Piercing, 245
Pituitary gland, 313
Planned behavior, theory of, 154
Planning, safety. *See* Safety planning
Plan of action
    commitment to, 92
    troubleshooting the, 92–93
Plaques, 292
PMR. *See* Progressive muscle relaxation
PMS (premenstrual syndrome), 326
Poddar, Prosenjit, 414–415
Poison, suicide by, 86
Policies, institutional, 365–366
Population-based strategies, 274–275
Posing a threat, 149–150
Positive view of self, 22
Postmortem studies, 263–267
Postpartum thyroiditis, 317
Posttraumatic Diagnostic Scale, 380
Posttraumatic growth, 18
Posttraumatic stress disorder (PTSD)
    assessment for, 380–381
    characteristics of, 378
    comorbidity with, 393, 436
    and interpersonal violence, 378–379
    and intimate partner violence, 191–192,
    194, 195, 197
    lifetime rate of, 18
    risk factors for, 172–173

Puryear, D. A., 25

Quadriplegia, 113
Quality management, 365–366
Quetiapine, 367

Race
    and violent victimization, 169
    and working-alliance formation, 36
Rape
    and alcohol use, 244
    of Kosovar women, 21–22
    marital, 391
    and violent victimization, 169–171
Rape crisis advocacy programs, 178
Reactions of others, 154
Reasonable care, duty to exercise, 409
"Reasonable professional" decisions, 150,
    413, 422
Reasonably foreseeable, 408
Reasonably identifiable victim requirement,
    416, 419
Reasoning abilities, 148
Reasons for Living Inventory for Adoles-
    cents, 89
Recidivism, 201
Reduplicative paramnesia, 296
Register of Hospitalization (Denmark), 110
Relapse prevention, with suicidal patients,
    93–94
Relationship conflict, 193–194, 196, 199
Relationship termination, 199–200
Relaxation training, 178, 385, 386
Release of patient, negligent, 412–413
Religiosity, 296, 298, 303
Religious belief, 68
Reminder cards, 177
Renal disease, 66, 108
Reproductive system disorders, 325–326
Residential treatment programs, 357
Resilience, 18, 167
Resistance, 60
Respect, 224
Respiratory disease, 107, 115
Responses of others, 154
Responsivity principle, 354
Restraints, 41–42, 138, 158, 367, 438
Retaliation, 176, 177
Revenge, 155
RICH (therapeutic contacts), 224–225
Risk analysis, 140
Risk assessment data, 423

Risk assessment interview, 44–50
    for adolescent suicide, 88–89
    case formulation development, 49–50
    chief complaint, 44
    current functional status, 45
    lethality potential, 46–47
    limits of, 50
    medical problems, 45
    medications, 45–46
    mental health/substance use history, 45
    mental status exam, 47–49
    precipitating factors, 44–45
    validity of information, 47
Risk–need–responsivity (RNR), 354–359
Risk prediction, limits of, 50
Risk principle, 354
Risperidone, 40, 367, 368
RNR. See Risk–need–responsivity
Rorschach Comprehensive System, 71
Rorschach Inkblot method, 71
Roth, S., 216
Runyon v. Smith, 426

Safe School Initiative, 155
Safety issues
    physical location of interview, 136–137
    with potentially violent patients, 39–42
    with violent patients, 137, 138
    with youth violence assessment, 150–
        151
Safety planning, 139, 155, 177
Same-sex couples, 192, 193
Sanctions, 406
Santa Barbara MHC, 364
SARA (Spousal Assault Risk Assessment),
    201
Scale for Suicide Ideation, 89
Schedule for Affective Disorders and Schizo-
    phrenia for School-Age Children,
    Present and Lifetime Version, 87–
    88
Schemas, 439
Schizoid personality disorder, 258, 266, 267,
    269, 272, 272n., 276
Schizophrenia
    antipsychotic agents for, 367–368
    disordered speech of, 304
    with Huntington's disease, 301
    as suicide risk factor, 64
    and violence, 128
Schizotypal personality disorder, 269, 271,
    272n.

Transient ischemic attacks, 291
Trauma(s)
    bodily effects of, 227–228
    multiple, 173, 176
    physiology of, 218–220
    preliminary practice guidelines for treat-
        ing, 173–174
    self-injury as adaptation to, 211–212,
        216–220
    Type I vs. Type II, 17
    vicarious, 229
Trauma Adaptive Recovery Group Educa-
    tion and Therapy (TARGET), 228
Trauma Assessment for Adults—Self-Report,
    380
Trauma narrative, 391
Traumatic brain injury, 109–110, 301–303
Traumatic events, 16, 18
Traumatic stress, 15–16
    literature on, 17–18
    PTSD vs., 16–17
Traumatic Stress Institute Belief Scale, 439
Treatment adherence
    and suicidal behavior treatments, 346,
        348
    and therapeutic alliance, 135
    and violence risk, 132
Treatment as usual (TAU), 361
Treatment considerations, 50–52
    hospitalization, 51–52
    intensity of treatment, 138
    outpatient management, 50–51
Treatment records, 423–424
Treatment-seeking patients, 276, 277
Tremors, 292, 298
Triiodothyronine (T3), 316
TSH (thyroid-stimulating hormone), 316
Tsunami in Southeast Asia, 17
Turkey, 259
Turner v. Jordan, 427
Type 1 (insulin-dependent) diabetes, 322–
    324
Type 2 diabetes, 322–324
Type II trauma, 17
Type I trauma, 17

UCC. See Urgent care clinic
Underdiagnosing, 424
Unintended victims, 416–417
United Nations, 251
United Network for Organ Sharing, 108
United States

diabetes in, 323–324
hypercortisolism in, 314
reports of child abuse/neglect in, 216
self-inflicted gunshot in, 65
suicide in, 67, 432
United States Renal Data System (USRDS),
    108
Universal strategies, 274
University of California, 414–415
Urgent care clinic (UCC), 9, 237
Urine tests, 238, 247
U.S. Department of Education, 155
U.S. Department of Justice, 199
U.S. National Comorbidity Survey, 245
U.S. Secret Service, 155
U.S. Surgeon General, 149
USRDS (United States Renal Data System),
    108
Utah, 420
Utilization of medical services, 66

VA. See Veterans Administration
Vagus nerve stimulation, 109
Validity, of patient information, 47
Van der Kolk, B. A., 216
Verbal abuse, 194
Verbal aggression, 151
Verbal de-escalation, 366
Verbal intervention, 137
Verbal limits, 39
Vermont, 427
Veterans, 18, 195, 245, 250, 443
Veterans Administration (VA), 365–366,
    418–419
Viagra, 250
Vicarious trauma (VT), 229, 439, 440
Victims of interpersonal violence, treatments
        for, 382–394
    anxiety management training, 384–386
    cognitive processing therapy, 390–392
    cognitive therapy, 388
    components of, 382–383
    exposure therapy, 386–387
    multiple-channel exposure therapy, 393
    prolonged exposure, 388–390
    psychoeducation, 383–384
    stress inoculation training, 392
Victims of violence, 167–181
    acute interventions for, 173–180
    availability of potential, 131
    and clinician's self-care, 435–436, 439–
        440, 443

ABOUT THE EDITOR

Phillip M. Kleespies, PhD, was awarded his doctoral degree in clinical psychology from Clark University in 1971. He is an assistant clinical professor of psychiatry at Boston University School of Medicine. As a clinical psychologist in the Department of Veterans Affairs (DVA) Boston Healthcare System, he has over 35 years of experience working in emergency department, urgent care clinic, and inpatient psychiatric settings with patients who are at risk of such behavioral emergencies as suicidal behavior, violence, and victimization. During those years, he has been an active supervisor and teacher to psychology interns and postdoctoral fellows with an interest in evaluating and managing patients at risk to self or others. His research interests have included the development of a database for the study of self-injurious and suicidal behavior in veterans and the impact of patient suicide and suicidal behavior on the treating clinician.

In 2006, Dr. Kleespies was awarded a DVA Kizer Award Recognition grant for his work on developing a monitoring system for patient self-injurious behavior in DVA Boston. He has authored or coauthored many publications and has made numerous presentations on behavioral emergencies and related topics. He is the editor of the book *Emergencies in Mental Health Practice: Evaluation and Management* (1998) and the author of *Life and Death Decisions: Psychological and Ethical Considerations in End-of-Life Care* (American Psychological Association [APA], 2004). He is a member of the VA Boston Ethics Case Consultation Team and the VA Boston Palliative Care Consult Team.

Dr. Kleespies is a diplomate in clinical psychology of the American Board of Professional Psychology and a fellow of APA. He was the founding president of Clinical Emergencies and Crises, Section VII of APA Division 12 (Society of Clinical Psychology), and he remains involved with the section as chair of its advisory board. He resides in Cambridge, Massachusetts.